Cancer Nanomedicine

Cancer Nanomedicine

Editor

Clare Hoskins

MDPI • Basel • Beijing • Wuhan • Barcelona • Belgrade • Manchester • Tokyo • Cluj • Tianjin

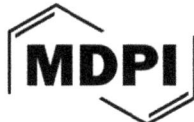

Editor
Clare Hoskins
University of Strathclyde
UK

Editorial Office
MDPI
St. Alban-Anlage 66
4052 Basel, Switzerland

This is a reprint of articles from the Special Issue published online in the open access journal *Cancers* (ISSN 2072-6694) (available at: https://www.mdpi.com/journal/cancers/special_issues/Cancer_Nanomedicine).

For citation purposes, cite each article independently as indicated on the article page online and as indicated below:

LastName, A.A.; LastName, B.B.; LastName, C.C. Article Title. *Journal Name* **Year**, *Article Number*, Page Range.

Volume 1
ISBN 978-3-03943-058-1 (Hbk)
ISBN 978-3-03943-059-8 (PDF)

Volume 1-2
ISBN 978-3-03943-106-9 (Hbk)
ISBN 978-3-03943-107-6 (PDF)

© 2020 by the authors. Articles in this book are Open Access and distributed under the Creative Commons Attribution (CC BY) license, which allows users to download, copy and build upon published articles, as long as the author and publisher are properly credited, which ensures maximum dissemination and a wider impact of our publications.

The book as a whole is distributed by MDPI under the terms and conditions of the Creative Commons license CC BY-NC-ND.

Contents

About the Editor vii

Preface to "Cancer Nanomedicine" ix

Clare Hoskins
Cancer Nanomedicine
Reprinted from: *Cancers* **2020**, *12*, 2127, doi:10.3390/cancers12082127 1

Fu-Ying Shih, Wen-Ping Jiang, Xiaojie Lin, Sheng-Chu Kuo, Guan-Jhong Huang, Yu-Chi Hou, Chih-Shiang Chang, Yang Liu and Yi-Ting Chiang
A Novel pH-Tunable Secondary Conformation Containing Mixed Micellar System in Anticancer Treatment
Reprinted from: *Cancers* **2020**, *12*, 503, doi:10.3390/cancers12020503 5

Karina Ovejero Paredes, Diana Díaz-García, Victoria García-Almodóvar, Laura Lozano Chamizo, Marzia Marciello, Miguel Díaz-Sánchez, Sanjiv Prashar, Santiago Gómez-Ruiz and Marco Filice
Multifunctional Silica-Based Nanoparticles with Controlled Release of Organotin Metallodrug for Targeted Theranosis of Breast Cancer
Reprinted from: *Cancers* **2020**, *12*, 187, doi:10.3390/cancers12010187 29

Jin Ah Kim, Dong Youl Yoon and Jin-Chul Kim
Oxidation-Triggerable Liposome Incorporating Poly(Hydroxyethyl Acrylate-*co*-Allyl methyl sulfide) as an Anticancer Carrier of Doxorubicin
Reprinted from: *Cancers* **2020**, *12*, 180, doi:10.3390/cancers12010180 53

Monica Argenziano, Casimiro Luca Gigliotti, Nausicaa Clemente, Elena Boggio, Benedetta Ferrara, Francesco Trotta, Stefania Pizzimenti, Giuseppina Barrera, Renzo Boldorini, Federica Bessone, Umberto Dianzani, Roberta Cavalli and Chiara Dianzani
Improvement in the Anti-Tumor Efficacy of Doxorubicin Nanosponges in In Vitro and in Mice Bearing Breast Tumor Models
Reprinted from: *Cancers* **2020**, *12*, 162, doi:10.3390/cancers12010162 71

Daniele Di Mascolo, Serena Varesano, Roberto Benelli, Hilaria Mollica, Annalisa Salis, Maria Raffaella Zocchi, Paolo Decuzzi and Alessandro Poggi
Nanoformulated Zoledronic Acid Boosts the Vδ2 T Cell Immunotherapeutic Potential in Colorectal Cancer
Reprinted from: *Cancers* **2020**, *12*, 104, doi:10.3390/cancers12010104 91

Alexander Winter, Svenja Engels, Philipp Goos, Marie-Christin Süykers, Stefan Gudenkauf, Rolf-Peter Henke and Friedhelm Wawroschek
Accuracy of Magnetometer-Guided Sentinel Lymphadenectomy after Intraprostatic Injection of Superparamagnetic Iron Oxide Nanoparticles in Prostate Cancer: The SentiMag Pro II Study
Reprinted from: *Cancers* **2020**, *12*, 32, doi:10.3390/cancers12010032 117

Jelena Kolosnjaj-Tabi, Slavko Kralj, Elena Griseti, Sebastjan Nemec, Claire Wilhelm, Anouchka Plan Sangnier, Elisabeth Bellard, Isabelle Fourquaux, Muriel Golzio and Marie-Pierre Rols
Magnetic Silica-Coated Iron Oxide Nanochains as Photothermal Agents, Disrupting the Extracellular Matrix, and Eradicating Cancer Cells
Reprinted from: *Cancers* **2019**, *11*, 2040, doi:10.3390/cancers11122040 129

Stefano Palazzolo, Mohamad Hadla, Concetta Russo Spena, Isabella Caligiuri, Rossella Rotondo, Muhammad Adeel, Vinit Kumar, Giuseppe Corona, Vincenzo Canzonieri, Giuseppe Toffoli and Flavio Rizzolio
An Effective Multi-Stage Liposomal DNA Origami Nanosystem for In Vivo Cancer Therapy
Reprinted from: *Cancers* **2019**, *11*, 1997, doi:10.3390/cancers11121997 . . . . **151**

Nina Filipczak, Anna Jaromin, Adriana Piwoni, Mohamed Mahmud, Can Sarisozen, Vladimir Torchilin and Jerzy Gubernator
A Triple Co-Delivery Liposomal Carrier That Enhances Apoptosis via an Intrinsic Pathway in Melanoma Cells
Reprinted from: *Cancers* **2019**, *11*, 1982, doi:10.3390/cancers11121982 . . . . **163**

Francisco Fabian Razura-Carmona, Alejandro Pérez-Larios, Napoleón González-Silva, Mayra Herrera-Martínez, Luis Medina-Torres, Sonia Guadalupe Sáyago-Ayerdi and Jorge Alberto Sánchez-Burgos
Mangiferin-Loaded Polymeric Nanoparticles: Optical Characterization, Effect of Anti-topoisomerase I, and Cytotoxicity
Reprinted from: *Cancers* **2019**, *11*, 1965, doi:10.3390/cancers11121965 . . . . **191**

Alexis Loiseau, Julien Boudon, Alexandra Oudot, Mathieu Moreau, Romain Boidot, Rémi Chassagnon, Nasser Mohamed Saïd, Stéphane Roux, Céline Mirjolet and Nadine Millot
Titanate Nanotubes Engineered with Gold Nanoparticles and Docetaxel to Enhance Radiotherapy on Xenografted Prostate Tumors
Reprinted from: *Cancers* **2019**, *11*, 1962, doi:10.3390/cancers11121962 . . . . **209**

Thierry Michy, Thibault Massias, Claire Bernard, Laetitia Vanwonterghem, Maxime Henry, Mélanie Guidetti, Guy Royal, Jean-Luc Coll, Isabelle Texier, Véronique Josserand and Amandine Hurbin
Verteporfin-Loaded Lipid Nanoparticles Improve Ovarian Cancer Photodynamic Therapy In Vitro and In Vivo
Reprinted from: *Cancers* **2019**, *11*, 1760, doi:10.3390/cancers11111760 . . . . **231**

Ana Santos-Rebelo, Pradeep Kumar, Viness Pillay, Yahya E. Choonara, Carla Eleutério, Mariana Figueira, Ana S. Viana, Lia Ascensão, Jesús Molpeceres, Patrícia Rijo, Isabel Correia, Joana Amaral, Susana Solá, Cecília M. P. Rodrigues, Maria Manuela Gaspar and Catarina Pinto Reis
Development and Mechanistic Insight into the Enhanced Cytotoxic Potential of Parvifloron D Albumin Nanoparticles in EGFR-Overexpressing Pancreatic Cancer Cells
Reprinted from: *Cancers* **2019**, *11*, 1733, doi:10.3390/cancers11111733 . . . . **251**

Manpreet Sambi, Alexandria DeCarlo, Cecile Malardier-Jugroot and Myron R. Szewczuk
Next-Generation Multimodality of Nanomedicine Therapy: Size and Structure Dependence of Folic Acid Conjugated Copolymers Actively Target Cancer Cells in Disabling Cell Division and Inducing Apoptosis
Reprinted from: *Cancers* **2019**, *11*, 1698, doi:10.3390/cancers11111698 . . . . **275**

Celia Nieto, Milena A. Vega, Jesús Enrique, Gema Marcelo and Eva M. Martín del Valle
Size Matters in the Cytotoxicity of Polydopamine Nanoparticles in Different Types of Tumors
Reprinted from: *Cancers* **2019**, *11*, 1679, doi:10.3390/cancers11111679 . . . . **295**

Fanchao Meng, Yating Sun, Robert J. Lee, Guiyuan Wang, Xiaolong Zheng, Huan Zhang, Yige Fu, Guojun Yan, Yifan Wang, Weiye Deng, Emily Parks, Betty Y.S. Kim, Zhaogang Yang, Wen Jiang and Lesheng Teng
Folate Receptor-Targeted Albumin Nanoparticles Based on Microfluidic Technology to Deliver Cabazitaxel
Reprinted from: *Cancers* **2019**, *11*, 1571, doi:10.3390/cancers11101571 311

Guosheng Wang, Weilei Hu, Haiqiong Chen, Xin Shou, Tingting Ye and Yibing Xu
Cocktail Strategy Based on NK Cell-Derived Exosomes and Their Biomimetic Nanoparticles for Dual Tumor Therapy
Reprinted from: *Cancers* **2019**, *11*, 1560, doi:10.3390/cancers11101560 329

Ilya Yakavets, Marie Millard, Laureline Lamy, Aurelie Francois, Dietrich Scheglmann, Arno Wiehe, Henri-Pierre Lassalle, Vladimir Zorin and Lina Bezdetnaya
Matryoshka-Type Liposomes Offer the Improved Delivery of Temoporfin to Tumor Spheroids
Reprinted from: *Cancers* **2019**, *11*, 1366, doi:10.3390/cancers11091366 345

Barbara Cortese, Stefania D'Amone, Mariangela Testini, Patrizia Ratano and Ilaria Elena Palamà
Hybrid Clustered Nanoparticles for Chemo-Antibacterial Combinatorial Cancer Therapy
Reprinted from: *Cancers* **2019**, *11*, 1338, doi:10.3390/cancers11091338 361

Irina Naletova, Lorena Maria Cucci, Floriana D'Angeli, Carmelina Daniela Anfuso, Antonio Magrì, Diego La Mendola, Gabriella Lupo and Cristina Satriano
A Tunable Nanoplatform of Nanogold Functionalised with Angiogenin Peptides for Anti-Angiogenic Therapy of Brain Tumours
Reprinted from: *Cancers* **2019**, *11*, 1322, doi:10.3390/cancers11091322 379

Md. Tanvir Hasan, Elizabeth Campbell, Olga Sizova, Veronica Lyle, Giridhar Akkaraju, D. Lynn Kirkpatrick and Anton V. Naumov
Multi-Drug/Gene NASH Therapy Delivery and Selective Hyperspectral NIR Imaging Using Chirality-Sorted Single-Walled Carbon Nanotubes
Reprinted from: *Cancers* **2019**, *11*, 1175, doi:10.3390/cancers11081175 409

Ana Latorre, Alfonso Latorre, Milagros Castellanos, Ciro Rodriguez Diaz, Ana Lazaro-Carrillo, Tania Aguado, Mercedes Lecea, Sonia Romero-Pérez, Macarena Calero, José María Sanchez-Puelles, Ángeles Villanueva and Álvaro Somoza
Multifunctional Albumin-Stabilized Gold Nanoclusters for the Reduction of Cancer Stem Cells
Reprinted from: *Cancers* **2019**, *11*, 969, doi:10.3390/cancers11070969 427

Ki-Hyun Bang, Young-Guk Na, Hyun Wook Huh, Sung-Joo Hwang, Min-Soo Kim, Minki Kim, Hong-Ki Lee and Cheong-Weon Cho
The Delivery Strategy of Paclitaxel Nanostructured Lipid Carrier Coated with Platelet Membrane
Reprinted from: *Cancers* **2019**, *11*, 807, doi:10.3390/cancers11060807 445

Nikola Bugárová, Zdenko Špitálsky, Matej Mičušík, Michal Bodík, Peter Šiffalovič, Martina Koneracká, Vlasta Závišová, Martina Kubovčíková, Ivana Kajanová, Miriam Zaťovičová, Silvia Pastoreková, Miroslav Šlouf, Eva Majková and Mária Omastová
A Multifunctional Graphene Oxide Platform for Targeting Cancer
Reprinted from: *Cancers* **2019**, *11*, 753, doi:10.3390/cancers11060753 461

Loujin Houdaihed, James Christopher Evans and Christine Allen
In Vivo Evaluation of Dual-Targeted Nanoparticles Encapsulating Paclitaxel and Everolimus
Reprinted from: *Cancers* **2019**, *11*, 752, doi:10.3390/cancers11060752 481

About the Editor

Clare, Hoskins, Ph.D., Dr Clare Hoskins is a Reader in the School of Pure and Applied Chemistry. She has published >40 peer reviewed articles and filed 1 patent. Her research has been supported with over £2M by national (e.g., EPSRC, BBSRC/FAPESP, Wellcome Trust) and international (e.g., Newton-Bhabha & British Council, Iraqi Ministry of Higher Education and Scientific Research) research funding. Clare is the Elected Secretary to the Royal Society of Chemistry, Chemical Nanosciences and Nanotechnology Network, she is a committee member of the UK and Ireland Controlled Release Society and she sits on the British Council Grant Review Panel for Newton Grants. In 2019 Clare was awarded the Academy of Pharmaceutical Sciences 'Emerging Scientist' sponsored by Pfizer and also the North Staffordshire Medical Institute Researcher Award. Clare sits on the editorial board of numerous journals in her field, she leads a vibrant interdisciplinary research group within the them of Bionanotechnology and Analytical Chemistry within the Technology Innovation Centre. The focus of her research is the development of a range of multifunctional nanoparticles and their translation into medical therapies and agricultural products.

Preface to "Cancer Nanomedicine"

Welcome to the special issue on Cancer Nanomedicine within Cancers. It has been a real delight to edit this special edition bringing together cutting edge research within the field with insightful reviews and opinions reflecting our community.

Cancer nanomedicine is a large umbrella under which researchers spanning the physical, chemical and biological sciences. I think this is well reflected in this edition.

Cancer treatments are often hindered by the lack of drug specificity, poor physicochemical properties of active pharmaceutical ingredients, poor penetration ability and drug resistance. With the discovery and characterization of an increasing number of cancer types with little improvement of the ability to diagnose, treatment options or patient prognosis, more advanced technologies are urgently required. Nanotechnology defines particulates within the 1×10^{-9} m range. Particulates within the nano-sized domain often exhibit unique properties compared to their larger size scale. These can be exploited in biomedicine for applications such as imaging, cell sorting, drug delivery and targeting. Cancer nanomedicine is rapidly becoming one of the leading areas of promise for cancer therapy, with first-generation treatments already available to patients.

The exciting advances within this field have lead to cancer nanomedicines already been used clinically today. Sceptics would argue that the translation of nanotechnologies into the clinic have not matched the initial hype, however, I believe moving forward more and more commercial success will be achieved. It is estimated that the global nanomedicine market will be worth US$334 billion by 2025, with cancer nanomedicine dominating in this field. As the science develops and leads us down new avenues, the findings and their meaning are closely scrutinised and debated within the community. This all leads to a thriving and exciting field in which to work.

I hope you enjoy reading the manuscripts within this special edition, since it has been such a great success with 46 papers being accepted for publication. In order to continue to showcase work in our strong field, a Topical Collection has been permanently opened within Cancers, and I invite you all to consider submitting your next manuscripts into this.

Clare Hoskins
Editor

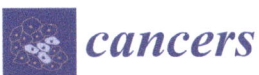 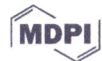

Editorial
Cancer Nanomedicine

Clare Hoskins

School of Pure and Applied Chemistry, University of Strathclyde, Glasgow G1 1RD, UK; clare.hoskins@strath.ac.uk

Received: 28 July 2020; Accepted: 29 July 2020; Published: 31 July 2020

Keywords: cancer nanomedicine; therapeutics; diagnostics; imaging; theranostics; Immunotherapy; tumour microenvironment

---

This Special Issue on Cancer Nanomedicine within *Cancers* brings together 46 cutting-edge papers covering research within the field along with insightful reviews and opinions reflecting our community. Cancer nanomedicine is a large umbrella under which researchers explore the physical, chemical and biological sciences. I think this is well reflected in this edition. Cancer treatments are often hindered by the lack of drug specificity, poor physicochemical properties of active pharmaceutical ingredients, poor penetration ability and drug resistance. With the discovery and characterization of an increasing number of cancer types with little improvement of the ability to diagnose, treatment options or patient prognosis, more advanced technologies are urgently required. Nanotechnology defines particulates within the 1×10^{-9} m range. Particulates within the nano-sized domain often exhibit unique properties compared to their larger size scale. These can be exploited in biomedicine for applications such as imaging, cell sorting, drug delivery and targeting. Cancer nanomedicine is rapidly becoming one of the leading areas of promise for cancer therapy, with first-generation treatments already available to patients.

Within this Special Issue, a diverse range of cancer nanomedicines have been discussed, including the more traditional organic-based systems, such as lipid [1–6], polymer [7–11] and cyclodextrin-based [12] particulates. Additionally, there are multiple studies from the growing area of inorganic systems, such as carbon nanomaterials (such as graphene oxide [13,14] and carbon nanotubes [15]) as well as other more established metallic nanomaterials, such as gold [16,17], iron oxide [18,19] and silica-based [20,21] systems. Interest into such inorganic systems has boomed over the last ten years, largely down to their multifunctional capabilities, in imaging [15], photothermal ability [22,23] or use in radiation enhancement [24]. Within this arena, a new class of nanoplatform has also developed, which is gaining traction. These platforms can be used for combined diagnostics and therapy, known as theranostics. The theranostic community is growing rapidly and in this issue a review of theranostics under development [25] as well a scientific paper [20] have been included.

One of the major challenges in cancer nanomedicine is tumour targeting and penetration. Conjugation of surface targetingligands, peptides and other molecules are of major focus within this field [26], including the use of TAT peptides [27], vitamins such as riboflavin [28], integrins [29] and antibodies [30]. Other issues such as tumour microenvironment also contribute to such challenges, and discussion on nanomedicine uptake looking at mechanistic evaluations such as shear stress [31], a hypoxic environment [32] and in overexpressing cell lines [33] have also been included.

Rapid clearance via the immune system has been another barrier historically faced by nanotechnologies. As such, nanomedicines have been developed that are inspired by or mimetic of biological systems such as extracellular vesicles [34] and exosomes [35] that exploit the naturally occurring nano vehicles produced inside the body to extract and repurpose as drug delivery systems. Other clever systems utilise other biomolecules in order to protect their nanoparticle payload, such as cloaking with cell membranes [36]. Other systems seek to deliver biomolecules such as siRNA [37,38] or to elicit an immune response in order to combat cancer [37–41].

Combination therapy has shown major improvement in chemotherapy compared with monotherapy. With improved tumour retardation, reduced drug resistance and better patient prognosis. As such, nanomedicines are under development incorporating combination therapies [30,42] in the hope to further enhance the findings found in small molecule trials, with the protective capabilities of nanomedicines through targeting techniques in order to reduce the toxic side effects of the potent compounds attributed to systemic circulation.

As the benefits of nanomedicine for cancer therapy have been realised, the incorporation of such nanotechnologies has been incorporated into larger-scale macromolecular systems. One such example is in the use of microbubbles [43]. Here, the nanotechnologies are conjugated onto the microbubble surfaces and ultrasonic energy is used as a means to cavitate the tumour tissue, allowing for deeper penetration of the nanomedicines in order for them to deliver their payload at the site of need.

As many of the cancer nanomedicines under development translate further towards the clinic, investigation on reliable scale-up and manufacture is explored. One technique that is currently dominating this field, particularly in liposomal development, is microfluidics. In this issue, we highlight its use in the manufacture of folate conjugated albumin particles incorporating Cabazitaxel [44]. The highly engineered mixing techniques and continuous flow parameters make such technology ideal for the formulation of cancer nanomedicines in the large batches required for trials and beyond. Work is ongoing globally into the evaluation of whether microfluidics can be exploited for other nanomedicine development and formulation.

The exciting advances within this field have led to cancer nanomedicines already being used clinically today. Sceptics would argue that the translation of nanotechnologies into the clinic have not matched the initial hype, with opinion included on the current state of the cancer nanomedicine field [45]. I believe, moving forward, more and more commercial success will be achieved. It is estimated that the global nanomedicine market will be worth USD 334 billion by 2025, with cancer nanomedicine dominating in this field. As the science develops and leads us down new avenues, the findings and their meaning are closely scrutinised and debated within the community. This issue includes 32 scientific manuscripts, 13 review articles and 1 case report reflecting the hot topics within this area [1–46].

Funding: This research received no external funding.

Conflicts of Interest: The author declares no conflict of interest.

References

1. Michy, T.; Massias, T.; Bernard, C.; Vanwonterghem, L.; Henry, M.; Guidetti, M.; Royal, G.; Coll, J.; Texier, I.; Josserand, V.; et al. Verteporfin-Loaded Lipid Nanoparticles Improve Ovarian Cancer Photodynamic Therapy In Vitro and In Vivo. *Cancers* **2019**, *11*, 1760. [CrossRef] [PubMed]
2. Kim, J.; Yoon, D.; Kim, J. Oxidation-Triggerable Liposome Incorporating Poly (Hydroxyethyl Acrylate-co-Allyl methyl sulfide) as an Anticancer Carrier of Doxorubicin. *Cancers* **2020**, *12*, 180. [CrossRef] [PubMed]
3. Bang, K.; Na, Y.; Huh, H.; Hwang, S.; Kim, M.; Kim, M.; Lee, H.; Cho, C. The Delivery Strategy of Paclitaxel Nanostructured Lipid Carrier Coated with Platelet Membrane. *Cancers* **2019**, *11*, 807. [CrossRef] [PubMed]
4. Palazzolo, S.; Hadla, M.; Russo Spena, C.; Caligiuri, I.; Rotondo, R.; Adeel, M.; Kumar, V.; Corona, G.; Canzonieri, V.; Toffoli, G.; et al. An Effective Multi-Stage Liposomal DNA Origami Nanosystem for In Vivo Cancer Therapy. *Cancers* **2019**, *11*, 1997. [CrossRef] [PubMed]
5. Yakavets, I.; Millard, M.; Lamy, L.; Francois, A.; Scheglmann, D.; Wiehe, A.; Lassalle, H.; Zorin, V.; Bezdetnaya, L. Matryoshka-Type Liposomes Offer the Improved Delivery of Temoporfin to Tumor Spheroids. *Cancers* **2019**, *11*, 1366. [CrossRef] [PubMed]
6. Filipczak, N.; Jaromin, A.; Piwoni, A.; Mahmud, M.; Sarisozen, C.; Torchilin, V.; Gubernator, J. A Triple Co-Delivery Liposomal Carrier That Enhances Apoptosis via an Intrinsic Pathway in Melanoma Cells. *Cancers* **2019**, *11*, 1982. [CrossRef]
7. Mahmoud, B.; AlAmri, A.; McConville, C. Polymeric Nanoparticles for the Treatment of Malignant Gliomas. *Cancers* **2020**, *12*, 175. [CrossRef]

8. Nieto, C.; Vega, M.; Enrique, J.; Marcelo, G.; Martín del Valle, E. Size Matters in the Cytotoxicity of Polydopamine Nanoparticles in Different Types of Tumors. *Cancers* **2019**, *11*, 1679. [CrossRef]
9. Sambi, M.; DeCarlo, A.; Malardier-Jugroot, C.; Szewczuk, M. Next-Generation Multimodality of Nanomedicine Therapy: Size and Structure Dependence of Folic Acid Conjugated Copolymers Actively Target Cancer Cells in Disabling Cell Division and Inducing Apoptosis. *Cancers* **2019**, *11*, 1698. [CrossRef]
10. Razura-Carmona, F.; Pérez-Larios, A.; González-Silva, N.; Herrera-Martínez, M.; Medina-Torres, L.; Sáyago-Ayerdi, S.; Sánchez-Burgos, J. Mangiferin-Loaded Polymeric Nanoparticles: Optical Characterization, Effect of Anti-topoisomerase I. and Cytotoxicity. *Cancers* **2019**, *11*, 1965. [CrossRef]
11. Shih, F.; Jiang, W.; Lin, X.; Kuo, S.; Huang, G.; Hou, Y.; Chang, C.; Liu, Y.; Chiang, Y. A Novel pH-Tunable Secondary Conformation Containing Mixed Micellar System in Anticancer Treatment. *Cancers* **2020**, *12*, 503. [CrossRef] [PubMed]
12. Argenziano, M.; Gigliotti, C.; Clemente, N.; Boggio, E.; Ferrara, B.; Trotta, F.; Pizzimenti, S.; Barrera, G.; Boldorini, R.; Bessone, F.; et al. Improvement in the Anti-Tumor Efficacy of Doxorubicin Nanosponges in In Vitro and in Mice Bearing Breast Tumor Models. *Cancers* **2020**, *12*, 162. [CrossRef] [PubMed]
13. Tabish, T.; Pranjol, M.; Horsell, D.; Rahat, A.; Whatmore, J.; Winyard, P.; Zhang, S. Graphene Oxide-Based Targeting of Extracellular Cathepsin D and Cathepsin L As A Novel Anti-Metastatic Enzyme Cancer Therapy. *Cancers* **2019**, *11*, 319. [CrossRef] [PubMed]
14. Bugárová, N.; Špitálsky, Z.; Mičušík, M.; Bodík, M.; Šiffalovič, P.; Koneracká, M.; Závišová, V.; Kubovčíková, M.; Kajanová, I.; Zaťovičová, M.; et al. A Multifunctional Graphene Oxide Platform for Targeting Cancer. *Cancers* **2019**, *11*, 753. [CrossRef]
15. Hasan, M.; Campbell, E.; Sizova, O.; Lyle, V.; Akkaraju, G.; Kirkpatrick, D.; Naumov, A. Multi-Drug/Gene NASH Therapy Delivery and Selective Hyperspectral NIR Imaging Using Chirality-Sorted Single-Walled Carbon Nanotubes. *Cancers* **2019**, *11*, 1175. [CrossRef]
16. Naletova, I.; Cucci, L.; D'Angeli, F.; Anfuso, C.; Magrì, A.; La Mendola, D.; Lupo, G.; Satriano, C. A Tunable Nanoplatform of Nanogold Functionalised with Angiogenin Peptides for Anti-Angiogenic Therapy of Brain Tumours. *Cancers* **2019**, *11*, 1322. [CrossRef]
17. Latorre, A.; Latorre, A.; Castellanos, M.; Rodriguez Diaz, C.; Lazaro-Carrillo, A.; Aguado, T.; Lecea, M.; Romero-Pérez, S.; Calero, M.; Sanchez-Puelles, J.; et al. Multifunctional Albumin-Stabilized Gold Nanoclusters for the Reduction of Cancer Stem Cells. *Cancers* **2019**, *11*, 969. [CrossRef]
18. Nana, A.; Marimuthu, T.; Kondiah, P.; Choonara, Y.; Du Toit, L.; Pillay, V. Multifunctional Magnetic Nanowires: Design, Fabrication, and Future Prospects as Cancer Therapeutics. *Cancers* **2019**, *11*, 1956. [CrossRef]
19. Winter, A.; Engels, S.; Goos, P.; Süykers, M.; Gudenkauf, S.; Henke, R.; Wawroschek, F. Accuracy of Magnetometer-Guided Sentinel Lymphadenectomy after Intraprostatic Injection of Superparamagnetic Iron Oxide Nanoparticles in Prostate Cancer: The SentiMag Pro II Study. *Cancers* **2020**, *12*, 32. [CrossRef]
20. Ovejero Paredes, K.; Díaz-García, D.; García-Almodóvar, V.; Lozano Chamizo, L.; Marciello, M.; Díaz-Sánchez, M.; Prashar, S.; Gómez-Ruiz, S.; Filice, M. Multifunctional Silica-Based Nanoparticles with Controlled Release of Organotin Metallodrug for Targeted Theranosis of Breast Cancer. *Cancers* **2020**, *12*, 187. [CrossRef]
21. Wu, Z.; Lee, C.; Lin, H. Hyaluronidase-Responsive Mesoporous Silica Nanoparticles with Dual-Imaging and Dual-Target Function. *Cancers* **2019**, *11*, 697. [CrossRef] [PubMed]
22. Ali, M.; Farghali, H.; Wu, Y.; El-Sayed, I.; Osman, A.; Selim, S.; El-Sayed, M. Gold Nanorod-Assisted Photothermal Therapy Decreases Bleeding during Breast Cancer Surgery in Dogs and Cats. *Cancers* **2019**, *11*, 851. [CrossRef] [PubMed]
23. Kolosnjaj-Tabi, J.; Kralj, S.; Griseti, E.; Nemec, S.; Wilhelm, C.; Plan Sangnier, A.; Bellard, E.; Fourquaux, I.; Golzio, M.; Rols, M. Magnetic Silica-Coated Iron Oxide Nanochains as Photothermal Agents, Disrupting the Extracellular Matrix and Eradicating Cancer Cells. *Cancers* **2019**, *11*, 2040. [CrossRef] [PubMed]
24. Loiseau, A.; Boudon, J.; Oudot, A.; Moreau, M.; Boidot, R.; Chassagnon, R.; Mohamed Saïd, N.; Roux, S.; Mirjolet, C.; Millot, N. Titanate Nanotubes Engineered with Gold Nanoparticles and Docetaxel to Enhance Radiotherapy on Xenografted Prostate Tumors. *Cancers* **2019**, *11*, 1962. [CrossRef]
25. Mukherjee, A.; Paul, M.; Mukherjee, S. Recent Progress in the Theranostics Application of Nanomedicine in Lung Cancer. *Cancers* **2019**, *11*, 597. [CrossRef]
26. Yoo, J.; Park, C.; Yi, G.; Lee, D.; Koo, H. Active Targeting Strategies Using Biological Ligands for Nanoparticle Drug Delivery Systems. *Cancers* **2019**, *11*, 640. [CrossRef]

27. Moku, G.; Layek, B.; Trautman, L.; Putnam, S.; Panyam, J.; Prabha, S. Improving Payload Capacity and Anti-Tumor Efficacy of Mesenchymal Stem Cells Using TAT Peptide Functionalized Polymeric Nanoparticles. *Cancers* **2019**, *11*, 491. [CrossRef]
28. Darguzyte, M.; Drude, N.; Lammers, T.; Kiessling, F. Riboflavin-Targeted Drug Delivery. *Cancers* **2020**, *12*, 295. [CrossRef]
29. Wu, P.; Opadele, A.; Onodera, Y.; Nam, J. Targeting Integrins in Cancer Nanomedicine: Applications in Cancer Diagnosis and Therapy. *Cancers* **2019**, *11*, 1783. [CrossRef]
30. Houdaihed, L.; Evans, J.; Allen, C. In Vivo Evaluation of Dual-Targeted Nanoparticles Encapsulating Paclitaxel and Everolimus. *Cancers* **2019**, *11*, 752. [CrossRef]
31. Shurbaji, S.G.; Anlar, G.A.; Hussein, E.; Elzatahry, A.C.; Yalcin, H. Effect of Flow-Induced Shear Stress in Nanomaterial Uptake by Cells: Focus on Targeted Anti-Cancer Therapy. *Cancers* **2020**, *12*, 1916. [CrossRef] [PubMed]
32. Feng, J.; Byrne, N.; Al Jamal, W.; Coulter, J. Exploitng Current Understanding of Hypoxia Mediated Tumour Progression for Nanotherapeutic Development. *Cancers* **2019**, *11*, 1989. [CrossRef] [PubMed]
33. Santos-Rebelo, A.; Kumar, P.; Pillay, V.; Choonara, Y.; Eleutério, C.; Figueira, M.; Viana, A.; Ascensão, L.; Molpeceres, J.; Rijo, P.; et al. Development and Mechanistic Insight into the Enhanced Cytotoxic Potential of Parvifloron D Albumin Nanoparticles in EGFR-Overexpressing Pancreatic Cancer Cells. *Cancers* **2019**, *11*, 1733. [CrossRef] [PubMed]
34. Susa, F.; Limongi, T.; Dumontel, B.; Vighetto, V.; Cauda, V. Engineered Extracellular Vesicles as a Reliable Tool in Cancer Nanomedicine. *Cancers* **2019**, *11*, 1979. [CrossRef]
35. Wang, G.; Hu, W.; Chen, H.; Shou, X.; Ye, T.; Xu, Y. Cocktail Strategy Based on NK Cell-Derived Exosomes and Their Biomimetic Nanoparticles for Dual Tumor Therapy. *Cancers* **2019**, *11*, 1560. [CrossRef]
36. Harris, J.; Scully, M.; Day, E. Cancer Cell Membrane-Coated Nanoparticles for Cancer Management. *Cancers* **2019**, *11*, 1836. [CrossRef]
37. Ben-David-Naim, M.; Dagan, A.; Grad, E.; Aizik, G.; Nordling-David, M.; Morss Clyne, A.; Granot, Z.; Golomb, G. Targeted siRNA Nanoparticles for Mammary Carcinoma Therapy. *Cancers* **2019**, *11*, 442. [CrossRef]
38. Kamaruzman, N.; Aziz, N.; Poh, C.; Chowdhury, E. Oncogenic Signaling in Tumorigenesis and Applications of siRNA Nanotherapeutics in Breast Cancer. *Cancers* **2019**, *11*, 632. [CrossRef]
39. Sau, S.; Petrovici, A.; Alsaab, H.; Bhise, K.; Iyer, A. PDL-1 Antibody Drug Conjugate for Selective Chemo-Guided Immune Modulation of Cancer. *Cancers* **2019**, *11*, 232. [CrossRef]
40. Kerstetter-Fogle, A.; Shukla, S.; Wang, C.; Beiss, V.; Harris, P.; Sloan, A.; Steinmetz, N. Plant Virus-Like Particle In Situ Vaccine for Intracranial Glioma Immunotherapy. *Cancers* **2019**, *11*, 515. [CrossRef]
41. Di Mascolo, D.; Varesano, S.; Benelli, R.; Mollica, H.; Salis, A.; Zocchi, M.; Decuzzi, P.; Poggi, A. Nanoformulated Zoledronic Acid Boosts the Vδ2 T Cell Immunotherapeutic Potential in Colorectal Cancer. *Cancers* **2020**, *12*, 104. [CrossRef]
42. Cortese, B.; D'Amone, S.; Testini, M.; Ratano, P.; Palamà, I. Hybrid Clustered Nanoparticles for Chemo-Antibacterial Combinatorial Cancer Therapy. *Cancers* **2019**, *11*, 1338. [CrossRef] [PubMed]
43. Lee, J.; Moon, H.; Han, H.; Lee, I.; Kim, D.; Lee, H.; Ha, S.; Kim, H.; Chung, J. Antitumor Effects of Intra-Arterial Delivery of Albumin-Doxorubicin Nanoparticle Conjugated Microbubbles Combined with Ultrasound-Targeted Microbubble Activation on VX2 Rabbit Liver Tumors. *Cancers* **2019**, *11*, 581. [CrossRef] [PubMed]
44. Meng, F.; Sun, Y.; Lee, R.; Wang, G.; Zheng, X.; Zhang, H.; Fu, Y.; Yan, G.; Wang, Y.; Deng, W.; et al. Folate Receptor-Targeted Albumin Nanoparticles Based on Microfluidic Technology to Deliver Cabazitaxel. *Cancers* **2019**, *11*, 1571. [CrossRef]
45. Salvioni, L.; Rizzuto, M.; Bertolini, J.; Pandolfi, L.; Colombo, M.; Prosperi, D. Thirty Years of Cancer Nanomedicine: Success, Frustration, and Hope. *Cancers* **2019**, *11*, 1855. [CrossRef] [PubMed]
46. Pantshwa, J.; Kondiah, P.; Choonara, Y.; Marimuthu, T.; Pillay, V. Nanodrug Delivery Systems for the Treatment of Ovarian Cancer. *Cancers* **2020**, *12*, 213. [CrossRef]

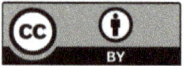

© 2020 by the author. Licensee MDPI, Basel, Switzerland. This article is an open access article distributed under the terms and conditions of the Creative Commons Attribution (CC BY) license (http://creativecommons.org/licenses/by/4.0/).

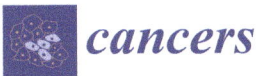

Article

A Novel pH-Tunable Secondary Conformation Containing Mixed Micellar System in Anticancer Treatment

Fu-Ying Shih [1,†], Wen-Ping Jiang [2,3,†], Xiaojie Lin [4], Sheng-Chu Kuo [5], Guan-Jhong Huang [3], Yu-Chi Hou [6], Chih-Shiang Chang [6], Yang Liu [2] and Yi-Ting Chiang [6,*]

1. Program for Biotech Pharmaceutical Industry, School of Pharmacy, China Medical University, Taichung 404, Taiwan; u106308001@cmu.edu.tw
2. The Metal Industries Research & Development Centre (MIRDC), Kaohsiung City 811, Taiwan; u101053651@cmu.edu.tw (W.-P.J.); yangliu@mail.mirdc.org.tw (Y.L.)
3. Department of Chinese Pharmaceutical Sciences and Chinese Medicine Resources, China Medical University, Taichung 404, Taiwan; gjhuang@mail.cmu.edu.tw
4. Department of Chemical Engineering, University of Washington, Seattle, WA 98195, USA; xjlin@uw.edu
5. Chinese Medicine Research Center, China Medical University, Taichung 404, Taiwan; sckuo@mail.cmu.edu.tw
6. School of Pharmacy, China Medical University, Taichung 404, Taiwan; houyc@mail.cmu.edu.tw (Y.-C.H.); chihshiang@mail.cmu.edu.tw (C.-S.C.)
* Correspondence: ytchiang@mail.cmu.edu.tw
† These authors contributed equally to this work.

Received: 10 January 2020; Accepted: 18 February 2020; Published: 21 February 2020

Abstract: In this study, for the first time, we precisely assembled the poly-γ-benzyl-l-glutamate and an amphiphilic copolymer d-α-tocopherol polyethylene glycol succinate into a mixed micellar system for the embedment of the anticancer drug doxorubicin. Importantly, the intracellular drug-releasing behaviors could be controlled by changing the secondary structures of poly-γ-benzyl-l-glutamate via the precise regulation of the buffer's pH value. Under neutral conditions, the micellar architectures were stabilized by both α-helix secondary structures and the microcrystalline structures. Under acidic conditions (pH 4.0), the interior structures transformed into a coil state with a disordered alignment, inducing the release of the loaded drug. A remarkable cytotoxicity of the Dox-loaded mixed micelles was exhibited toward human lung cancer cells in vitro. The internalizing capability into the cancer cells, as well as the intracellular drug-releasing behaviors, were also identified and observed. The secondary structures containing Dox-loaded mixed micelles had an outstanding antitumor efficacy in human lung cancer A549 cells-bearing nude mice, while little toxicities occurred or interfered with the hepatic or renal functions after the treatments. Thus, these pH-tunable α-helix-containing mixed micelles are innovative and promising for controlled intracellular anticancer drug delivery.

Keywords: secondary structure; mixed micelle; pH responsive; drug delivery system

1. Introduction

Poly-γ-benzyl-l-glutamate (PBLG), whose structure contains a polypeptide backbone and benzyl side chains, has attracted extensive interest for its biocompatibility and biodegradability [1]. For drug or gene delivery systems, PBLG has commonly been conjugated with hydrophilic polymers into amphiphilic copolymers, where PBLG segments are employed as hydrophobic motifs to stabilize the carriers [2,3]. Notably, the ordered secondary structure driven by the polypeptide backbone is an important feature for PBLG [4]. The α-helix and β-sheet secondary structures are discovered under different conditions. For example, the high molecular weight of PBLG is favored in α-helix structures, while PBLG with a low degree of polymerizations tends towards β-sheet alignment [5]. In fact, these secondary structures are the consequences of the intermolecular or intramolecular hydrogen bond interactions, and thus the conformations of PBLG would be affected by the environmental milieus. It has been reported that the solution polarity strongly influences the helix structures of PBLG [6], and that PBLG showed a helix-coil transformation in different solvents in the presence of an acid, such as trifluoroacetic acid [7–9]. Notably, the polymers blended with PBLG have the ability to influence the secondary conformations of PBLG, through either hydrogen bonds or π–π stacking interactions [10,11]. Those performances of the secondary structures would furthermore alter the crystalline alignment of PBLG and play a critical role in the physical properties of PBLG [12,13].

As PBLG has a high biosafety and unique secondary structures, for the first time we directly organized the hydrophobic PBLG (M.W. 30–70k Da) with an amphiphilic copolymer d-α-tocopherol polyethylene glycol 1000 succinate (TPGS) into mixed micelles to convey the anticancer drug doxorubicin (Dox). In neutral milieus, such as in the blood or physiological conditions after intravenously administration, the secondary conformation of PBLG within the micellar system is expected to be present, while in mimetic endo/lysosome acidic condition (pH 4.0), the secondary arrangement would undergo transitions into a random coil state (Scheme 1). The interior secondary conformations have been proved by Y. Mochida to stabilize the micellar structures from abrupt disintegration [14]. The micellar density would be regulated as the transitions of the interior secondary structures occurred, representing the potential manner of controlling drug delivery [15], and the interior secondary conformation transitions led to the micelle–vehicle transitions [16]. M. Choi et al. have prepared β-sheet silk nanofilm and controlled the drug liberation via regulating the secondary structure contents, identifying the feasibility of a secondary conformational drug delivery system [17].

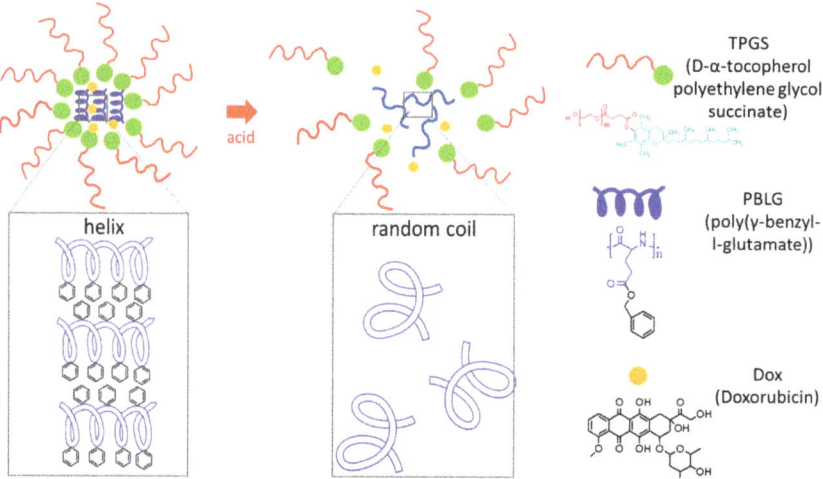

Scheme 1. A pH tunable secondary structure containing mixed micelles. The mixed micelles comprising d-α-tocopherol polyethylene glycol 1000 succinate and poly-γ-benzyl-l-glutamate, have interior helix secondary structures due to the polypeptide backbone of PBLG in the neutral conditions. The inner helix structures in the neutral condition enabled to stabilize the micellar structures and encapsulate the anticancer drug doxorubicin. In acidic environment, the secondary structures of mixed micelles would undergo helix-coil transformation to release drug.

This work is the first study that introduces PBLG into an artificially mixed micelle system for controlled intracellular anticancer drug delivery. As we have illustrated previously, the amphiphilic phenolic TPGS and the encapsulated Dox definitely have a predominant impact on both the secondary structures and the crystalline alignment of PBLG within the micellar system. In addition, the terminus of PBLG has a lack of intrahelical hydrogen bonds [8] and is physically incorporated inside the micellar system, thus the response of PBLG toward external pH environments and the releasing profiles needs to be comprehensively investigated. Here, the intracellular drug-releasing and the cytotoxicity toward human cancer cells will also be studied to evaluate the feasibility of these mixed micelles as a novel pH-responsive drug delivery system.

2. Results

2.1. Preparation and Characterization of pH-Responsive Secondary Structure Contained Mixed Micelles

PBLG and TPGS were weighed at various ratios and dissolved into the N, N-dimethylacetamide (DMAc). The mixed micelles were thereafter prepared via the solvent exchange method. The particle sizes and distributions were measured using dynamic laser scattering (DLS) and the results are shown in Table 1. The critical micellar concentration (CMC) values were also determined using the pyrene probes, also shown in Table 1. The particle sizes of TPL, comprising the highest ratios of the TPGS, were 184.0 ± 0.7 nm, and the particle sizes of the mixed micelles which had the lowest ratios of the TPGS (TPH) were 148.7 ± 1.3 nm. The mixed micelles whose particle sizes were 157.0 ± 3.0 nm presented equal weight ratios of the PBLG and TPGS. All the micelles exhibited low polydispersity (PDI) value, representing the monodispersity of these micelles. TPH micelles exhibited not only the smallest particle size but also the lowest CMC value (5.68×10^{-4} mg/mL). The CMC value of TPM (3.22×10^{-3} mg/mL) was slightly higher than that of TPL mixed micelles (1.29×10^{-3} mg/mL). The CMC value was considered as the majority in the stability of the mixed micelles [18]. Therefore, the stability of these mixed micelles at 37 °C was evaluated through the hydrodynamic diameter changes, and the results are shown in Figure 1a. TPL micelles, whose CMC was higher than TPH mixed micelles, exhibited relatively significant particle size changes, and the particle size increased until around 205 nm, after incubation at 37 °C for 24 h. The hydrodynamic diameters of TPM and TPH did not show obvious particle size changes, indicating that the TPM and TPH mixed micelles showed a high stability at 37 °C. It is worth noting that the CMC value of the TPM micelle was five times higher than that of the TPH micelle and even also higher than TPL mixed micelles, while the hydrodynamic diameters did not significantly increase upon incubation. PBLG was previously reported as folding into specific secondary structures and the inner secondary structures of the micelles have been identified related to the particle stability [14,19]. Since the stability was more connected with the PBLG contents, instead of the CMC value, the role of PBLG in the mixed micellar system was investigated in our study.

Table 1. The particle sizes and distributions of the mixed micelles with various compositions.

Code	Composition (wt%)		Size (nm)	PDI	CMC (mg/mL)
	TPGS	PBLG			
TPH	25	75	148.73 ± 1.27	0.09 ± 0.03	5.68×10^{-4}
TPM	50	50	157.03 ± 3.00	0.09 ± 0.02	3.22×10^{-3}
TPL	75	25	184.00 ± 0.72	0.07 ± 0.04	1.29×10^{-3}

Note: The particle sizes and PDI (polydispersity) were determined by the dynamic laser scattering (DLS) and CMC (critical micellar concentration) values were determined by pyrene probe methods.

For the hierarchical conformation analysis of PBLG in these mixed micelles, circular dichroism (CD) spectroscopy was further applied from the wavelength of 190 to 250 nm to identify the PBLG participation and its secondary folding. The CD spectra of these mixed micelles with or without incubation at 37 °C for 24 h is shown in Figure 1b. Before incubation at 37 °C, the mixed micelles all exhibited a negative band around 222 nm, as well as a positive band at approximately 195 nm. The valley around 222 nm represented the α-helix conformation. However, another characteristic negative peak for α-helix conformation was not observed at 208 nm in the CD spectrum because the randomly coiled polypeptides also existed [9]. The single minimum spectrum was also observed in all groups, while the magnitudes of the 2 bands within the mixed micelles were dependent upon the TPGS and PBLG ratios. The α-helix conformation contents increased with the increasing PBLG ratios within the mixed micelles, evidencing the PBLG folding inside the micelles with helical folding, whereas the increasing TPGS ratios would lead to the random coil state within the inner micellar structures. TPH exhibited the highest α-helix content among all the micelles, due to the strong magnitude of the valley at 222 nm. The mixed micelles were further incubated at 37 °C for 24 h. The CD spectrum, also shown in Figure 1b, revealed the weakened magnitude of the negative peak at 222 nm because of the lowering of the α-helix conformational contents. In particular, for TPL, the random-coiled state was almost dominant, whereas the helical domains still could be detectable in TPH and TPM mixed micelles. The results clearly point out that the secondary folding may have the main role in stability.

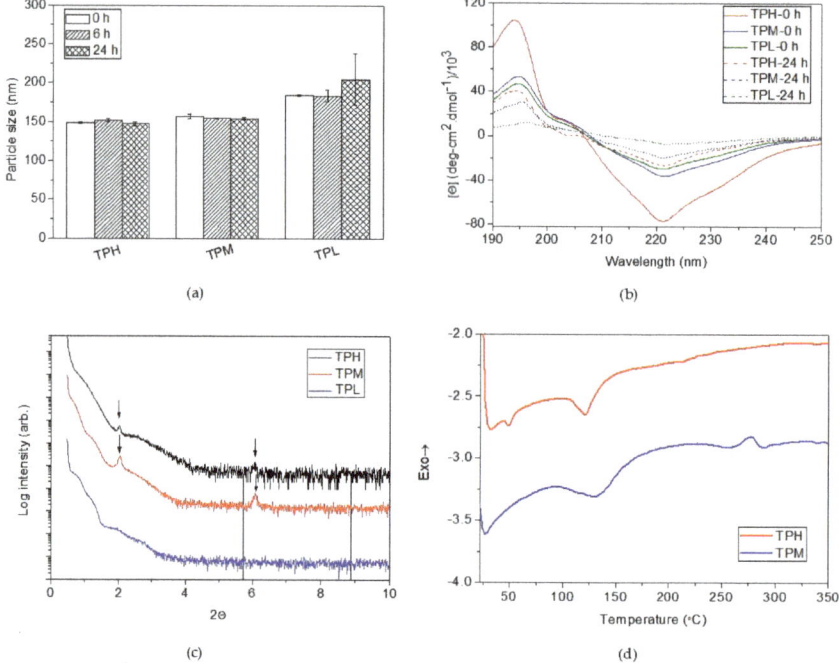

Figure 1. Stability tests of the mixed micelles incubated at 37 °C. (**a**) The changes of particle sizes and distribution at both 6 h and 24 h. (**b**) The CD spectrum of micelles at 24 h for determination of the secondary structures of the mixed micelles. (**c**) The XRD pattern and (**d**) differential scanning calorimetry analysis of micelles for crystalline alignment evaluation.

Based on the results of the particle sizes and secondary structure featuring in the CD spectrum, we focused on TPH and TPM mixed micelles to investigate their inner microstructure. The mixed micellar structures were mainly identified with differential scanning calorimetry (DSC) thermograms after mixed micelles were incubated at 37 °C for 24 h. In the TPGS thermograms in Figure S1 in the Supporting Information, two endothermal peaks at 40 and 317 °C can be observed, representing, respectively, the melting point (T_m) and the decomposition temperature. The PBLG thermogram shows one sharp endothermal peak at 311 °C, indicating its T_m. However, for TPH and TPM mixed micelles, after incubation at 37 °C for 24 h, the endothermal peaks at 317 and 311 °C were undetectable, which could be attributed to the micelle formation. These results show that the secondary structures within the micellar structures play a crucial role in micellar stability.

Despite TPH and TPM mixed micelles having adequate stability in the mimetic physiological environment, they exhibited subtle distinctions after incubation at 37 °C for 24 h according to the transmission electron microscopy (TEM) images with phosphotungstic acid (PTA) staining (Figure S2 in the Supporting Information). The core–shell structures could be observed in both TPH and TPM mixed micelles. However, TPM mixed micelles were observed with relatively loose structures, due probably to the lower α-helical conformation contents and higher CMC value (Figure 1b). The regular secondary structures may lead to the formation of liquid crystalline structures [20]; crystalline structures have been reported in the microphase of PBLG [21] and they would affect the strength and stability of the micelles [22]. Thus, the crystalline structure induced by helix conformation within the TPH and TPM mixed micelles was investigated in our study. The crystalline structure within the mixed micelles was analyzed using an X-ray diffractometer (XRD) and DSC. The XRD pattern of TPH and TPM mixed micelles in Figure 1c showed 2 peaks at $2\theta = 2$ and 6, while no peak was detectable for TPL mixed micelles. The results could be reasonably explained by the secondary architectures. The ordered α-helix structures in TPH and TPM mixed micelles enabled the formation of the inner crystalline structure and led to a higher stability. The distinctions of the crystalline microphase between TPH and TPM mixed micelles from TEM images after incubation at 37 °C for 24 h were further identified via the DSC thermograms in Figure 1d. TPH mixed micelles exhibited 2 sharp endothermal peaks around 50 and 120 °C that indicate the melting temperature, respectively, demonstrating the highly crystalline structure. The TPM thermogram showed one broad endothermal peak around 132 °C and a sharp endothermal peak at 277 °C, demonstrating the interior semicrystalline structure within TPM mixed micelles. TPH mixed micelles possessed high crystalline alignments, even after being incubated at 37 °C, indicating that micellar structures still could be maintained; although the secondary structure of TPM mixed micelles still could be detected, only the semicrystalline structure was aligned within the TPM mixed micelles, inducing the looser structures after 37 °C incubation. The secondary structure could regulate the interior crystalline behaviors of the mixed micelles and further affect the micellar stability.

2.2. pH Responsiveness of the pH-Responsive Secondary Structure Contained Mixed Micelles

The secondary structure of PBLG was reported as having a responsive ability toward the protons in solutions. [23]. The pH-responsive behaviors of PBLG could be assumed by tuning the secondary structures. Since TPH and TPM mixed micelles exhibited little particle size change and high stability, the pH responsiveness was investigated to evaluate the potential for a pH responsive drug delivery system. First, the hydrodynamic diameters of TPH and TPM mixed micelles at pH 4.0 condition in 37 °C were examined using DLS, as shown in Figure 2a. TPM mixed micelles increased in particle size upon incubation. After 6 h incubation, the particle sizes enlarged from around 155 nm to 193.33 ± 1.10 nm, and the particle sizes kept increasing to 199.30 ± 2.93 nm at 24 h post-incubation. Conversely, TPH micelles did not exhibit significant particle size changes, even after being incubated for 24 h. The CD spectrum shown in Figure 2b revealed that the helix conformation of TPH still remained after 24 h of acidic treatment, while the α-helix structures were undetectable for the TPM micelles. TPM mixed micelles were also incubated at pH 6.5 condition, which was imitate the tumor tissue environment, and the CD spectrum were also investigated, shown in Figure S3 in the Supporting Information. The valley at 222 nm of TPM mixed micelles incubated at pH 6.5 was intermediate between that of mixed micelles incubated at pH 7.4 and pH 4.0, while the valley was closer than the position of mixed micelles incubated at pH7.4. The results further identified TPM mixed micelles were sensitive to outer milieus but in mimetic tumor environment (pH 6.5), TPM mixed micelles possessed similar inner structures to those in pH 7.4 condition. The XRD pattern was also examined in Figure 2c. The peaks at $2\theta = 2$ and 6 were canceled in the TPM micelles, while they were still detectable in the TPH micelles. The DSC thermograms were also evaluated, as shown in Figure S4 in the Supporting Information. For TPM mixed micelles, the combinational endothermal peaks from 310 to 323 °C were detected, resulting from the TPGS decomposition and the Tm of PBLG. This evidenced the loss of interactions between polymers within micelles and the crumbling of the TPM mixed micelles; for TPH mixed micelles, only one peak at 297 °C was observed, possibly showing that only fractional crystalline domains were disordered.

The crumbling of the TPM mixed micelles was further directly observed using a cryoTEM. The images are shown in Figure 2d,e. Figure 2d shows the TPM mixed micelles without acid treatment and the complete micelles can be observed, demonstrating that TPM micelles after incubation at 37 °C in pH 7.4 for 24 h can still maintain their architectures. The cryoTEM images in Figure 2e indicate that TPM micelles collapse after acidic treatment. In addition, the XRD pattern images, as shown in Figure 2f, also indicate that, after incubation at the neutral condition for 24 h, the spot-like crystalline diffractions could be discovered within the TPM mixed micelles. The diffraction pattern of the TPM mixed micelles is represented in the ordered crystalline structure, aligning with the out-of-plane direction [24]. The crystalline spots disappeared in the XRD pattern image of the acid-treated TPM micelles in Figure 2g, demonstrating that the crystalline nanodomains in TPM mixed micelles would be disordered at pH 4.0, in harmony with the results of the XRD pattern in Figure 2c. The gel permeation chromatogram (GPC) in Figure S5 in the Supporting Information shows that the molecular weight of the mixed micelles did not change after acidic treatment for 24 h, demonstrating that neither TPGS nor PBLG in the mixed micelles were degraded by acids. The disordered alignment of PBLG and the inducing micellar deformation were the main cause for the pH responsiveness of the mixed micelles, whereas the pH sensitivity of PBLG, however, was mostly neglected in other polymeric micellar systems [1,23,25]. The pH-tunable secondary structure containing mixed micelles was further studied in application as a novel drug delivery system.

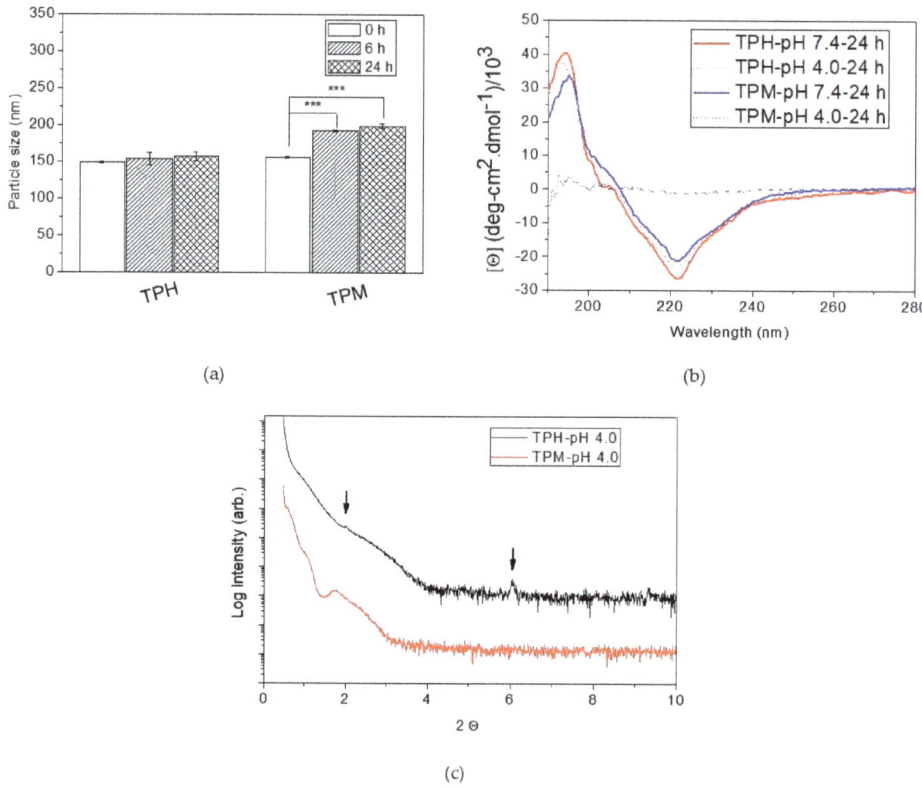

Figure 2. *Cont.*

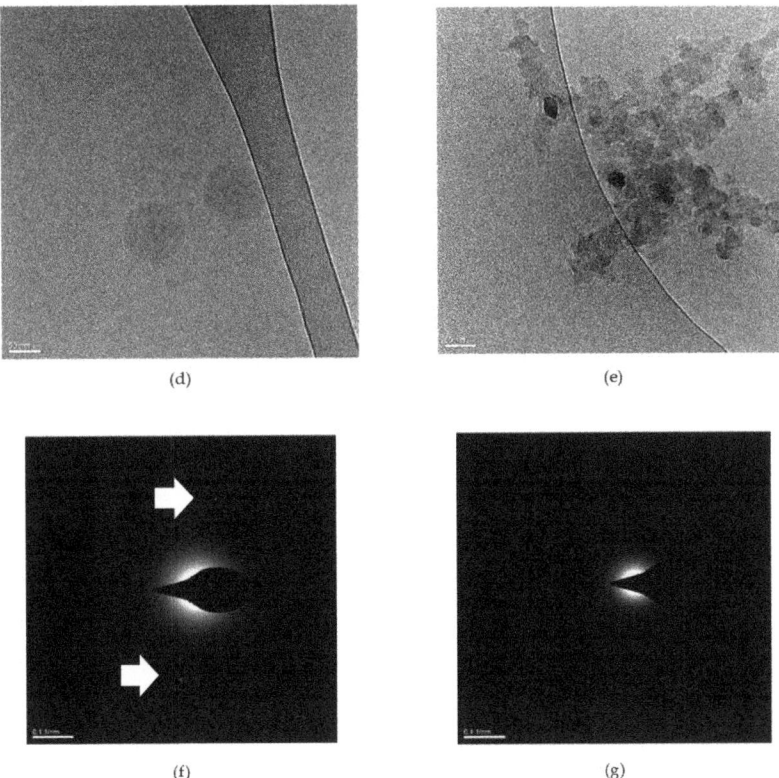

Figure 2. pH-Responsiveness of the mixed micelles. (**a**) The particle sizes of the TPH and TPM mixed micelles were measured by DLS in pH 4.0 condition after incubation at 37 °C for 6 and 24 h. (**b**) The CD spectrum of micelles were conducted to determine their secondary structures. (**c**) XRD patterns of the TPH and TPM mixed micelles after acidic treatment for 24 h. A cryoTEM was utilized for morphological observation of TPM micelles after incubation at pH 7.4 (**d**) and 4.0 (**e**) for 24 h. The diffraction images of TPM mixed micelles at pH 7.4 (**f**) and pH 4.0 (**g**) were simultaneous undergone to further conduct the crystalline alignment. Asterisk markers indicate significant difference in statistics (*** $p < 0.005$).

2.3. Doxorubicin-Loaded Secondary Conformation Contained Mixed Micelles Preparation and Drug-Releasing Behaviors

TPM mixed micelles have been identified as stable at 37 °C and pH responsive at pH 4.0, qualities which are considered to be underlying principles for a drug delivery system in anticancer therapy. TPH mixed micelles exhibited high stability at pH 7.4 condition, also indicating potential as a drug delivery system. Both TPH and TPM mixed micelles were herein chosen to encapsulate the anticancer drug doxorubicin (Dox) for further study. The anticancer drug doxorubicin hydrochloride was first reacted with triethylamine (TEA) in DMAc and then dissolved together with PBLG and TPGS, forming the doxorubicin-loaded mixed micelles (Dox-loaded mixed micelles) through the solvent exchange procedure. In order to optimize the loading efficiency and drug contents in the mixed micelles, the various doxorubicin concentrations (50, 100, 250, and 500 μg/mL) were fed into the polymer–DMAc mixtures for mixed micelles preparation, and the loading doxorubicin was determined using an ultraviolet–visible light spectrometer (UV-vis spectrometer). The drug contents and loading efficiencies of TPH and TPM mixed micelles are respectively shown in Figure 3a,b. The drug contents in TPH mixed micelles remained steadily around 3%, even as the increasing levels of Dox were employed, while their loading efficiencies decreased along with the loading concentration. The maximum loading efficiency was 91.5% when 50 µg/mL of Dox was added. For TPM mixed micelles, the maximum drug loading efficiency was approximately 80% when 50 µg/mL of Dox was applied, while the drug contents were 0.5%. The maximum drug content of TPM mixed micelles was almost 2% when 250 µg/mL of Dox was introduced, while the loading efficiency reduced to less than 10%.

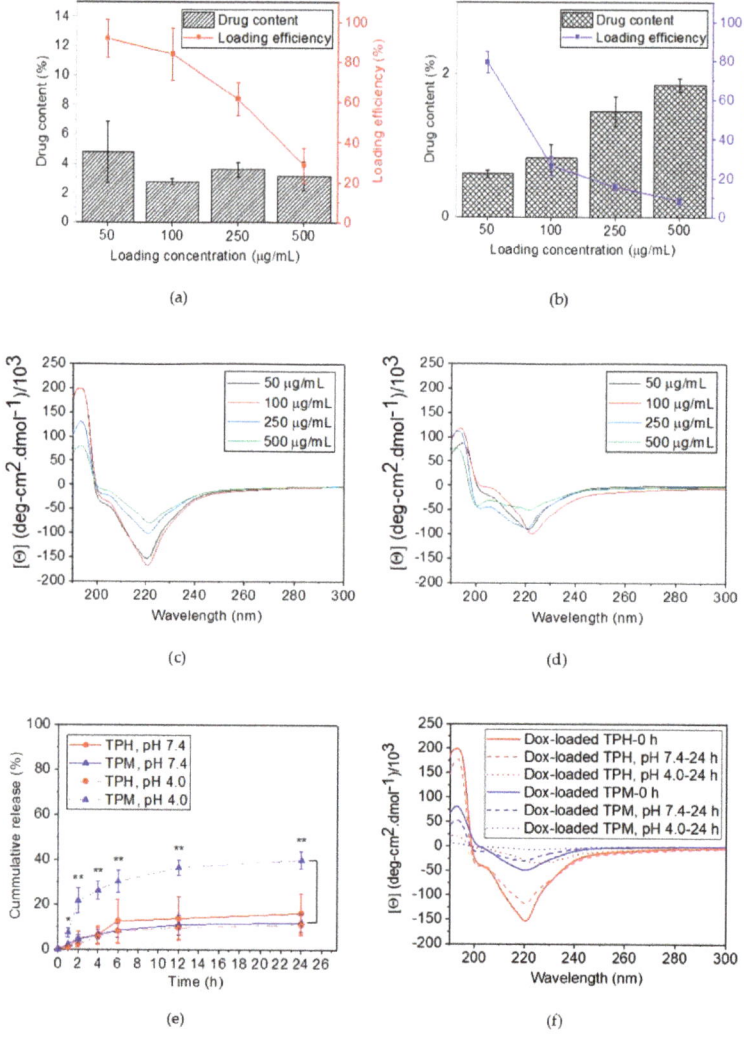

Figure 3. Drug loading and releasing behaviors. The anticancer drug doxorubicin (Dox) was encapsulated into TPH and TPM polymeric mixed micelles. To optimize the drug loading efficiency, various amounts of the doxorubicin were in-feed and the drug contents and efficiency of TPH (**a**) and TPM mixed micelles (**b**) were determined by a UV-vis spectrum. Simultaneously, CD spectrum of TPH (**c**) and TPM (**d**) micelles were also detected. The drug releasing profiles of these mixed micelles at 37 °C in pH 7.4 and 4.0 conditions were also determined using a UV-vis spectrum (**e**). The CD spectrum of the mixed micelles after incubation at pH 7.4 and 4.0 conditions for 24 h were also investigated (**f**). Asterisk markers represent significant difference in statistics (** $p < 0.01$).

The CD spectrum also indicates that the secondary conformations within the TPH and TPM mixed micelles changed with the loading concentration of Dox in Figure 3c,d, respectively. With respect to the TPH mixed micelles in Figure 3c, the helix–coil hybrids were detected in various Dox loading concentrations. However, the helical contents, determined by the valley at 221 nm, decrease along with the loading concentration. The CD spectrum of TPM mixed micelles in Figure 3d exhibits distinguishing characteristic peaks upon the addition of Dox loading solutions. Figure 3d shows the results of when 50 µg/mL of Dox infeed solution was treated with the mixed micelles of an α-helix conformation, whose valley was detected at 221 nm. As the loading Dox concentration increased to 100 µg/mL, a helix–coil conformation still could be determined, while the negative peak slightly moved to 222 nm. As the Dox concentration further increased, toward 250 and 500 µg/mL, the mixed micelle exhibited two negative peaks at 200 and 220 nm and one positive peak at 192 nm, indicating the fairly large number of random-coil structures [9]. Considering the loading efficiency as well as the secondary structures of Dox-loaded mixed micelles, eventually, we chose the 50 µg/mL of Dox in the feed concentration to fabricate the Dox-loaded TPH and TPM mixed micelles to further study their drug-releasing profiles.

Figure 3e presents the drug-releasing profiles of Dox-loaded TPH and TPM micelles at 37 °C in pH 7.4 and 4.0 conditions. At pH 7.4, both the mixed micelles released low levels of Dox. After being incubated at pH 7.4 for 24 h, only approximately 10% of Dox was liberated from TPM mixed micelles, and 15% of Dox was released from TPH mixed micelles. Meanwhile, Dox-loaded TPM mixed micelles at pH 4.0 exhibited an abrupt releasing behavior within the first two hours and a continuous releasing curve until 24 h post-incubation. A total of 40% of the Dox was released from the TPM mixed micelle in acidic conditions. Regarding the TPH mixed micelles, the drug-releasing behavior at pH 4.0 condition was nearly close to that at pH 7.4 condition, demonstrating the lack of pH responsiveness of TPH mixed micelles. The drug-releasing behaviors were considered relevant to the secondary conformation. The CD spectrum of Dox-loaded TPM mixed micelles in Figure 3f shows that at pH 7.4 for 24 h, the α-helix conformation remained dominant. After acidic treatment for 24 h, the proportions of the random coil state increased. The CD spectrum of Dox-loaded TPH mixed micelles also exhibited the pH responsive alternation in magnitude. However, after acidic treatment for 24 h, the helical domains of TPH mixed micelles remained more than those of TPH mixed micelles. The result identified that the alteration of secondary conformation within TPM mixed micelles at various pH conditions could lead to facilitating drug releasing, whereas the remaining secondary structures of TPH mixed micelles halt the rapid drug release at acidic condition.

2.4. In Vitro Tests

In this study, we exploited the toxicity of free Dox, Dox-loaded TPH and TPM micelles toward 2 different genomes of human lung cancer cells, including lung squamous cancer cell CH27 and human adenocarcinomic A549 cells. The cell viabilities of the cells after free Dox and Dox-loaded mixed micelles treatment was determined using a (3-(4,5-dimethylthiazol-2-yl)-2,5-diphenyltetrazolium bromide (MTT) assay, presented in Figure 4a,b. The cell growth was not inhibited with Dox-loaded TPH mixed micelles, whereas the cells after treatment with free Dox and Dox-loaded TPM mixed micelles revealed dose-dependent inhibition. The half-maximal inhibitory concentration (IC_{50}) of free Dox toward A549 and CH27 cells was approximately 4 µg/mL. The IC_{50} values of the Dox-loaded TPM mixed micelles toward A549 and CH27 cells were 4.28 and 6.37 µg/mL, respectively. The bare polymeric mixed micelles were also treated with human normal fibroblast cells (Detroit 551 cells). The treated concentration of the bare polymeric mixed micelles was adjusted based on the drug contents, and the cell viability of the bare polymeric mixed micelles was also determined using MTT assay. The results of TPH and TPM mixed micelles, in Figure 4c and Figure S6 in the Supporting Information, point out that very low toxicity of the mixed micelles was detected. The cell death was less than 10% when the cells were treated with 1 mg/mL of the bare TPM mixed micelles. When the cells were treated with 2 mg/mL of the bare TPM mixed micelles, the cell viability was still over 85%. Detroit 551 cells exhibited 90%

survival rate after being treated with 0.36 mg/mL of bare TPH mixed micelles, and when the cells were treated with lower levels of bare TPH mixed micelles, the cytotoxicity was hardly detected. In order to confirm the cytotoxicity of the Dox-loaded TPH and TPM micelles, another carcinoma was also tested. The cytotoxicity of human colon cancer cells HCT116 was detected to evaluate the doxorubicin efficacy toward cancer cells with an MTT assay, shown in Figure S7 in the Supporting Information. Dox-loaded TPH mixed micelles still exhibited very low toxicity toward cancer cells. The IC$_{50}$ of the HCT116 cells given with free Dox and Dox-loaded TPM mixed micelles was around 10 mg/mL, higher than that of the human lung cancer cells. Cancerous cells tolerated the anticancer agent doxorubicin distinctly from other cellular types. Therefore, this result firmly indicates that the doxorubicin was physically encapsulated into TPM micelles and dominated the tumor inhibitory effects toward different cancer cellular type, instead of the TPM mixed micelles. In this study, the human lung cancer cells A549 exhibited a great response to free Dox and Dox-loaded TPM mixed micelles. Herein, the human lung cancer cells A549 were primarily tested in our advancing assessment.

The in vitro cytotoxic tests show interesting results in Dox-loaded TPH and TPM mixed micelles. Dox-loaded TPM mixed micelles exhibited tumor inhibitory effects in lung and colon cancer cell lines, while Dox-loaded TPH mixed micelles did not show any cytotoxicity, even when the same Dox concentration within the mixed micelles was given. To further investigate the cytotoxic mechanism, the endocytosis and intracellular drug-release behavior were evaluated. For internalizing the investigation into cancer cells, a fluorescent dye, 5,6-carboxyfluorescein succinimidyl ester (Fluorescein-NHS ester), was conjugated onto the TPH and TPM mixed micelles and treated with the human lung cancer cells A549, and the intracellular fluorescence was determined using flow cytometry. Prior to Fluorescein conjugation, the TPGS was first modified into TPGS-NH$_2$. The terminal hydroxyl group of TPGS reacted with the carboxylic groups in cysteine via ester linkage, as Figure S8a in the Supporting Information presents. After purification, the modified TPGS-NH$_2$ was characterized by a hydrogen nuclear magnetic resonance (^{1}H-NMR) and Fourier transform infrared spectroscopy (FTIR), shown in Figure S8b in the Supporting Information. The conversion rate of the TPGS-NH$_2$ was around 72.2%, calculating from the ethylene groups (-CH$_2$CH$_2$-) on the PEG segments in TPGS at 3.5–3.65 ppm and the methyl group (-CH$_2$-) on the cysteine at 3–3.1 ppm. The FTIR spectrum in Figure S8c in the Supporting Information shows a peak at 1541 cm^{-1}, representing the N–H bending at the modified TPGS-NH$_2$ polymer [26]. The amine groups were thus successfully modified onto the TPGS for fluorescent dye labeling.

The TPGS-NH$_2$ polymer was assembled with PBLG into TPH and TPM polymeric mixed micelles using the solvent exchange method, as mentioned above. The amide bonds in these mixed micelles were reacted with the NHS ester groups in Fluorescein. In order to dismiss the cell abnormality and fluorescent interference from Dox, only bare TPH and TPM mixed micelles were labeled with Fluorescein dye. After removal of the excess Fluorescein dye, the fluorescence in TPH and TPM mixed micelles was adjusted until it was the same, and the Fluorescein-labeled TPH and TPM mixed micelles were treated with human lung cancer A549 cells for 1 and 3 h. The result in Figure 4d shows that the fluorescence intensity increased with the incubation time. The fluorescence intensity increased by 10 times after the cells were treated with Fluorescein-labeled TPM mixed micelles for 1 h, whereas 19-fold fluorescence intensity was detected in cells when treated with Fluorescein-labeled TPH mixed micelles. The fluorescence intensity increased to 13-fold at 3 h post-treatment with Fluorescein-labeled TPM mixed micelles, and the increasing fluorescence intensity represented the internalization of mixed micelles into lung cancer cells. The fluorescence within A549 cells slightly increased when the cells were treated with Fluorescein-labeled TPH mixed micelles and incubated for 3 h. The overall fluorescence intensity of cells treated with TPH mixed micelles was higher than that of cells treated with TPM mixed micelles.

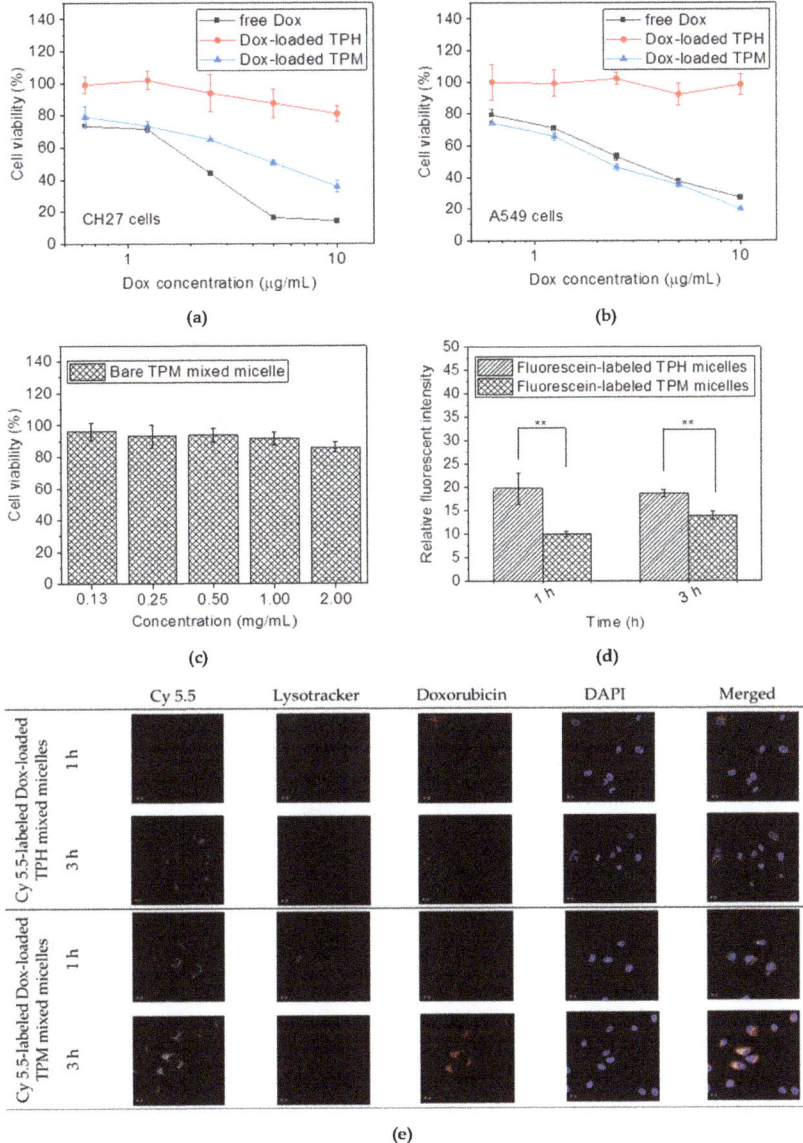

Figure 4. In vitro tests for Dox-loaded micelles contained secondary structures. Inhibitory effects of the free Dox, Dox-loaded TPM and Dox-loaded TPH micelles after incubation with human lung cancer CH27 (**a**) and A549 cells (**b**) after 24 h. (**c**) Cytotxicity of the bare TPM micelles toward human normal cells Detroit 551. (**d**) Fluorescent intensity of Fluorescein-labeled Doxed-loaded mixed micelles within human lung cancer cells A549. (**e**) The intracellular drug releasing behaviors of Cy 5.5-labeled Dox-loaded TPM micelles in human lung cancer A549 cells were also observed. The fluorescent dye Cy 5.5-labeled Dox-loaded TPM mixed micelles were co-cultured with A549 cancer cells. After 1 and 3 h treatment, the cells were washed with PBS. The lysosomes and cell nucleus were respectively labeled with fluorescent dye lysotracker and DAPI. The fluorescence within cancer cells after 1 and 3 h incubation was detected using a confocal laser scanning microscopy (CLSM). The Dox and Cy 5.5 fluorescences were respectively present in red and grey in the CLSM images, and the fluorescences of lysotracker and DAPI were shown in green and blue (**$p < 0.01$).

Since the mixed micelles have the ability to be internalized into human lung cancer A549 cells, and cytotoxicity toward cancer cells caused from TPH and TPM mixed micelles is totally different, the intracellular drug-release behaviors in our study are further discussed. The Dox intracellular releasing was observed using confocal laser scanning microscopy (CLSM). The modified polymer TPGS-NH$_2$ was assembled with PBLG and the anticancer drug Dox. Later, the fluorescent dye cyanine 5.5 (Cy 5.5) was labeled onto the Dox-loaded mixed micelles following the previous methods. Before treatment, the Cy 5.5-labeled Dox-loaded TPH and TPM mixed micelles were adjusted based on the Dox concentration. Thereafter, Cy 5.5-labeled Dox-loaded mixed micelles were treated with A549 cells for 1 and 3 h. The cells were further stained with fluorescent dye, including lysotracker Red DND-99 and 4′,6-diamidino-2-phenylindole (DAPI), to respectively symbolize the cellular lysosomes and nuclei. The fluorescence of Cy 5.5 dye and the anticancer drug doxorubicin is presented in grey and red colors, respectively, in Figure 4e, whereas the fluorescence for determining lysosome and cellar nuclei is presented in green and blue colors, respectively. Figure 4e shows the Cy 5.5 fluorescence overlapping with the lysosome fluorescence after 1 h incubation, in agreement with the internalization of Dox-loaded TPH and TPM mixed micelles. The higher fluorescence intensity of Cy 5.5 fluorescence was observed in cells treated with Cy 5.5-labeled Dox-loaded mixed micelles because the higher levels of modified TPGS-NH$_2$, which enabled conjugation with fluorescent dye Cy 5.5 and the TPM micelles. After Cy 5.5-labeled Dox-loaded TPM mixed micelles were co-cultured with cells for 3 h, the red colors can be significantly observed as overlapping with the fluorescence of Cy 5.5 (grey) and lysosomes (green). This demonstrates that mixed micelles moved toward lysosomes and the Dox was released. The Dox-loaded TPM mixed micelles were able to release their payloads at the acidic environment (pH 4.0), as the acidity of the lysosome may lead to the secondary conversion, intracellularly liberating the Dox. However, the intracellular drug-releasing behavior was not witnessed in cells incubated with Cy 5.5-labeled Dox-loaded TPH mixed micelles for 3 h. Weak Dox fluorescence (red) overlaps with the fluorescence of the lysosome (green), indicating only little Dox was released from TPH mixed micelles, even though the Cy 5.5 fluorescence on TPH mixed micelles increased upon incubation time. The CLSM images could clearly interpret the different intracellular drug-releasing behaviors between the TPH and TPM mixed micelles that primarily affect the cytotoxicity of Dox-loaded mixed micelles toward cancer cells. The severe cytotoxicity of Dox-loaded TPM mixed micelles determined from MTT assay could be recognized as the consequence of the internalization and intracellular drug-releasing behaviors of the Dox-loaded mixed micelles. Eventually, Dox-loaded TPM mixed micelles, which have ability to inhibit cancer cell growth by intracellular drug releasing, were selected to further perform the in vivo tests for anticancer feasibility.

2.5. Tumor Accumulation and In Vivo Antitumor Efficacy

The tumor accumulating behaviors were surveyed in this study by A549 cells-bearing nude mice models. Human lung cancer A549 cells were xenografted onto the back of the 4 week old female nude mice. Mice were provided by National Laboratory Animal Center (NLAC), NARLabs, Taiwan. When the tumor volume reached 50–100 mm^3, the mice were intravenously injected with Cy 5.5-labled TPM mixed micelles. At 30 min and 6 h post-injection, the Cy 5.5 fluorescence in mice was observed using IVIS, shown in Figure 5a. The Cy 5.5 fluorescence was observed spreading over the A549 bearing nude mice after 30 min injection. At 6 h post-administration, the Cy 5.5 fluorescence was mainly deposited in the tumor sites, showing that the TPM micelles were stably prone to accumulating in the tumors.

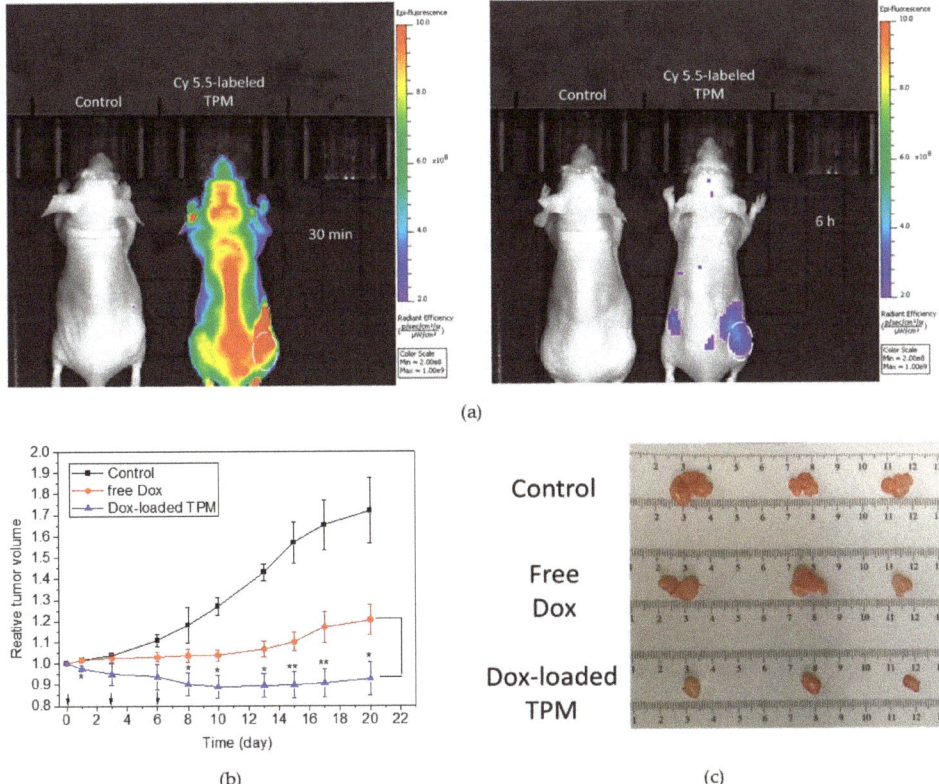

Figure 5. In vivo evaluation of the secondary structure contained mixed micelles. (**a**) The optical florescence of human lung cancer A549 bearing nude mice at post 30 min and 6 h injection with Cy5.5-labeled TPM micelles. The fluorescent intensity of the tumor marked. (**b**) Antitumor efficacy in A549 cells-inoculating nude mice. The tumor-bearing nude mice were divided into 3 groups and independently intravenously administered with PBS, doxorubicin and Dox-loaded mixed micelles at a 10 mg/kg/mL of Dox equivalent dosage each time. Total three dosages were given, present in arrows. The tumor sizes were monitored and the comparison with each group was statically analysis. The asterisk markers represented the statically significant differences (*$p < 0.05$ and **$p < 0.01$). (**c**) After 20 d treatment, the mice were sacrifice and the tumor tissues were collected and photographed.

The A549 cells-bearing nude mice models were also employed to realize the tumor inhibition of Dox-loaded TPM mixed micelles in vivo. When the tumor volume grew to 50 mm^3, the tumor-inoculated mice were separated into 3 groups, with 3 mice per group. The mice in these 3 groups were independently intravenously injected with PBS (named control), free Dox (10 mg/kg) and Dox-loaded TPM micelles (10 mg/kg, adjusted on the Dox concentration) at days 0, 3, and 6. The tumor sizes of these mice were measured and recorded, as presented in Figure 5b. The tumor sizes of the mice in the control group increased over time. Twenty days later, the average tumor sizes grew two times bigger than those at day 0. The tumor growth in those mice treated with free Dox was retarded at first. At day 3 and 6, the tumor sizes approached those in mice administered with Dox-loaded TPM micelles. However, the rates of tumor growth increased when free Dox was not affordable to those mice and, after day 8, the tumor sizes were significantly larger than those in mice treated with Dox-loaded TPM micelles. At 20 d post-first injection, the tumor sizes enlarged 1.2-fold. The tumor growths of those mice applied with Dox-loaded TPM mixed micelles were inhibited during these 20 days. Before day 10, the tumor sizes dramatically reduced due to the continuous Dox-loaded micelles administration. Thereafter, the tumor sizes slightly increased, but the tumors grew slowly. The tumors were collected and photographed after the mice were sacrificed at day 20, in Figure 5c. The tumors from the mice treated with Dox-loaded TPM micelles were the smallest among all the specimens. That could be explained by the efficient tumor deposit of the Dox-loaded TPM micelles and Dox intracellularly release.

The body weights of all the mice were also monitored and the results did not exhibit the statistical significance. However, in order to further evaluate the biosafety, blood samples were also collected at day 20 and the biochemical indexes were examined, in particular for renal and hepatic functions. The hepatic functions could be evaluated through glutamic–oxalocetic transaminase (GOT) and glutamic–pyruvic transaminase (GPT) indexes, whereas the renal functions could be assessed with blood urea nitrogen (BUN) and creatinine values. The examination results are shown in Table 2. The normal references for GOT and GPT in mice were 28–132 U/L and 59–247 U/L, respectively [27]. The GOT values in mice with a PBS injection (control group) were 216 ± 43 U/L on average, whereas the GOT average values in mice applied with free Dox were 225 ± 50 U/L and those in mice with Dox-loaded TPM miceller treatment were 187 ± 43 U/L. The GOT values were all higher than the normal indexes. The GPT values for the mice in the control, free Dox and Dox-loaded TPM micelles groups were 91 ± 21, 95 ± 11, and 90 ± 26 U/L, respectively. The BUN values of all the mice in the control, free Dox and Dox-loaded TPM micelles groups were approximately 31 mg/dL on average. Nevertheless, the normal value of the BUN ranged from 17 to 28 mg/dL [27] and the BUN of all mice was a little higher than the normal range. Another biochemical index creatinine was utilized to evaluate the renal function. The creatinine values in all mice were around 0.4 mg/dL, while the normal creatinine value is 0.2–0.8 mg/dL [27]. According to the renal and hepatic functional indexes and the body weight, Dox-loaded TPM micelles did not cause severe damage to the kidney and liver, which are considered to be affected by nanoparticles [28,29].

Table 2. Hepatic and renal function evaluation.

Code	Hepatic Function		Renal Function	
	GOT (U/L)	GPT (U/L)	BUN (mg/dL)	Creatinine (mg/dL)
Control	216 ± 43	91 ± 21	32 ± 3	0.42 ± 0.03
Free Dox	226 ± 50	95 ± 11	31 ± 3	0.39 ± 0.06
Dox-loaded TPM micelle	187 ± 42	90 ± 26	31 ± 2	0.36 ± 0.05

3. Discussion

In this study, the mixed micelles containing secondary structures were prepared. The secondary conformation of PBLG has been reported as being affected by blended polymers via hydrogen or π–π stacking interactions [10,11]. In a mixed micellar system, R. Mondal et al. further identified amphiphilic copolymers to have the ability to influence the secondary structures [30]. J. Atkinson illustrated that amphiphiles assist the secondary folding [31]. S. Kuo et al. also indicated that phenolic polymers induce the intramolecular hydrogen interaction formation and affected the helix ratios when blending with PBLG polymers in solid state [10]. In our study, the mixed micelles were identified by the DSC analysis, as shown in the Supporting Information, identifying the participation of the amphiphilic TPGS and hydrophobic PBLG in the micelles. The CD spectrum in Figure 1b showed the helix-coil characteristic peaks of all mixed micelles, representing that PBLG still could fold into secondary structures in existence with amphiphilic TPGS in a mixed micellar system. The magnitude of the 222 nm valley negatively increased upon the introduction of the PBLG to the mixed micellar system, indicating that the helix structures dominantly came from PBLG and the insertion of TPGS may interfere the helical arrangement in our mixed micellar system.

Generally, the lower CMC value may increase the stability of the micelles. In this study, the highest contents of the PBLG in mixed micelles exhibited the lowest CMC value and better stability (TPH mixed micelles), because of the highest ratio of the helical conformation, in consistency with the results from J. Ding et al. [32]. However, TPM mixed micelles, having the lowest CMC value, rather exhibited high stability, due to the α-helix conformation. The ordered secondary structures may facilitate the crystalline alignment, as S. Funari et al. reported, due to the reduction of the elastic properties in polymers [33], whereas the crystalline microphase of the hydrophobic segments plays a determinant role in micellar stability [34]. The concentrated PBLG, as comprising in a micellar system, induced the crystalline alignment [35]. Therefore, it is not surprising to discover the crystalline formations by XRD analysis within a mixed micellar system, in Figure 2c,f [35]. In our case, the crystalline structure would align in a lamellar manner and grow out-of-plane [24]. WARD results show that 2 θ = 2 and 6, showing that the distances between the α-helices of the PBLG and the pitch length of α-helices were 4.415 and 1.472 nm, respectively. The latter value was close to that reported by S. Kuo et al., identifying the α-helix conformation of PBLG in the mixed micelles; the former was much larger than that reported by S. Kuo et al., resulting from the TPGS random coil insertion into the mixed micelles [35]. Although the crystallinity and secondary structures were embedded inside the mixed micelles, based on pevious studies from S. Funari et al., the crystalline core of the mixed micelles still could respond to outer temperature stimuli [10]. Y. Mochida et al. also announced that the helix core bundled inside the micelles could still release the payload in response to the external conditions [14]. The reducing or disappearing secondary structures and core crystalline as R. Sallach et al. indicated, led to a loosening of the density of the micellar core and the releasing of the payloads [15]. In Figure 1b, the mixed micelles could be discovered their rearrangement of inner structures in response to outer temperature by the alternation in magnitude of secondary structure. Further, in Figure 2b,c, the inner secondary structures as well as crystallinity responded to the pH values of outer environment. For PBLG, the secondary structures or crystalline alignments were reported being influenced by the protonation toward the environments, though the mechanism is not completely clear [8,9]. Nevertheless, the pH sensitivity of PBLG was mostly neglected or seldom discussed in other polymeric micellar systems [1,23,25]. This might be because the terminus of PBLG was modified or conjugated onto another hydrophilic polymer in most drug or gene delivery systems. T. Itoh et al. indicated that the terminus of PBLG and the neighboring carboxylic or amine regions lack intrahelical hydrogen bonds, leading to the helix coil interconversion in response to the environment [8]. In our study, the terminals were embedded within the micellar structure, hence exerting significantly pH-responsive properties in the mixed micelles.

Small molecules of doxorubicin were encapsulated in the mixed micelles. The effect of the small molecules on the secondary structures was inconclusive [36,37]. Small amount of Dox led to the negatively increments in magnitude at 222 nm in the CD spectrum, showing the helix contents increased after Dox loading into the mixed micelles, in comparison of the bare mixed micellar carrier. That could be attributed to the π–π stacking interactions between the doxorubicin and the hydrophobic core of the mixed micelles. However, the CD spectrum in Figure 3c,d also indicates that high levels of Dox encapsulation led to the reduction of helical alignment within the mixed micelles. In our study, only a little Dox leaked from the mixed micelles at pH 7.4, according to the drug releasing profiles, as shown in Figure 3e, while in most mixed micellar system, particularly composed of TPGS, burst release occurred within the first 4 h [38,39]. Less drug leakage of our mixed micellar system in neutral conditions could be attributed to the crystalline core [34,40,41], aligned from the PBLG's secondary conformation. In a pH 4.0 environment, the secondary structures in Dox-loaded TPM mixed micelles, as well as the crystalline alignments, were driven into disorder. Dox-loaded TPH mixed micelles, which possessed highly crystalline alignment at the core, however, did less response to the environmental pH values, because their crystallinity could not be regulated by the environmental pH, probably. The crystalline microphase inside a drug carrier, as J. Jeong et al. reported, would reduce the Dox diffusion out of the drug carriers and hence retard the drug release [42]. Consequently, the drug could be released from the semicrystalline mixed micelles (TPM mixed micelles) in pH 4.0 faster than in pH 7.4.

Doxorubicin is currently applied in lung and colon cancers in clinic [43–45]. In our study, the cytotoxicities of the Dox-loaded mixed micelles toward human lung cancer cell lines A549, CH27, and human colon cancer cell line HCT116 were independently evaluated by MTT assay. Among all the cells tests, A549 cells superiorly sensitize with Dox-loaded TPM mixed micelles, while the IC$_{50}$ values of the both human lung cancer cell lines were similar, as shown in Figure 4b. The reason for this might be the rapid internalization or the fast-intracellular drug release. Human colon cancer HCT116 cells, which are considered to be less response to doxorubicin [45], exhibited the lowest cell death among the three cell lines (in the Supporting Information). The results prove that the doxorubicin was physically encapsulated into mixed micelles. Considering the future application, we focus on the A549 cell line, which was the most sensitive cells among these three cell lines to deeply investigate. Notably, Dox-loaded TPH mixed micelles were also treated with these cell lines, while almost no cytotoxicity was shown and the reasons were further studied. The internalization of the mixed micelles into A549 cells was investigated. Numerous studies have revealed that a well-defined conformation peptide chain exhibited a cell penetrating ability [46–48]. The mixed micelles in this study could be detected as rapidly entering into cancer cells by flow cytometry, as Figure 4d shows. TPH mixed micelles, having high contents of the helical structures, showed faster uptake into A549 cells than TPM micelles. M. Oba et al. further identified that the secondary conformation is altered during endocytosis [49], demonstrating that the inner secondary structures within the mixed micelles are altered with the pH values during internalization. The CLSM images in Figure 4e show that the doxorubicin is liberated from TPM mixed micelles during endocytosis, due to the disordered secondary folding and the disruption of the crystalline alignment in response to pH values. However, Figure 4e indicates that little Dox could be released from TPH mixed micelles in the process of internalization. This could account for their lack of secondary structure regulation and crystallinity. The in vitro results pictured show that the Dox-loaded mixed micelles could be taken up by cancer cells and the payloads would be intracellularly released.

The tumor accumulating behaviors of the mixed micelles were also investigated. The mixed micelles were able to rapidly accumulate in tumor tissue, while at 6 h post-administration, most mixed micelles were observed as being eliminated from mice. Y. Noguchi demonstrated that N-(2-hydroxypropyl) methacrylamide (HPMA) macromolecules also revealed a rapid tumor deposit within 10 min. After 6 h, some of them, in particular lower molecular weights of the macromolecules, would be totally perfused into the blood and clearance [50], while the higher molecular weight copolymers, which were later proved as having better tumor anti-proliferation [51], accumulate mainly at the tumor site. Our secondary conformation containing mixed micelles which were mainly observed as being deposited in the tumor tissues after 6 h treatment, illustrating their potential in antitumor treatment. The in vivo antitumor inhibition identified the efficient antitumor effects. After treatment, although the hepatic index GOT and the renal index BUN of all mice were higher than the normal references, there was, notably, no significant difference between the groups, showing that the abnormalities were not launched from the Dox treatment. In our system, the crystalline core efficiently prohibited the burst release [38,39], retaining more active drugs being transported into the tumors. As the mixed micelles containing the secondary structures have shown exceptional antineoplastic efficacy in vitro and in vivo with low toxicity, the novel micelles would be worth being further developed.

4. Materials and Methods

4.1. Materials

Poly-γ-benzyl-L-glutamate (PBLG) (M.W. 30,000–70,000), d-α-tocopherol polyethylene glycol 1000 succinate (TPGS), triethylamine (TEA), 1-ethyl-3-(3-dimethylaminopropyl) carbodiimide (EDC) and MTT reagents were obtained from Sigma-Aldrich Co., LTD (St. Louis, MO, USA). ACS-grade organic solvents including N, N-dimethylacetamide (DMAc) and tetrahydrofuran (THF) were respectively purchased from Duksan pure chemicals (Ansan City, South Korea) and Merck (Darmstadt, Germany).

Chemical reagent 4-dimethylaminopyridine (DMAP) was purchased from Alfa Aesar (Lancashire, UK) and doxorubicin hydrochloride (Dox-HCl) was purchased from Tokyo Chemical Industry Co., LTD (Tokyo, Japan). Phosphotungstic acid (PTA) for TEM staining was prepared from sodium phosphotungstate hydrate, which was acquired from Acros Organics (Geel, Belgium). Fluorescent dye lysotracker Red DND-99 and 5,6-carboxyfluorescein succinimidyl ester (Fluorescein-NHS ester) were both purchased from Thermo Fisher Co., Ltd. (Waltham, MA, USA). The other fluorescent dye cyanine 5.5 NHS ester (Cy 5.5-NHS ester) was obtained from Lumiprobe (Hunt Valley, MD, USA). Fluorescence 4′,6-diamidino-2-phenylindole contained mounting medium (DAPI-containing mounting medium) was purchased from Cisbio (Parc Marcel Boiteux, France). The animal tests were approved by Institutional Animal Care and Use Committee (IACUC approval number: CMUIACUC-2018-154-1) in China Medical University. The materials in our animal tests, including Matrigel and isoflurane were respectively obtained from Merck (Darmstadt, Germany) and Panion and BF Biotech. Inc. (Taiwan).

4.2. Preparation and Characterizations of TPGS/PBLG Polymeric Mixed Micelles

Polymers including PBLG and TPGS were weighed at various ratios and dissolved with DMAc (8 mL totally). The solutions were placed into the dialysis bags (M.W. C.O. 1k) and dialyzed against deionized water at room temperature with changing water for 6 times, forming TPGS/PBLG polymeric mixed micelles. After dialysis, the particle sizes of TPGS/PBLG polymeric mixed micelles were determined using dynamic laser scattering (DLS) (Malvern ZS90).

Hydrophobic fluorescent probe pyrene was dissolved into acetone (6×10^{-5} M) and diluted with deionized water until it reached 1.2×10^{-6} M. The organic solvent acetone was evaporated using a rotary evaporation machine. Simultaneously, polymers including PBLG and TPGS were, dissolved into THF and prepared into 2 mg/mL of polymer solutions. The solution was slowly added into the deionized water and the organic solvent THF was eliminated using a rotary evaporation machine. The PBLG and TPGS solution were thereafter diluted and mixed together under the ratios of micellar components. The polymers were serially diluted from 0.5 to 9.6×10^{-4} mg/mL. The diluted polymer solution was then taken and mixed with the equal volume of the pyrene solution. After being stored in a dark place for 1 d, the fluorescence intensities of these solutions were measured with a fluorescence reader (SpectraMax iD3). The wavelengths at 337 nm (I_{337}) and 335 nm (I_{335}) were utilized for excitation and the fluorescence wavelength at 393 nm was detected.

The secondary structures of the TPGS/PBLG polymeric mixed micelles were characterized by the circular dichroism spectrum (CD spectrum) (JASCO J-815 spectropolarimeter). The crystalline alignment was characterized using a high-resolution x-ray diffractometer (HRXRD) (Bruker D8 SSS) and assessed by a differential scanning calorimetry (DSC) (Netzsch 200F3) from 30 °C to 350 °C with the nitrogen flow.

4.3. Stability and pH Responsive Behaviors

The polymeric mixed micelles were independently incubated at 37 °C in pH 7.4 and pH 4.0 conditions. At 6 h and 24 h later, the hydrodynamic diameters of the polymeric mixed micelles were measured by DLS. The chemical or physical interactions within micelles were also determined by gel permeation chromatography (GPC) after incubation at different pH value after 24 h. The secondary structures after 6 h and 24 h incubation were simultaneously predicted using the CD spectrum. The crystalline alignment was determined by HRXRD and DSC analysis. The polymeric mixed micelles were incubated with pH 7.4 and pH 4.0 conditions, respectively. After 24 h, the polymeric mixed micelles were dropped onto the copper grid and stained by 1 wt% of phosphotungstic acid (PTA). After the removal of the excess sample and staining reagents, the copper grids were dried and stored at room temperature. The morphologies of the polymeric mixed micelles were observed using transmission electron microscopy (TEM) (JEOL JEM-1400) with the accelerated voltages. The samples were also frozen with liquid methane and observed using cryo-electron microscopy (CryoEM) (FEI Tecnai G2 F20 TWIN).

4.4. Drug Loading and Releasing Behavior Study

The anticancer drug doxorubicin (1 mmole) was dissolved into DMAc and TEA was added into the solutions. The solutions were stirred and reacted for 2 h. After 2 h, the anticancer drug doxorubicin was weighed and dissolved into DMAc with the TPGS and PBLG. The solutions were thereafter placed into the dialysis bags (M.W. C.O. 1k) and dialyzed against deionized water. After dialysis, the Dox-loaded polymeric mixed micelles were collected and stored at 4 °C.

Dox-loaded mixed micelles were placed into an ultracentrifugal tube (M.W.C.O 10 k) (Pall Corporation, Port Washington, NY, USA) and their pH values were adjusted to 7.4 or 4.0 using 0.1 M of HCl aqueous solution. The ultracentrifugal tube was placed at 37 °C under shaking. At 1, 2, 4, 6, 12 and 24 h post-incubation, the releasing doxorubicin was collected after centrifugation. The concentration of doxorubicin was detected using an ELISA reader (Biotek Synergy HT) at 488 nm wavelength. The secondary conformation of the Dox-loaded mixed micelles was also monitored using CD spectroscopy.

4.5. In Vitro Cytotoxicity Assessment

The cytotoxicity toward human cancer cells was assessed using MTT assay. Human squamous lung cancer CH27, epithelial lung cancer A549 and colon cancer HCT116 cells (1×10^5 cells/mL) were seeded each well in a 96-well plate and incubated at 37 °C with 5% CO_2 supply. As the cells attached, the cells were treated with predetermined concentrations from 10.00 to 0.63 µg/mL of free Dox and Dox-loaded mixed micelles with sequential dilutions 0.63, 1.25, 2.5, 5.00, and 10.00 µg/mL. After being co-cultured for 24 h, the excess free Dox solution and Dox-loaded mixed micelles were removed and the cells were washed with PBS twice. The MTT reagent was applied and the enzyme-linked immunosorbent assay (ELISA) reader (Biotek Synergy HT) was utilized for cell viability determination.

In addition, the cytotoxicity of the bare polymeric mixed micelles was also determined by MTT assay. Human normal fibroblast cells Detroit 551 were (1×10^5 cells/mL) seeded each well in a 96-well plate and placed at 37 °C with 5% CO_2 supply. When the cells attached onto the plate, the bare TPM polymeric mixed micelles (0.13, 0.25, 0.5, 1.00, and 2.00 mg/mL) and TPH (0.02, 0.05, 0.09, 0.18, and 0.36 mg/mL) micelles were treated with Detroit 551 cells and the cells were incubated at 37 °C with 5% CO_2 supply. Twenty-four hours later, the bare polymeric mixed micelles were eliminated and cells were washed with PBS twice. The MTT assay was also utilized for cytotoxic assessment.

4.6. Internalization and Intracellular Drug Releasing Observation

In order to label the fluorescence, TPGS was modified into amine groups after reacting with the cysteine via ester bond conjugation. The modification of TPGS was performed by the following method: TPGS (1 mmole) and cysteine (1 mmole) were weighed and dissolved with deionized water in sample vials. DMAP (0.1 mmole) and EDC (0.3 mmole) were also dissolved into deionized water and slowly added into the TPGS and cysteine mixtures. After stirring at 25 °C for 24 h, the TPGS solution was passed through the PD-10 desalting column for purification. The products were characterized by ^{1}H-NMR and FT-IR.

The prepared TPGS-NH_2 and PBLG were dissolved into the DMAc. The solutions were prepared for polymeric mixed micelles using solvent exchange methods, as mentioned above. The polymeric mixed micelle solutions were collected and mixed with the fluorescent dye Fluorescein-NHS ester at 25 °C for 24 h. Afterwards, the micellar solution was placed into a dialysis bags (M.W.C.O 6–8 k) and dialyzed against deionized water for purification. The Fluorescein-labeled polymeric mixed micelles were collected and stored at 4 °C.

Human lung cancer cells A549 (1×10^6 cells/mL) were seeded onto the 6-well plate. As the cells attached onto the plate, the Fluorescein-loaded polymeric mixed micelles were treated with the A549 cells at 37 °C with 5% CO_2 supply. After 1 and 3 h incubation [52], the excess Fluorescein-loaded polymeric mixed micelles were removed and the cells were washed with phosphate buffering saline (PBS) twice. The cells were thereafter collected using centrifugation. The harvested cells were placed into testing tubes on ice. Thereafter, 1×10^4 cells were randomly chosen and the Fluorescein intensity was determined using flow cytometry (BD FACS Canto, East Rutherford, NJ, USA) [53] to evaluate the internalization of the mixed micelles.

TPGS-NH$_2$ was further assembled into polymeric mixed micelles with PBLG and doxorubicin, following the methods described above. After the dialysis, the polymeric mixed micelles were mixed with the fluorescent dye Cy 5.5-NHS ester at 37 °C with stirring for 24 h. The excess Cy 5.5-NHS ester was eliminated by dialysis. Human lung cancer cells A549 were seeded onto a 6-well plate. As the cells attached, the Cy 5.5-labeled Dox-loaded polymeric mixed micelles were incubated with the cells at 37 °C with 5% CO_2 supply. At 1 and 3 h post-treatment, the Cy 5.5-labeled Dox-loaded polymeric mixed micelles were removed and the cells were washed with PBS thrice. The fluorescent dye lysotracker Red DND-99 (1 µM) was treated with A549 cells for 1 h at 37 °C with 5% CO_2 supply. After treatment, the excess lysotracker fluorescent dye was removed. After washing the cells using PBS thrice, the cells were fixed with 4% of paraformaldehyde. Twenty min later, the cells were washed with PBS and the cells were mounted with DAPI-containing mounting medium. The cells were observed using confocal laser scanning microscopy (CLSM) (Leica TCS SP 8, Germany). The fluorescences of Cy 5.5 and lysotracker Red DND-99 were detected using the excitation wavelength at 633 nm and 570 nm and the emission wavelength at 650 nm and 590 nm, respectively. The fluorescence of doxorubicin was observed at the excitation wavelength of 488 nm and the emission wavelength of 520 nm. DAPI was observed using the approximate excitation and emission wavelength, preset in the equipment.

4.7. Tumor Deposit and In Vivo Antitumor Efficacy

The xenografted human lung cancer A549 cells nude mice model was established to assess the tumor accumulating behaviors and the in vivo antitumor efficacy. Human lung cancer A549 cells (1×10^7 cells/mL) were homogenously mixed with an equal volume of Matrigel solution and the mixture (0.1 mL) was subcutaneously transplanted into the back of each mouse. As the tumor volume achieved 500 mm^3 or above, the tumor-inoculated nude mice were intravenously administered with Cy 5.5-labeled TPM mixed micelles. At 30 min and 6 h post-injection, the mice were anesthetized with 1.5% of isoflurane and the optical fluorescence was observed using an in vivo imaging system (IVIS) (Lumina LT system) with an excitation length at 640 nm and a Cy 5.5 filter channel.

The A549 tumor-bearing mice model was also exploited in antitumor assessment, following the abovementioned methods. When the tumor volume grew to 500 mm^3, the mice were randomly divided into 3 groups, with 3 mice per group. The mice in each group were independently injected with PBS, 10 mg/kg of free Dox and 10 mg/kg of Dox-loaded TPM micelles (the concentration was previously adjusted according to the Dox concentration) via their tail veins at day 0, 2, and 6. The tumor sizes and weights were monitored every 2 or 3 days. The tumor sizes were measured using a caliper and calculated as the following formula: Tumor size (mm^3) = ab^2/2, where a and b, respectively, represent the length and width of the tumor. Twenty days later, all of the mice were sacrificed, and CO_2 and blood samples were taken. The blood was centrifuged under 3000 r.p.m. for 10 min and the supernatant serum was obtained to analyze the hepatic and renal functions by an automatic analyzer (Hitachi-7150, Japan) with the commercial kits provided by DiaSys Diagnostic Systems GmbH (Germany). The glutamic–oxalocetic transaminase (GOT) and glutamic–pyruvic transaminase (GPT) indexes were utilized to evaluate the hepatic functions, whereas the renal functions were presented by the blood urea nitrogen (BUN) and creatinine (CRE) indexes, according to the manufacturer's instructions.

4.8. Statistical Analysis

All results are shown in average values and standard deviation, presented in mean ± S.D. (standard deviation). All data were statistically analyzed using Student's t-test (Microsoft Excel 2000). The significant differences were considered when the *p*-value was less than 0.05 ($p < 0.05$). The significant differences are shown in star marks (*$p < 0.05$; **$p < 0.01$ and ***$p < 0.001$).

5. Conclusions

For the first time, we revealed and fabricated a pH-tunable secondary structure containing mixed micelles (TPGS and PBLG) for controlled intracellular anticancer drug delivery. Importantly, the drug loading and releasing using these micelles could be precisely controlled through the regulation of the pH value, via the embedded PBLG. In the neutral condition, α-helix conformations of PBLG formed the crystalline structures to stabilize the mixed micelles with the loaded anticancer drug Dox; meanwhile, in acidic milieus (pH 4.0), the secondary conformation would transform into a random-coil state and disorder the inner crystalline alignment in the mixed micelles, allowing the drug release. The Dox-loaded pH-tunable mixed micelles would be internalized into cells, causing intracellular drug release and leading to cell death. The mixed micelles were also deposited in the primary tumor and the antitumor efficacy of the Dox-loaded mixed micelles was identified in vivo. The novel pH-tunable secondary conformation containing mixed micelles are, therefore, valuable for future clinical study.

Supplementary Materials: The following are available online at http://www.mdpi.com/2072-6694/12/2/503/s1, Figure S1: DSC analysis of TPGS, PBLG, TPH and TPM, Figure S2: TEM images of TPH (a) and TPM (b) mixed micelles after incubation at 37 °C for 24 h, Figure S3: The CD spectrum of TPM mixed micelles at pH 7.4, 6.5 and 4.0 conditions after incubation at 37 °C for 24h, Figure S4: DSC analysis of TPGS, PBLG, TPH and TPM at pH4.0, Figure S5: Gel permeation chromatography (GPC) of TPM at different pH values (7.4 and 4.0) after incubation at 37 °C for 6 and 24 h, Figure S6: Cell viability of bare TPH mixed micelles in human normal cells Detroit 551, Figure S7: The cytotoxicity assay of free Dox, Dox-loaded TPH and TPM micelles was independently conducted on human colon carcinoma cell lines HCT 116, Figure S8: Characterization of TPGS-NH$_2$.

Author Contributions: Y.-T.C. conceived the concepts and designed experiments; Y.-T.C. and X.L. analyzed the results and wrote the manuscript; F.-Y.S. prepared and characterized the mixed micelles, including the particle size measurements, TEM morphologic observation, drug releasing behavior studies, internalization and intracellular drug releasing behaviors; W.-P.J. performed the cytotoxicity evaluation and animal tests under the supervision by G.-J.H.; S.-C.K. and Y.-C.H. provided funding and the cell culture room for in vitro tests; C.-S.C. and Y.L. provided the consultant of XRD. All authors have read and agreed to the published version of the manuscript.

Funding: This work is funded mainly by Ministry of Science and Technology (MOST) (MOST 107-2314-B-039-013) in Taiwan, in Republic of China (R.O.C.). And the research was also financially supported by the "Chinese Medicine Research Center, China Medical University" from the Featured Areas Research Center Program within the framework of the Higher Education Sprout Project by the Ministry of Education (MOE) in Taiwan (CMRC-CHM-5) and a grant from China Medical University in Taiwan (R.O.C.).

Acknowledgments: The authors appreciated Ministry of Science and Technology (MOST) (MOST 107-2314-B-039-013) in Taiwan (R.O.C.), China Medical University and Ministry of Education (MOE) in Taiwan (CMRC-CHM-5) for financial supports. The authors would also like to appreciate Mr. Ju-Chun Tai for the technical assistance with CLSM and flow cytometry in China Medical University. The authors are also grateful for the measuring assistance with the TEM and XRD in National Chung Hsing University and with the cryoTEM operation in Academic Sinica Cryo-EM center.

Conflicts of Interest: The authors declare no conflict of interest.

Abbreviations

PBLG	poly-γ-benzyl-l-glutamate
TPGS	d-α-tocopherol polyethylene glycol succinate
Dox	doxorubicin
DMAc	dimethylacetamide
DLS	dynamic laser scattering
CD spectrum	circular dichroism spectrum
DSC	differential scanning calorimetry
T_m	melting point
XRD	x-ray diffractometer
TEM	transmission electron microscopy
PTA	phosphotungstic acid
GPC	gel permeation chromatogram
UV–vis spectrometer	ultraviolet–visible light spectrometer
Fluorescein	5,6-carboxyfluorescein succinimidyl ester
CLSM	confocal laser scanning microscopy

References

1. Tian, H.; Deng, C.; Lin, H.; Sun, J.; Deng, M.; Chen, X.; Jing, X. Biodegradable cationic PEG–PEI–PBLG hyperbranched block copolymer: Synthesis and micelle characterization. *Biomaterials* **2005**, *26*, 4209–4217. [CrossRef] [PubMed]
2. Tian, H.; Xiong, W.; Wei, J.; Wang, Y.; Chen, X.; Jing, X.; Zhu, Q. Gene transfection of hyperbranched PEI grafted by hydrophobic amino acid segment PBLG. *Biomaterials* **2007**, *28*, 2899–2907. [CrossRef] [PubMed]
3. Li, S.; Wang, A.; Jiang, W.; Guan, Z. Pharmacokinetic characteristics and anticancer effects of 5-fluorouracil loaded nanoparticles. *BMC Cancer* **2008**, *8*, 103. [CrossRef]
4. Vandermeulen, G.W.; Klok, H.A. Peptide/protein hybrid materials: Enhanced control of structure and improved performance through conjugation of biological and synthetic polymers. *Macromol. Biosci.* **2004**, *4*, 383–398. [CrossRef] [PubMed]
5. Papadopoulos, P.; Floudas, G.; Klok, H.-A.; Schnell, I.; Pakula, T. Self-Assembly and Dynamics of Poly (γ-benzyl-L-glutamate) Peptides. *Biomacromolecules* **2004**, *5*, 81–91. [CrossRef] [PubMed]
6. Bradbury, E.; Crane-Robinson, C.; Hartman, P. Effect of polydispersity on the nmr spectra of poly (γ-benzyl-l-glutamate) through the helix→ coil transition. *Polymer* **1973**, *14*, 543–548. [CrossRef]
7. Novotná, P.; Urbanová, M. Vibrational circular dichroism study of solvent-and temperature-induced conformational changes in poly-γ-benzyl-l-glutamate and poly-β-benzyl-l-aspartate. *Vib. Spectrosc.* **2013**, *66*, 1–7. [CrossRef]
8. Itoh, T.; Hatanaka, T.; Ihara, E.; Inoue, K. Helix–coil transformation of poly (γ-benzyl-L-glutamate) with polystyrene attached to the N or C terminus in trifluoroacetic acid–chloroform mixtures. *Polym. J.* **2012**, *44*, 189. [CrossRef]
9. Inomata, K.; Itoh, M.; Nakanishi, E. Helix–Coil Transition and Micellar Structure of Poly (ethylene glycol)-block-Poly [N 5-(2-hydroxyethyl) L-glutamine] in Cyclohexanol/Water Mixed Solvents. *Polym. J.* **2005**, *37*, 404. [CrossRef]
10. Kuo, S.-W.; Chen, C.-J. Using hydrogen-bonding interactions to control the peptide secondary structures and miscibility behavior of poly (L-glutamate) s with phenolic resin. *Macromolecules* **2011**, *44*, 7315–7326. [CrossRef]
11. Kuo, S.-W.; Chen, C.-J. Functional polystyrene derivatives influence the miscibility and helical peptide secondary structures of poly (γ-benzyl l-glutamate). *Macromolecules* **2012**, *45*, 2442–2452. [CrossRef]
12. Niehoff, A.; Mantion, A.; McAloney, R.; Huber, A.; Falkenhagen, J.; Goh, C.M.; Thünemann, A.F.; Winnik, M.A.; Menzel, H. Elucidation of the structure of poly (γ-benzyl-L-glutamate) nanofibers and gel networks in a helicogenic solvent. *Colloid Polym. Sci.* **2013**, *291*, 1353–1363. [CrossRef] [PubMed]
13. Rajan, V.; Woo, C.-W. Liquid-crystalline properties and reentrance phenomena in PBLG solutions. *Phys. Rev. A* **1980**, *21*, 990. [CrossRef]
14. Mochida, Y.; Cabral, H.; Miura, Y.; Albertini, F.; Fukushima, S.; Osada, K.; Nishiyama, N.; Kataoka, K. Bundled assembly of helical nanostructures in polymeric micelles loaded with platinum drugs enhancing therapeutic efficiency against pancreatic tumor. *ACS Nano* **2014**, *8*, 6724–6738. [CrossRef]
15. Sallach, R.E.; Wei, M.; Biswas, N.; Conticello, V.P.; Lecommandoux, S.; Dluhy, R.A.; Chaikof, E.L. Micelle density regulated by a reversible switch of protein secondary structure. *J. Am. Chem. Soc.* **2006**, *128*, 12014–12019. [CrossRef]
16. Liu, H.; Wang, R.; Wei, J.; Cheng, C.; Zheng, Y.; Pan, Y.; He, X.; Ding, M.; Tan, H.; Fu, Q. Conformation-directed micelle-to-vesicle transition of cholesterol-decorated polypeptide triggered by oxidation. *J. Am. Chem. Soc.* **2018**, *140*, 6604–6610. [CrossRef]
17. Choi, M.; Choi, D.; Hong, J. Multilayered controlled drug release silk fibroin nanofilm by manipulating secondary structure. *Biomacromolecules* **2018**, *19*, 3096–3103. [CrossRef]
18. Owen, S.C.; Chan, D.P.; Shoichet, M.S. Polymeric micelle stability. *Nano Today* **2012**, *7*, 53–65. [CrossRef]
19. Mason, A.F.; Buddingh', B.C.; Williams, D.S.; van Hest, J.C. Hierarchical self-assembly of a copolymer-stabilized coacervate protocell. *J. Am. Chem. Soc.* **2017**, *139*, 17309–17312. [CrossRef]
20. McGill, M.; Holland, G.P.; Kaplan, D.L. Experimental methods for characterizing the secondary structure and thermal properties of silk proteins. *Macromol. Rapid Commun.* **2019**, *40*, 1800390. [CrossRef]

21. Ndukwe, I.E.; Wang, X.; Pelczer, I.; Reibarkh, M.; Williamson, R.T.; Liu, Y.; Martin, G.E. PBLG as a versatile liquid crystalline medium for anisotropic NMR data acquisition. *Chem. Commun.* **2019**, *55*, 4327–4330. [CrossRef] [PubMed]
22. Müller-Goymann, C. Physicochemical characterization of colloidal drug delivery systems such as reverse micelles, vesicles, liquid crystals and nanoparticles for topical administration. *Eur. J. Pharm. Biopharm.* **2004**, *58*, 343–356. [CrossRef] [PubMed]
23. Huang, W.; Wang, W.; Wang, P.; Tian, Q.; Zhang, C.; Wang, C.; Yuan, Z.; Liu, M.; Wan, H.; Tang, H. Glycyrrhetinic acid-modified poly (ethylene glycol)–b-poly (γ-benzyl l-glutamate) micelles for liver targeting therapy. *Acta Biomater.* **2010**, *6*, 3927–3935. [CrossRef] [PubMed]
24. Hashimoto, Y.; Sato, T.; Goto, R.; Nagao, Y.; Mitsuishi, M.; Nagano, S.; Matsui, J. In-plane oriented highly ordered lamellar structure formation of poly (N-dodecylacrylamide) induced by humid annealing. *RSC Adv.* **2017**, *7*, 6631–6635. [CrossRef]
25. Wang, Z.; Sheng, R.; Luo, T.; Sun, J.; Cao, A. Synthesis and self-assembly of diblock glycopolypeptide analogues PMAgala-b-PBLG as multifunctional biomaterials for protein recognition, drug delivery and hepatoma cell targeting. *Polym. Chem.* **2017**, *8*, 472–484. [CrossRef]
26. Chew, N.G.P.; Zhao, S.; Malde, C.; Wang, R. Superoleophobic surface modification for robust membrane distillation performance. *J. Membr. Sci.* **2017**, *541*, 162–173. [CrossRef]
27. Lu, P.-L.; Chen, Y.-C.; Ou, T.-W.; Chen, H.-H.; Tsai, H.-C.; Wen, C.-J.; Lo, C.-L.; Wey, S.-P.; Lin, K.-J.; Yen, T.-C. Multifunctional hollow nanoparticles based on graft-diblock copolymers for doxorubicin delivery. *Biomaterials* **2011**, *32*, 2213–2221. [CrossRef]
28. Zhang, Y.-N.; Poon, W.; Tavares, A.J.; McGilvray, I.D.; Chan, W.C. Nanoparticle–liver interactions: Cellular uptake and hepatobiliary elimination. *J. Control. Release* **2016**, *240*, 332–348. [CrossRef]
29. Du, B.; Yu, M.; Zheng, J. Transport and interactions of nanoparticles in the kidneys. *Nat. Rev. Mater.* **2018**, *3*, 358–374. [CrossRef]
30. Mondal, R.; Ghosh, N.; Paul, B.K.; Mukherjee, S. Triblock-copolymer-assisted mixed-micelle formation results in the refolding of unfolded protein. *Langmuir* **2017**, *34*, 896–903. [CrossRef]
31. Atkinson, J.; Clarke, M.W.; Warnica, J.M.; Boddington, K.F.; Graether, S.P. Structure of an intrinsically disordered stress protein alone and bound to a membrane surface. *Biophys. J.* **2016**, *111*, 480–491. [CrossRef] [PubMed]
32. Ding, J.; Xiao, C.; Zhao, L.; Cheng, Y.; Ma, L.; Tang, Z.; Zhuang, X.; Chen, X. Poly (L-glutamic acid) grafted with oligo (2-(2-(2-methoxyethoxy) ethoxy) ethyl methacrylate): Thermal phase transition, secondary structure, and self-assembly. *J. Polym. Sci. Part A* **2011**, *49*, 2665–2676. [CrossRef]
33. Funari, S.S.; Nuscher, B.; Rapp, G.; Beyer, K. Detergent-phospholipid mixed micelles with a crystalline phospholipid core. *Proc. Natl. Acad. Sci. USA* **2001**, *98*, 8938–8943. [CrossRef] [PubMed]
34. Lu, Y.; Zhang, E.; Yang, J.; Cao, Z. Strategies to improve micelle stability for drug delivery. *Nano Res.* **2018**, *11*, 4985–4998. [CrossRef]
35. Kuo, S.-W.; Lee, H.-F.; Huang, W.-J.; Jeong, K.-U.; Chang, F.-C. Solid state and solution self-assembly of helical polypeptides tethered to polyhedral oligomeric silsesquioxanes. *Macromolecules* **2009**, *42*, 1619–1626. [CrossRef]
36. Mao, J.; DeSantis, C.; Bong, D. Small molecule recognition triggers secondary and tertiary interactions in DNA folding and hammerhead ribozyme catalysis. *J. Am. Chem. Soc.* **2017**, *139*, 9815–9818. [CrossRef]
37. Ryan, T.M.; Friedhuber, A.; Lind, M.; Howlett, G.J.; Masters, C.; Roberts, B.R. Small amphipathic molecules modulate secondary structure and amyloid fibril-forming kinetics of Alzheimer disease peptide Aβ1–42. *J. Biol. Chem.* **2012**, *287*, 16947–16954. [CrossRef]
38. Cagel, M.; Bernabeu, E.; Gonzalez, L.; Lagomarsino, E.; Zubillaga, M.; Moretton, M.A.; Chiappetta, D.A. Mixed micelles for encapsulation of doxorubicin with enhanced in vitro cytotoxicity on breast and ovarian cancer cell lines versus Doxil®. *Biomed. Pharmacother.* **2017**, *95*, 894–903. [CrossRef]
39. Mu, L.; Elbayoumi, T.; Torchilin, V. Mixed micelles made of poly (ethylene glycol)–phosphatidylethanolamine conjugate and d-α-tocopheryl polyethylene glycol 1000 succinate as pharmaceutical nanocarriers for camptothecin. *Int. J. Pharm.* **2005**, *306*, 142–149. [CrossRef]
40. Boyd, B.J.; Whittaker, D.V.; Khoo, S.-M.; Davey, G. Lyotropic liquid crystalline phases formed from glycerate surfactants as sustained release drug delivery systems. *Int. J. Pharm.* **2006**, *309*, 218–226. [CrossRef]

41. Kim, H.K.; Park, T.G. Comparative study on sustained release of human growth hormone from semi-crystalline poly (L-lactic acid) and amorphous poly (D, L-lactic-co-glycolic acid) microspheres: Morphological effect on protein release. *J. Control. Release* **2004**, *98*, 115–125. [CrossRef] [PubMed]
42. Jeong, J.-C.; Lee, J.; Cho, K. Effects of crystalline microstructure on drug release behavior of poly (ε-caprolactone) microspheres. *J. Control. Release* **2003**, *92*, 249–258. [CrossRef]
43. Seymour, L.W.; Ferry, D.R.; Kerr, D.J.; Rea, D.; Whitlock, M.; Poyner, R.; Boivin, C.; Hesslewood, S.; Twelves, C.; Blackie, R. Phase II studies of polymer-doxorubicin (PK1, FCE28068) in the treatment of breast, lung and colorectal cancer. *Int. J. Oncol.* **2009**, *34*, 1629–1636. [CrossRef] [PubMed]
44. Roth, B.J.; Johnson, D.H.; Einhorn, L.H.; Schacter, L.P.; Cherng, N.C.; Cohen, H.J.; Crawford, J.; Randolph, J.A.; Goodlow, J.L.; Broun, G.O. Randomized study of cyclophosphamide, doxorubicin, and vincristine versus etoposide and cisplatin versus alternation of these two regimens in extensive small-cell lung cancer: A phase III trial of the Southeastern Cancer Study Group. *J. Clin. Oncol.* **1992**, *10*, 282–291. [CrossRef]
45. Sliwinska, M.A.; Mosieniak, G.; Wolanin, K.; Babik, A.; Piwocka, K.; Magalska, A.; Szczepanowska, J.; Fronk, J.; Sikora, E. Induction of senescence with doxorubicin leads to increased genomic instability of HCT116 cells. *Mech. Ageing Dev.* **2009**, *130*, 24–32. [CrossRef]
46. Gellman, S.H. Foldamers: A manifesto. *Acc. Chem. Res.* **1998**, *31*, 173–180. [CrossRef]
47. Potocky, T.B.; Menon, A.K.; Gellman, S.H. Effects of conformational stability and geometry of guanidinium display on cell entry by β-peptides. *J. Am. Chem. Soc.* **2005**, *127*, 3686–3687. [CrossRef]
48. Wada, S.-I.; Urase, T.; Hasegawa, Y.; Ban, K.; Sudani, A.; Kawai, Y.; Hayashi, J.; Urata, H. Aib-containing peptide analogs: Cellular uptake and utilization in oligonucleotide delivery. *Bioorg. Med. Chem.* **2014**, *22*, 6776–6780. [CrossRef]
49. Oba, M.; Nagano, Y.; Kato, T.; Tanaka, M. Secondary structures and cell-penetrating abilities of arginine-rich peptide foldamers. *Sci. Rep.* **2019**, *9*, 1349. [CrossRef]
50. Noguchi, Y.; Wu, J.; Duncan, R.; Strohalm, J.; Ulbrich, K.; Akaike, T.; Maeda, H. Early phase tumor accumulation of macromolecules: A great difference in clearance rate between tumor and normal tissues. *Jpn. J. Cancer Res.* **1998**, *89*, 307–314. [CrossRef]
51. Seymour, L.; Ulbrich, K.; Steyger, P.; Brereton, M.; Subr, V.; Strohalm, J.; Duncan, R. Tumour tropism and anti-cancer efficacy of polymer-based doxorubicin prodrugs in the treatment of subcutaneous murine B16F10 melanoma. *Br. J. Cancer* **1994**, *70*, 636. [CrossRef] [PubMed]
52. Chiang, Y.-T.; Cheng, Y.-T.; Lu, C.-Y.; Yen, Y.-W.; Yu, L.-Y.; Yu, K.-S.; Lyu, S.-Y.; Yang, C.-Y.; Lo, C.-L. Polymer–liposome complexes with a functional hydrogen-bond cross-linker for preventing protein adsorption and improving tumor accumulation. *Chem. Mater.* **2013**, *25*, 4364–4372. [CrossRef]
53. Banerjee, K.; Gautam, S.K.; Kshirsagar, P.; Ross, K.A.; Spagnol, G.; Sorgen, P.; Wannemuehler, M.J.; Narasimhan, B.; Solheim, J.C.; Kumar, S. Amphiphilic polyanhydride-based recombinant MUC4β-nanovaccine activates dendritic cells. *Genes Cancer* **2019**, *10*, 52. [PubMed]

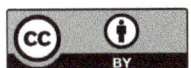

© 2020 by the authors. Licensee MDPI, Basel, Switzerland. This article is an open access article distributed under the terms and conditions of the Creative Commons Attribution (CC BY) license (http://creativecommons.org/licenses/by/4.0/).

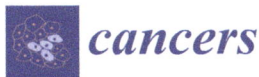 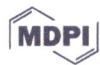

Article

Multifunctional Silica-Based Nanoparticles with Controlled Release of Organotin Metallodrug for Targeted Theranosis of Breast Cancer

Karina Ovejero Paredes [1,2], Diana Díaz-García [3], Victoria García-Almodóvar [1,3], Laura Lozano Chamizo [1,2], Marzia Marciello [1], Miguel Díaz-Sánchez [3], Sanjiv Prashar [3], Santiago Gómez-Ruiz [3,] and Marco Filice [1,2,*]

1. Nanobiotechnology for Life Sciences Group, Department of Chemistry in Pharmaceutical Sciences, Faculty of Pharmacy, Universidad Complutense de Madrid (UCM), Plaza Ramón y Cajal s/n, E-28040 Madrid, Spain; kovejero@ucm.es (K.O.P.); v.garciaalm@alumnos.urjc.es (V.G.-A.); laurloza@ucm.es (L.L.C.); marmarci@ucm.es (M.M.)
2. Microscopy and Dynamic Imaging Unit, Fundación Centro Nacional de Investigaciones Cardiovasculares Carlos III (CNIC), Calle Melchor Fernandez Almagro 3, E-28029 Madrid, Spain
3. COMET-NANO Group. Department of Biology and Geology, Physics and Inorganic Chemistry, ESCET, Universidad Rey Juan Carlos, Calle Tulipán s/n, E-28933 Móstoles (Madrid), Spain; diana.diaz@urjc.es (D.D.-G.); miguel.diaz@urjc.es (M.D.-S.); sanjiv.prashar@urjc.es (S.P.)
* Correspondence: santiago.gomez@urjc.es (S.G.-R.); mfilice@ucm.es (M.F.)

Received: 4 November 2019; Accepted: 8 January 2020; Published: 12 January 2020

Abstract: Three different multifunctional nanosystems based on the tethering onto mesoporous silica nanoparticles (MSN) of different fragments such as an organotin-based cytotoxic compound $Ph_3Sn\{SCH_2CH_2CH_2Si(OMe)_3\}$ (MSN-AP-Sn), a folate fragment (MSN-AP-FA-Sn), and an enzyme-responsive peptide able to release the metallodrug only inside cancer cells (MSN-AP-FA-PEP-S-Sn), have been synthesized and fully characterized by applying physico-chemical techniques. After that, an in vitro deep determination of the therapeutic potential of the achieved multifunctional nanovectors was carried out. The results showed a high cytotoxic potential of the MSN-AP-FA-PEP-S-Sn material against triple negative breast cancer cell line (MDA-MB-231). Moreover, a dose-dependent metallodrug-related inhibitory effect on the migration mechanism of MDA-MB-231 tumor cells was shown. Subsequently, the organotin-functionalized nanosystems have been further modified with the NIR imaging agent Alexa Fluor 647 to give three different theranostic silica-based nanoplatforms, namely, MSN-AP-Sn-AX (AX-1), MSN-AP-FA-Sn-AX (AX-2), and MSN-AP-FA-PEP-S-Sn-AX (AX-3). Their in vivo potential as theranostic markers was further evaluated in a xenograft mouse model of human breast adenocarcinoma. Owing to the combination of the receptor-mediated site targeting and the specific fine-tuned release mechanism of the organotin metallodrug, the nanotheranostic drug MSN-AP-FA-PEP-S-Sn-AX (AX-3) has shown targeted diagnostic ability in combination with enhanced therapeutic activity by promoting the inhibition of tumor growth with reduced hepatic and renal toxicity upon the repeated administration of the multifunctional nanodrug.

Keywords: triple negative breast cancer; organotin; mesoporous silica nanoparticles; MDA-MB-231; theranostic nanomaterials; nanobiotechnology; molecular imaging

1. Introduction

Breast cancer is the most common cancer in women worldwide and also the leading cause of cancer death in women (15.0%) [1–3]. Within all the possible different subtypes, triple negative breast cancer (TNBC) is the most aggressive subclass and it is characterized by having the worst prognosis with a high risk of relapse [2,4–6]. TNBCs are characterized by the absence of estrogen and progesterone receptors, as well as by having normal levels of HER2 (human epidermal growth factor receptor 2). For these reasons, hormone therapies and treatments targeting the HER2 receptor cannot be used to treat this type of cancer [7].

To tackle this issue and increase the specificity of the treatment, it is important to identify a proper receptor that meets some crucial parameters: it must be overexpressed, should not be released into circulation [8], and must become active on the target cell surface, as quickly as possible, in order to recognize more drug, to finally enhance the treatment efficiency [9]. Within the receptor that meet these criteria, the folate receptor alpha (a glycosylphosphatidylinositol (GPI) anchored cell surface glycoprotein that is able to bind free folate with high affinity) represents a good candidate being overexpressed by many cancer tissues (ovarian, epithelial, cervical, lung, kidney, brain, colorectal, and breast tumors) [10–12]. More specifically, the folate receptor alpha is overexpressed in many TNBCs cells, including the MDA-MB-231 cell line [13–16].

Dating from the approval of cisplatin from FDA (1978), the use of metal-based drugs in cancer chemotherapy has considerably increased [17–19]. Although cisplatin derivatives have been extensively used as chemotherapeutics, the onset of tumor drug-resistance has been observed upon treatment with these compounds [20]. In addition, other reported side-effects as low bioavailability and poor solubility in physiological media are still hampering the definitive application of these chemotherapeutic drugs [21]. Therefore, the search for alternative metallodrugs bearing different elements such as gallium, titanium, palladium, gold, cobalt, ruthenium, or tin could represent an interesting strategy to overcome the cisplatin-related drawbacks previously detailed [22,23]. Within the possible alternatives, organotin(IV) derivatives are getting attention as promising chemotherapeutics because of their cytotoxicity [21,24]. In addition, organotin(IV) compounds are interesting because of their potential ability to overcome resistance [25] and because they are not substrates of the P-glycoprotein 1 (permeability glycoprotein, or Pgp, also known as multidrug resistance protein 1 (MDR1)), a cell membrane transporter protein (responsible for the out of cell efflux of most of the anticancer drugs in particular) [22]. Despite its promising potential, even the organotin-based drugs present some limitations that make mandatory the use of a proper vector for their biomedical application. In this sense, nanomaterials can act as suitable vectors for metallodrug delivery by (i) protecting the active species from degradation, (ii) enhancing their therapeutic activity [26], (iii) increasing drug bioavailability and specificity, or (iv) increasing the solubility [23,27–30]. Because of its synthetic flexibility and biocompatibility, mesoporous silica-based nanostructured materials (MSN) represent one of the most used nanovectors in biomedicine, with special importance in metallodrug-based drug delivery systems [23,31–38]. Consequently, the MSNs have stood out in different biomedical fields such as molecular imaging (fluorescence and magnetic resonance imaging) and drug delivery [39–45]. Especially in this last research area, MSN have shown a lots of benefits [46] such as a variable and controllable particle and pore size, a large surface area that can be selectively functionalized for drug delivery or high biocompatibility [47–49] or the possibility of combining several functionalities in a single nanosystem [50]. In this sense, one of these possible combinations is represented by the *theranosis* or the generation of a single nanoentity able to combine therapeutic and diagnostic features at the same time [28,51–55]. In general, nanovectors may deliver their therapeutic cargo via two possible pathways: enhanced permeability and retention (EPR) effect [56] or receptor-mediated transcytosis [57]. In comparison with EPR, the receptor-mediated strategy is able to promote a more efficient and selective delivery of therapeutic drugs, for example, to tumoral cells.

Besides the theranostic behavior and the selective targeting ability, an ideal multifunctional nanosystem should be also able to release its therapeutic cargo in a controlled manner, for example, upon precise endogenous stimuli. Consequently, the drugs will only be accumulated in the targeted site and in a selective manner, thus, avoiding adverse side effects related to a possible off-target toxicity. For this purpose, in the last decade, stimuli-responsive "smart" nanomaterials have attracted great attention as promising materials in comparison to the conventional ones [58,59]. Within all the available "smart" materials, the enzyme-responsive ones, or the materials whose chemical structures or physical properties are responsive to the biocatalytic action of specific enzymes, have attracted great attention [59,60]. Because of dysregulation of enzyme expression in many diseases, these dysregulated enzymes can be turned into promising and selective biological triggers in therapeutics [58,61,62].

Thus, in our study, we have designed, synthesized, and fully characterized in vitro and in vivo a theranostic silica-based nanoplatform bearing therapeutic (organotin(IV) complex), diagnostic (Alexa Fluor 647) and targeting (folate fragment) moieties potentially useful in TNBCs treatment. Furthermore, we have also evaluated the effect of a site-selective controlled delivery of the metallodrug, based on the specific activation of an enzyme-responsive linker that can be cleaved only after tumor cell uptake. The synthesized materials have been fully characterized by chemical and physical techniques. The nanovectors showing the best properties have been used for in vitro toxicity evaluation. Finally, the best candidates have been assessed in vivo as theranostic agents for the metallodrug-based treatment of triple negative human breast adenocarcinoma generated in murine models. The overall achieved results were very promising paving the way for a more extensive application of these nanovectors for cancer theranosis.

2. Results and Discussion

2.1. Synthesis of the Different MSN-Based Multifunctional Nanomaterials

To prepare and assess the different silica-based multifunctional nanomaterials, first, mesoporous silica nanoparticles, as common nanoplatform, were synthesized as previously described and detailed here in Supporting Information. After that, the achieved MSN material was dehydrated by treatment at 150 °C under vacuum for 6 h for the subsequent surface functionalization with 3-(aminopropyl)triethoxysilane (AP) to give the MSN-AP material. For the further functionalization steps, the MSN-AP material was then functionalized with an organotin-based metallodrug by using three different strategies, one for the creation of each required moiety (Scheme 1).

In more details, the first designed method consisted in the direct tethering reaction of MSN-AP with $Ph_3Sn\{SCH_2CH_2CH_2Si(OMe)_3\}$ complex via protonolysis and elimination of methanol groups to obtain the material MSN-AP-Sn (Scheme 1, route a). The resulting material is likely to be cytotoxic, as our group has demonstrated that Sn-functionalized silica-based nanostructured show interesting cytotoxic properties in other cancer cell lines [34,36]. The second strategy expected the incorporation of the organotin metallodrug after the previous functionalization of MSN-AP material with a folate fragment, in order to study the impact of the potential receptor-mediated active targeting ability on the biological properties of the nanomaterial (Scheme 1, route b). The incorporation reaction of targeting moiety was carried out by coupling the folic acid with the amino groups of the MSN-AP owing to the carbodiimide chemistry and using EDAC as coupling agent. The material with folic acid (MSN-AP-FA) was subsequently reacted with $Ph_3Sn\{SCH_2CH_2CH_2Si(OMe)_3\}$ in a tethering reaction to give the material MSN-AP-FA-Sn via the elimination of methanol groups of the tin compound. Again, this material is expected to show cytotoxic activity because of the incorporation of the highly cytotoxic $SnPh_3$ moiety and the potential higher uptake due to the incorporation of the folic acid fragment.

Finally, the third strategy was designed in order to anchor the metallodrug to the nanovector surface by means of an enzyme responsive linker (ERL) based on a specific peptide sequence. The selected GFLG tetrapeptide linker (highly sensitive to the lysosomal cysteine protease cathepsin B that is overexpressed in breast adenocarcinoma) [63] will presumably permit the release of the therapeutic cargo (organotin(IV) metallodrug), once the theranostic nanovector is uptaken by the cancer cells [64,65]. Toward this scope, the MSN-AP material was treated simultaneously with folic acid and the Fmoc-GFLG-COOH protected peptide by an EDAC-assisted coupling reaction in order to achieve the material MSN-AP-FA-PEP. Subsequently, the terminal amino group of the peptide was deprotected with pyrrolidine and reacted with 3-mercaptopropionic acid to give the thiol-pendant system MSN-AP-FA-PEP-S. Thus, the latter was finally reacted with $Ph_3Sn\{SCH_2CH_2CH_2Si(OMe)_3\}$ complex in the presence of an excess of triethylamine to give the final material MSN-AP-FA-PEP-S-Sn

(Scheme 1, route c). In this material, the triphenyltin fragments are present both directly attached to the silica-material (as in the case of MSN-AP-Sn and MSN-AP-FA-Sn systems) and also attached to the modified peptide via a Sn-S bond formed with the thiol group of the added mercaptopropionic acid.

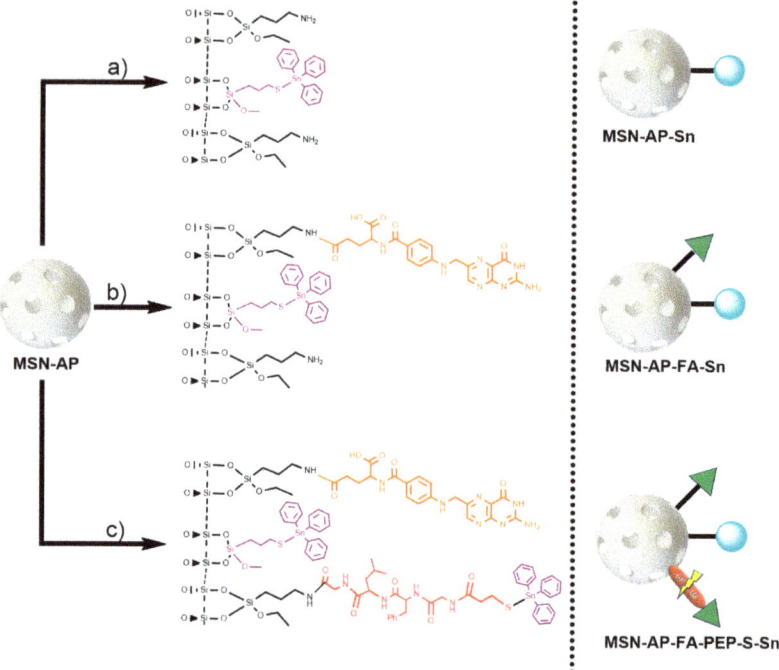

Scheme 1. General synthetic strategy for the preparation of mesoporous silica nanoparticles (MSN) materials. Route (**a**): preparation of MSN modified with organotin metallodrug; Route (**b**): preparation of MSN modified with organotin metallodrug and folate targeting group; Route (**c**): preparation of MSN modified with organotin metallodrug, folate targeting group, and organotin metallodrug linked to enzyme-responsive peptide GFLG.

2.2. Physical and Chemical Characterization of the Different MSN-Based Multifunctional Nanomaterials

For the characterization of the silica-based nanomaterials, different solid-state techniques were used. First, FT-IR studies were carried out to identify each fragment attached to the silica system during the modifications. Thus, for example, the IR spectrum of the nanomaterial functionalized with the organotin complex and folic acid (MSN-AP-FA-Sn, Figure S1 of Supporting Information) shows the typical bands of a functionalized silica-based nanoparticle, namely, a broadband between 3500–3200 cm^{-1} attributed to the O-H bonds of free silanol groups and the absorbed water in the silica. In addition, a strong band at 1100 cm^{-1} corresponding to the silanol groups (Si-O-Si) was observed. Furthermore, a medium intensity band at 900 cm^{-1} was presented and assigned to the stretching bands of Si-O bonds. Interestingly, a set of different low intensity bands were observed between ca. 3100 and 2800 cm^{-1} and attributed to the C-H and N-H vibrations of the different ligands (AP and FA). Finally, between 1700 and 1300 cm^{-1} and 680–740 cm^{-1} low intensity different bands associated with all the amido and carbonyl groups were also observed confirming the presence of the different functionalizing fragments. A similar spectrum was also observed for the material MSN-AP-FA-PEP-S-Sn (Figure S2 of Supporting Information).

The functionalized materials were also characterized by diffuse reflectance ultraviolet spectroscopy (DR-UV), an especially useful technique for the characterization of the absorption of the different functionalizing ligands or metallodrugs in silica-based systems in solid state (Figure 1). In all cases, the tin-containing materials showed a very intense peak between 200 and 220 nm due to the amino ligand AP and at ca. 260 nm due to the functionalization with the organotin derivative. Interestingly, the DR-UV spectra of both MSN-AP-FA-Sn and MSN-AP-FA-PEP-S-Sn showed an additional low intensity shoulder at ca. 320 nm, which is attributed to the anchored folic acid of the material (Figure 1).

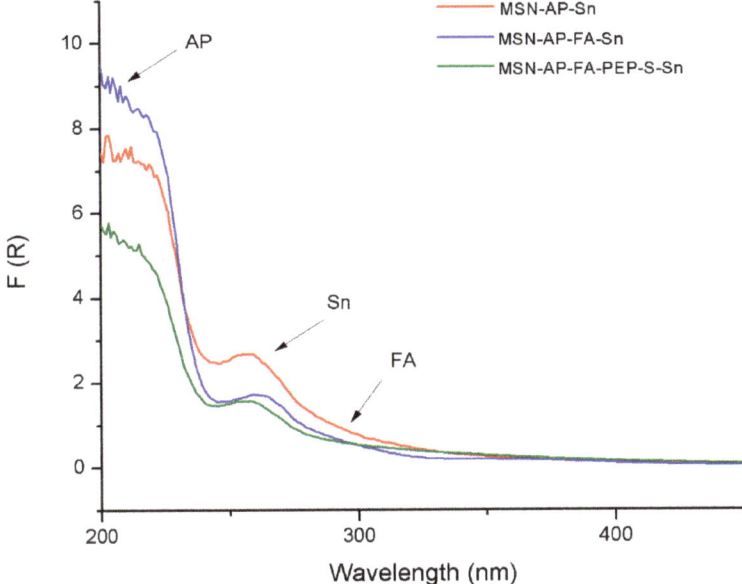

Figure 1. Diffuse reflectance ultraviolet spectroscopy (DR-UV) spectra of the tin-functionalized materials MSN-AP-Sn, MSN-AP-FA-Sn, and MSN-AP-FA-PEP-S-Sn.

For the quantification of the amount of functionalization, TG studies were carried out for all the functionalized materials, showing a similar mass loss close to 14% between 110 °C and 700 °C, which indicates a similar functionalization degree (Table S1 and Figure S3 of Supporting Information). In addition, XRF studies of the tin-containing materials showed that, relying on the observed S:Sn ratio of approximately 1:5, it seems that not all the tin is linked to MSN through the mercaptopropyl ligand in MSN-AP-Sn and MSN-AP-FA-Sn, but the migration of $SnPh_3^+$ fragments and formation of species of the type $Si-O-SnPh_3$ also occurred. Interestingly, in the case of MSN-AP-AF-PEP-S-Sn material, the S:Sn ratio lowered up to 1:2.7 indicating that the formation of the $Si-O-SnPh_3$ species is minimized and the $SnPh_3$ complex is reacting with both the mercaptopropyl group and the thiol group of the modified peptide (Table S2 of Supporting Information).

The MSN-AP-AF-Sn (Figure 2) and MSN-AP-AF-PEP-S-Sn (Figure S4) were also characterized by ^{119}Sn MAS NMR spectroscopy. In both cases, the spectra are characterized by the appearance of two broad signals at ca. −52 ppm and 40 ppm. The signal recorded at −52 ppm corresponds to the tin atom bound to the S of either the mercaptopropyl ligand or of the thiol-modified peptide, while the signal at ca. 40 ppm is due to the tin atoms of the $Si-O-SnPh_3$ species.

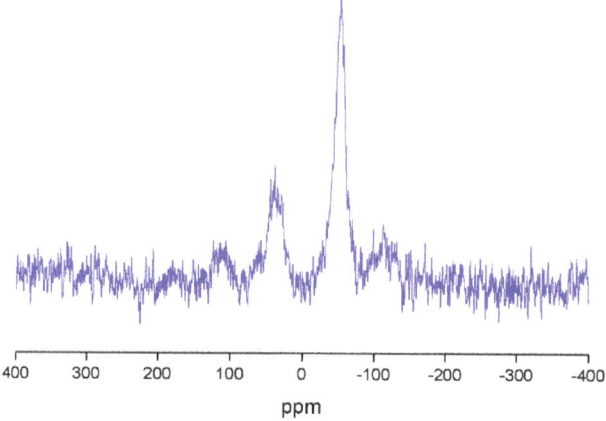

Figure 2. ^{119}Sn MAS NMR spectrum of MSN-AP-FA-Sn.

In addition, ^{29}Si MAS NMR spectroscopy was used for the characterization of the tin-containing material MSN-AP-FA-PEP-S-Sn (Figure 3). The spectrum mainly shows the signals of the silicon atoms of the structure, such as [Si(OSi)$_2$] (the highest peak (Q^4)) at −112.7 ppm), [Si(OSi)$_2$(OH)] (a very intense peak Q^3 at −105.3 ppm), [Si(OSi)$_2$(OH)$_2$] (a low intensity peak (Q^2) at −95.3 ppm), and the [Si(OSi)(OH)$_3$] (Q^1, very difficult to observe at −86.2 ppm because of its low intensity). The high intensity of Q^4 and Q^3 is in agreement with the expected for the mesoporous nature of the synthesized silica nanoparticles. In addition, at ca. −69 and −62 ppm, the T^2 ((SiO)$_2$SiOH–R) and T^3 ((SiO)$_3$Si–R) peaks of very low intensity were also observed. In addition, the different spectra of the intermediate materials MSN-AP (Figure S5 of Supporting Information) and MSN-AP-FA-PEP (Figure S6 of Supporting Information), show slight changes on the intensity of the different Q^4, Q^3, and Q^2 peaks, as well as the T^2 and T^3 peaks. This indicates that the different functionalization reactions do not have a strong influence on the chemical environment associated with the silicon atoms of the material.

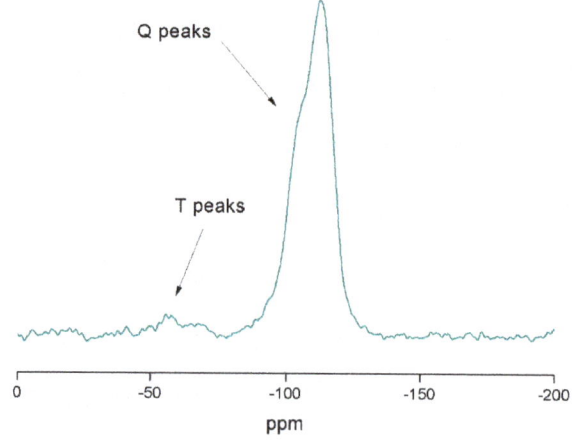

Figure 3. ^{29}Si MAS NMR spectrum of MSN-AP-FA-PEP-S-Sn.

Beside a deep physico-chemical characterization, the tin-containing synthesized materials were also characterized in terms of size and morphological appearance by transmission electron microscopy (TEM), as well as by dynamic light scattering (DLS).

The TEM micrograph retrieved oval-shaped nanoparticles with a mean particle size distribution of 116.15 ± 3.67 nm (Figure 4).

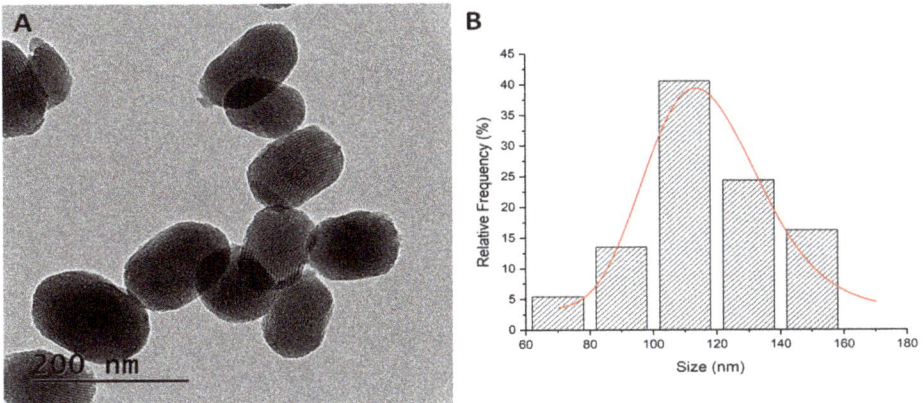

Figure 4. TEM micrograph of MSN-AP-AF-Sn (**A**) and mean size distribution (**B**).

The DLS-mediated hydrodynamic size measurements of the MSN multifunctional nanomaterials were 290 (PDI: 0.287), 312 (PDI: 0.274) and 323 (PDI: 0.282) nm for MSN-AP-Sn, MSN-AP-FA-Sn, and MSN-AP-FA-PEP-S-Sn, respectively. The surface ζ-potential of the MSN nanomaterials resulting from each synthetic step was in agreement with the expected values (Figure 5). As general consideration, all the synthesized nanomaterials showed an isoelectric point (pI) value lower than the physiological pH (≈7.4) (Table S3, Supporting Information). For example, the pI values for the final MSN-AP-FA-Sn and MSN-AP-FA-PEP-S-Sn materials were 5.1 and 6.4 respectively. This behavior will grant a surface negative charge of metallodrug-functionalized silica-based nanomaterials once administered in physiological environment. The latter is a crucial requirement in order to confer a good colloidal stability to the nanoparticles.

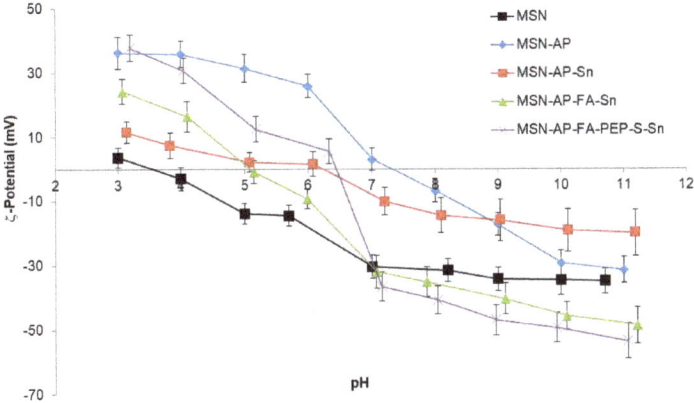

Figure 5. Z-Potential of the different functionalized nanoparticles.

2.3. In Vitro Characterization of the Different MSN-Based Multifunctional Nanomaterials

After the successful deep characterization of all the achieved multifunctional MSN materials, their newly generated therapeutic properties were characterized in a different set of in vitro analyses. First, the MTT cell viability assay was carried out in order to assess the ability of all MSN materials to inhibit the viability of MDA-MB-231 human breast cancer cells as a function of the concentration (Figure 6). The results clearly indicate that, at all the tested concentrations, the MSN-AP-FA-PEP-S-Sn material functionalized with the ERL-peptide was able to reduce the cell viability in a more efficient manner in comparison with the nanoparticles showing the metallodrug directly linked to the silica material (Figure 6). Furthermore, it can also be observed that the viability decreased in an inverse proportional manner with respect of the tin concentration rise. Thus, these results clearly confirmed the correct design of the peptide-based controlled delivery system created for this multifunctional silica-based nanodrug. In fact, the anti-proliferative activity enhancement of organotin metallodrug MSNs was achieved only in the case of interaction with tumor cells from breast adenocarcinoma that have been described overexpressing both folate receptor alpha and the cathepsin B enzyme, being this last the responsible of peptide cleavage and the metallodrug release [59,66,67].

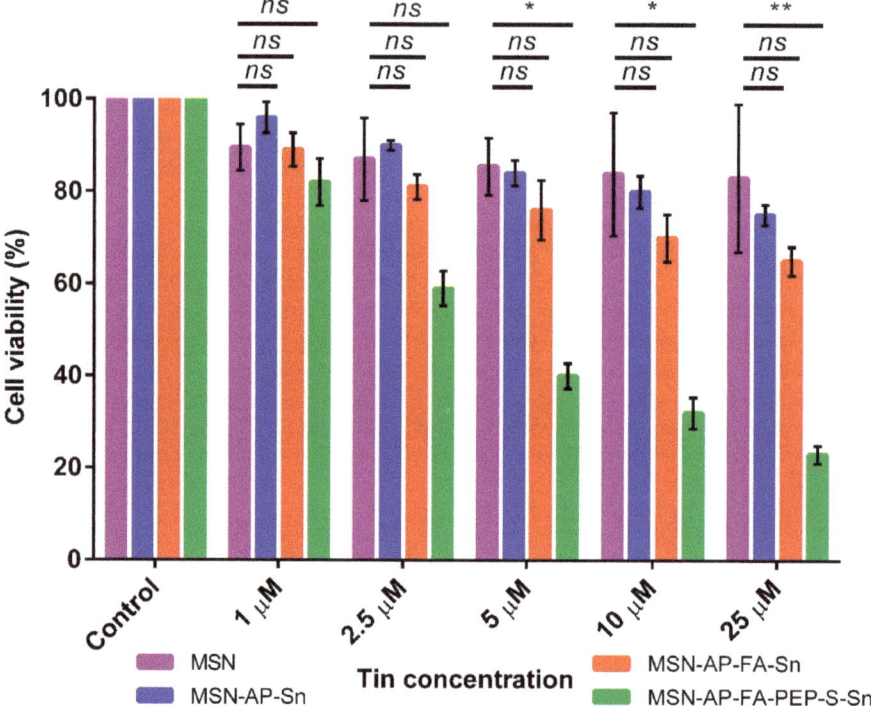

Figure 6. MTT viability assay of MDA-MB-231 cells after incubation with different concentrations of the MSN nanomaterials. All the results were expressed as % of control (mean ± SD, n = 3 independent experiments and 3 replicates/experiment). Significance was calculated by one-way ANOVA Tukey's test. ns: $p > 0.05$ or not significant statistical difference between the groups of data; *: $p < 0.05$ or significant statistical difference between the groups of data; **: $p < 0.01$ or significant statistical difference between the groups of data.

Besides the antiproliferative activity, we decided to evaluate also the potential inhibition of migration ability of MDA-MB-231 cells by means of wound healing assay (Figure 7). This is a standard in vitro technique for probing collective cell migration in two dimensions that is also known as sheet migration. This migration behavior typically occurs in diverse processes such as cancer metastasis [68–70], embryonic morphogenesis [71], and tissue injury [72]. In order to ensure the characterization of the potential anti-migration ability without promoting cell death, based on the results achieved previously, we decided to carry out this assay using 1 µM tin concentration per well or the lowest toxic concentration identified by MTT assay (Figure 6). The results obtained with this assay indicate a general positive trend about the inhibition of cell migration related to the use of each material (Figure 7). The obtained relative inhibition percentage has been calculated by comparing the residual scar areas after 24 h edge progression vs. the initial gap area. As reported in Figure 7, the cells incubated with bare MSN and only tin-functionalized nanomaterials are able to promote the wound healing in major percentage (63.55% and 62% for MSN and MSN-AP-Sn, respectively) in comparison with the control cells. In other terms, in absence of folate targeting, the MDA-MB-231 cell migration is only moderately inhibited. Conversely, the cells treated with both folate-functionalized materials are much more inhibited during their gap closure. In fact, especially in the case of MSN-AP-FA-PEP-S-Sn material, the wound healing after 24 h was almost completely negligible indicating a clear inhibitory effect on the migration mechanism of MDA-MB-231 tumor cells that is directly related to the overall design of our nanodrug (combination of active targeting *plus* ERL-mediated controlled release mechanisms) (Figure 7).

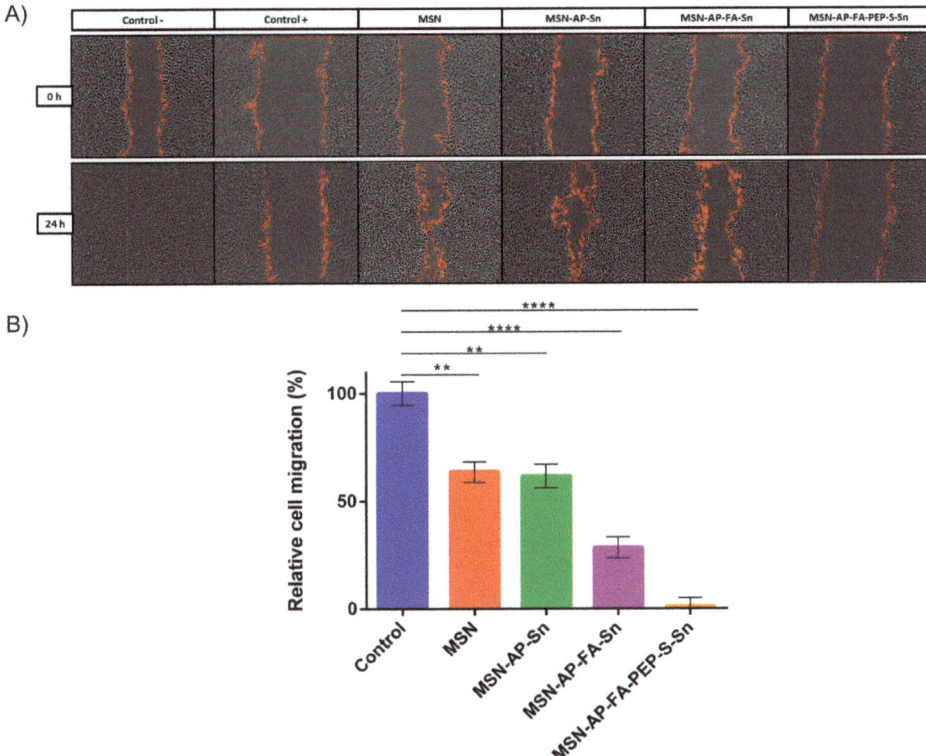

Figure 7. Wound healing assay of MDA-MB-231 cells incubated with the MSN nanoparticles. (**A**) Phase contrast microscopy images of wells. The edges of the scar are marked in red. Positive control (control +): cells incubated with DMSO (complete migration inhibition); negative control (control −): cells grown in culture media (complete migration and wound healing). (**B**) Quantification of cell migration. The results were expressed as % of the initial scar area (mean ± SD, n = 2 independent experiments and 2 replicates/experiment). Significance was calculated by unpaired t-test of one-way ANOVA. **: $p < 0.01$ or significant statistical difference between the two groups of data; ****: $p < 0.0001$ or highly significant statistical difference between the two groups of data.

After the positive evaluation of therapeutic potential of our metallodrug-based MSN nanoplatform, we decided to go further and evaluate its imaging ability, a crucial requirement for the potential in vivo application. Toward this scope, we functionalized the nanomaterials with Alexa Fluor 647 dye (AX), in order to enable NIR fluorescence imaging in vivo. The chemical anchoring of the dye was carried out by carbodiimide chemistry as per the manufacturer's instructions, in a reaction of the different tin-functionalized materials MSN-AP-Sn, MSN-AP-FA-Sn, or MSN-AP-FA-PEP-S-Sn to give AX-1, AX-2, and AX-3 materials, respectively (Schemes 2 and 3).

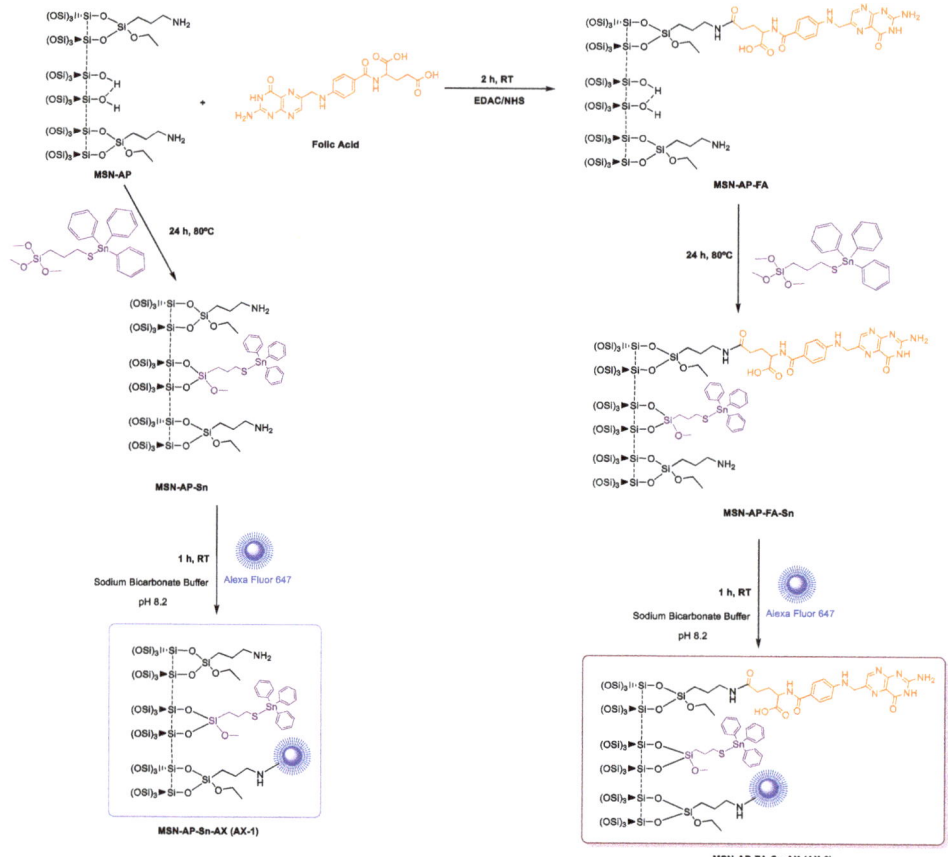

Scheme 2. Reactions of the formation of the theranostic tin-functionalized materials AX-1 and AX-2.

The outcome of the dye functionalization reaction was successfully verified by FTIR (Figure S2 of Supporting Information) and DR-UV spectroscopy (Figure S7 of Supporting Information) of labeled nanoparticles. In addition, fluorescence imaging of MSN nanomaterials after coupling reaction with NIR dye Alexa Fluor 647 was carried out to confirm the correct incorporation of the fluorophore (Figure S8 of Supporting Information).

Thus, to assess effectively the in vitro imaging ability in biological environment, the MDA-MB-231 cells were incubated 24 h with AX-labeled nanoparticles of MSN-AP-FA-PEP-S-Sn-AX nanoparticles (AX-3) and the cell uptake was analyzed by confocal laser scanning microscopy (CLSM) (Figure 8). The 2D and 3D images show a clear internalization of AX-3 nanoparticles inside the tumor cells (Figure 8A,B). In addition, based on the 3D image analysis (Figure 8B), the presence of inner circular accumulations of nanoparticles can be observed. Considering the size, shape, and localization, these repetitive structures should correspond to the lysosome vesicles that are promoting the MSN cell internalization and metallodrug activation mediated by peptide cleavage at the same time [64,65].

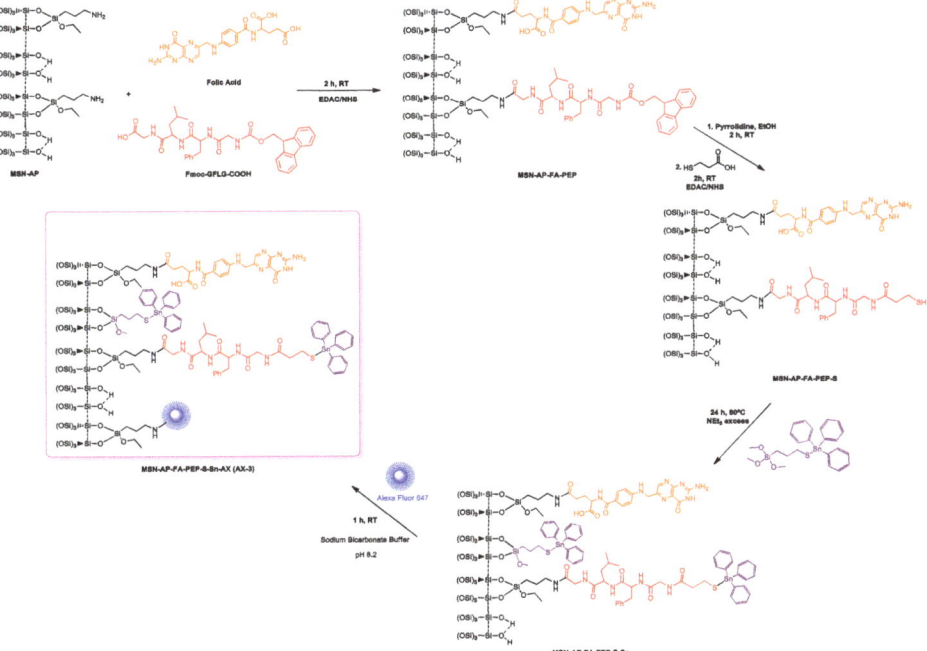

Scheme 3. Reactions of the formation of the tin-functionalized material AX-3.

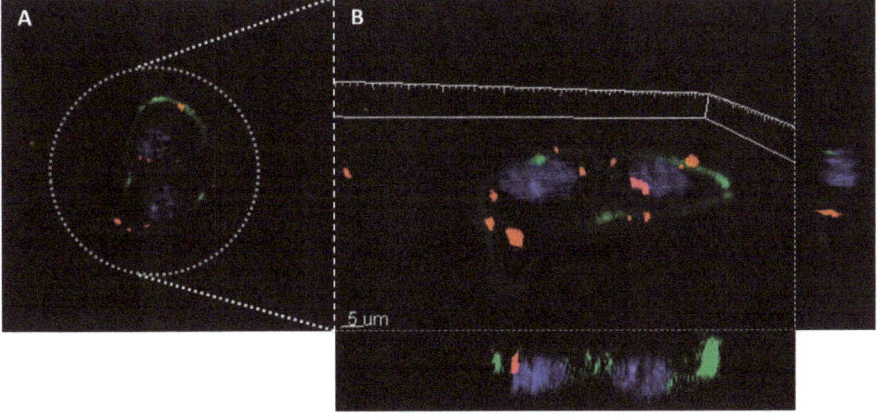

Figure 8. Confocal laser scanning microscope images of the MDA-MB-231 cells incubated overnight with the nanomaterial AX-3 (**A**): 2D image; (**B**): 3D reconstruction. Colors legend: MSN nanoparticles are in red (Alexa Fluor 647, Ex.650/Em.665 nm), cellular nucleus are in blue (DAPI staining, Ex.358/Em.461) and actin filaments are in green (Phalloidin staining, Ex.495/Em.519 nm).

2.4. In Vivo Evaluation of Theranostic Properties of Metallodrug Based MSN Nanomaterials on Breast Adenocarcinoma Mice Models

After the in vitro evaluation of the therapeutic and imaging properties of MSN nanoplatforms, the assessment of their potential theranostic activity in vivo was carried out. Toward this scope, human breast adenocarcinoma bearing mice were used. The mice were randomized in four different groups ($n = 3$ each group) in order to assess (i) the active targeting contribution vs. passive tumor adsorption mediated by the EPR effect, (ii) the therapeutic activity of Sn directly linked on MSN surface vs. (iii) the controlled delivery of organotin metallodrug promoted by lysosomal cleavage of ERL-peptide and (iv) a control group treated with saline. The different MSN nanomaterials were administered 5 times during 10 days by tail vein injection by following the posology timeline reported in Figure 9.

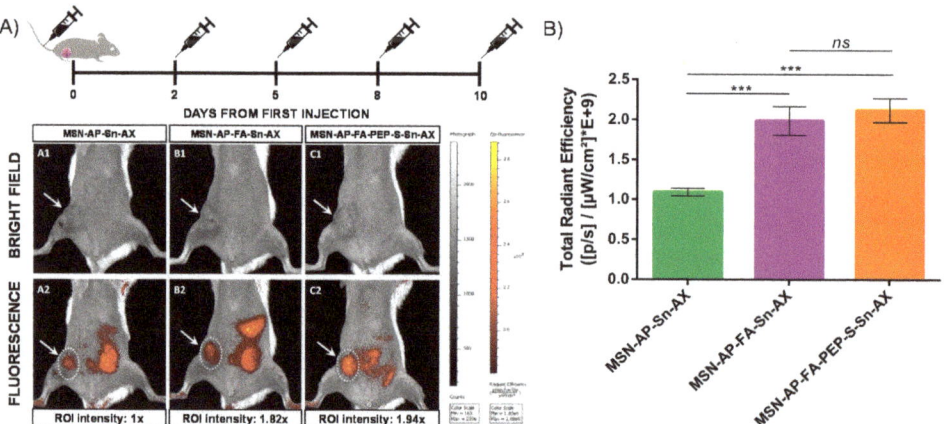

Figure 9. (**A**) In vivo fluorescence imaging of mice treated with different nanoparticles at endpoint: A: MSN-AP-Sn-AX (AX-1); B: MSN-AP-FA-Sn-AX (AX-2); C: MSN-AP-FA-PEP-S-Sn-AX (AX-3). Row 1 (A1, B1, and C1) corresponds to representative bright field images to visualize the tumor area (white arrows) and row 2 (A2, B2, and C2) corresponds to representative fluorescence images acquired 2 h post-injection of nanoparticles. The applied ROI areas used for signal intensities comparison are all equal and marked with white dotted lines. (**B**) Total in vivo fluorescence accumulated in the mice tumor treated with different nanomaterials at end point ($n = 3$ for each group). The applied ROI area was the same in each case. Significance was calculated by unpaired t-test of one-way ANOVA. ns: $p > 0.05$ or not significant statistical difference between the groups of data; ***: $p < 0.001$ or highly significant statistical difference between the two groups of data.

First, the diagnostic properties were evaluated by tracking the nanoparticle biodistribution 2 h post-injection of each dose by in vivo fluorescence imaging (IVIS) of mice full body (Figure 9A). The representative images of mice treated with the three different MSN theranostic nanoparticles (MSN-AP-Sn-AX (AX-1), MSN-AP-FA-Sn-AX (AX-2), and MSN-AP-FA-PEP-S-Sn-AX (AX-3)) and acquired at the end of the whole treatment showed clearly an accumulation within the tumor mass (white arrows) as well as in the liver and in the bowel, confirming the preferential excretion route. After analyzing and normalizing the intensities of the same region-of-interest (ROI) areas centered on the tumor zones for each treated mouse (white spotted line), the accumulation efficiency is almost two folds higher for both folate-targeted nanoparticles (AX-2 and AX-3) in comparison with the passively diffused ones (AX-1)(Figure 9B). These results confirmed the successful folate receptor-targeted activity of the organotin-based MSN nanovectors.

After assessing successfully the targeted diagnostic ability of MSN nanomaterials, we then evaluated also their therapeutic potential. In this sense, the tumor mass growth of the mice groups treated with all the MSN nanomaterials was analyzed by checking their dimensions during the entire treatment. The achieved results, reported as the relative volume increase of all the tumor mass at the end of each treatment and normalized according to the initial tumor mass at the beginning of each treatment, are summarized in Figure 10A.

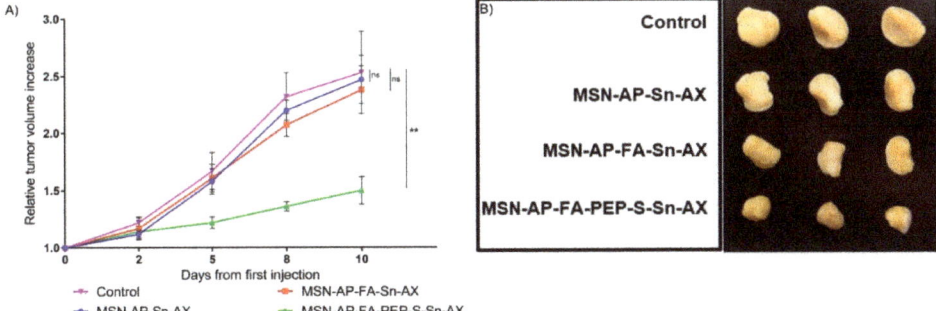

Figure 10. (**A**) Relative tumor volume increase over the course of the treatment with the nanomaterials or saline (control) (n = 3 mice/group). Significance was calculated by unpaired t-test of one-way ANOVA. ns: $p > 0.05$ or not significant statistical difference between the groups of data; **: $p < 0.01$ or significant statistical difference between the two groups of data; (**B**) ex vivo tumor images for all mice treated with different MSN nanomaterials or saline (control).

After 10 days of nanoparticle administration, the tumor mice groups treated with saline or the MSN-AP-FA-Sn-AX underwent an average tumor mass increase by 2.5 and 2.4 folds respectively in comparison with the volume of each tumor mass measured at the beginning of the nanotherapy. Conversely, the breast tumors of the mice treated with MSN-AP-FA-PEP-S-Sn-AX nanoparticles only increased their volumes by 1.5 folds on average (Figure 10A). The Figure 10B shows the ex vivo images of the tumor proceeding by each experimental group (saline, MSN-AP-Sn-AX, MSN-AP-FA-Sn-AX, and MSN-AP-FA-PEP-S-Sn-AX nanoparticle, respectively) after postmortem excision. Photographs and weight of excised tumor at endpoint confirmed that only MSN-AP-FA-PEP-S-Sn-AX (AX-3) treatment inhibited tumor growth (Figure 10B and Figure S9).

Altogether, all these results successfully demonstrate the therapeutic potential against breast adenocarcinoma of the organotin-based theranostic nanoplatform as well as the effectiveness and relevance of the overall nanoplatform design. In fact, the concomitant use of folate as targeting agent together with ERL-peptide for controlled drug delivery has been demonstrated to be crucial in order to allow the cytotoxic organotin fragment to be cleaved from the nanostructure selectively inside the tumoral cell and then to exert its chemotherapeutic effect.

Finally, the long-term in vivo toxicity of the nanomaterials was checked by monitoring the possible effects on the liver and kidney functions both being the principal excretion routes. To this scope, the serum level of alanine aminotransferase (ALT), aspartate aminotransferase (AST), alkaline phosphatase (AKP), albumin (ALB), and blood urea nitrogen (BUN) were monitored before and after each treatment (Figure S10). The quantification of these enzymes in serum is generally considered a useful biomarker to control the hepatic and renal functionalities. In fact, increased levels of these biomarkers are generally associated to acute and/or chronic liver and kidney injuries. As reported in Figure S10, the treated vs. control serum levels of all hepatic and renal biomarkers were kept constant or slightly decreased for all the mice groups at the end of each nanotherapy. Consequently, these results indicate that no liver or kidney damage has been caused in vivo because of the administration of the organotin metallodrug over the course of the treatment. Nevertheless, we are aware about the necessity to deeply analyze in forthcoming works especially the potential liver injury risk in humans. Nonetheless, based on the achieved overall results, our hypothesis of the potentially limited in vivo toxicity thanks to the combination of the targeting ability of the nanosystem *plus* the selective enzymatic metallodrug activation, has been successfully confirmed in our mouse model.

3. Materials and Methods

3.1. Synthesis of Nanomaterials

3.1.1. General Conditions

All reactions were performed using standard Schlenk tube techniques in an inert atmosphere of dry nitrogen. Solvents were distilled from the appropriate drying agents and degassed before use. The reagents used in the preparation of the starting material (MSN), tetraethyl orthosilicate (TEOS) and hexadecyltrimethylammonium bromide (CTAB) were purchased from Sigma Aldrich and Acros Organics, respectively. The ligand 3-(aminopropyl)triethoxysilane (AP) was purchased from Sigma Aldrich, and 3-mercaptopropyltrimethoxysilane (MP) from Fluorochem. 3-Mercaptopropionic acid, triphenyltin chloride, folic acid, and all the reagents necessary for EDAC coupling, were purchased from Sigma Aldrich. AlexaFluor[TM] 647 NHS ester, tris(trithlamonium salt) from Invitrogen. The Fmoc-GFLG-COOH peptide was custom made synthesized by Biomedal (Sevilla, Spain).

3.1.2. Synthesis of the Starting Material: Mesoporous Silica Nanoparticles (MSN)

The synthesis of MSN was carried out from a modification of the experimental procedure reported by Zhao et al. [73], using CTAB (1 g, 2.74 mmol) as surfactant in a basic solution of nanopure water and TEOS (5 mL, 22.4 mmol) as silicon source. The reaction was carried out during 2 h at 80 °C. After that time, the precipitate was dried and calcined to 550 °C for 16 h to obtain the starting mesoporous material MSN.

3.1.3. Functionalization with Amino Ligands. Preparation of MSN-AP Material

The functionalization with amino ligands was carried out with a slight modification of reported procedures [74]. In brief, the starting material (MSN) was dehydrated at 80 °C under vacuum for 24 h. Subsequently, MSN was suspended in dry toluene and a defined amount of the amino ligand (AP) was added to the mixture. The suspension was then stirred at 110 °C for 48 h. Afterwards the mixture was then centrifuged, washed with toluene (2 × 10 mL) and diethylether (2 × 10 mL).

3.1.4. Functionalization with the Cytotoxic Agent (Sn). Synthesis of MSN-AP-Sn

First, the formation of the organotin derivate $Ph_3Sn\{SCH_2CH_2CH_2Si(OMe)_3\}$ was carried out via the reaction of triphenyltin(IV) chloride and 3-mercaptopropyltrimethoxysilane (Scheme 4). In a Schlenk tube, $SnPh_3Cl$ (284.1 mg) was dissolved in dry toluene in a proportion of 20% wt Sn/SiO_2. Subsequently, 3-mercaptopropyltrimethoxysilane (178.1 µL) and triethylamine (205.5 µL) was added in a relation of 1:1:2 molar respectively regarding the organotin compound. The solution was kept under stirring and nitrogen atmosphere during 24 h at 80 °C. After that time, the stirring was stopped, and the compound was filtered and added, under nitrogen and with a cannula, to a toluene suspension of the silica material MSN-AP. The reaction mixture was stirred at 80 °C for 24 h. The material was then filtered and washed with toluene (2 × 10 mL) and diethylether (2 × 10 mL).

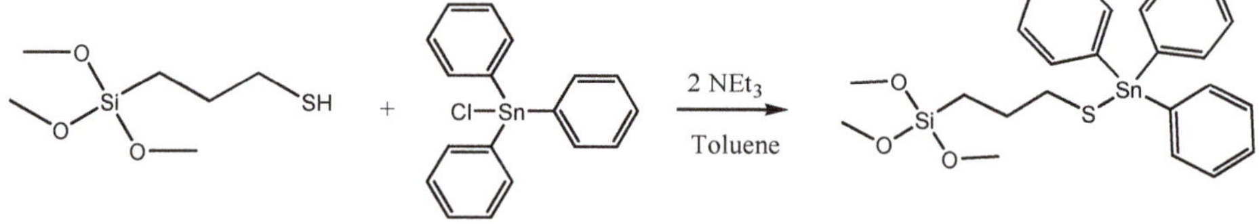

Scheme 4. Reaction of the formation of the cytotoxic organotin(IV) derivative.

3.1.5. Incorporation of Folic Acid (FA). Synthesis of MSN-AP-FA

For the incorporation of folic acid in the amino-functionalized material MSN-AP an EDAC coupling reaction was carried out (Scheme 2). In a general method, 18.4 mg of folic acid (5% weight with respect to the quantity of MSN-AP) was dissolved in dimethylsulfoxide (DMSO) and subsequently added to 35 mL of a 0.1 M of MES buffer. EDAC (14 mg) and NHS (21 mg) were added to the mixture and reacted under vigorous stirring for 15 min at room temperature. Subsequently, 350 mg of MSN-AP was added to the EDAC solution and reacted at room temperature under stirring. Then, 2-mercaptoethanol (55.5 µL) was added to the mixture and the suspension was stirred for 2 additional hours. Finally, the reaction mixture was centrifuged, washed with DMSO, ethanol, water, and dried overnight in a stove at 80 °C. Finally, 300 mg of the material MSN-AP-FA was obtained.

3.1.6. Functionalization with the Cytotoxic Agent (Sn). Synthesis of MSN-AP-FA-Sn

The functionalization with the cytotoxic tin agent $Ph_3Sn\{SCH_2CH_2CH_2Si(OMe)_3\}$ as described previously for material MSN-AP-Sn (Scheme 2), but using the following quantities: $SnPh_3Cl$ (243.54 mg), 3-mercaptopropyltriethoxysilane (152.62 µL) and triethylamine (176.12 µL)) and MSN-AP-FA (300 mg) (Scheme 3). Finally, 280 mg of the material MSN-AP-FA-Sn was obtained.

3.1.7. Simultaneous Incorporation of Folic Acid (FA) and Targeting Peptide (Fmoc-Gly-Phe-Leu-Gly-COOH). Synthesis of MSN-AP-FA-Pep

For the simultaneous functionalization of the amino-functionalized material MSN-AP with folic acid and the peptide Fmoc-Gly-Phe-Leu-Gly-COOH (Fmoc-GFLG-COOH), an EDAC coupling reaction was performed (Scheme 3). In a general method, a quantity of folic acid (11 mg, 5% weight with respect to the quantity of MSN-AP) and Fmoc-GFLG-COOH (11 mg, 5% weight with respect to the quantity of MSN-AP) were dissolved in DMSO using an ultrasound bath and the solution was added to 42 mL 0.1 M of MES buffer. EDAC (16.8 mg) and NHS (25.2 mg) were added to the mixture and reacted under vigorous stirring for 15 min at room temperature. Subsequently, MSN-AP (210 mg) was added to the EDAC solution and reacted at room temperature under stirring. Then, 2-mercaptoethanol (74.3 µL) was added to the mixture and the suspension stirred for 2 additional hours. Finally, the reaction mixture was centrifuged, washed with DMSO (2 × 10 mL), ethanol (2 × 10 mL), water (2 × 10 mL) and dried in a stove at 80 °C overnight. Finally, 210 mg of the material MSN-AP-FA-PEP was obtained.

3.1.8. Incorporation of 3-Mercaptopropionic Acid (MS). Synthesis of MSN-AP-FA-PEP-S

Before the coupling of MS, the Fmoc deprotection is needed. For the deprotection reaction a 1:3 molar suspension peptide:pyrrolidine (210 mg MSN-AP-FA-PEP and 9.3 µL of pyrrolidine) in 20 mL of ethanol was reacted during 2 h at room temperature. The solid was centrifuged, washed with ethanol, and kept in cold. For the incorporation of MS, an EDAC coupling was carried out using a very similar method than that of the synthesis of MSN-AP-FA. The synthesis consisted of the addition of one equivalent of MS for each equivalent of the anchored peptide (210 mg of deprotected MSN-AP-FA-PEP and 3.2 µL of 3-mercaptopropionic acid (MS)), in the presence of 21 mL 0.1 M of MES buffer. EDAC (8.4 mg) and NHS (12.6 mg) were also used (Scheme 3). The obtained solid was washed with DMSO (2 × 10 mL), ethanol (2 × 10 mL) and water (2 × 10 mL). The solid was then dried in a stove at 80 °C. Finally, 200 mg of the material MSN-AP-FA-MS was obtained.

3.1.9. Functionalization with the Cytotoxic Agent (Sn). Synthesis of MSN-AP-FA-PEP-S-Sn

The functionalization with the cytotoxic tin agent was carried out by the addition of the $SnPh_3$ moiety from the compound $Ph_3Sn\{SCH_2CH_2CH_2Si(OMe)_3\}$ which was prepared as described previously for material MSN-AP-Sn, but using the following quantities: $SnPh_3Cl$ (97.4 mg), 3-mercaptopropyltrimethoxysilane (61.1 µL) and triethylamine (176.1 µL). The compound $Ph_3Sn\{SCH_2CH_2CH_2Si(OMe)_3\}$ prepared in situ was added to a suspension of MSN-AP-FA-PEP-S

(120 mg) in toluene in the presence of excess of triethylamine. The reaction mixture was stirred for 24 h at 80 °C (Scheme 4). The excess of triethylamine allows the deprotonation of the thiol group of the peptide and the formation of the S-SnPh$_3$ moiety by an exchange reaction with the compound Ph$_3$Sn{SCH$_2$CH$_2$CH$_2$Si(OMe)$_3$} leading to the formation of the material MSN-AP-FA-PEP-S-Sn. The material was filtered and washed with toluene (2 × 10 mL), ethanol (2 × 10 mL), and water (2 × 10 mL). Finally, 110 mg of the material MSN-AP-FA-PEP-S-Sn was obtained.

3.1.10. Incorporation of the Imaging Agent Alexa Fluor 647. Preparation of AX Materials

For the incorporation of the fluorophore, 100 µg of Alexa-Fluor 647 were dissolved in 100 µL of dimethylsulfoxide (DMSO) and the solution was added to 50 mg of the materials functionalized with tin MSN-AP-Sn, MSN-AP-FA-Sn, or MSN-AP-FA-PEP-S-Sn dispersed in 5 mL of 0.1 M sodium bicarbonate buffer at pH 8.2. The mixture was reacted for 1 h at room temperature under dark conditions. Finally, the solid was centrifuged and washed with DMSO (2 × 5 mL) and water (2 × 5 mL) to give MSN-AP-Sn-AX (AX-1), MSN-AP-FA-Sn-AX (AX-2) or MSN-AP-FA-PEP-S-Sn-AX (AX-3), respectively.

3.2. General Remarks on Chemico-Physical Characterization of the Materials

X-ray diffraction (XRD) pattern of the systems were obtained on a Philips Diffractometer model PW3040/00 X'Pert MPD/MRD at 45 kV and 40 mA, using a wavelength Cu Kα (λ = 1.5418 Å). Sn wt% determination by X-ray fluorescence were carried out with an X-ray fluorescence spectrophotometer Philips MagiX with an X-ray source of 1 kW and a Rh anode using a helium atmosphere. Thermogravimetry analyses (TG) were obtained on a Shimadzu mod. DSC-50Q (Shimadzu, Kioto, Japan) operating up to 700 °C (ramp 20 °C/min) at an intensity of 50 A. IR spectra were prepared using KBr pellets with a spectrophotometer Termo Nicolet Avatar 380 FT-IR with a Michelson filter interferometer. DR UV-Vis measurements were carried out on a Varian Cary-500 spectrophotometer equipped with an integrating sphere and polytetrafluoroethylene (PTFE) as reference. ^{119}Sn MAS NMR and ^{29}Si MAS NMR spectra, were recorded on a Varian-Infinity Plus Spectrometer at 400 MHz for proton frequency (4 µs 90° pulse, 4000 transients, spinning speed of 6 MHz, contact time 3 ms, pulse delay 1.5 s). Transmission electron microscopy (TEM) was carried out on a JEOL JEM 1400, operating at 100 kV. Dynamic light scattering (DLS) measurements were carried out on a Zetasizer Nano Zen 3600 (Malvern, UK), diluting samples in potassium nitrate (KNO$_3$, 10^{-2}M).

3.3. In Vitro Studies

3.3.1. Cell lines and Culture Condition

The human breast adenocarcinoma cell line MDA-MB-231 was grown in DMEM-F12 (Lonza, Basel, Switzerland) supplemented with 10% FBS (Sigma, St. Louis, MO, USA), 1% non-essential amino acids (NEAA, Hyclone, South Logan, UT, USA), 1% sodium pyruvate 100 mM (Hyclone, South Logan, UT, USA), and 1% penicillin/streptomycin (Lonza, Basel, Switzerland).

Culture was maintained at 37 °C in a humidified atmosphere with 5% CO$_2$. The cells were subcultured every 2 to 3 days by treatment with TrypLE™ Express Enzyme (Gibco) for MDA-MB-231.

3.3.2. Nanodrug Preparation

Suspensions of the functionalized materials were prepared in culture media, without phenol red, at different concentrations depending on the experiments, always sonicating repeatedly before cellular incubation.

3.3.3. Viability Assay

1×10^4 cells were seeded per well in a 96-well culture plate for 48 h. After that, cells were incubated 24 h at 37 °C with dispersions of each MSN-functionalized material in culture medium without phenol red at different final tin concentrations (1 µM, 2.5 µM, 5 µM, 10 µM, and 25 µM). MSN bare material was incubated at the same silica concentration of the other organotin-bearing materials to evaluate the potential cytotoxicity of the material itself. After incubation, these solutions were discarded and replaced by 100 µL of medium, without phenol red and without serum, and 10 µL of a 12 mM MTT (dimethylthiazolyl-diphenyl-tetrazolium bromide) solution (in PBS 1X pH 7.4) was added to each well and mixed. After 3 h of incubation, all the supernatants less 25 µL were removed and 100 µL DMSO was added to each well to dissolve the formazan, leaving it 15 min to react. Cell viability was estimated by measuring absorbance at 570 nm using a *Unicam W-500 UV-Vis* plate reader. The absorbance values obtained were subtracted from the absorbance value of the "white wells" (only medium with MTT, no cells). The percentage of viability was calculated taking as 100% of viability the absorbance of the negative control wells (cells without material), and also positive control wells (cells incubated with DMSO) were studied.

3.3.4. Cellular Uptake

Total of 2.5×10^4 MDA-MB-231 cells were seeded in a 6-well culture plate and incubated overnight with the nanomaterial (MSN-AP-FA-PEP-S-Sn-AX) in a 1 µM final tin concentration. Then cells were fixed with 4% paraformaldehyde (PFA) pH = 7.4 for 15 min at RT. After that, cells were washed three times with PBS 1X (5 min each) and permeabilized with 0.1% Triton X-100 in PBS for 5 min. Cells were rinsed three times with PBS 1X (5 min each) and then incubated for 20 min at RT with a blocking solution of 1% FBS in PBS 1X. Cells were rinsed again three times with PBS 1X (5 min each) and finally they were treated for 45 min at RT with a F-actin specific stain, AlexaFluor 488 Phalloidin (1:500 in PBS). Cells were washed with PBS and stained with DAPI (0.1% in PBS) for 5 min. The images were taken using a confocal microscope Zeiss LSM 780 (20×) under 37 °C and 5% CO_2 and they were processed with ImageJ Fiji and Imaris software.

3.3.5. Wound Healing Assay

1×10^5 MDA-MB-231 cells were seeded per well in a 24-well culture plate for 48 h, until a cell monolayer was created. The monolayer was scratched with a pipette tip, the medium was absorbed with vacuum and the wells were cleaned twice with PBS without Ca or Mg. Then, the cells were incubated with the different nanomaterials at different concentrations (1 µM, 2.5 µM, 5 µM, and 10 µM) and the migration into the gap was imaged 0 and 24 h later using a Nikon Time Lapse microscope.

3.4. In Vivo Studies

3.4.1. Animals and Ethics

Mice were housed in specific facilities (pathogen-free for mice) at the Spanish National Center for Cardiovascular Research (CNIC, Madrid, Spain). All animal experiments were carried out after previous approval by the ethics and animal welfare committee at CNIC and were in agreement with the Spanish Legislation and UE Directive 2010/63/EU.

3.4.2. Breast Cancer Mouse Model

The breast cancer was generated by injecting subcutaneously 5×10^5 MDA-MB-231 cells (in a 20 µL mixture of PBS 1X and Matrigel, 1.86:1 v/v) into 8 week old NOD Scid IL2 receptor gamma chain KO female mice, in their fourth left breast. Animals were housed at 22 °C, under a 12 h light/dark cycle with freely available water and food. The tumor was generally generated within the next 15–20 days after the injection.

3.4.3. Treatment with Nanoparticles and in Vivo Fluorescence Imaging

Mice (n = 3/group) were injected i.v. into the tail vein every 2–3 days with 150 µL of the materials solutions at 420 µM over 10 days (5 injections). This therapeutic regimen was chosen based on our and others' previous studies [50,52,75,76]. Two hours following the last injection, in vivo fluorescence imaging of Alexa Fluor 647 was performed on mice anesthetized with isoflurane gas. Murine models without nanoparticles treatment were used as control. Fluorescence in vivo imaging was performed with the IVIS Imaging System 200 series (Xenogen) (acquisition parameters: Cy5.5 ex/em filter, high level, BIN-HR, FOV: 6.6, f8). The region-of-interest (ROI) comparison was carried out by applying a constant ROI area to each image and processed using the Living Image software version 4.4 from Caliper Life Sciences. Fluorescence intensity was quantified as radiant efficiency accumulated over the 10 days treatment with MSN-based nanomaterials.

3.4.4. Tumor Measurement

In order to evaluate the tumor growth, all mice were monitored by caliper measurements of tumor width (W) and length (L). Tumor volume was determined using the formula $V = (L \times (W^2))/2$ and volumes were normalized and compared with respect to the initial volumes.

3.4.5. Statistic and Analysis

Data analysis was performed using the Prism 6 software (GraphPad, San Diego, CA, USA), and all chart data were expressed as mean ± standard deviation (Mean ± SD).

4. Conclusions

Triple negative breast cancer (TNBC) is the most aggressive subclass within human breast adenocarcinoma type and the development of a suitable therapeutic paradigm is still a great challenge. Toward this scope, in this work, we have successfully demonstrated that mesoporous silica nanoparticles are suitable nanoplatforms enabling the creation of a controlled delivery system of a metallodrug together with imaging abilities in order to promote the targeted theranosis of breast cancer. In more detail, a targeted nanodrug candidate functionalized with organotin(IV) complex (therapeutic), Alexa Fluor 647 NIR dye (diagnostic), and folate fragment (active targeting) moieties useful for the theranosis of human breast adenocarcinoma in mice models has been achieved. Furthermore, the application of an enzyme-responsive GFGL peptide linker for the site-selective controlled delivery of the metallodrug and triggered only after tumor cell uptake has been designed and successfully applied. Thanks to the combination of the receptor-mediated site targeting and the specific fine-tuned release mechanism, the MSN-AP-FA-PEP-S-Sn-AX (AX-3) nanotheranostic drug has showed enhanced therapeutic activity and reduced off-target toxicity after in vitro as well as in vivo applications in orthotopic mouse model of human TNBC. Considering the achieved results, the intrinsic flexibility of MSN materials and the possibility to couple other complementary therapeutic protocols, we are fully confident that our proposed strategy can pave the way toward the development of a more powerful generation of engineered nanotheranostics for the multitherapeutic treatment of triple negative breast cancers.

Supplementary Materials: The following are available online at http://www.mdpi.com/2072-6694/12/1/187/s1, Figure S1: FT-IR spectrum of the functionalized materials MSN-AP and MSN-AP-FA-Sn, Figure S2. FT-IR spectrum of the functionalized materials MSN-AP-FA-PEP-S-Sn and AX-3, Figure S3. TG of the materials MSN, MSN-AP-Sn, MSN-AP-FA-Sn and MSN-AP-FA-PEP-S-Sn, Figure S4. 119Sn MAS NMR spectrum of MSN-AP-FA-PEP-S-Sn, Figure S5. 29Si MAS NMR spectrum of MSN-AP, Figure S6. 29Si MAS NMR spectrum of MSN-AP-FA-PEP, Figure S7. DR-UV spectra of the Alexa Fluor-functionalized materials MSN-AP-FA-AX (AX-1), MSN-AP-FA-Sn-AX (AX-2) and MSN-AP-FA-PEP-S-Sn-AX (AX-3), Figure S8. Fluorescence imaging of MSN nanomaterials after coupling reaction with NIR dye Alexa Fluor 647, Figure S9. Tumor mass weight comparison after post mortem excision. Figure S10. Serum levels of alanine aminotransferase (ALT), aspartate aminotransferase (AST), alkaline phosphatase (AKP), albumin (ALB) and blood urea nitrogen (BUN) before (blue) and after (red) 10 days of different nanotherapies (n=3). Table S1. Mass loss (110 °C-700 °C) from thermogravimetry analyses, Table S2. Molar ratio S:Sn and Si:Sn obtained by XRF analyses., Table S3. Surface ζ-potential of the MSN nanomaterials.

Author Contributions: Conceptualization of the work: M.F. and S.G.-R., supervision of the synthesis and characterization of the nanomaterials: S.G-R, M.F. and S.P, experimental part related to the synthesis and characterization of nanomaterials: D.D.-G., M.D.-S., V.G.-A., K.O.P., M.M., L.L.C; data analysis and interpretation: M.F., S.G-R and S.P, in vitro characterization of nanomaterials: K.O.P., L.L.C. V.G.-A., in vivo experiments: K.O.P. preparation of the manuscript: M.F., S.G.-R., S.P., D.D.-G., M.M. and K.O.P. All authors have read and agreed to the published version of the manuscript.

Funding: The CNIC is supported by MINECO and the Pro-CNIC Foundation and is a Severo Ochoa Center of Excellence (SEV-2015-0505). M.F. would like to thank MINECO for the research grant no. SAF2014-59118-JIN co-funded by Fondo Europeo de Desarrollo Regional (FEDER) and COST Action CA1520: "European Network on NMR Relaxometry-EURELAX." M.F. acknowledges the Comunidad Autonoma de Madrid for research project no. 2017-T1/BIO-4992 ("Atracción de Talento" Action) also cofunded by Universidad Complutense de Madrid. M.F. and K.O.P. are grateful to ICTS-ReDIB. M.M and M.F. are grateful to the Comunidad Autónoma de Madrid and FEDER for the I+D collaborative Programme in Biomedicine NIETO-CM (Project reference B2017-BMD3731). We would also like to thank the Ministerio de Ciencia, Innovación y Universidades of Spain (grants numbers RTI2018-094322-B-I00 and CTQ2017-90802-REDT) for the funding and Dirección General de Investigación e Innovación, Consejería de Educación e Investigación de la Comunidad de Madrid for the predoctoral grant PEJD-2017-PRE/AMB-4047 (M.D.-S.).

Conflicts of Interest: The authors declare no conflict of interest

References

1. Bray, F.; Ferlay, J.; Soerjomataram, I.; Siegel, R.L.; Torre, L.A.; Jemal, A. Global cancer statistics 2018: GLOBOCAN estimates of incidence and mortality worldwide for 36 cancers in 185 countries. *CA Cancer J. Clin.* **2018**, *68*, 394–424. [CrossRef] [PubMed]
2. Lee, K.L.; Kuo, Y.C.; Ho, Y.S.; Huang, Y.H. Triple-Negative Breast Cancer: Current Understanding and Future Therapeutic Breakthrough Targeting Cancer Stemness. *Cancers* **2019**, *11*, 1334. [CrossRef] [PubMed]
3. Sanchez-Collado, J.; Lopez, J.J.; Jardin, I.; Camello, P.J.; Falcon, D.; Regodon, S.; Salido, G.M.; Smani, T.; Rosado, J.A. Adenylyl Cyclase Type 8 Overexpression Impairs Phosphorylation-Dependent Orai1 Inactivation and Promotes Migration in MDA-MB-231 Breast Cancer Cells. *Cancers* **2019**, *11*, 1624. [CrossRef] [PubMed]
4. Mustacchi, G.; De Laurentiis, M. The role of taxanes in triple-negative breast cancer: Literature review. *Drug Des. Dev. Ther.* **2015**, *9*, 4303–4318. [CrossRef]
5. Liedtke, C.; Mazouni, C.; Hess, K.R.; Andre, F.; Tordai, A.; Mejia, J.A.; Symmans, W.F.; Gonzalez-Angulo, A.M.; Hennessy, B.; Green, M.; et al. Response to neoadjuvant therapy and long-term survival in patients with triple-negative breast cancer. *J. Clin. Oncol.* **2008**, *26*, 1275–1281. [CrossRef]
6. Thomas, E.S.; Gomez, H.L.; Li, R.K.; Chung, H.C.; Fein, L.E.; Chan, V.F.; Jassem, J.; Pivot, X.B.; Klimovsky, J.V.; de Mendoza, F.H.; et al. Ixabepilone plus capecitabine for metastatic breast cancer progressing after anthracycline and taxane treatment. *J. Clin. Oncol.* **2007**, *25*, 5210–5217. [CrossRef]
7. Ramadan, W.S.; Vazhappilly, C.G.; Saleh, E.M.; Menon, V.; AlAzawi, A.M.; El-Serafi, A.T.; Mansour, W.; El-Awady, R. Interplay between Epigenetics, Expression of Estrogen Receptor- alpha, HER2/ERBB2 and Sensitivity of Triple Negative Breast Cancer Cells to Hormonal Therapy. *Cancers* **2018**, *11*, 13. [CrossRef]
8. Fernandez, M.; Javaid, F.; Chudasama, V. Advances in targeting the folate receptor in the treatment/imaging of cancers. *Chem. Sci.* **2018**, *9*, 790–810. [CrossRef]
9. Srinivasarao, M.; Galliford, C.V.; Low, P.S. Principles in the design of ligand-targeted cancer therapeutics and imaging agents. *Nat. Rev. Drug Discov.* **2015**, *14*, 203–219. [CrossRef]
10. Parker, N.; Turk, M.J.; Westrick, E.; Lewis, J.D.; Low, P.S.; Leamon, C.P. Folate receptor expression in carcinomas and normal tissues determined by a quantitative radioligand binding assay. *Anal. Biochem.* **2005**, *338*, 284–293. [CrossRef]
11. Zwicke, G.L.; Mansoori, G.A.; Jeffery, C.J. Utilizing the folate receptor for active targeting of cancer nanotherapeutics. *Nanotechnol. Rev.* **2012**, *3*, 18496. [CrossRef] [PubMed]
12. Quici, S.; Casoni, A.; Foschi, F.; Armelao, L.; Bottaro, G.; Seraglia, R.; Bolzati, C.; Salvarese, N.; Carpanese, D.; Rosato, A.; et al. Folic acid-conjugated europium complexes as luminescent probes for selective targeting of cancer cells. *J. Med. Chem.* **2015**, *58*, 2003–2014. [CrossRef] [PubMed]
13. Babaer, D.; Amara, S.; Ivy, M.; Zhao, Y.; Lammers, P.E.; Titze, J.M.; Tiriveedhi, V. High salt induces P-glycoprotein mediated treatment resistance in breast cancer cells through store operated calcium influx. *Oncotarget* **2018**, *9*, 25193–25205. [CrossRef] [PubMed]
14. Gueder, N.; Allan, G.; Telliez, M.S.; Hague, F.; Fernandez, J.M.; Sanchez-Fernandez, E.M.; Ortiz-Mellet, C.; Ahidouch, A.; Ouadid-Ahidouch, H. sp^2-Iminosugar alpha-glucosidase inhibitor 1-C-octyl-2-oxa-3-oxocastanospermine specifically affected breast cancer cell migration through Stim1, beta1-integrin, and FAK signaling pathways. *J. Cell. Physiol.* **2017**, *232*, 3631–3640. [CrossRef] [PubMed]

15. Hammadi, M.; Chopin, V.; Matifat, F.; Dhennin-Duthille, I.; Chasseraud, M.; Sevestre, H.; Ouadid-Ahidouch, H. Human ether a-gogo K(+) channel 1 (hEag1) regulates MDA-MB-231 breast cancer cell migration through Orai1-dependent calcium entry. *J. Cell. Physiol.* **2012**, *227*, 3837–3846. [CrossRef]
16. Necela, B.M.; Crozier, J.A.; Andorfer, C.A.; Lewis-Tuffin, L.; Kachergus, J.M.; Geiger, X.J.; Kalari, K.R.; Serie, D.J.; Sun, Z.; Moreno-Aspitia, A.; et al. Folate receptor-alpha (FOLR1) expression and function in triple negative tumors. *PLoS ONE* **2015**, *10*, e0122209.
17. Díaz-Garcia, D.; Cenariu, D.; Pérez, Y.; Cruz, P.; Del Hierro, I.; Prashar, S.; Fischer-Fodor, E.; Gómez-Ruiz, S. Modulation of the mechanism of apoptosis in cancer cell lines by treatment with silica-based nanostructured materials functionalized with different metallodrugs. *Dalton Trans.* **2018**, *47*, 12284–12299. [CrossRef]
18. Ott, I.; Gust, R. Non platinum metal complexes as anti-cancer drugs. *Arch Pharm Weinh.* **2007**, *340*, 117–126. [CrossRef]
19. Rosenberg, B.; Van Camp, L.; Krigas, T. Inhibition of Cell Division in Escherichia coli by Electrolysis Products from a Platinum Electrode. *Nature* **1965**, *205*, 698–699. [CrossRef]
20. Markus, G.; Michael, A.J.; Bernhard, K.K. Update of the Preclinical Situation of Anticancer Platinum Complexes: Novel Design Strategies and Innovative Analytical Approaches. *Curr. Med. Chem.* **2005**, *12*, 2075–2094.
21. Ellahioui, Y.; Prashar, S.; Gómez-Ruiz, S. Anticancer Applications and Recent Investigations of Metallodrugs Based on Gallium, Tin and Titanium. *Inorganics* **2017**, *5*, 4. [CrossRef]
22. Mjos, K.D.; Orvig, C. Metallodrugs in medicinal inorganic chemistry. *Chem. Rev.* **2014**, *114*, 4540–4563. [CrossRef] [PubMed]
23. Wani, W.A.; Prashar, S.; Shreaz, S.; Gómez-Ruiz, S. Nanostructured materials functionalized with metal complexes: In search of alternatives for administering anticancer metallodrugs. *Coord. Chem. Rev.* **2016**, *312*, 67–98. [CrossRef]
24. Kaluderovic, G.N.; Kommera, H.; Hey-Hawkins, E.; Paschke, R.; Gómez-Ruiz, S. Synthesis and biological applications of ionic triphenyltin(IV) chloride carboxylate complexes with exceptionally high cytotoxicity. *Metallomics* **2010**, *2*, 419–428. [CrossRef] [PubMed]
25. Rocamora-Reverte, L.; Carrasco-García, E.; Ceballos-Torres, J.; Prashar, S.; Kaluderovic, G.N.; Ferragut, J.A.; Gómez-Ruiz, S. Study of the anticancer properties of tin(IV) carboxylate complexes on a panel of human tumor cell lines. *ChemMedChem* **2012**, *7*, 301–310. [CrossRef] [PubMed]
26. Lovejoy, K.S.; Lippard, S.J. Non-traditional platinum compounds for improved accumulation, oral bioavailability, and tumor targeting. *Dalton Trans.* **2009**, *28*, 10651–10659. [CrossRef]
27. Siccardi, M.; Martin, P.; McDonald, T.O.; Liptrott, N.J.; Giardiello, M.; Rannard, S.; Owen, A. Research Spotlight: Nanomedicines for HIV therapy. *Ther. Deliv.* **2013**, *4*, 153–156. [CrossRef]
28. Marciello, M.; Pellico, J.; Fernandez-Barahona, I.; Herranz, F.; Ruiz-Cabello, J.; Filice, M. Recent advances in the preparation and application of multifunctional iron oxide and liposome-based nanosystems for multimodal diagnosis and therapy. *Interface Focus* **2016**, *6*, 20160055. [CrossRef]
29. Filice, M.; Palomo, J.M. Cascade Reactions Catalyzed by Bionanostructures. *ACS Catal.* **2014**, *4*, 1588–1598. [CrossRef]
30. Filice, M.; Marciello, M.; Morales, M.d.P.; Palomo, J.M. Synthesis of heterogeneous enzyme–metal nanoparticle biohybrids in aqueous media and their applications in C–C bond formation and tandem catalysis. *Chem. Commun.* **2013**, *49*, 6876–6878. [CrossRef]
31. Erami, R.S.; Ovejero, K.; Meghdadi, S.; Filice, M.; Amirnasr, M.; Rodríguez-Diéguez, A.; De La Orden, M.U.; Gómez-Ruiz, S. Applications of Nanomaterials Based on Magnetite and Mesoporous Silica on the Selective Detection of Zinc Ion in Live Cell Imaging. *Nanomaterials* **2018**, *8*, 434. [CrossRef] [PubMed]
32. Pérez-Quintanilla, D.; Gómez-Ruiz, S.; Zizak, Z.; Sierra, I.; Prashar, S.; Hierro, I.; Fajardo, M.; Juranic, Z.; Kaluđerović, G. A New Generation of Anticancer Drugs: Mesoporous Materials Modified with Titanocene Complexes. *Chem. Eur. J.* **2009**, *15*, 5588–5597. [CrossRef] [PubMed]
33. Ceballos-Torres, J.; Virag, P.; Cenariu, M.; Prashar, S.; Fajardo, M.; Fischer-Fodor, E.; Gómez-Ruiz, S. Anti-cancer Applications of Titanocene-Functionalised Nanostructured Systems: An Insight into Cell Death Mechanisms. *Chem. Eur. J.* **2014**, *20*, 10811–10828. [CrossRef] [PubMed]
34. Bulatović, M.; Maksimovic-Ivanic, D.; Bensing, C.; Gómez-Ruiz, S.; Steinborn, D.; Schmidt, H.; Mojić, M.; Korac, A.; Golic, I.; Pérez-Quintanilla, D.; et al. Organotin(IV)-Loaded Mesoporous Silica as a Biocompatible Strategy in Cancer Treatment. *Angew. Chem. Int. Ed. Engl.* **2014**, *53*, 5982–8987. [CrossRef]

35. Ceballos-Torres, J.; Prashar, S.; Fajardo, M.; Chicca, A.; Gertsch, J.; Pinar, A.B.; Gómez-Ruiz, S. Ether-Substituted Group 4 Metallocene Complexes: Cytostatic Effects and Applications in Ethylene Polymerization. *Organometallics* **2015**, *34*, 2522–2532. [CrossRef]
36. Bensing, C.; Mojic, M.; Gómez-Ruiz, S.; Carralero, S.; Dojcinovic, B.; Maksimovic-Ivanic, D.; Mijatovic, S.; Kaluđerović, G. Evaluation of functionalized mesoporous silica SBA-15 as a carrier system for $Ph_3Sn(CH_2)_3OH$ against A2780 ovarian carcinoma cell line. *Dalton Trans.* **2016**, *45*, 18984–18993. [CrossRef]
37. Gómez-Ruiz, S.; García-Peñas, A.; Prashar, S.; Rodríguez-Diéguez, A.; Fischer-Fodor, E. Anticancer Applications of Nanostructured Silica-Based Materials Functionalized with Titanocene Derivatives: Induction of Cell Death Mechanism through TNFR1 Modulation. *Materials* **2018**, *11*, 224. [CrossRef]
38. Ellahioui, Y.; Patra, M.; Mari, C.; Kaabi, R.; Karges, J.; Gasser, G.; Gómez-Ruiz, S. Mesoporous silica nanoparticles functionalised with a photoactive ruthenium(II) complex: Exploring the formulation of a metal-based photodynamic therapy photosensitiser. *Dalton Trans.* **2019**, *48*, 5940–5951. [CrossRef]
39. Lee, C.-H.; Cheng, S.-H.; Wang, Y.-J.; Chen, Y.-C.; Chen, N.-T.; Souris, J.; Chen, C.-T.; Mou, C.-Y.; Yang, C.-S.; Lo, L.-W.; et al. Near-Infrared Mesoporous Silica Nanoparticles for Optical Imaging: Characterization and In Vivo Biodistribution. *Adv. Funct. Mater.* **2009**, *19*, 215–222. [CrossRef]
40. Guillet-Nicolas, R.; Laprise-Pelletier, M.; Nair, M.M.; Chevallier, P.; Lagueux, J.; Gossuin, Y.; Laurent, S.; Kleitz, F.; Fortin, M.A. Manganese-impregnated mesoporous silica nanoparticles for signal enhancement in MRI cell labelling studies. *Nanoscale* **2013**, *5*, 11499–11511. [CrossRef]
41. Chen, Y.; Yin, Q.; Ji, X.; Zhang, S.; Chen, H.; Zheng, Y.; Sun, Y.; Qu, H.; Wang, Z.; Li, Y.; et al. Manganese oxide-based multifunctionalized mesoporous silica nanoparticles for pH-responsive MRI, ultrasonography and circumvention of MDR in cancer cells. *Biomaterials* **2012**, *33*, 7126–7137. [CrossRef] [PubMed]
42. Brevet, D.; Gary-Bobo, M.; Raehm, L.; Richeter, S.; Hocine, O.; Amro, K.; Loock, B.; Couleaud, P.; Frochot, C.; Morere, A.; et al. Mannose-targeted mesoporous silica nanoparticles for photodynamic therapy. *Chem. Commun. Camb.* **2009**, *28*, 1475–1477. [CrossRef] [PubMed]
43. Ahmadi, E.; Dehghannejad, N.; Hashemikia, S.; Ghasemnejad, M.; Tabebordbar, H. Synthesis and surface modification of mesoporous silica nanoparticles and its application as carriers for sustained drug delivery. *Drug Deliv.* **2014**, *21*, 164–172. [CrossRef] [PubMed]
44. Wang, Y.; Zhao, Q.; Han, N.; Bai, L.; Li, J.; Liu, J.; Che, E.; Hu, L.; Zhang, Q.; Jiang, T.; et al. Mesoporous silica nanoparticles in drug delivery and biomedical applications. *Nanomedicine* **2015**, *11*, 313–327. [CrossRef] [PubMed]
45. Vallet-Regí, M.; Rámila, A.; del Real, R.P.; Pérez-Pariente, J. A New Property of MCM-41: Drug Delivery System. *Chem. Mater.* **2001**, *13*, 308–311. [CrossRef]
46. Kesse, S.; Boakye-Yiadom, K.O.; Ochete, B.O.; Opoku-Damoah, Y.; Akhtar, F.; Filli, M.S.; Asim Farooq, M.; Aquib, M.; Maviah Mily, B.J.; Murtaza, G.; et al. Mesoporous Silica Nanomaterials: Versatile Nanocarriers for Cancer Theranostics and Drug and Gene Delivery. *Pharmaceutics* **2019**, *11*, 77. [CrossRef] [PubMed]
47. Huang, X.; Young, N.P.; Townley, H.E. Characterization and Comparison of Mesoporous Silica Particles for Optimized Drug Delivery. *Nanomater. Nanotechnol.* **2014**, *4*, 1. [CrossRef]
48. Tang, F.; Li, L.; Chen, D. Mesoporous silica nanoparticles: Synthesis, biocompatibility and drug delivery. *Adv. Mater.* **2012**, *24*, 1504–1534. [CrossRef]
49. Hu, Q.; Li, J.; Qiao, S.; Hao, Z.; Tian, H.; Ma, C.; He, C. Synthesis and hydrophobic adsorption properties of microporous/mesoporous hybrid materials. *J. Hazard. Mater.* **2009**, *164*, 1205–1212. [CrossRef]
50. Sanchez, A.; Ovejero Paredes, K.; Ruiz-Cabello, J.; Martinez-Ruiz, P.; Pingarron, J.M.; Villalonga, R.; Filice, M. Hybrid Decorated Core@Shell Janus Nanoparticles as a Flexible Platform for Targeted Multimodal Molecular Bioimaging of Cancer. *ACS Appl. Mater. Interfaces* **2018**, *10*, 31032–31043. [CrossRef]
51. Jaidev, L.R.; Chellappan, D.R.; Bhavsar, D.V.; Ranganathan, R.; Sivanantham, B.; Subramanian, A.; Sharma, U.; Jagannathan, N.R.; Krishnan, U.M.; Sethuraman, S. Multi-functional nanoparticles as theranostic agents for the treatment & imaging of pancreatic cancer. *Acta Biomater.* **2017**, *49*, 422–433. [PubMed]
52. Lazaro-Carrillo, A.; Filice, M.; Guillén, M.J.; Amaro, R.; Viñambres, M.; Tabero, A.; Paredes, K.O.; Villanueva, A.; Calvo, P.; del Puerto Morales, M.; et al. Tailor-made PEG coated iron oxide nanoparticles as contrast agents for long lasting magnetic resonance molecular imaging of solid cancers. *Mater. Sci. Eng. C* **2020**, *107*, 110262. [CrossRef] [PubMed]
53. Talelli, M.; Aires, A.; Marciello, M. Protein-Modified Magnetic Nanoparticles for Biomedical Applications. *Curr. Org. Chem.* **2015**, *19*, 1. [CrossRef]

54. Filice, M.; Ruiz-Cabello, J. *Nucleic Acid Nanotheranostics: Biomedical Applications*; Elsevier Science: Amsterdam, The Netherlands, 2019.
55. Xie, J.; Lee, S.; Chen, X. Nanoparticle-based theranostic agents. *Adv. Drug Deliv. Rev.* **2010**, *62*, 1064–1079. [CrossRef]
56. Torchilin, V. Tumor delivery of macromolecular drugs based on the EPR effect. *Adv. Drug Deliv. Rev.* **2011**, *63*, 131–135. [CrossRef]
57. Foroozandeh, P.; Aziz, A.A. Insight into Cellular Uptake and Intracellular Trafficking of Nanoparticles. *Nanoscale Res. Lett.* **2018**, *13*, 339. [CrossRef]
58. Hu, Q.; Katti, P.S.; Gu, Z. Enzyme-responsive nanomaterials for controlled drug delivery. *Nanoscale* **2014**, *6*, 12273–12286. [CrossRef]
59. Zelzer, M.; Todd, S.J.; Hirst, A.R.; McDonald, T.O.; Ulijn, R.V. Enzyme responsive materials: Design strategies and future developments. *Biomater. Sci.* **2013**, *1*, 11–39. [CrossRef]
60. Andresen, T.L.; Thompson, D.H.; Kaasgaard, T. Enzyme-triggered nanomedicine: Drug release strategies in cancer therapy. *Mol. Membr. Biol.* **2010**, *27*, 353–363. [CrossRef]
61. Ruan, J.; Zheng, H.; Rong, X.; Rong, X.; Zhang, J.; Fang, W.; Zhao, P.; Luo, R. Over-expression of cathepsin B in hepatocellular carcinomas predicts poor prognosis of HCC patients. *Mol. Cancer* **2016**, *15*, 17. [CrossRef]
62. Dufresne, M.; Jane, D.; Theriault, A.; Adeli, K. Expression of cathepsin B and aryl hydrocarbon hydroxylase activities, and of apolipoprotein B in human hepatoma cells maintained long-term in a serum-free medium. *Vitr. Cell. Dev. Biol. Anim.* **1993**, *29A*, 873–878. [CrossRef] [PubMed]
63. Poreba, M.; Groborz, K.; Vizovisek, M.; Maruggi, M.; Turk, D.; Turk, B.; Powis, G.; Drag, M.; Salvesen, G.S. Fluorescent probes towards selective cathepsin B detection and visualization in cancer cells and patient samples. *Chem. Sci.* **2019**, *10*, 8461–8477. [CrossRef] [PubMed]
64. Szpaderska, A.; Frankfater, A. An intracellular form of cathepsin B contributes to invasiveness in cancer. *Cancer Res.* **2001**, *61*, 3493–3500. [PubMed]
65. Ruan, H.; Hao, S.; Young, P.; Zhang, H. Targeting Cathepsin B for Cancer Therapies. *Horiz. Cancer Res.* **2015**, *56*, 23–40. [PubMed]
66. Barwal, I.; Kumar, R.; Kateriya, S.; Dinda, A.K.; Yadav, S.C. Targeted delivery system for cancer cells consist of multiple ligands conjugated genetically modified CCMV capsid on doxorubicin GNPs complex. *Sci. Rep.* **2016**, *6*, 37096. [CrossRef]
67. Xing, L.; Xu, Y.; Sun, K.; Wang, H.; Zhang, F.; Zhou, Z.; Zhang, J.; Zhang, F.; Caliskan, B.; Qiu, Z.; et al. Identification of a peptide for folate receptor alpha by phage display and its tumor targeting activity in ovary cancer xenograft. *Sci. Rep.* **2018**, *8*, 8426. [CrossRef]
68. Lecomte, N.; Njardarson, J.T.; Nagorny, P.; Yang, G.; Downey, R.; Ouerfelli, O.; Moore, M.A.S.; Danishefsky, S.J. Emergence of potent inhibitors of metastasis in lung cancer via syntheses based on migrastatin. *Proc. Natl. Acad. Sci. USA* **2011**, *108*, 15074–15078. [CrossRef]
69. Hai, J.; Zhu, C.Q.; Bandarchi, B.; Wang, Y.H.; Navab, R.; Shepherd, F.A.; Jurisica, I.; Tsao, M.S. L1 cell adhesion molecule promotes tumorigenicity and metastatic potential in non-small cell lung cancer. *Clin. Cancer Res.* **2012**, *18*, 1914–1924. [CrossRef]
70. Fujisawa, T.; Rubin, B.; Suzuki, A.; Patel, P.S.; Gahl, W.A.; Joshi, B.H.; Puri, R.K. Cysteamine suppresses invasion, metastasis and prolongs survival by inhibiting matrix metalloproteinases in a mouse model of human pancreatic cancer. *PLoS ONE* **2012**, *7*, e34437. [CrossRef]
71. Scarpa, E.; Mayor, R. Collective cell migration in development. *J. Cell Biol.* **2016**, *212*, 143–155. [CrossRef]
72. Reinhart-King, C.A. Chapter 3 Endothelial Cell Adhesion and Migration. In *Methods in Enzymology*; Academic Press: Cambridge, MA, USA, 2008; Volume 443, pp. 45–64.
73. Zhao, Y.; Trewyn, B.G.; Slowing, I.I.; Lin, V.S.Y. Mesoporous Silica Nanoparticle-Based Double Drug Delivery System for Glucose-Responsive Controlled Release of Insulin and Cyclic AMP. *J. Am. Chem. Soc.* **2009**, *131*, 8398–8400. [CrossRef] [PubMed]
74. Bollu, V.S.; Barui, A.K.; Mondal, S.K.; Prashar, S.; Fajardo, M.; Briones, D.; Rodriguez-Dieguez, A.; Patra, C.R.; Gómez-Ruiz, S. Curcumin-loaded silica-based mesoporous materials: Synthesis, characterization and cytotoxic properties against cancer cells. *Mater. Sci. Eng. C Mater. Biol. Appl.* **2016**, *63*, 393–410. [CrossRef] [PubMed]

75. Li, E.; Yang, Y.; Hao, G.; Yi, X.; Zhang, S.; Pan, Y.; Xing, B.; Gao, M. Multifunctional Magnetic Mesoporous Silica Nanoagents for in vivo Enzyme-Responsive Drug Delivery and MR Imaging. *Nanotheranostics* **2018**, *2*, 233–242. [CrossRef] [PubMed]
76. Rosenholm, J.; Mamaeva, V.; Sahlgren, C.; Lindén, M. Nanoparticles in targeted cancer therapy: Mesoporous silica nanoparticles entering preclinical development stage. *Nanomed. Lond. Engl.* **2012**, *7*, 111–120. [CrossRef] [PubMed]

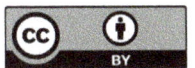

© 2020 by the authors. Licensee MDPI, Basel, Switzerland. This article is an open access article distributed under the terms and conditions of the Creative Commons Attribution (CC BY) license (http://creativecommons.org/licenses/by/4.0/).

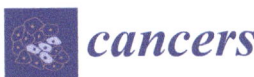

Article

Oxidation-Triggerable Liposome Incorporating Poly(Hydroxyethyl Acrylate-*co*-Allyl methyl sulfide) as an Anticancer Carrier of Doxorubicin

Jin Ah Kim, Dong Youl Yoon and Jin-Chul Kim *

Department of Medical Biomaterials Engineering, College of Biomedical Science and Institute of Bioscience and Biotechnology, Kangwon National University, 192-1, Hyoja 2 dong, Chuncheon, Kangwon-do 200-701, Korea
* Correspondence: jinkim@kangwon.ac.kr; Tel.: +82-033-250-6561

Received: 30 October 2019; Accepted: 8 January 2020; Published: 10 January 2020

Abstract: Since cancer cells are oxidative in nature, anti-cancer agents can be delivered to cancer cells specifically without causing severe normal cell toxicity if the drug carriers are designed to be sensitive to the intrinsic characteristic. Oxidation-sensitive liposomes were developed by stabilizing dioleoylphosphatidyl ethanolamine (DOPE) bilayers with folate-conjugated poly(hydroxyethyl acrylate-co-allyl methyl sulfide) (F-P(HEA-AMS)). The copolymer, synthesized by a free radical polymerization, was surface-active but lost its surface activity after AMS unit was oxidized by H_2O_2 treatment. The liposomes with F-P(HEA-AMS) were sensitive to H_2O_2 concentration (0%, 0.5%, 1.0%, and 2.0%) in terms of release, possibly because the copolymer lost its surface activity and its bilayer-stabilizing ability upon oxidation. Fluorescence-activated cell sorting (FACS) and confocal laser scanning microscopy (CLSM) revealed that doxorubicin (DOX)-loaded liposomes stabilized with folate-conjugated copolymers markedly promoted the transport of the anti-cancer drug to cancer cells. This was possible because the liposomes were readily translocated into the cancer cells via receptor-mediated endocytosis. This liposome would be applicable to the delivery carrier of anticancer drugs.

Keywords: dioleoylphosphatidylethanolamine; liposomes; poly(hydroxyethyl acrylate-co-allyl methyl sulfide) copolymer; folate; oxidation-sensitive release; doxorubicin; cellular interaction; in vitro anti-cancer activity

---

1. Introduction

Phospholipids are amphiphilic molecules and they were self-assembled in aqueous phase by an entropy-driven process [1–5]. Phosphatidylcholine (PC) is cylindrical in shape and its packing parameter is about 1, so it can be assembled into bilayer vesicles (i.e., liposome). Phosphatidylethanolamine (PE) is conical and its packing parameter is larger than 1, thus it can constitute non-bilayer assemblies (i.e., reversed hexagonal phase). If amphiphilic complementary molecules are inserted in between the head groups of PE molecules, liposomes can be formed [6–8]. Hydrophobically modified poly(*N*-isopropylacrylamide) was adopted as a stabilizer for the formation of dioleoylphophatidylethanolamine (DOPE) liposomes [9,10]. If the liposomes encounter a temperature higher than the phase transition temperature of the polymer, the polymer chains can contract and the bilayer domain they can cover and stabilize would decrease, leading to the disintegration of liposomes and the thermally triggered release of its payload. Cholesteryl hemisuccinate (CHEMS) was used as a complementary molecule for the stabilization of DOPE liposomes [11–13]. If the liposome suspension is acidified, the head group of CHEMS (i.e., carboxyl group) becomes unionized, its effective size decreases, thus the complementary molecule can lose its ability to stabilize DOPE bilayers, resulting in acidification-triggered release. Hydrophobically modified immunoglobulin G (HmIgG) could stabilize

DOPE bilayer and it was claimed to be used as a targetable drug carrier [14]. If the liposomes come in contact with their target site, the HmIgG molecules are supposed to diffuse on the liposomal surface toward antigens and cause the disintegration of the liposomes. Glucose oxidase was immobilized on the surface of the DOPE liposome stabilized with CHEMS to render the liposome sensitive to glucose [15]. The enzyme can convert glucose to gluconic acid and acidify the medium, triggering the release from the pH-sensitive liposomes.

In this study, oxidation-sensitive and cancer cell-targetable liposomes were prepared by stabilizing DOPE liposomes with folate-conjugated poly(hydroxyl ethyl acrylate-co-allyl methyl sulfide) (F-P(HEA-AMS)). Since HEA is hydrophilic and AMS is lipophilic, P(HEA-AMS) is a kind of amphiphilic polymer. AMS can act as a hydrophobic anchor and be hydrophobically intercalated into the bilayers with HEA segments orienting toward aqueous bulk phase. Thus, the copolymer would be able to stabilize DOPE liposomes (Figure 1A). Owing to folate conjugated to the copolymer, the liposomes can target cancer cells that mostly are known to overexpress folate receptors and they would be readily internalized into the cells via receptor mediated endocytosis. Doxorubicin (DOX) was loaded in the liposomes as an anti-cancer drug. DOX is known to kill cancer cells by being inserted between DNA double strands and suppressing the biosynthesis of proteins. It is also known that oxygen free radicals are formed by DOX within cancer cells and they peroxidize the cellular membrane lipids and exterminate the cancer cells [16]. In addition to inherent intracellular ROS, DOX-induced oxygen free radicals would also cause the methyl sulfide of AMS of the copolymer to be oxidized. Once oxidized within cells, AMS would hardly act as a hydrophobic anchor. As a result, the polymeric stabilizer would be desorbed from the liposomal membrane and it would cause the disintegration of liposomes and trigger the release of DOX from the liposomes (Figure 1B).

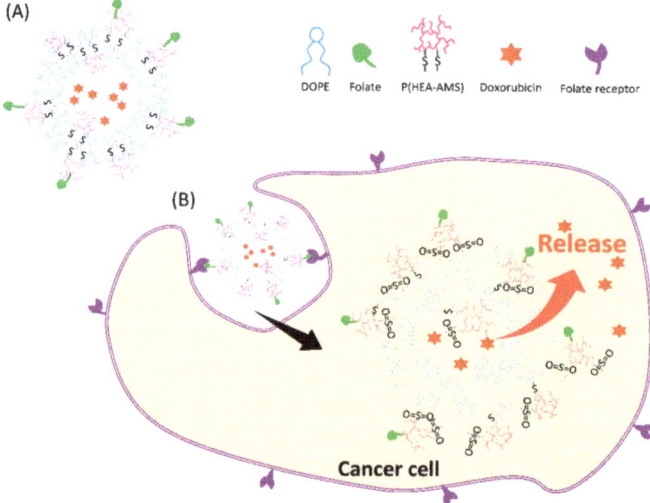

Figure 1. Scheme of oxidation-sensitive dioleoylphophatidylethanolamine (DOPE) liposomes stabilized with liposome incorporating folate-conjugated poly(hydroxyethyl acrylate-co-allyl methyl sulfide) (F-P(HEA-AMS)). AMS can act as a hydrophobic anchor and be hydrophobically intercalated into the bilayers with HEA segments orienting toward aqueous bulk phase. Thus, the copolymer would be able to stabilize DOPE liposomes (**A**). If the liposomes are exposed to an oxidative condition, the methyl sulfide of AMS can be oxidized to methyl sulfone and it would hardly act as a hydrophobic anchor. As a result, the polymeric stabilizer would be desorbed from the liposomal membrane and it would cause the disintegration of liposomes and trigger the release from the liposomes (**B**).

2. Results and Discussion

2.1. ^1H NMR Spectroscopy

The ^{1}H NMR spectrum of poly(hydroxyethyl acrylate-co-butyl methacrylate) (P(HEA-BMA)), poly(hydroxyethyl acrylate-co-allyl methyl sulfide) (P(HEA-AMS)), folate-conjugated poly(hydroxyethyl acrylate-co-butyl methacrylate) (F-P(HEA-BMA)) and folate-conjugated poly(hydroxyethyl acrylate-co-allyl methyl sulfide) (F-P(HEA-AMS)) are shown in Figure 2. In the ^{1}H NMR spectrum of P(HEA-BMA), the methyl group of BMA was found in the range of 0.92–1.06 ppm, two methylene groups next to the methyl group in the range of 1.35–2.14 ppm, the methylene group next to ester bond at 2.41 ppm, the methyl group next to quaternary carbon in the range of 1.35–2.14 ppm, the vinyl methylene group in the range of 1.35–2.14 ppm, the hydroxyl group of HEA at 4.80 ppm, the methylene group next to hydroxyl group at 3.76 ppm, the methylene group next to ester bond at 4.16 ppm, the methine group around 2.41 ppm, and the vinyl methylene group in the range of 1.35–2.14 ppm. The signal of the methyl group of BMA did not overlap with any other signals and the signal of the methylene group next to the hydroxyl group of HEA did not either. Using the area of those signals, the molar ratio of HEA to BMA was calculated to be 100 ÷ 3.5. In the ^{1}H NMR spectrum of P(HEA-AMS), the methyl group of AMS was found in the range of 1.63–1.99 ppm, the methylene group next to the sulfur at 2.69 ppm, and the methine group at 2.42 ppm. The signals of HEA of P(HEA-AMS) appeared at almost the same position as those of HEA of P(HEA-BMA). The signal of the methylene group of AMS did not overlap with any other signals and the signal of the methylene group next to the hydroxyl group of HEA did not either. Using the area of those signals, the molar ratio of HEA to AMS was calculated to be 100 ÷ 5.2. The aromatic protons of folate were found at 6.78 ppm, 7.66 ppm and 7.99 ppm, and the units (i.e., HEA, BMA, and AMS unit) of folate-conjugated copolymers were found at almost the same position as those of folate-free copolymers. In the spectrum of F-P(HEA-BMA), the area of the aromatic ring signals was 2.0, and that of the ethyl group signals of HEA unit was 56.9. Thus, the molar ratio of folate to HEA unit was calculated to be about 1 ÷ 14, indicating that folate was conjugated to every 14 HEA units. Since the molar ratio of HEA to BMA was 100 ÷ 3.5, the molar ratio of folate:HEA:BMA of F-P(HEA-BMA) was calculated to be 6.7 ÷ 93.3 ÷ 3.5. In the spectrum of F-P(HEA-AMS), the area of the aromatic ring signals was 3.6, and that of the ethyl group signals of HEA unit was 109.8. Therefore, the molar ratio of folate to HEA unit was calculated to be about 1 ÷ 15. Since the molar ratio of HEA to AMS was 100 ÷ 5.2, the molar ratio of folate/HEA/AMS of F-P(HEA-AMS) was calculated to be 6.2 ÷ 93.8 ÷ 5.2.

2.2. Examination of Oxidation of Copolymers by XPS

Figure 3 shows the XPS spectrum of P(HEA-AMS) and H_2O_2-P(HEA-AMS). A strong peak around 163.5 eV was found in the spectrum of P(HEA-AMS) and it could be ascribed to the sulfur signal of the sulfide moiety (i.e., the AMS unit). H_2O_2-P(HEA-AMS) showed a relatively broad peak centered at 168 eV with a shoulder at 166 eV. Those signals could be assigned to the sulfur electron of the sulfone moiety and that of the sulfoxide one, respectively. Thus, it could be said that the AMS unit was readily oxidized by H_2O_2 under our experimental condition.

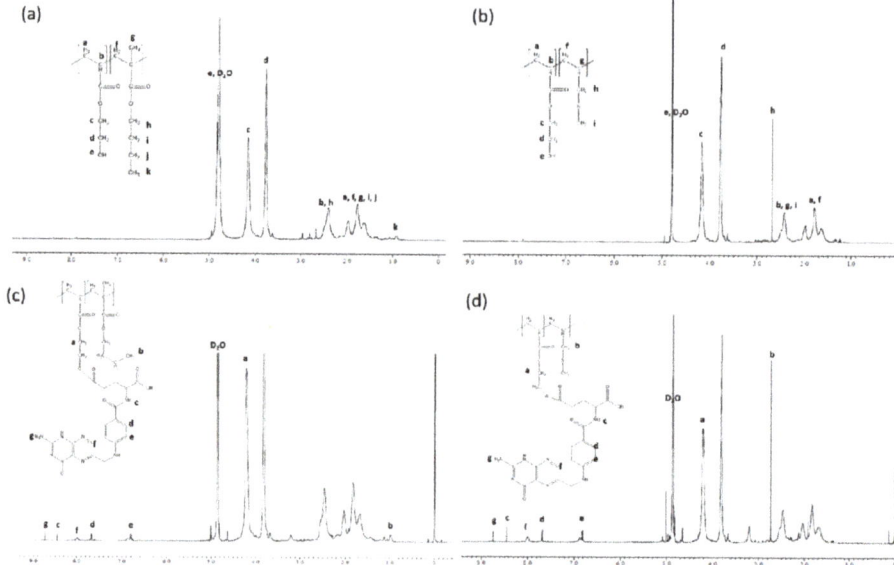

Figure 2. ^{1}H NMR spectrum of P(HEA-BMA) (**a**) and P(HEA-AMS) (**b**), F-P(HEA-BMA) (**c**) and F-P(HEA-AMS) (**d**).

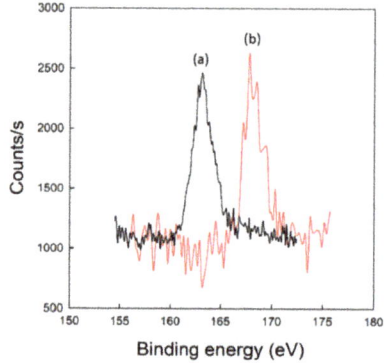

Figure 3. XPS spectrum of P(HEA-AMS) (**a**) and H_2O_2-P(HEA-AMS) (**b**).

2.3. Measurement of Interfacial Tension

Figure 4 shows the air/water interfacial tension of P(HEA-BMA), H_2O_2-P(HEA-BMA), P(HEA-AMS), and H_2O_2-P(HEA-AMS) solution. The interfacial tension of P(HEA-BMA) solution decreased steeply from 73 dyne/cm to 57 dyne/cm with an increasing concentration in the range of 0–0.02 mg/mL, it decreased gradually from 57 dyne/cm to 56 dyne/cm in the range of 0.02–0.5 mg/mL, and no more decrease was observed in the remaining concentration range. An L type of interfacial tension profile is typical of a surface-active agent [17,18]. The concentration where two tangential lines intersect each other can be assumed to be the critical micellization concentration (CMC) [18–20]. The CMC was estimated to be 0.0156 mg/mL. BMA is a hydrophobic monomer and its copolymerization with a hydrophilic monomer (i.e., HEA) would result in the formation of an amphiphilic and interface-active copolymer. Owing to its amphiphilicity, the copolymer chains would be aligned at air/water interface with HEA segments being in water and BMA residue facing air to reduce the interfacial tension. The interfacial tension profile of H_2O_2-P(HEA-BMA) solution was almost the same as that of P(HEA-BMA) solution. This suggested that the interfacial activity of P(HEA-BMA) was little changed after treated with H_2O_2. In fact, P(HEA-BMA) had no oxidizable groups and its chemical structure would hardly be affected by the oxidizing agent treatment. P(HEA-AMS) solution also exhibited an L type of interfacial tension profile. The plateau interfacial value was about 61 dyne/cm and it was higher than that of P(HEA-BMA), indicating that P(HEA-AMS) was less interface-active than P(HEA-BMA). The ^{1}H NMR spectroscopy revealed that the molar content of the hydrophobic monomer (i.e., AMS) of the former copolymer was about 4.9% and it was more than that of the hydrophobic monomer (i.e., BMA) of the latter copolymer, 3.4%. Nevertheless, P(HEA-AMS) was less interface-active. AMS has methylene methyl sulfide (CH_3-S-CH_2-) on the side of vinyl group and BMA has butoxy carbonyl group (CH_3-$(CH_2)_3$-O-C=O-) and methyl group on the side. Thus, AMS seemed to be less hydrophobic than BMA and to be less effective in causing the copolymer to be amphiphilic. This could explain why the interfacial activity of P(HEA-AMS) was lower than that of P(HEA-BMA). The CMC of P(HEA-AMS), estimated by the crossing point of two tangential lines, was about 0.025 mg/mL, and it was higher than that of P(HEA-BMA), about 0.0156 mg/mL. This also indicated that P(HEA-AMS) was less surface-active and less amphiphilic. The interfacial tension of H_2O_2-P(HEA-AMS) solution slightly decreased to 68.0 dyne/cm when the concentration increased to 1.0 mg/mL, and it was higher than that of P(HEA-AMS) solution in the full concentration tested. Since a saturation type of decrease pattern in the interfacial tension disappeared and the interfacial tension was reduced only by 4 dyne/cm when increased up to the maximum concentration, it was concluded that P(HEA-AMS) lost most of its interfacial activity after treated with H_2O_2. XPS revealed that the sulfide of AMS unit was oxidized to the sulfoxide and the sulfone upon the oxidizing agent treatment (Figure 3). Once P(HEA-AMS) was oxidized, the copolymer would lose its amphiphilicity and its interfacial activity because AMS unit became hydrophilic.

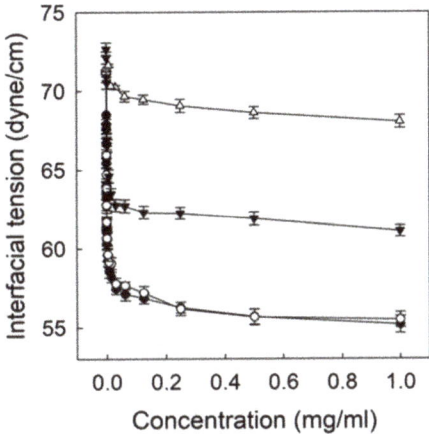

Figure 4. Air/water interfacial tension of P(HEA-BMA) (●), H_2O_2-P(HEA-BMA) (○), P(HEA-AMS) (▼), and H_2O_2-P(HEA-AMS) solution (△).

2.4. Characterization of DOPE Liposomes Stabilized with Copolymers

Figure 5 shows the TEM photo of liposome/F-P(HEA-BMA)(200/1), liposome/F-P(HEA-BMA)(100/1), liposome/F-P(HEA-BMA)(50/1), liposome/F-P(HEA-AMS)(200/1), liposome/F-P(HEA-AMS)(100/1), and liposome/F-P(HEA-AMS)(50/1) that 200/1, 100/1 and 50/1 refer to dioleoylphophatidylethanolamine (DOPE)/copolymer mass ratio. The liposomes were multi-lamellar vesicles regardless of whether the stabilizer was F-P(HEA-BMA) or F-P(HEA-AMS). DOPE is conical because the head (i.e., ethanolamine) is much smaller than the tail (i.e., dioleoyl group) and its packing parameter is more than 1. When dispersed in aqueous solution, DOPE molecules are assembled into reversed hexagonal phase [21,22]. An amphiphilic molecule having a large hydrophilic head and a small hydrophobic tail can be used as a complementary molecule to have DOPE molecules assembled into liposomal bilayers [23,24]. The hydrophobic tail of complementary molecule is likely to be inserted in between the tails of DOPE molecules through hydrophobic interaction while the hydrophilic head would fill the space between the heads of DOPE molecules. F-P(HEA-BMA) and F-P(HEA-AMS) were thought to act as a complementary molecule to stabilize the DOPE liposomal bilayers. The HEA segments of the copolymers would be able to fill the space between the heads of DOPE molecules while the hydrophobic anchors (i.e., BMA and AMS) being anchored in between the tails. This would be a mechanism by which the copolymers could have DOPE molecules assembled into the liposomal bilayers. The quenching % of calcein enveloped in liposomes decreased with increasing the amount of the copolymers. For example, the quenching % of calcein enveloped in liposome/F-P(HEA-BMA)(200/1), liposome/F-P(HEA-BMA)(100/1), and liposome/F-P(HEA-BMA)(50/1) were 55.6%, 51.0%, and 46.2%, respectively. The quenching % of calcein enveloped in liposome/F-P(HEA-AMS)(200/1), liposome/F-P(HEA-AMS)(100/1), and liposome/F-P(HEA-AMS)(50/1) were 57.7%, 55.6%, and 53.9%, respectively.

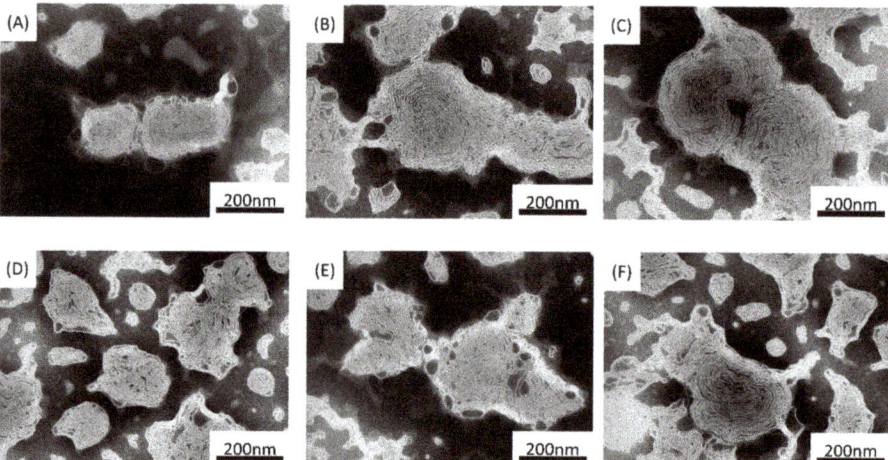

Figure 5. TEM micrograph of liposome/F-P(HEA-BMA)(200/1) (**A**), liposome/F-P(HEA-BMA)(100/1) (**B**), liposome/F-P(HEA-BMA)(50/1) (**C**), liposome/ F-P(HEA-AMS)(200/1) (**D**), liposome/F-P(HEA-AMS)(100/1) (**E**), and liposome/F-P(HEA-AMS)(50/1) (**F**). The magnification was 80,000 times, and bar on each micrograph corresponds to 200 nm.

The specific loading percentages of doxorubicin (DOX) loaded in liposome/F-P(HEA-BMA)(200/1), liposome/F-P(HEA-BMA)(100/1), liposome/F-P(HEA-BMA)(50/1) were 1.82%, 2.35%, and 2.39%, respectively. It seemed that the specific loading % was greater at a lower mass ratio of DOPE to copolymer. This was possibly because the specific loading % of a water-soluble drug is proportional to the size of liposome [25,26]. In fact, the mean hydrodynamic diameter of the liposomes was larger when the DOPE to copolymer mass ratio was lower. The specific loading percentages of DOX loaded in liposome/F-P(HEA-AMS)(200/1), liposome/F-P(HEA-AMS)(100/1), and liposome/F-P(HEA-AMS)(50/1) were 1.85%, 1.98%, 2.21%, respectively. The same reason would be applicable in explaining why the specific loading % was greater at a lower mass ratio of DOPE to copolymer.

The mean diameter of liposomes increased with increasing the amount of the copolymers. For example, the hydrodynamic mean diameter of liposome/F-P(HEA-BMA)(200/1), liposome/F-P(HEA-BMA)(100/1), and liposome/F-P(HEA-BMA)(50/1) were about 163 nm, 273 nm, and 283 nm, respectively. The hydrodynamic mean diameter of liposome/F-P(HEA-AMS)(200/1), liposome/F-P(HEA-AMS)(100/1), and liposome/F-P(HEA-AMS)(50/1) were about 169 nm, 176 nm, and 262 nm, respectively. If the amount of copolymers increases, the amount of DOPE bilayers formed would increase because the copolymers could stabilize DOPE bilayer. An increase in the amount of bilayer would lead to increase in the number of liposomal particle or increase in the number of bilayer per one liposomal particle. Since the mean diameter was proportional to the amount of copolymers, the latter case was likely to take place more favorably than the former case. In fact, as the amount of copolymers was higher, the diameter seemed to be larger and the number of bilayer per one liposomal particle seemed to be greater (Figure 5).

2.5. Observation of Oxidation-Sensitive Release

The H_2O_2 concentration-dependent release profiles of calcein enveloped in liposome/F-P(HEA-BMA)(200/1), liposome/F-P(HEA-BMA)(100/1), and liposome/F-P(HEA-BMA)(50/1) were presented in Figure S1. The release % of the fluorescence dye enveloped in liposome/F-P(HEA-BMA)(200/1) did not increase markedly with time lapse regardless of what the H_2O_2 concentration was and it did not strongly depend on H_2O_2 concentration either. For example, the maximum release % obtained when H_2O_2 concentration was 0%, 0.5%, 1.0%, and 2.0% was about 0.2%, 3.4%, 5.8%, and 7.8%, respectively. The small increase in the release % with increasing H_2O_2 concentration was probably because of the H_2O_2-caused oxidation of DOPE molecules. Two double bonds are in the tail of the phospholipid and they are subjected to oxidation [27,28]. Upon the H_2O_2-caused oxidation, the double bond of DOPE can be broken down and the hydrophobic chain (i.e., oleoyl group) can be shortened, resulting in the destabilization of DOPE bilayers and the release of the dye. F-P(HEA-BMA) had no oxidation-sensitive groups and it would hardly affect the H_2O_2 concentration-dependent release. The H_2O_2 concentration-dependent release profile and the release percentages of calcein enveloped in liposome/F-P(HEA-BMA)(100/1) and liposome/F-P(HEA-BMA)(50/1) were almost the same as those of the dye enveloped in liposome/F-P(HEA-BMA)(200/1). This implied that the copolymer had little effect on the H_2O_2 concentration-dependent release. In fact, there were no oxidation-sensitive groups in the copolymer.

Figure 6 shows the H_2O_2 concentration-dependent release profiles of calcein enveloped in liposome/F-P(HEA-AMS)(200/1), liposome/F-P(HEA-AMS)(100/1), and liposome/F-P(HEA-AMS)(50/1). Liposome/F-P(HEA-AMS)(200/1) showed no appreciable release during the whole period of release experiment (i.e., 60 s) when no H_2O_2 was contained in the release medium, indicating that the liposomes were stable in the buffer solution free of the oxidizing agent. When the concentration of oxidizing agent was 0.5%, the liposomes released their content rapidly for the first few seconds and slowly during the remaining period. Specifically, the release degree was about 25% in 5 s and it increased slowly to about 35% for the remaining 55 s. The hydrophobic side chain (i.e., methylene methyl sulfide) of the copolymer would be able to be anchored in between DOPE molecules through hydrophobic interaction while the hydrophilic HEA segments orienting toward aqueous bulk phase. This was thought to be a mechanism with which DOPE liposomes were stabilized by the copolymer. If the copolymer is exposed to an oxidative condition, the sulfide can be oxidized to become sulfoxide and sulfone (Figure 3) [29,30]. Upon the oxidation, the hydrophobic anchor was likely to become hydrophilic, it would hardly be kept to be anchored into the liposomal bilayers and the copolymers would be removed from the liposomal bilayers, leading to the disintegration of the liposomes and the triggered release of the liposomal content. In fact, the copolymer lost its interfacial activity after treated with H_2O_2 (Figure 4). However, the release degree was higher at the two highest H_2O_2 concentrations during the whole period of release experiment. Thus, the maximum release degree at the concentration of 1.0% was about 78.0% and when H_2O_2 concentration was 2.0%, the release degree was about 78.4%, almost the same. As H_2O_2 concentration was higher, the sulfide copolymer was likely to be oxidized more readily and DOPE liposomes would be destabilized more extensively, leading to higher release degree. The oxidation degree of the sulfide copolymer at the concentration of 1.0% seemed to be already high enough to disintegrate the liposomes completely. The H_2O_2 concentration-dependent release profiles of dye enveloped in liposome/F-P(HEA-AMS)(100/1) were like those of dye enveloped in liposome/F-P(HEA-AMS)(200/1). Liposome/F-P(HEA-AMS)(100/1) exhibited no significant release when the release medium was free of H_2O_2. But it showed a triggered release when the release medium contained the oxidizing agent. For example, the maximum release degree was about 0.5%, 60.6%, 79.3%, and 80.2%, respectively, when the concentration of the oxidizing agent was 0%, 0.5%, 1.0%, and 2.0%. As in case of liposome/F-P(HEA-AMS)(200/1), the release degree at the concentration of 1.0% was higher than that observed at the concentration of 0.5% and no significant difference was found between the release degree at the concentration of 1.0 % and that at 2.0%, suggesting that the oxidation at 1.0% was already high enough to induce the complete disintegration of the liposomes. At the concentration of 0.5%, liposome/F-P(HEA-AMS)(100/1) exhibited higher release degree than liposome/F-P(HEA-AMS)(200/1). Since the former liposomes incorporate more sulfide copolymer for a fixed amount of DOPE than the latter liposomes, they would be subjected more readily to the oxidation-induced destabilization. The H_2O_2 concentration-dependent release profiles of dye for liposome/F-P(HEA-AMS)(50/1) were quite different. The maximum release degree was about 0.6%, 77.2%, 83.2%, and 83.7%, when the H_2O_2 concentration was 0%, 0.5%, 1.0%, and 2.0%, respectively. The liposome/F-P(HEA-AMS)(50/1) showed higher release degree at the H_2O_2 concentration 0.5% than the other liposomes and there was no significant difference between the release degree at H_2O_2 concentrations of 0.5%, 1.0% and 2.0%. These indicated that liposome/F-P(HEA-AMS)(50/1) was the most sensitive to H_2O_2 among the liposomes tested. Since liposome/F-P(HEA-AMS)(50/1) was incorporating higher amount of the sulfide copolymer than the other two kinds of liposomes, the amount of copolymer which can undergo oxidation would also be greater and the liposome was likely to be more susceptible to destabilization in an oxidative condition. This could be a reason why liposome/F-P(HEA-AMS)(50/1) was more sensitive to the oxidizing agent than liposome/F-P(HEA-AMS)(200/1) and liposome/F-P(HEA-AMS)(100/1).

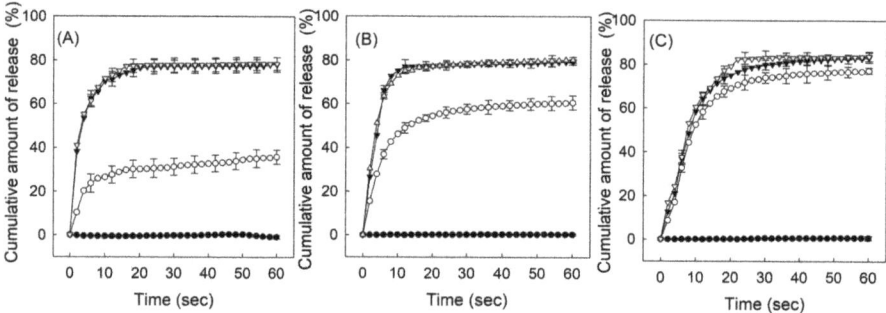

Figure 6. H_2O_2 concentration-dependent release profiles of calcein enveloped in liposome/P(HEA-AMS)(200/1) (**A**), liposome/P(HEA-AMS)(100/1) (**B**), and liposome/ P(HEA-AMS)(50/1) (**C**) at 0 % (●), 0.5 % (○), 1.0 % (▼), and 2.0 % (▽) H_2O_2 concentration.

2.6. Observation of Interaction of Liposomes and Cancer Cell and Tumor Cells

Figure 7 shows the fluorescence intensity distribution obtained using flow cytometry (FACS) of KB cells (a human cancer cell type originating from the cervix) (A) and LN229 cells (human glioma cell line) (B) treated with free DOX, liposome/P(HEA-BMA)(100/1)/DOX, liposome/F-P(HEA-BMA)(100/1)/DOX, liposome/P(HEA-AMS)(100/1)/DOX, and liposome/F-P(HEA-AMS)(100/1)/DOX. When the cells were treated with free DOX, the fluorescence intensity at the maximum cell count was about 10 and it was the lowest among the test samples tested. When the cells were treated with liposome/P(HEA-BMA)(100/1)/DOX, the fluorescence intensity at the maximum cell count was about 9000 and it was higher than that obtained with the cells treated with free DOX. This suggested that the liposomal DOX was internalized into the cells more efficiently than free DOX. It was reported that particulate matters including liposomes were translocated into the cells via particulate endocytosis and small solutes including DOX were taken up by the cells via pinocytosis [31,32]. Small solutes would also be able to be internalized into the cells via simple diffusion. Since DOX was loaded and localized in the liposomes (specific loading %: 1.82–2.39), the cellular uptake of liposomes seemed to transport DOX to the cells more effectively than the molecular level transport phenomena (i.e., pinocytosis). The cellular uptake would be a reason why the fluorescence intensity of the cells treated with liposome/P(HEA-BMA)(100/1)/DOX was stronger than that of the cells treated with free DOX. When the cells were treated with liposome/F-P(HEA-BMA)(100/1)/DOX, the fluorescence intensity at the maximum cell count was about 1.5×10^3 and it was much stronger than that obtained with the cells treated with liposome/P(HEA-BMA)(100/1)/DOX. Folate-receptor was reported to be overexpressed on the surface of KB cells and LN229 cells [33–36]. Thus, the folate-conjugated liposome would readily be able to bind to the cancer cells and tumor cells through receptor-ligand interaction then the liposome would be likely to be internalized into the cells via receptor-mediated endocytosis. The strong fluorescence intensity of the cancer cells and tumor cells treated with the folate-conjugated liposomes could be ascribed to the receptor-mediated uptake. The cancer cells and the tumor cell treated with liposome/P(HEA-AMS)(100/1)/DOX and liposome/F-P(HEA-AMS)(100/1)/DOX showed similar fluorescence intensity distributions to the cancer cells and tumor cells treated with liposome/P(HEA-BMA)(100/1)/DOX and liposome/F-P(HEA-BMA)(100/1)/DOX, respectively. This indicates that the former liposomes were as potent as the latter ones in terms of their translocation into the cancer cells and tumor cells.

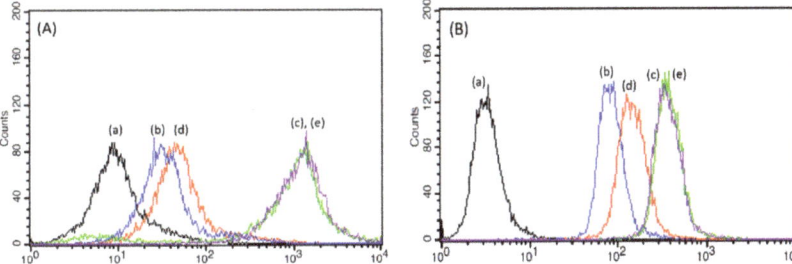

Figure 7. Fluorescence intensity distribution of KB cells (**A**) and LN229 cells (**B**) treated with free DOX (**a**), liposome/P(HEA-BMA)(100/1)/DOX (**b**), liposome/F-P(HEA-BMA)(100/1)/DOX (**c**), liposome/P(HEA-AMS)(100/1)/DOX (**d**), and liposome/F-P(HEA-AMS)(100/1)/DOX (**e**).

Figure 8 shows the confocal laser scanning microscopy (CLSM) micrograph of KB cells (A) and LN229 cells (B) treated with free DOX, liposome/P(HEA-BMA)(100/1)/DOX, liposome/F-P(HEA-BMA)(100/1)/DOX, liposome/P(HEA-AMS)(100/1)/DOX, and liposome/F-P(HEA-AMS)(100/1)/DOX. When the cancer cells and tumor cells were treated with free DOX, DAPI-dyed nuclei (blue circular objects) were found with no trace of DOX (red color). When treated with liposome/P(HEA-BMA)(100/1)/DOX, weak DOX fluorescence appeared within and around the nuclei, suggesting that DOX was taken up by the cancer cells and tumor cells. As described above, the endocytosis of the liposome into the cells would promote the cellular internalization of DOX. When treated with liposome/F-P(HEA-BMA)(100/1)/DOX, DOX fluorescence was found within and near by the nuclei and the intensity was much stronger than that of the cells treated with the folate-free liposomes. Possibly due to the specific interaction of folate and its receptor, the endocytosis of the liposomes would be expedited, leading to a promoted cellular internalization of DOX. The cancer cells and tumor cells treated with liposome/P(HEA-AMS)(100/1)/DOX and liposome/F-P(HEA-AMS)(100/1)/DOX exhibited similar DOX fluorescence intensities to the cancer cells and tumor cells treated with liposome/P(HEA-BMA)(100/1)/DOX and liposome/F-P(HEA-BMA)(100/1)/DOX, respectively. This suggests that the feasibility of the cellular uptake of the former liposomes was as high as that of the latter ones.

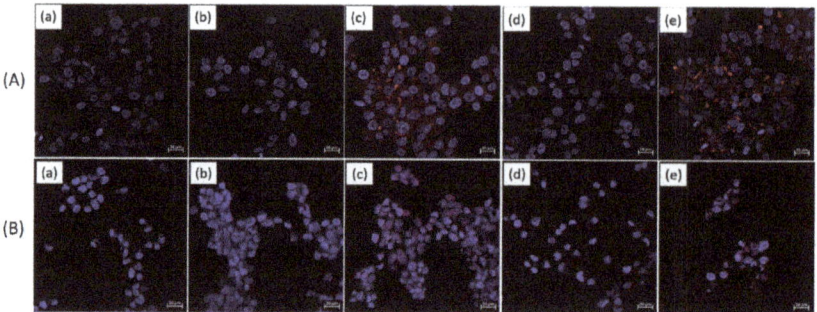

Figure 8. CLSM micrograph of KB cells (**A**) and LN229 cells (**B**) treated with free DOX (**a**), liposome/P(HEA-BMA)(100/1)/DOX (**b**), liposome/F-P(HEA-BMA)(100/1)/DOX (**c**), liposome/P(HEA-AMS)(100/1)/DOX (**d**), and liposome/F-P(HEA-AMS)(100/1)/DOX (**e**). In all cases, cells were also treated with DAPI to dye the nuclei.

2.7. Observation of In Vitro Anti-Cancer Cellular Efficacy

Figure 9 shows the viability of KB cells (A) and LN229 cells (B) treated with liposome/F-P(HEA-BMA)(100/1), liposome/F-P(HEA-AMS)(100/1), free DOX, liposome/P(HEA-BMA)(100/1)/DOX, liposome/F-P(HEA-BMA)(100/1)/DOX, liposome/P(HEA-AMS)(100/1)/DOX, and liposome/F-P(HEA-AMS)(100/1)/DOX. When treated with liposomes without DOX (i.e., liposome/F-P(HEA-BMA)(100/1) and liposome/F-P(HEA-AMS)(100/1)), the viability of cancer cell and tumor cell fluctuated near 100% in the full range of concentration tested, suggesting that the liposomes exhibited no appreciable in vitro cytotoxicity under present experimental condition. The viability of the cancer cell and tumor cell treated with free DOX gradually decreased to about 43% in KB cells and 53% in LN229 cells when the concentration increased to 4 μg/mL. The viability of the cancer cell and tumor cell treated with liposome/P(HEA-BMA)(100/1)/DOX decreased to about 40% in KB cells and 48% in LN229 cells in the same concentration range and it was not significantly different from that of cells treated with free DOX. On the other hand, the viability of the cancer cell and tumor cell treated with liposome/F-P(HEA-BMA)(100/1)/DOX was significantly lower than that of cells treated with free DOX. For example, the viability of cells treated with the folate-conjugated liposome was about 33% in KB cells and 38% in LN229 cells at the DOX concentration of 4 μg/mL and it was lower than that of cells treated with DOX. The folate-conjugated liposomes would be targeted to the cancer cell and tumor cell through the specific interaction of folate and its receptor. In fact, FACS and CLSM revealed that liposome/F-P(HEA-BMA)(100/1) and liposome/F-P(HEA-AMS)(100/1) markedly promoted the delivery of DOX to the cancer cell and tumor cell. This could account for why the in vitro anti-cancer efficacy of liposome/F-P(HEA-BMA)(100/1)/DOX was significantly higher than that of free DOX. Meanwhile, the viability of cells treated with liposome/P(HEA-AMS)(100/1)/DOX was significantly lower than that of cells treated with liposome/P(HEA-BMA)(100/1)/DOX. For example, the viability of cells treated with the former liposome was about 35% in KB cells and 43% in LN229 cells at the DOX concentration of 4 μg/mL and it was lower than that of cells treated with the latter one. According to the results of FACS shown in Figure 7, liposome/P(HEA-AMS)(100/1) seemed to promote the intracellular delivery of DOX to almost the same degree as liposome/P(HEA-BMA)(100/1). However, liposome/P(HEA-AMS)(100/1) released its content in an oxidation responsive manner but liposome/P(HEA-BMA)(100/1) did not (Figure 6 and Figure S1). If the oxidation-sensitive liposomes are taken up by the cancer cell and tumor cell, P(HEA-AMS) chains would be oxidized and the liposomes would be able to destabilized, leading to the promoted release of their payload because the intracellular space of the cancer cell and tumor cell is in a high ROS level [37,38]. It is also known that oxygen free radicals are formed by DOX within the cancer cell and tumor cell and they peroxidize the cellular membrane lipids and exterminate the cancer cell and tumor cell [39–41]. The oxidation-sensitive liposomes would also be destabilized by the oxygen free radicals produced by DOX. This would be a reason why liposome/P(HEA-AMS)(100/1)/DOX was more efficacious than liposome/P(HEA-BMA)(100/1)/DOX in killing the cancer cell and tumor cell. The viability of cells treated with liposome/F-P(HEA-AMS)(100/1)/DOX markedly decreased to about 16% in KB cells, 31% in LN229 cells when the concentration increased to 4 µg/mL. Overall, LN229 cells showed less anticancer efficacy than KB cells, because the internalization was less than KB cells, as shown by FACS and CLSM (Figures 7 and 8). Liposome/F-P(HEA-AMS)(100/1)/DOX exhibited the highest in vitro anti-cancer efficacy among the liposomes tested. According to the results of FACS and CLSM study shown, liposome/F-P(HEA-AMS)(100/1)/DOX seemed to be efficiently translocated into the cancer cell and tumor cell. In addition, the liposome could release its payload actively in an oxidative condition (Figure 6). These results could explain why liposome/F-P(HEA-AMS)(100/1)/DOX was so effective in killing the cancer cell and tumor cell.

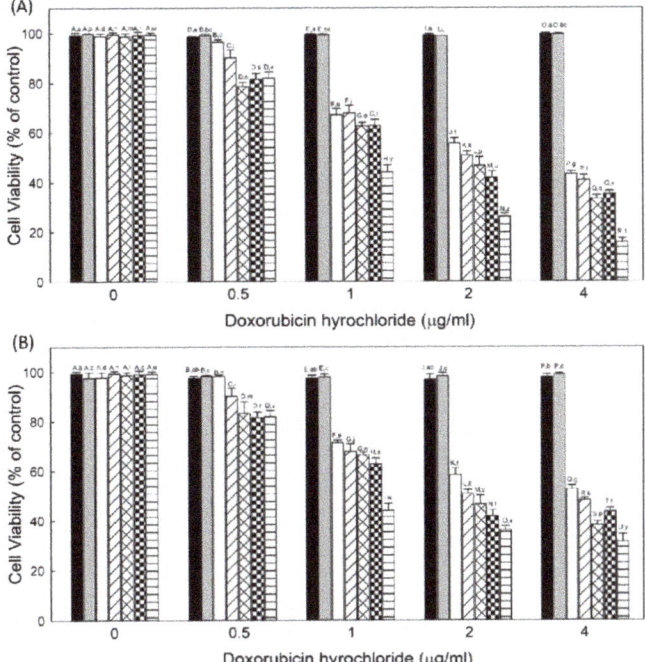

Figure 9. Viability of KB cells (**A**) and LN229 cells (**B**) treated with liposome/F-P(HEA-BMA)(100/1) (black bar), liposome/F-P(HEA-AMS)(100/1) (gray bar), free DOX (white bar), liposome/P(HEA-BMA)(100/1)/DOX (hashed bar), liposome/F-P(HEA-BMA)(100/1)/DOX (cross hatched bar), liposome/P(HEA-AMS)(100/1)/DOX (checkered bar), and liposome/F-P(HEA-AMS)(100/1)/DOX (striped bar).

3. Materials and Methods

3.1. Materials

1,2-Dioleoyl-sn-Glycero-3-Phosphoethanolamine (DOPE), 2-hydroxyethyl acrylate (HEA), butyl methacrylate (BMA), allyl methyl sulfide (AMS), folic acid (FA), dicyclohexylcarbodiimide (DCC), N,N-dimethylformamide (DMF), deoxycholic acid (DOC, sodium salt), calcein, Triton X-100, phosphate buffer solution (PB), phosphotungstic acid (PTA), thiazolyl blue tetrazolium bromide (MTT), fluoroshield^{TM} with DAPI, doxorubicin hydrochloride (DOX) and deuterium oxide (D_2O) were purchased from Sigma-Aldrich Co. (St. Louis, MO, USA). Azobisisobutyronitrile (AIBN) was purchased from Junsei Chemical Co. (Tokyo, Japan). Phosphate buffered saline (PBS), RPMI 1640 medium (no folic acid), fetal bovine serum (FBS), penicillin-streptomycin, and trypsin-EDTA (0.25%) were purchased from Gibco™ (Dublin, Ireland). Phosphorus pentoxide (P_2O_5) was purchased from Kanto Chemical Co., Inc. (Tokyo, Japan). Diethyl ether, dimethyl sulfoxide (DMSO), 4-dimethylaminopyridine (DMAP) and hydrogen peroxide (H_2O_2) were purchased from Daejung Chemical & Metals Co. Ltd. (Gyeonggi-do, Korea). Sephadex G-100 was provided by GE Healthcare (Uppsala, Sweden). Human nasopharyngeal epidermoid carcinoma cell line (KB) was purchased from the Korean cell line bank (Seoul, Korea). Human glioma cell line (LN229) was obtained from the American Type Culture Collection (ATCC, Manassas, VA, USA). All other reagents were of analytical grade.

3.2. Preparation of HEA Copolymers

Poly (HEA-co-AMS) (P(HEA-AMS)) and poly (HEA-co-BMA) (P(HEA-BMA)) were prepared by free radical reaction. In total, 5 g of HEA was dissolved in 50 mL of DMF in a 250 mL 3-neck round bottom flask. A hydrophobic comonomer (AMS and BMA) was dissolved in the HEA solution so that the HEA to comonomer molar ratio was 80:20. 40 mg of AIBN was added to the mixture monomer solution and the reaction mixture was purged with nitrogen gas for 30 min. The monomers were copolymerized at 75 °C with reflux for 12 h. After standing the flask containing reaction mixture until the temperature reached room temperature (20–23 °C), the copolymers were precipitated using diethyl ether as a non-solvent and they were purified by re-precipitation. The precipitates were separated by filtration and dried at room temperature.

3.3. Preparation of Folate-Conjugated HEA Copolymers

FA (0.320 g), DCC (1.534 g), and DMAP (0.904 g) were co-dissolved in 10 mL of DMSO contained in a 30 mL round bottom flask and the mixture solution was stirred using a magnetic bar at 30 °C for 2 h under dark condition and N_2 atmosphere. In total, 0.856 g each of P(HEA-AMS) and P(HEA-BMA) was dissolved in 10 mL of DMSO, it was poured into FA solution, and the reaction mixture was stirred at 30 °C for 24 h. The byproduct (i.e., dicyclohexylurea) was removed by filtration, the filtrate was centrifuged at 12,000 rpm for 30 min. Then, the supernatant was dialyzed against distilled water using a dialysis tube (MWCO 1000) to remove impurities and unreacted FA. The dialyzed reaction product was freeze-dried for further use. Folate-conjugated P(HEA-AMS) and folate–conjugated P(HEA-BMA) were abbreviated to F-P(HEA-AMS) and F-P(HEA-BMA), respectively.

3.4. ^{1}H NMR Spectroscopy

Residual solvent and water were removed by incubating copolymers with P_2O_5 in a vacuum incubator at 45 °C. Each of the dry copolymers was dissolved in D_2O and the copolymer solution was put in a 10 mm NMR tube and sealed with a cap. The ^{1}H NMR spectrum was obtained by scanning the copolymer solution on a NMR spectrophotometer (400 MHz, JNM-ECZ400S/L1, JEOL, Tokyo, Japan. installed in the Central Laboratory of Kangwon National University).

3.5. Treatment of Copolymers with H_2O_2

Each of copolymers (i.e., P(HEA-AMS) and P(HEA-BMA)) was dissolved in H_2O_2 solution (1% (v/v), in distilled water), the solutions were kept at room temperature (24 °C) for 10 min to oxidize the copolymers, and they were freeze-dried for further use. A copolymer treated with H_2O_2 solution was designated as H_2O_2 "copolymer name".

3.6. Examination of Oxidation of Copolymers by XPS

The binding energy spectrum of P(HEA-AMS) and H_2O_2-P(HEA-AMS) were obtained by X-ray photoelectron spectroscopy (XPS, K Alpha+, Thermo Scientific, Basingstoke, UK) using a 180° double focusing hemispherical analyzer with 128-channel position sensitive detector. The reference value used to determine the binding energy of atomic electrons was the observed binding energy of C 1 s (284.8 eV). The copolymers were exposed to an achromatic Al K-alpha (1286.6 eV) X-ray source with the power of 72 W and the spectrophotometer was operated at room temperature (20–23 °C) and at a pressure of less than 5×10^{-8} mbar.

3.7. Measurement of Interfacial Tension

The interfacial activity of H_2O_2-untreated and treated copolymers (i.e., P(HEA-AMS), H_2O_2-(HEA-AMS), P(HEA-BMA), and H_2O_2-P(HEA-BMA)) were examined by measuring the air/water interfacial tension of the copolymer solutions. Each of the copolymer solutions whose concentration was 0.01 mg/mL to 1.0 mg/mL was prepared by the continuous two times dilution of an aqueous copolymer solution (1.0 mg/mL). The interfacial tension was measured by a ring method on a tensiometer (DST 60, SEO, Suwon, Gyeonggi-do, Korea).

3.8. Preparation of DOPE Liposomes Stabilized with Copolymers

DOPE liposomes stabilized with F-P(HEA-BMA) and F-P(HEA-AMS) were prepared by a sonication and detergent removal method. The dry thin film of DOPE was prepared by removing the organic solvent from 2 mL of DOPE solution (10 mg/mL, in chloroform) contained in a 25 mL round bottom flask connected to a rotary evaporator operating at 150 rpm under reduced pressure. Variable amounts (0.02 mL, 0.04 mL, and 0.08 mL) of copolymer solution (5 mg/mL, in PB (10 mM, pH 7.4)), 0.09 mL of DOC solution (2% (w/v), in the same buffer solution), and 1 mL of calcein solution (100 mM, in the same buffer solution) were mixed in a 10 mL vial and the volume of the mixture solutions was made up to 2 mL by adding the buffer solution. When DOX-loaded liposomes were prepared, doxorubicin (DOX) solution (1 mL, 0.2% (w/v) in PBS (10 mM, pH 7.4)) was used instead of the calcein solution. In the mixture solutions, the concentration of copolymer was 0.05 mg/mL, 0.1 mg/mL or 0.2 mg/mL, and the concentration of DOC, calcein, and DOX were 0.09% (w/v), 50 mM, and 0.1%, respectively. 2 mL each of the mixture solutions was put in the round bottom flask containing dry DOPE film deposited on its inside wall and it was whirled by a hand to suspend the phospholipid in the mixture solution. The DOPE suspension was sonicated in a bath type of sonicator (VC 505, Sonic & Materials, Newtown, CT, USA) at room temperature for 20 min (pulse-on for 10 s and pulse-off for 10 s). DOPE liposomes containing calcein (or DOX) and copolymer were separated from unentrapped calcein (or DOX) and DOC by gel permeation chromatography using a Sephadex G-100 column. Liposome prepared from the mixture whose DOPE to copolymer mass ratio was x/y was termed as liposome/copolymer name (x/y) and the liposome containing DOX as liposome/copolymer name (x/y)/DOX.

3.9. Characterization of DOPE Liposomes Stabilized with Copolymers

The structure of DOPE liposomes stabilized with copolymers was investigated by transmission electron microscopy. In order to visualize the bilayer and the lamellar structure, the liposomes were negatively stained [42–44]. 100 µL of the liposome suspension was mixed with the same amount of phosphotungstic acid solution (2% (w/v)) and the mixture was stood at room temperature for 3 h for the staining of the liposomes. An aliquot amount of the stained liposome suspension was put on a formvar/copper-coated grid and it was dried overnight at room temperature. The replica was subjected to microscopy using a transmission electron microscope (TEM; LEO-912AB OMEGA, LEO, Germany; located in the Korea Basic Science Institute (KBSI), Kangwon, Chuncheon, Korea).

The fluorescence quenching of calcein enveloped in the liposome was determined using an Equation (1):

$$\text{Quenching (\%)} = (F_t - F_i) \div F_t \times 100 \quad (1)$$

where F_t is the fluorescence intensity after the liposomes were completely solubilized by Triton X-100 and F_i is the fluorescence intensity before solubilized [45,46]. The fluorescence intensity was measured at 514 nm with being excited at 495 nm using a fluorescence spectrophotometer (Hitachi F2500, Hitachi, Japan). The specific loading of DOX loaded in liposomes was determined as follows. DOX-loaded liposomes suspended in PBS (10 mM, pH 7.4) were solubilized using Triton X-100 and the fluorescence intensity of DOX in the solution was measured at 560 nm with being excited at 470 nm on a fluorescence spectrophotometer (Hitachi F2500, Hitachi, Japan). The amount of DOX was determined by reading the fluorescence intensity-corresponding concentration on a calibration curve. The calibration curve was set up by plotting the fluorescence intensity of DOX solutions (0–0.002 mg/mL, in PBS buffer (10 mM, pH 7.4)) versus the concentration. The specific loading % was calculated as the percent of the mass of DOX based on the mass of phospholipid. Dynamic light scattering method was used to measure the mean hydrodynamic diameter of DOPE liposomes stabilized with copolymers. The liposome suspensions were diluted with PB (10 mM, pH 7.4) to render the light scattering intensity to be 50–200 kcps, and the mean diameter was determined using a dynamic light scattering equipment (ZetaPlus 90, Brookhaven Instrument Co., Holtsville, NY, USA).

3.10. Observation of Oxidation-Sensitive Release

H_2O_2 (30%, v/v) was mixed with PB (10 mM, pH 7.4) so that the concentration was 0% (v/v), 0.5% (v/v), 1.0% (v/v), and 2.0% (v/v). 0.1 mL of liposome suspension was injected to 1.9 mL of H_2O_2 solution contained in a glass cuvette placed in the cuvette hold of a fluorescence spectrophotometer (Hitachi F2500, Hitachi, Japan). The fluorescence intensity was measured with time for 60 s. The excitation wavelength and emission one were 495 nm and 514 nm, respectively. The release % was calculated using the following Equation (2) [47,48]:

$$\text{Release \%} = (F_t - F_i) \div (F_f - F_i) \times 100 \quad (2)$$

where F_i was the initial fluorescence intensity of the liposome suspension, F_f was the fluorescence intensity after the liposomes were completely solubilized by Triton X100, and F_t was the fluorescence intensity of the liposome suspension at a given time.

3.11. Observation of Interaction of Liposomes and Cancer Cell and Tumor Cell

KB cell and LN229 cell suspension (1 mL) were seeded in a 12-well plate (3×10^4 cells/well) and cultured in a CO_2 incubator at 37 °C for 24 h. The culture medium was decanted off, cells were washed with PBS (10 mM, pH 7.4), FBS-free RPMI 1640 culture medium (0.1 mL) and an equi-volumetric amount of each of test samples (free DOX solution, liposome/P(HEA-BMA)(100/1)/DOX suspension, liposome/F-P(HEA-BMA)(100/1)/DOX suspension, liposome/P(HEA-AMS)(100/1)/DOX suspension, and liposome/F-P(HEA-AMS)(100/1)/DOX suspension) was added to wells, and they were incubated for 5 h. Free DOX and unbound liposome were washed off by rinsing the cells with the buffer solution after the culture medium was removed. The cells were detached and harvested from the well wall by adding trypsin/EDTA solution to the wells. The cell suspensions were contained in Eppendorf tubes, they were centrifuged, and the supernatant was removed. After re-suspended in 500 µL of PBS (10 mM, pH 7.4) of 4 °C, the fluorescence intensity distribution of the cells was obtained using a flow cytometer (FACS, FACS Calibur, Becton Dickinson, Franklin Lakes, NJ, USA, in the Central Laboratory Center of Kangwon National University). The excitation and the emission wave length used to measure the fluorescence intensity were 470 and 560 nm, respectively. The interaction of DOX-loaded liposomes with the cancer cell and the tumor cell was also investigated by confocal laser scanning microscopy (CLSM). The cell culture condition in FACS study was used in CLSM study too. The cells treated with free DOX and DOX-loaded liposomes were treated with 200 µL of formaldehyde solution (2.5% (v/v)) for their structural fixation. After the cells were rinsed with PBS (10 mM, pH 7.4), the nuclei of cells were dyed using DAPI, free dye was removed by washing the cells with the buffer solution, and the CLSM micrographs were taken on a confocal laser scanning microscope (LSM 880 with Airyscan, Carl Zeiss, Oberkochen, Germany; installed in the Central Laboratory of Kangwon National University).

3.12. Observation of In Vitro Anti-Cancer Efficacy

The DOX concentration of liposome suspensions was adjusted to 5, 10, 20, and 40 μg/mL by diluting the suspensions with PBS (10 mM, pH 7.4). DOX-free liposomes suspensions (i.e., liposome/F-P(HEA-BMA)(100/1) and liposome/F-P(HEA-AMS)(100/1)) were used as positive controls. The liposome content of the control suspensions was made to be the same as that of the DOX-loaded liposome suspensions. DOX solution (in PBS (10 mM. pH 7.4)) was used as an additional positive control and PBS (10 mM, pH 7.4) as a negative control. Each well of a 96-well plate was seeded with 200 μL of cell (1×10^4 cells/mL) and cultured at 37 °C for 24 h in a CO2 incubator. After the culture medium was taken off, RPMI free of FBS (180 μL) and each test sample (20 μL, DOX-loaded liposome suspensions, empty liposome suspensions, DOX solution, and blank PBS (10 mM, pH 7.4)) were put to each well, and incubated for 24 h in a CO_2 incubator thermostated at 37 °C. The culture medium was taken off, the residual was washed off from the cell by rinsing them with PBS (10 mM, pH 7.4)), MTT reagent (20 μL, 5 mg/mL) was put to each well, and stored at the incubator for 4 h to induce the production of formazan. The supernatant was decanted off and formazan was dissolved out by adding DMSO (200 μL) to each well. The optical density of formazan solution was measured at 540 nm on a microplate reader (N10588, Thermo Fisher Scientific, Waltham, MA, USA). The percent of the optical density of formazan obtained from cells treated with a test sample or a control with respect to the optical density of formazan obtained from cells treated with the empty buffer solution was represented as cell viability.

4. Conclusions

Novel oxidation-sensitive liposomes were developed by stabilizing DOPE bilayers with F-P(HEA-AMS) and oxidation-insensitive liposomes were prepared as controls using F-P(HEA-BMA). According to the air/water interfacial tension measurement, the copolymers were surface-active and lost its surface-activity upon oxidation. Regardless of DOPE to copolymer mass ratio (200:1, 100:1, and 50:1), the release degree in 60 s of calcein enveloped in DOPE liposomes stabilized with F-P(HEA-BMA) slightly increased from a few to several % when H_2O_2 concentration increased from 0–2%. Meanwhile, the oxidizing agent concentration had a great effect on the release degree of dye enveloped in DOPE liposomes stabilized with F-P(HEA-AMS). The hydrophobic anchor (i.e., methylene methyl sulfide group) of the copolymer was likely to be oxidized to become hydrophilic and it would be desorbed from DOPE bilayers, leading to the disintegration of the liposomes. According to the results of FACS and CLSM study, the transport of DOX to cancer cell and tumor cell was markedly enhanced by liposomes stabilized with folate-conjugated copolymers (i.e., F-P(HEA-BMA) and F-P(HEA-AMS)), possibly because the liposomes were readily translocated into the cancer cell and the tumor cell via receptor-mediated endocytosis. The feasibility of the cellular uptake of liposomes with F-P(HEA-BMA) seemed to be almost the same as that of liposomes with F-P(HEA-AMS). However, the latter liposomes promoted the in vitro anti-cancer efficacy of DOX much more effectively than the former ones. This was possibly because liposomes with F-P(HEA-AMS) could release their payload sensitively in an oxidative condition.

Supplementary Materials: The following are available online at http://www.mdpi.com/2072-6694/12/12/180/s1, Figure S1: H_2O_2 concentration-dependent release profiles of calcein.

Author Contributions: Conceptualization, D.Y.Y.; Data curation, J.A.K.; Formal analysis, J.A.K.; Funding acquisition, J.-C.K.; Investigation, J.A.K. and D.Y.Y.; Project administration, J.-C.K.; Resources, J.-C.K.; Software, J.A.K. and D.Y.Y.; Validation, D.Y.Y. and J.-C.K.; Visualization, J.A.K.; Writing–original draft, J.-C.K.; Writing–review & editing, J.-C.K. All authors have read and agreed to the published version of the manuscript.

Funding: This research was supported by the Basic Science Research Program through the National Research Foundation of Korea (NRF) funded by the Ministry of Education (NRF-2018R1D1A1B07043439) and Basic Science Research Program through the National Research Foundation of Korea (NRF) funded by the Ministry of Education (No. 2018R1A6A1A03025582).

Conflicts of Interest: The authors declare no conflict of interest.

References

1. Marsh, D. Thermodynamics of phospholipid self-assembly. *Biophys. J.* **2012**, *102*, 1079–1087. [CrossRef] [PubMed]
2. Alexandridis, P.; Lindman, B. *Amphiphilic Block Copolymers: Self-Assembly and Applications*; Elsevier: Amsterdam, The Netherlands, 2000.
3. Ng, C.C.; Cheng, Y.-L.; Pennefather, P.S. Properties of a self-assembled phospholipid membrane supported on lipobeads. *Biophys. J.* **2004**, *87*, 323–331. [CrossRef] [PubMed]
4. Noguchi, H.; Takasu, M. Self-assembly of amphiphiles into vesicles: A Brownian dynamics simulation. *Phys. Rev. E* **2001**, *64*, 041913. [CrossRef] [PubMed]
5. Li, J.; Wang, X.; Zhang, T.; Wang, C.; Huang, Z.; Luo, X.; Deng, Y. A review on phospholipids and their main applications in drug delivery systems. *Asian J. Pharm. Sci.* **2015**, *10*, 81–98. [CrossRef]
6. Kumar, V. Complementary molecular shapes and additivity of the packing parameter of lipids. *Proc. Natl. Acad. Sci. USA* **1991**, *88*, 444–448. [CrossRef]
7. Ho, R.J.; Rouse, B.T.; Huang, L. Target-sensitive immunoliposomes: Preparation and characterization. *Biochemistry* **1986**, *25*, 5500–5506. [CrossRef]
8. Sudimack, J.J.; Guo, W.; Tjarks, W.; Lee, R.J. A novel pH-sensitive liposome formulation containing oleyl alcohol. *Biochim. Biophys. Acta (BBA) Biomembr.* **2002**, *1564*, 31–37. [CrossRef]
9. Kim, J.-C.; Bae, S.K.; Kim, J.-D. Temperature-sensitivity of liposomal lipid bilayers mixed with poly (N-isopropylacrylamide-co-acrylic acid). *J. Biochem.* **1997**, *121*, 15–19. [CrossRef]
10. Kim, J.-C.; Kim, M.-S.; Kim, J.-D. Temperature-Sensitive releases from liposomes containing hydrophobically modified poly (N-isopropylacrylamide). *Korean J. Chem. Eng.* **1999**, *16*, 28–33. [CrossRef]
11. Chu, C.-J.; Dijkstra, J.; Lai, M.-Z.; Hong, K.; Szoka, F.C. Efficiency of cytoplasmic delivery by pH-sensitive liposomes to cells in culture. *Pharm. Res.* **1990**, *7*, 824–834. [CrossRef]
12. Ellens, H.; Bentz, J.; Szoka, F.C. pH-induced destabilization of phosphatidylethanolamine-containing liposomes: Role of bilayer contact. *Biochemistry* **1984**, *23*, 1532–1538. [CrossRef] [PubMed]
13. Lai, M.Z.; Vail, W.J.; Szoka, F.C. Acid-and calcium-induced structural changes in phosphatidylethanolamine membranes stabilized by cholesteryl hemisuccinate. *Biochemistry* **1985**, *24*, 1654–1661. [CrossRef]
14. Lee, E.-O.; Kim, J.-G.; Kim, J.-D. Induction of vesicle-to-micelle transition by bile salts for DOPE vesicles incorporating immunoglobulin G. *J. Biochem.* **1992**, *112*, 671–676. [CrossRef] [PubMed]
15. Jo, S.-M.; Lee, H.Y.; Kim, J.-C. Glucose-sensitive liposomes incorporating hydrophobically modified glucose oxidase. *Lipids* **2008**, *43*, 937–943. [CrossRef] [PubMed]
16. Goodman, J.; Hochstein, P. Generation of free radicals and lipid peroxidation by redox cycling of adriamycin and daunomycin. *Biochem. Biophys. Res. Commun.* **1977**, *77*, 797–803. [CrossRef]
17. Bąk, A.; Podgórska, W. Interfacial and surface tensions of toluene/water and air/water systems with nonionic surfactants Tween 20 and Tween 80. *Colloids Surf. A Physicochem. Eng. Asp.* **2016**, *504*, 414–425. [CrossRef]
18. Schick, M. Surface films of nonionic detergents—I. Surface tension study. *J. Colloid Sci.* **1962**, *17*, 801–813. [CrossRef]
19. Shinoda, K.; Nakagawa, T.; Tamamushi, B.-I. *Colloidal Surfactants: Some Physicochemical Properties*; Elsevier: Amsterdam, The Netherlands, 2016; Volume 12.
20. Patist, A.; Bhagwat, S.; Penfield, K.; Aikens, P.; Shah, D. On the measurement of critical micelle concentrations of pure and technical-grade nonionic surfactants. *J. Surfactants Deterg.* **2000**, *3*, 53–58. [CrossRef]
21. Johnsson, M.; Edwards, K. Phase behavior and aggregate structure in mixtures of dioleoylphosphatidylethanolamine and poly (ethylene glycol)-lipids. *Biophys. J.* **2001**, *80*, 313–323. [CrossRef]
22. Cullis, P.t.; Kruijff, B.d. Lipid polymorphism and the functional roles of lipids in biological membranes. *Biochimica Biophysica Acta (BBA) Rev. Biomembr.* **1979**, *559*, 399–420. [CrossRef]
23. Kono, K.; Zenitani, K.-I.; Takagishi, T. Novel pH-sensitive liposomes: Liposomes bearing a poly (ethylene glycol) derivative with carboxyl groups. *Biochim. Biophys. Acta (BBA) Biomembr.* **1994**, *1193*, 1–9. [CrossRef]
24. Ishida, T.; Kirchmeier, M.; Moase, E.; Zalipsky, S.; Allen, T. Targeted delivery and triggered release of liposomal doxorubicin enhances cytotoxicity against human B lymphoma cells. *Biochim. Biophys. Acta (BBA) Biomembr.* **2001**, *1515*, 144–158. [CrossRef]

25. Karavas, E.; Georgarakis, E.; Sigalas, M.P.; Avgoustakis, K.; Bikiaris, D. Investigation of the release mechanism of a sparingly water-soluble drug from solid dispersions in hydrophilic carriers based on physical state of drug, particle size distribution and drug–polymer interactions. *Eur. J. Pharm. Biopharm.* **2007**, *66*, 334–347. [CrossRef] [PubMed]
26. Ghadiri, M.; Fatemi, S.; Vatanara, A.; Doroud, D.; Najafabadi, A.R.; Darabi, M.; Rahimi, A.A. Loading hydrophilic drug in solid lipid media as nanoparticles: Statistical modeling of entrapment efficiency and particle size. *Int. J. Pharm.* **2012**, *424*, 128–137. [CrossRef]
27. Khandelia, H.; Mouritsen, O.G. Lipid gymnastics: Evidence of complete acyl chain reversal in oxidized phospholipids from molecular simulations. *Biophys. J.* **2009**, *96*, 2734–2743. [CrossRef]
28. Fruhwirth, G.O.; Loidl, A.; Hermetter, A. Oxidized phospholipids: From molecular properties to disease. *Biochim. Biophys. Acta (BBA) Mol. Basis Dis.* **2007**, *1772*, 718–736. [CrossRef]
29. Trost, B.M.; Curran, D.P. Chemoselective oxidation of sulfides to sulfones with potassium hydrogen persulfate. *Tetrahedron Lett.* **1981**, *22*, 1287–1290. [CrossRef]
30. Sato, K.; Hyodo, M.; Aoki, M.; Zheng, X.-Q.; Noyori, R. Oxidation of sulfides to sulfoxides and sulfones with 30% hydrogen peroxide under organic solvent-and halogen-free conditions. *Tetrahedron* **2001**, *57*, 2469–2476. [CrossRef]
31. Lee, K.D.; Nir, S.; Papahadjopoulos, D. Quantitative analysis of liposome-cell interactions in vitro: Rate constants of binding and endocytosis with suspension and adherent J774 cells and human monocytes. *Biochemistry* **1993**, *32*, 889–899. [CrossRef]
32. Cheng, L.; Huang, F.-Z.; Cheng, L.-F.; Zhu, Y.-Q.; Hu, Q.; Li, L.; Wei, L.; Chen, D.-W. GE11-modified liposomes for non-small cell lung cancer targeting: Preparation, ex vitro and in vivo evaluation. *Int. J. Nanomed.* **2014**, *9*, 921. [CrossRef]
33. Fernández, M.; Javaid, F.; Chudasama, V. Advances in targeting the folate receptor in the treatment/imaging of cancers. *Chem. Sci.* **2018**, *9*, 790–810. [CrossRef] [PubMed]
34. Lee, R.J.; Low, P.S. Folate-mediated tumor cell targeting of liposome-entrapped doxorubicin in vitro. *Biochimica Biophysica Acta (BBA) Biomembr.* **1995**, *1233*, 134–144. [CrossRef]
35. Siwowska, K.; Schmid, R.; Cohrs, S.; Schibli, R.; Müller, C. Folate receptor-positive gynecological cancer cells: In vitro and in vivo characterization. *Pharmaceuticals* **2017**, *10*, 72. [CrossRef] [PubMed]
36. Peters, T.; Grunewald, C.; Blaickner, M.; Ziegner, M.; Schütz, C.; Iffland, D.; Langguth, P. Cellular uptake and in vitro antitumor efficacy of composite liposomes for neutron capture therapy. *Radiat. Oncol.* **2015**, *10*, 52. [CrossRef] [PubMed]
37. Yang, H.; Villani, R.M.; Wang, H.; Simpson, M.J.; Roberts, M.S.; Tang, M.; Liang, X. The role of cellular reactive oxygen species in cancer chemotherapy. *J. Exp. Clin. Cancer Res.* **2018**, *37*, 266. [CrossRef] [PubMed]
38. Liou, G.-Y.; Storz, P. Reactive oxygen species in cancer. *Free. Radic. Res.* **2010**, *44*, 479–496. [CrossRef]
39. Kim, S.-Y.; Kim, S.-J.; Kim, B.-J.; Rah, S.-Y.; Chung, S.M.; Im, M.-J.; Kim, U.-H. Doxorubicin-induced reactive oxygen species generation and intracellular Ca2+ increase are reciprocally modulated in rat cardiomyocytes. *Exp. Mol. Med.* **2006**, *38*, 535. [CrossRef]
40. Asensio-López, M.C.; Soler, F.; Pascual-Figal, D.; Fernández-Belda, F.; Lax, A. Doxorubicin-induced oxidative stress: The protective effect of nicorandil on HL-1 cardiomyocytes. *PLoS ONE* **2017**, *12*, e0172803. [CrossRef]
41. Myers, C.E.; McGuire, W.P.; Liss, R.H.; Ifrim, I.; Grotzinger, K.; Young, R.C. Adriamycin: The role of lipid peroxidation in cardiac toxicity and tumor response. *Science* **1977**, *197*, 165–167. [CrossRef]
42. White, J.; Helenius, A. pH-dependent fusion between the Semliki Forest virus membrane and liposomes. *Proc. Natl. Acad. Sci. USA* **1980**, *77*, 3273–3277. [CrossRef]
43. Bangham, A.D.; Horne, R. Negative staining of phospholipids and their structural modification by surface-active agents as observed in the electron microscope. *J. Mol. Boil.* **1964**, *8*, 660–668. [CrossRef]
44. Yashroy, R. Lamellar dispersion and phase separation of chloroplast membrane lipids by negative staining electron microscopy. *J. Biosci.* **1990**, *15*, 93–98. [CrossRef]
45. Were, L.M.; Bruce, B.D.; Davidson, P.M.; Weiss, J. Size, stability, and entrapment efficiency of phospholipid nanocapsules containing polypeptide antimicrobials. *J. Agric. Food Chem.* **2003**, *51*, 8073–8079. [CrossRef] [PubMed]
46. Anabousi, S.; Kleemann, E.; Bakowsky, U.; Kissel, T.; Schmehl, T.; Gessler, T.; Seeger, W.; Lehr, C.-M.; Ehrhardt, C. Effect of PEGylation on the stability of liposomes during nebulisation and in lung surfactant. *J. Nanosci. Nanotechnol.* **2006**, *6*, 3010–3016. [CrossRef]

47. Hong, Y.J.; Kim, J.-C. pH-and calcium ion-dependent release from egg phosphatidylcholine liposomes incorporating hydrophobically modified alginate. *J. Nanosci. Nanotechnol.* **2010**, *10*, 8380–8386. [CrossRef]
48. Jo, S.-M.; Xia, Y.; Lee, H.Y.; Kim, Y.C.; Kim, J.-C. Liposomes incorporating hydrophobically modified glucose oxidase. *Korean J. Chem. Eng.* **2008**, *25*, 1221–1225. [CrossRef]

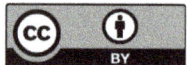

© 2020 by the authors. Licensee MDPI, Basel, Switzerland. This article is an open access article distributed under the terms and conditions of the Creative Commons Attribution (CC BY) license (http://creativecommons.org/licenses/by/4.0/).

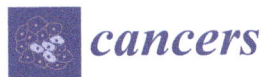

Article

Improvement in the Anti-Tumor Efficacy of Doxorubicin Nanosponges in In Vitro and in Mice Bearing Breast Tumor Models

Monica Argenziano [1], Casimiro Luca Gigliotti [2], Nausicaa Clemente [2], Elena Boggio [2], Benedetta Ferrara [1], Francesco Trotta [3], Stefania Pizzimenti [4], Giuseppina Barrera [4], Renzo Boldorini [2], Federica Bessone [1], Umberto Dianzani [2], Roberta Cavalli [1,*] and Chiara Dianzani [1]

[1] Dipartimento di Scienza e Tecnologia del Farmaco, University of Torino, 10125 Torino, Italy; monica.argenziano@unito.it (M.A.); benedetta.ferrara@unito.it (B.F.); f.bessone@unito.it (F.B.); chiara.dianzani@unito.it (C.D.)
[2] Department of Health Sciences and Interdisciplinary Research Center of Autoimmune Diseases (IRCAD), University of Eastern Piedmont (UPO), 28100 Novara, Italy; luca.gigliotti@med.uniupo.it (C.L.G.); nausicaa.clemente@med.uniupo.it (N.C.); elena.boggio@med.uniupo.it (E.B.); renzo.boldorini@med.uniupo.it (R.B.); umberto.dianzani@med.uniupo.it (U.D.)
[3] Department of Chemistry, University of Torino, 10125 Torino, Italy; francesco.trotta@unito.it
[4] Department of Clinical and Biological Sciences, University of Turin, 10125 Torino, Italy; stefania.pizzimenti@unito.it (S.P.); giuseppina.barrera@unito.it (G.B.)
* Correspondence: roberta.cavalli@unito.it; Tel.: +39-0116707190; Fax: +39-0116707162

Received: 19 December 2019; Accepted: 8 January 2020; Published: 9 January 2020

Abstract: Doxorubicin (DOX) is an anthracycline widely used in cancer therapy and in particular in breast cancer treatment. The treatment with DOX appears successful, but it is limited by a severe cardiotoxicity. This work evaluated the in vitro and in vivo anticancer effect of a new formulation of β-cyclodextrin nanosponges containing DOX (BNS-DOX). The BNS-DOX effectiveness was evaluated in human and mouse breast cancer cell lines in vitro in terms of effect on cell growth, cell cycle distribution, and apoptosis induction; and in vivo in BALB-neuT mice developing spontaneous breast cancer in terms of biodistribution, cancer growth inhibition, and heart toxicity. BNS-DOX significantly inhibited cancer cell proliferation, through the induction of apoptosis, with higher efficiency than free DOX. The breast cancer growth in BALB-neuT mice was inhibited by 60% by a BNS-DOX dose five times lower than the DOX therapeutic dose, with substantial reduction of tumor neoangiogenesis and lymphangiogenesis. Biodistribution after BNS-DOX treatment revealed a high accumulation of DOX in the tumor site and a low accumulation in the hearts of mice. Results indicated that use of BNS may be an efficient strategy to deliver DOX in the treatment of breast cancer, since it improves the anti-cancer effectiveness and reduces cardiotoxicity.

Keywords: β-cyclodextrin nanosponges; doxorubicin; breast cancer; BALB-neuT mice; EPR effect

---

1. Introduction

Doxorubicin (DOX) is one of the most effective anticancer drugs used against solid tumors of diverse origins and in particular against breast cancer. However, its use is associated with severe adverse effects including cardiotoxicity, myelosuppression and palmar plantar erythrodysenthesia, which impose a narrow therapeutic dose limiting DOX effectiveness [1]. Moreover, cancer cells frequently become resistant to DOX treatment and some conditions of the tumor microenvironment-such as hypoxia, acidity, defective vasculature, and lymphatic vessels-limit the DOX anticancer effectiveness [2].

Hence, there is necessity for an effective approach that limits DOX side effects by reducing DOX doses and modifying its bio-distribution to favor its concentration into the tumor site. To this aim, we evaluated the possibility of incorporating DOX into nanoparticles capable of favoring accumulation of the drug into the tumor site. In recent years, the development of nano-delivery systems for anticancer agents, with dimensions of less than 1000 nm have been found to be acceptable for intravenous administration, and have improved the therapeutic effectiveness of several compounds. Compared to conventional carriers, they report several advantages, such as capacity to solubilize hydrophobic drugs, reduction of total drug dose, and prevention of side effects [3]. When infused in the bloodstream, nanoparticles can accumulate in tumors owing to the enhanced permeability and retention (EPR) effect since the immature vasculature of tumors display fenestrations smaller than 200 nm, allowing for extravasation and entrapment of nanoparticles from the blood into the tumor tissue [4]. Recent studies showed that DOX and mitomycin C, co-loaded in polymer–lipid hybrid nanoparticles, inhibited the growth of sensitive and multidrug resistant human mammary tumor xenografts [2].

Many cyclodextrin (CD) derivatives have been proposed for drug delivery, and they have been shown to improve bioavailability, aqueous solubility, and stability of hosted drugs [5–8]. β-cyclodextrin nanosponges (BNS) are hyper-cross-linked polymers with CD units as the building blocks of the system and are a biocompatible and suitable nanosystem to carry drugs [9–11]. Different anticancer drugs-such as paclitaxel, camptothecin, and tamoxifen-have been efficiently incorporated in nanosponges, showing an improved antitumor effect [12]. In this study, DOX was loaded in β-cyclodextrin based nanosponges (BNS-DOX), and the effect of DOX and BNS-DOX was compared in vitro in human and mouse breast cancer cell lines, either sensitive or resistant to DOX, and in vivo in the growth of spontaneous mammary cancer in BALB-neuT mice, which mimics some of the most critical features of the human disease and represents a real model of human epidermal growth factor receptor 2 (HER2) positive breast cancer [13]. Results indicated that use of BNS may be an efficient strategy to deliver DOX in the treatment of breast cancer, since it improves the anti-cancer efficacy and reduces cardiotoxicity.

2. Results

The in vitro and in vivo results are listed below. Table 1 reports the physico-chemical characteristics of blank BNS and BNS loaded with DOX. BNS nanoformulations with an average diameter of about 300 nm and negative surface charge were obtained. Both the BNS nanoformulations displayed similar sizes. Doxorubicin was incorporated in the nanosponge nanostructure in a good extent. Indeed, the loading capacity and encapsulation efficiency of BNS-DOX were 16.4% and 98.5%, respectively. Notably, the drug loading did not affect the physico-chemical parameters of BNS and the physical stability of the nanosuspensions. The physical stability of BNS-DOX stored at 4 °C was confirmed up to 1 month.

Table 1. Physico-chemical characteristics of blank and doxorubicin (DOX)-loaded β-cyclodextrin nanosponges (BNS).

Formulation	Average Diameter ± SD (nm)	Polydispersity Index	Zeta Potential ± SD (mV)
Blank BNS	302.5 ± 4.6	0.20 ± 0.01	−35.2 ± 2.7
BNS-DOX	310.4 ± 5.7	0.21 ± 0.01	−29.8 ± 1.3

The spherical morphology of BNS-DOX and their nanometric sizes were shown by Transmission electron microscopy (TEM) analysis (Figure 1A).

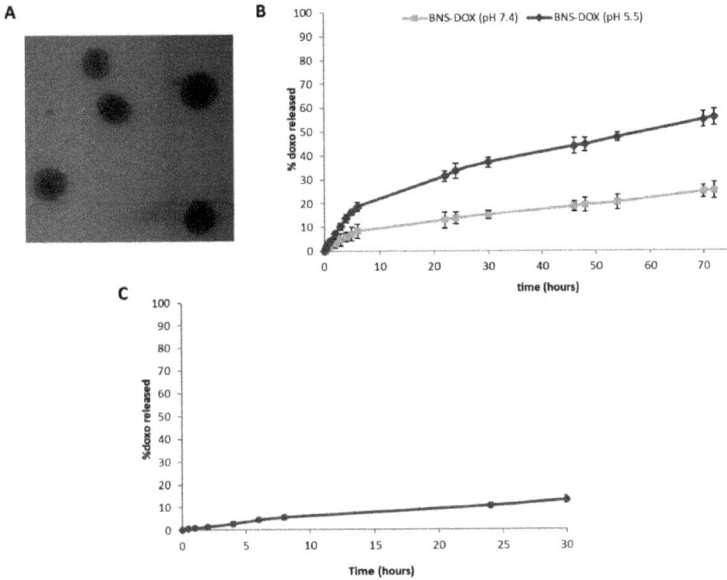

Figure 1. Characterization of β-cyclodextrin nanosponges containing doxorubicin (BNS-DOX). (**A**) Transmission electron microscopy image of BNS-DOX (scale bar 150 nm). (**B**) In vitro release kinetics of DOX from BNS-DOX at the two different pH levels (5.5 and 7.4). (**C**) In vitro release kinetics of DOX from BNS-DOX in rat plasma at 37 °C.

DOX was released from BNS-DOX with a prolonged release kinetics, without initial burst effect (Figure 1B). This in vitro release profile confirmed the DOX incorporation in BNS polymeric matrix. The percentage of DOX released was higher at acidic pH values. Indeed, it increased about 2.5 fold at pH 5.5 compared to that at pH 7.4 (Figure 1B). The slow and prolonged in vitro release profile of DOX from BNS-DOX was observed also in plasma and it was comparable to that of the one obtained in phosphate buffered saline (PBS) at pH 7.4 (Figure 1C). After 24 h, the percentage of DOX released from the BNS was 10.5% and 13% in plasma and in buffer (pH 7.4), respectively.

No changes in the BNS physico-chemical parameters and no aggregation phenomena were observed after incubation in plasma at 37 °C for 24 h, confirming the BNS-DOX stability.

In order to determine the BNS-DOX effect in tumor cell growth, (3-(4,5-Dimethylthiazol-2-yl)-2,5diphenyltetrazolium bromide (MTT) analysis was performed in breast tumor cells lines, which were human MDA-MB231 and MCF-7 cells (both DOX-sensitive), and mouse 4T1 (DOX-sensitive) and EMT6/AR10r (DOX-resistant) cells. MDA-MB231, 4T1, and EMT6/AR10r were chosen as models of triple negative tumors (TNBC)-i.e., negative for estrogen receptor (ER), progesterone receptor (PR), and HER2-while MCF-7 was chosen as a model of ER/PR positive tumors.

To assess the effect on cell viability, cells were cultured in the presence and absence of titrated concentrations (10^{-5}–10^{-9} M) of DOX or BNS-DOX and the MTT assay was performed after 72 h. Results showed that BNS-DOX inhibited cell viability in a concentration-dependent manner in all cell lines with higher efficacy than DOX (Figure 2).

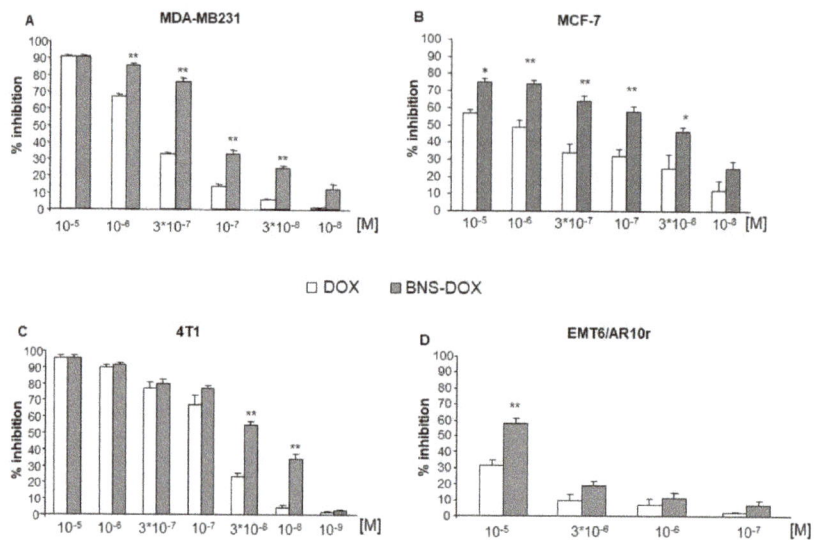

Figure 2. Percentage of cell survival following DOX and BNS-DOX treatment. (**A**,**B**) MDA-MB231 and MCF-7 human breast cancer cell lines and (**C**,**D**) 4T1 and EMR6/AR10r mouse breast cancer cell lines were treated with increasing concentrations of the drugs for 72 h. Results are expressed as % of viability inhibition of control shown as mean ± SEM ($n = 5$). Eight replicate wells were used to determine each data point, and five different experiments were performed. * $p < 0.05$, ** $p < 0.01$, significantly different from the same concentration of DOX.

In particular, EMT6/AR10r cells were quite resistant to both drug formulations and only the highest dose of BNS-DOX (10^{-5} M) substantially inhibited the cell growth. The empty BNS did not show any level of toxicity, even at high concentrations. Table 2 reports the half maximal inhibitory concentration (IC_{50}) obtained from these experiments and shows that BNS-DOX displays lower IC_{50} than DOX in all cell lines.

Table 2. Half maximal inhibitory concentration (IC_{50}) of BNS-DOX and DOX.

Cell Line	IC_{50} BNS-DOX	IC_{50} DOX	p-Value
MDA-MB231	$1.6 \pm 0.2 \times 10^{-7}$	$5 \pm 0.2 \times 10^{-7}$	0.001
4T1	$2.8 \pm 0.2 \times 10^{-8}$	$8.64 \pm 0.8 \times 10^{-8}$	0.0021
EMT6/AR10r	$5.3 \pm 0.67 \times 10^{-6}$	$29 \pm 0.9 \times 10^{-5}$	0.0045
MCF-7	$1.5 \pm 0.5 \times 10^{-8}$	$15 \pm 0.9 \times 10^{-7}$	0.001

Two-tailed p-value has been determined with unpaired t-test with Welch correction.

Results show that the inhibitory effect was exerted by BNS-DOX at a concentration always lower (3–10 times lower) than free DOX. Since a main limitation of DOX is its cardiotoxicity, we performed the same experiments on rat cardiomyocyte H9c2 cells, but results showed that BNS-DOX and DOX did not display a substantial difference in inhibiting cell viability of these cells.

In order to assess whether the effects on the cell viability are related to inhibition of cell cycle progression, a cell cycle analysis was performed after 72 h of culture in the presence and absence of titrated amounts of DOX or BNS-DOX (Figure 3).

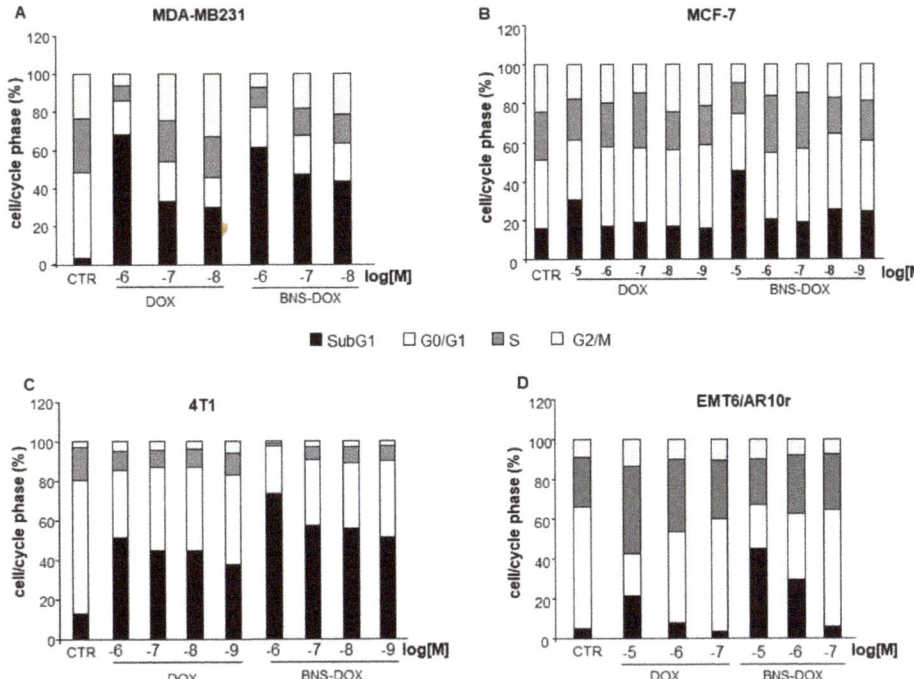

Figure 3. Effects of DOX and BNS-DOX treatment on cell cycle. (**A,B**) MDA-MB231 and MCF-7 human breast cancer cell lines and (**C,D**) 4T1 and EMR6/AR10r mouse breast cancer cell lines (1.5×10^5) were treated or not with DOX and BNS-DOX for 72 h and the cell cycle was then assessed by flow cytometry. Graphs represented the % of the quantification of cell cycle phases from three independent experiments.

The different cell lines showed distinct patterns of cell cycle distribution and BNS-DOX or DOX treatments showed variable effects, but the most consistent one was an increase of subG1 cells, induced to a higher extent by BNS-DOX compared to DOX.

These data suggest that the inhibition of cell growth induced by DOX or BNS-DOX can be due to induction of apoptosis. To verify this possibility, cells cultured for 72 h in the presence and absence of titrated amounts of DOX or BNS-DOX were stained with annexin-V and analyzed by flow cytometry to detect dying cells (Figure 4).

Results showed that treatment with DOX and BNS-DOX significantly increased the proportion of Annexin-V-positive cells, and BNS-DOX was significantly more effective than DOX in all cell lines, with patterns similar to those displayed by cell growth experiments.

To confirm the effect on cell apoptosis, we assessed caspase 3 activity on lysates of MDA-MB231, 4T1, and EMT6/AR10r cells cultured for 72 h in the presence and absence of titrated amounts of DOX or BNS-DOX. Results showed that both DOX and BNS-DOX activated caspase3 in all cell lines, and BNS-DOX was more effective than DOX (Figure 5).

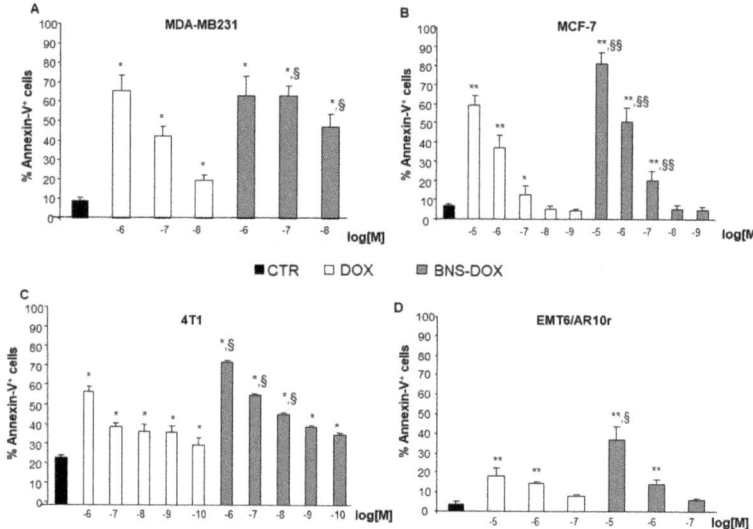

Figure 4. Effects of DOX and BNS-DOX treatment on cell death. Annexin-V positive cells were evaluated in (**A,B**) MDA-MB231 and MCF-7 human breast cancer cell lines and (**C,D**) 4T1 and EMR6/AR10r mouse breast cancer cell lines cultured for 72 h in the presence or absence of DOX or BNS-DOX. Results are expressed as % of positive cells from five independent experiments (* $p < 0.05$, ** $p < 0.01$, versus the control; § $p < 0.05$, §§ $p < 0.01$, versus the same concentration).

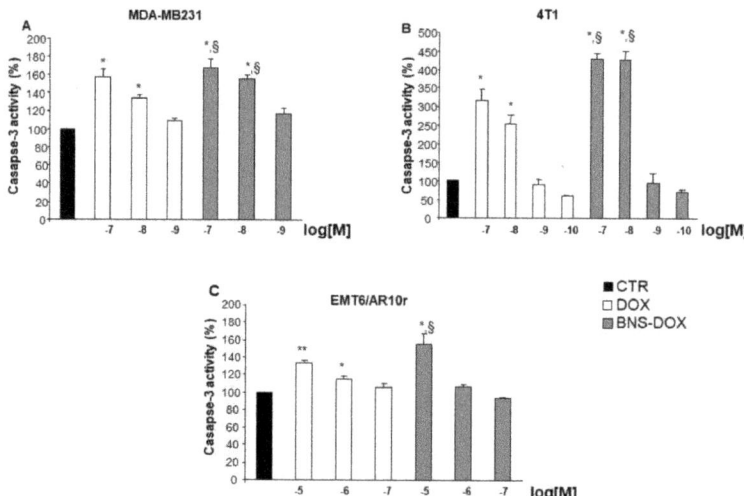

Figure 5. Levels of caspase3 activity after DOX and BNS-DOX treatment. Caspase-3 activity was evaluated in (**A**) MDA-MB231 human breast cancer cell lines and (**B,C**) 4T1 and EMR6/AR10r mouse breast cancer cell lines cultured for 72 h in the presence or absence of DOX or BNS-DOX. Results are expressed as % calculated as follows: (result displayed by each treatment/the results displayed by untreated cells) from five independent experiments (* $p < 0.05$, ** $p < 0.01$, versus the control; § $p < 0.05$ versus the same concentration).

Since MCF-7 cells do not express caspase3 [14,15] we did not evaluate its activity in this cell line. To further compare the effect of the two drug formulations on mammary cancer cell growth, we performed a clonogenic assay. Cells were treated for 3 h in the presence and absence of titrated amounts of BNS-DOX or DOX, then, the drug was removed and cells were cultured for 10 days. This approach was used in order to determine if the nanoparticles, once they penetrated inside the tumor cell, were able to function as a reservoir and release the drug during an extended period of time. Colony count at the end of the culture showed that, also in this case, BNS-DOX was more effective than free DOX in inhibiting cell growth in all cell lines (Figure 6).

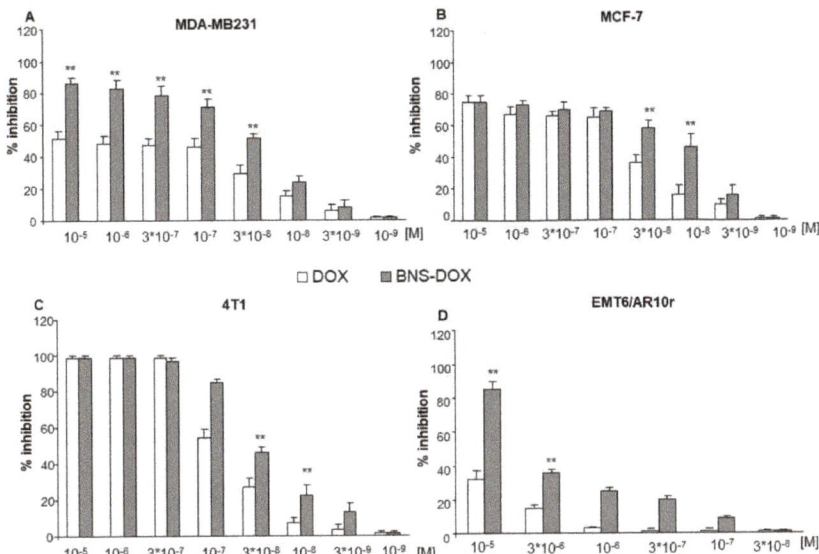

Figure 6. Effect of DOX and BNS-DOX on cell clonogenicity was tested by the colony forming assay. (**A**,**B**) MDA-MB231 and MCF-7 human breast cancer cell lines and (**C**,**D**) 4T1 and EMR6/AR10r mouse breast cancer cell lines were seeded in six-well plates and treated with each drug formulation at the indicated concentrations for 3 h. The medium was then changed and cells were cultured for an additional 10 days and subsequently fixed and stained with crystal violet. Graphs showed the % of clonogenicity inhibition (compared to controls) expressed as means ± SEM ($n = 5$). ** $p < 0.01$ significantly different from the same concentration of DOX.

To evaluate the cellular uptake of BNS-DOX in EMT6 cells confocal microscopy studies were carried out, exploiting the intrinsic red fluorescence of doxorubicin. BNS-DOX were easily internalized in cells, in agreement with our previous studies. Figure 7A reports the confocal microscopy images after 1 h and 3 h of incubation, showing the localization of BNS-DOX in cell cytoplasm around the nucleus. In contrast, a lower mean fluorescence intensity was observed for the cells treated with free DOX (Figure 7B).

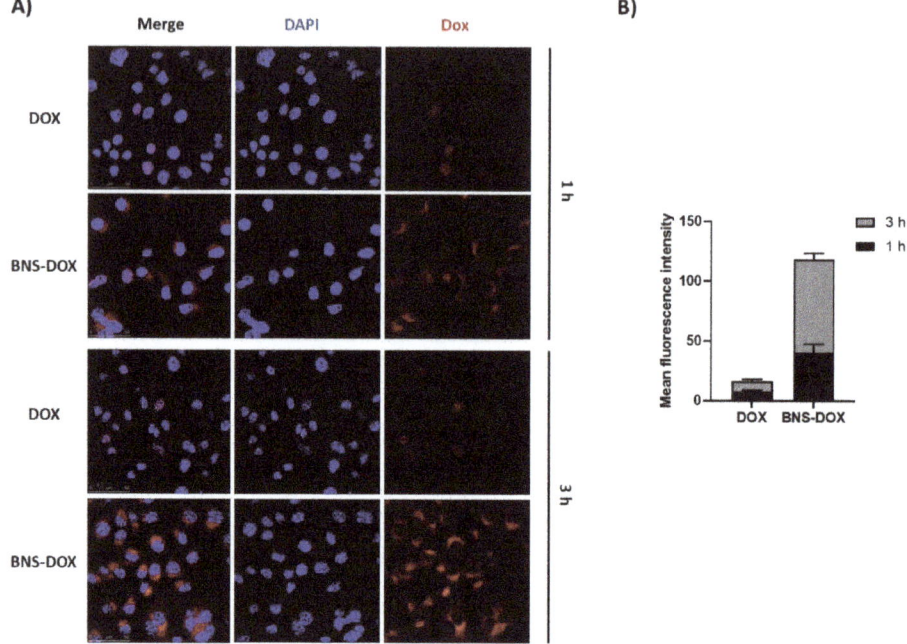

Figure 7. Cellular uptake studies. (**A**) BNS-DOX and DOX were incubated with EMT6 cells for 1 and 3 h. Exploiting doxorubicin (Dox) fluorescence, the cells were fixed and analyzed with Leica SPE confocal microscopy using a 63× oil lens. Images are representative of three field per condition ($n = 3$). (**B**) Quantification of Dox fluorescence inside the cells from images in panel A ($n = 3$).

To compare the effect of DOX and BNS-DOX on breast cancer cell growth, we used the BALB-neuT mice, which has a strong similarity with the human HER2-positive tumors. BALB-neuT females develop spontaneous breast tumors with 100% penetrance and a known kinetic: at 60 days from birth (9 week) they develop in situ carcinoma, at 120–150 days invasive tumors, and at 230 days cancerous extensive tumor masses involving all mammary glands [13,16–19]. The treatment with DOX and BNS-DOX began at 16–18 weeks from birth and mice were treated weekly with intravenous injections of DOX, BNS-DOX, empty nanoparticles (BNS), or PBS. The animal weight was of about 20 grams at time 0 (Figure 8B). At sacrifice, after 7 weeks from the beginning of the treatment, the tumor weights of mice treated with BNS-DOX were about 60% lower than those of mice treated with either PBS, DOX, or empty BNS (Figure 8A).

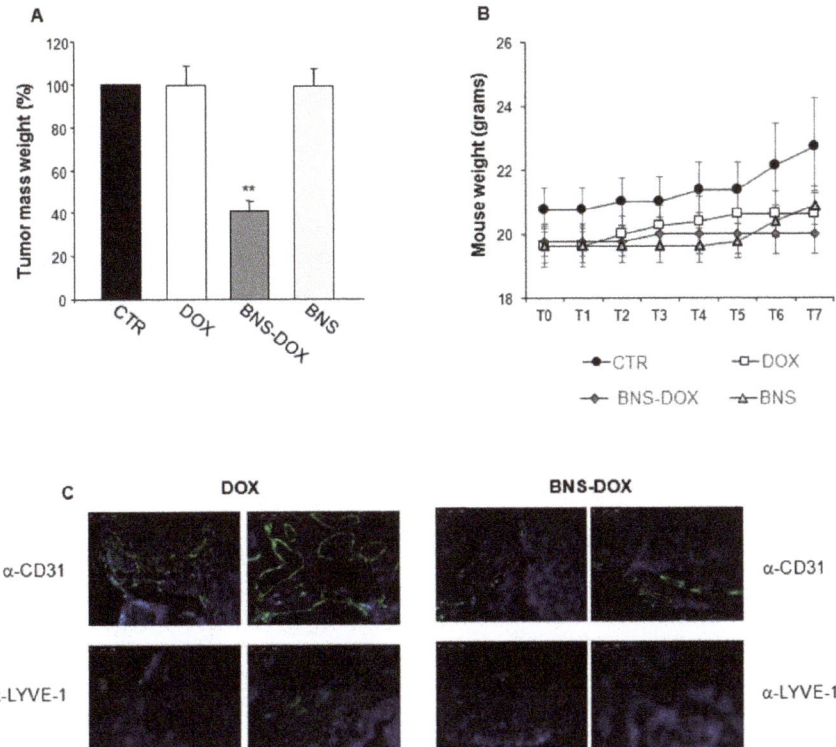

Figure 8. Effect of DOX and BNS-DOX on tumor growth in vivo. Thirteen-week-old female wt or BALB-neuT mice were treated with i.v. injection of 2 mg/kg DOX, or BNS-DOX, or BNS or the same volume of PBS as a control for six weeks (once every week). Mice were sacrificed at the seventh week after the first injection. (**A**) The graph shows an average of the tumor mass weight, expressed as % compared to the control group. (**B**) Weight of the animals was evaluated every week from the day of the first injection, performed at T0 (when the tumor was palpable); each treatment involved 8 mice. (**C**) Immunofluorescence staining of cluster of differentiation 31 (CD31) and lymphatic vessel endothelial hyaluronan receptor 1 (LYVE-1) of tumour tissue sections from of Neu-T mice treated with DOX or BNS-DOX. The slides were stained with either pAb rabbit α-mouse CD31 or pAb rabbit α-mouse LYVE-1 plus a secondary antibody α-rabbit conjugated with Alexa Fluor® 488. Representative images of three independent experiments are shown (scale bar 100 μm), ** $p < 0.01$.

To assess the effect of treatments on tumor neoangiogenesis and lymphangiogenesis, we analyzed the expression of CD31 marking blood vessels and LYVE-1 marking lymphoid vessels by immunofluorescence in cryostat sections cut in OCT, which allows optimal retention of the structural micro-architecture. Results showed that tumors from mice treated with BNS-DOX and DOX displayed substantially fewer areas of active angiogenesis and lymphatic vasculature than the tumors from mice treated with DOX (Figure 8C).

Since DOX is highly lipophilic and systemically distributes among all tissues, we compared the tissue biodistribution of doxorubicin in the tumors and several organs of BALB-neuT mice treated with either BNS-DOX or DOX at sacrifice by HLPC analysis. Analysis of the tumors showed that those from mice treated with BNS-DOX contained significantly more doxorubicin than those tumors from mice treated with DOX. Analysis of the organs showed that mice treated with BNS-DOX and DOX did not display substantial differences in the drug content of lungs, liver, kidneys, spleen, and brain, whereas the drug content of the heart was significantly lower (5 times lower) in BNS-DOX mice than in DOX mice (Figure 9A).

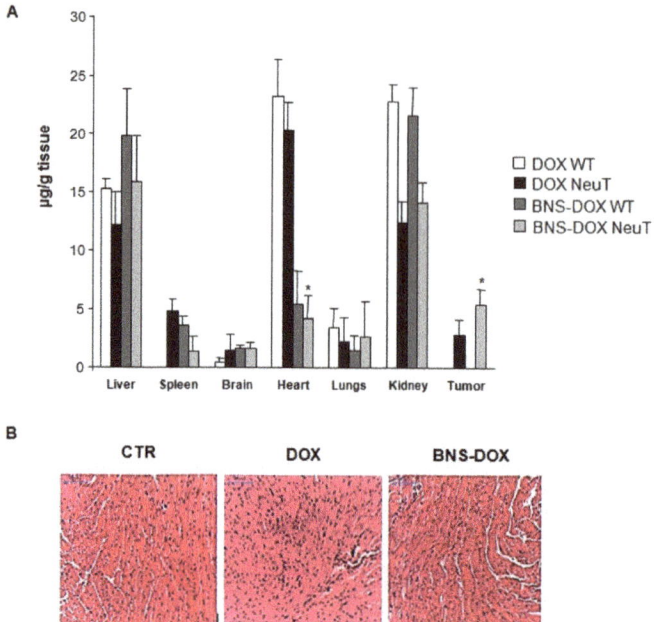

Figure 9. (**A**) Tissue biodistribution of DOX (expressed as µg/g tissue) after i.v. administration to BALB-neuT and BALB mice of 2 mg/kg of DOX or BNS-DOX. (**B**) Histopathologic analysis of the heart. Hematoxylin and eosin (H&E) stained were observed with 20× magnification (scale bar 100 µm). Representative image of heart tissue from Neu-T mice treated with phosphate buffered saline (PBS), DOX, or BNS-DOX. * $p < 0.05$.

Similar results were obtained by analyzing DOX distribution in control wild type BALB/c mice (not developing mammary tumors) receiving the same BNS-DOX and DOX treatment as BALB/neuT mice. In both BALB/c and BALB/neuT, treatment with BNS and DOX did not affect the weights of mice and organs compared with those of untreated mice.

Since these data suggest that BNS-DOX might be less cardiotoxic than DOX, we analyzed tissue sections stained with hematoxylin and eosin (H&E) staining obtained from the heart of mice treated with either BNS-DOX or DOX. Microscopic analysis showed that BNS-DOX did not affect the integrity and histology of the heart tissue, whereas DOX caused cardiotoxicity characterized by necrosis with red blood cells extravasation and moderate eosinophil infiltration (Figure 9B).

3. Discussion

DOX is widely used as a chemotherapy agent for the treatment of breast cancer [1]. Its cytotoxic and antiproliferative effects are exerted through several mechanisms, but the best known is in the poisoning of topoisomerases II cleavage complexes [20,21], causing G1 and G2 cell cycle arrest and induction of apoptosis. Other effects of DOX include its intercalation into DNA and the generation of free radicals causing DNA damage and lipid peroxidation [22].

Lack of specificity with inability to discriminate between malignant and noncancerous cells are the main causes of the side effects typical of standard DOX formulations, which limit doses and effectiveness of the drug. Moreover, DOX (or its derivatives) use is limited by cardiac and kidney toxicity and frequent onset of drug resistance in numerous tumor cell types [1]. In breast cancer cells, emergence of multidrug resistance (MDR) mainly involves upregulation of efflux transporters that are either located in the plasma or the nuclear membrane, which decrease the intracellular drug concentration [23].

Among them, the most extensively studied MDR transporters include P-glycoprotein (P-gp/ABCB1), multidrug resistance protein-1 (MRP1/ABCC1), and breast cancer resistance protein (BCRP, ABCG2) [24], all involved in drug inactivation and extrusion. Another possible feature of cancer cells is ability to escape apoptosis, caused by alterations in the apoptosis pathways [25,26].

To overcome these problems, several delivery systems have been proposed as carriers for DOX, but only liposomal DOX (Doxil®) achieved FDA approval in 1995 for treatment of Kaposi's sarcoma [27]. Although Doxil® is able to decrease cardiotoxicity in metastatic breast cancer patients [28], this formulation presents some limitations, such as fixed functionality, leakage of encapsulated agent, and high cost of manufacturing [29]. Moreover, although Doxil® improves the pharmacokinetic properties of DOX, it does not increase the pharmacological efficacy of DOX because of the insufficient cell uptake of liposomes [30]. In this context, other types of DOX nanocarriers have been proposed [31], such as poly(lactic-co-glycolic acid) (PLGA) nanoparticles [32], solid lipid nanoparticles [33] or nanosponges with different structures [34–37].

Here, we investigated a new type of β-cyclodextrin nanosponges for the in vitro and in vivo delivery of doxorubicin. The doxorubicin BNS formulation prepared for this study is capable of incorporating a good amount of drug, forming a reservoir which allows the DOX release in a prolonged manner. Notably, DOX incorporation in the polymer nanoparticles can be attributed to hydrophilic and hydrophobic interactions. It is worth noting that nanosponges present multiple domains, i.e., the hydrophobic β-CD cavities and the hydrophilic nanochannels in the polymer network. Moreover, further electrostatic interactions between DOX amino groups and carboxylic groups of polymer matrix may occur. This nanostructure feature can increase the effectiveness of the drug loading. The loading capacity obtained in this study (16.4 w%) was in line with other nanosponge formulations previously designed by our group [36,37]. This result is particularly promising taking into account also the DOX incorporation in other kinds of nanocarriers reported in literature [33,38–41] Therefore, DOX-BNS was further investigated both in vitro and in vivo.

In vitro studies showed the physical stability of BNS-DOX aqueous nanosuspension in plasma without aggregation phenomena. The in vivo physical stability and safety of BNS-DOX after i.v. administration are two key parameters to be taken into account for a nanoformulation [42]. As far as concern the cytotoxicity, no toxic effects were observed with empty BNS.

Our in vitro experiments showed that BNS-DOX displays increased ability to decrease the growth of both the ER/PR+ and the TNBC cell lines, and even of the DOX-resistant EMT6/AR10r cells, compared to the free DOX. The similar efficacy between DOX and BNS-DOX, that was observed in 4T1 cells at higher drug concentrations, was probably linked to the relatively high sensitivity of this cell line to DOX treatment. This observation was in agreement with the higher number of SubG1 cells found in 4T1 DOX-treated cells. The proportion of subG1 cells after DOX treatment depended on the sensitivity of the different cell lines. Similar results were obtained in MCF-7 and MCF-7 DOX-resistant human breast cancer cells by De et al. 2014 [43]. Moreover, results obtained from the clonogenic assay demonstrated that a short term exposure of cells to BNS-DOX is sufficient to elicit subsequent inhibition of colony formation, possibly because of a rapid internalization of the drug into the cancer cells, followed by sustained release and decreased extrusion by MDR mechanisms, such as the energy-dependent Pg-p type efflux pumps which decrease the drug concentration in the cell and its effectiveness. Clonogenic experiments showed that DOX inhibited cell proliferation at higher doses, because it can enter inside the cells, thanks to its lipophilic characteristics, but it can easily extruded by the cells by MDR mechanism. Carcinoma of colon, kidney, pancreas, and liver express high P-gp levels, while lung, ovary, and breast carcinoma, melanoma, and lymphomas express low P-gp levels, which often increase after chemotherapy causing acquired drug resistance [44]. Probably, BNS-DOX are internalized through endocytosis [45] and DOX is then slowly released in the cytoplasm far from these efflux pumps, reducing drug elimination. Indeed, cell uptake studies by confocal microscopy showed the internalization of BNS-DOX into the cells and their localization in the cytoplasm around the cell nucleus. Therefore, BNS-DOX could act as a drug reservoir inside the cells, that slowly release the drug.

The inhibitory effect on cell growth are mainly ascribable to induction of cell apoptosis, as indicated by the increase of the sub-G1 cell population detected by cell cycle analysis, of the proportion of dying cells stained by AnnexinV and of capsase3 activation.

The in vivo studies confirm the higher anticancer effect of BNS-DOX compared to DOX. Particularly relevant was the choice of the murine BALB-neuT model, which recapitulates several features of human tumors displaying mutations of the *ERBB2* proto-oncogene coding for receptor tyrosine-protein kinase erbB-2, also known as *HER2* (from human epidermal growth factor receptor 2) or *HER2/neu* [46]. HER2 is a member of the epidermal growth factor receptors (EGFR) family that has a crucial role in cell proliferation, apoptosis, adhesion, and cellular death; a mutation or an over expression of this gene can lead to carcinogenesis [47]. Results show that BNS-DOX reduces by 60% the tumor growth compared to DOX, at a 2 mg/kg dose that is 5-fold lower than the DOX therapeutic one (10 mg/kg). Indeed, at this dose, the free DOX is almost ineffective. This outcome might be related to the enhanced permeability and retention (EPR) effect. The irregular formation of blood and lymphatic vessels in the tumor, favored the extravasation and entrapment of the nanoparticles in the target site. In line with this possibility, our analysis of drug biodistribution detected higher levels of doxorubicin in the tumors of the mice treated with BNS-DOX than in those treated with DOX.

Besides these effects, the increased therapeutic effect of BNS-DOX may be partly ascribed to inhibition of tumor neoangiogenesis and lymphangiogenesis, detected by the immunohistological analysis of cancer tissue sections, which would limit nutrients and oxygen available to the tumor, and also tumor metastatic spread. Moreover, decreased lymphangiogenesis would favor entrapment of BNS-DOX in the tumor. This behavior was already observed with paclitaxel loaded in BNS in melanoma cell models [48].

Furthermore, the in vivo experiments did not detect severe toxic side effects of BNS-DOX, as a matter of fact it did not affect the aspect of the fur, weight, consumption of food and water, and viability of the animals. Interestingly, the drug biodistribution analysis showed drug levels in heart tissue of mice treated with BNS-DOX are 5-fold lower than those detected in mice treated with DOX, which may be relevant in decreasing the cardiotoxic side effects of DOX, being this effect the main limitation of the drug. In line with this observation, histological analysis of heart tissue sections detected signs of cardiac damage in the DOX-treated mice, but not in those treated with BNS-DOX. A further point is that, in vitro too, BNS-DOX display less toxicity than DOX on cultures of rat cardiomyocytes. The low level of heart accumulation might depend on the size (about 300 nm of diameter) and chemical structure of our BNS, capillary filtration and modality of internalization into cells [49]. This capability of doxorubicin loaded in nanosponges to reduce the cardiotoxicity was already observed with other nanosponge formulations [37].

Taken together, all these results underline the promising features of BNS-DOX to improve the therapeutic outcome of the drug.

4. Materials and Methods

4.1. Materials

The β-CDs were a kind gift from Roquette Italia (Cassano Spinola, Italy). All reagents were of analytical grade. The laboratory reagents were from Sigma-Aldrich, unless otherwise specified. The cell culture reagents were purchased from Gibco/Invitrogen (Life Technologies, Paisley, UK), unless otherwise indicated.

4.2. Preparation of Doxorubicin-Loaded Nanosponges

BNS were synthetized using β-cyclodextrins as building block and pyromellitic anhydride as crosslinking agent in 1:4 molar ratio (CD/cross-linker). The synthesis was carried out according our previous works [48,50].

A blank BNS aqueous nanosuspension (10 mg/mL) was prepared by homogenizing the BNS coarse powder suspended in saline solution (NaCl 0.9% w/v) firstly with a high-shear homogenizer (Ultra-Turrax, IKA, Konigswinter, Germany, 10 min, 24,000 rpm) and then with a high-pressure homogenizer (EmulsiFlex C5, Avastin, Mannheim, Germany, 90 min, 500 bar) to further reduce the BNS size.

Then, doxorubicin was added to the blank BNS nanosuspension to obtain doxorubicin loaded BNS (BNS-DOX) at a concentration of 2 mg/mL. The sample was incubated under stirring for 24 h at room temperature in the dark, to promote the loading. A dialysis step was performed to eliminate the unloaded doxorubicin.

4.3. Characterization of Doxorubicin-Loaded Nanosponges

BNS and BNS-DOX samples were in vitro characterized by determining their average diameter, polidispersity index, and zeta potential with dynamic light scattering (90 Plus particle sizer, Brookhaven Instruments Corporation, Holtsville, NY, USA). The samples were diluted with water (1:30 v/v) immediately prior the measurements, carried out at a fixed angle of 90° and at a temperature of 25 °C. Transmission electron microscopy (TEM) analysis was performed using a Philips CM 10 transmission electron microscope to observe the morphology of BNS-DOX. The BNS nanosuspensions were sprayed on Formvar coated copper grid and air-dried before observation.

A weighted amount of freeze-dried BNS-DOX was dispersed in 5 mL of water and sonicated for 15 min. The sample was then centrifuged (10 min, 15,000 rpm) and after the supernatant was analyzed by High Performance Liquid Cromatography (HPLC), to determine the DOX concentration in the BNS.

The loading capacity of BNS-DOX was calculated according to: Loading capacity (%) = [amount of DOX/weight of BNS-DOX] × 100. The encapsulation efficiency of BNS-DOX was determined using the formula: Encapsulation efficiency (%) = [amount of DOX loaded/total amount of DOX] × 100.

The physical stability of BNS-DOX stored at 4 °C was assessed up to 1 month, by checking the physicochemical parameters over time.

4.4. In Vitro Release Studies

The in vitro release kinetics of DOX from BNS-DOX was evaluated with a multi-compartment rotating cell, using a cellulose membrane (Spectrapore, cut-off = 12,000 Da) to separate the donor from the receiving compartment. The in vitro drug release studies were performed at two different pH values (5.5 and 7.4). Samples of receiving phase (phosphate buffered saline, PBS at pH 5.5 or 7.4) were withdrawn at fixed times and analyzed by HPLC to quantify the amount of drug released from BNS-DOX over time. DOX was detected using a fluorescence detector at excitation and emission wavelengths of 480 and 560 nm, respectively.

4.5. Stability and In Vitro Release Studies in Plasma

The stability of BNS-DOX was investigated in plasma, determining their size and DOX concentration over time after BNS-DOX incubation in plasma at 37 °C for 24 h. The in vitro release kinetics of DOX from BNS-DOX in plasma was also studied. For this purpose 50 microliters of BNS-DOX were incubated at 37 °C with rat plasma diluted with PBS at pH = 7.4 (1:3 v/v). At fixed time 200 microliters of the sample were withdrawn, centrifuged using a centrifugal filter device (Amicon® Ultra, 20,000 rpm, 10 min) and then the filtrate was analyzed by HPLC to quantify the amount of DOX released from BNS-DOX over time.

4.6. Cell Culture Conditions

Cancer cell lines were obtained from the American Type Culture Collection (ATCC; Manassas, VA, USA). MDA-MB231, MCF-7, H9c2 were grown in culture dishes as a monolayer in Dulbecco's Modified Eagle (DMEM) medium (Invitrogen, Burlington, ON, Canada), 4T1 in RPMI 1640, and EMT6/AR10r DOX resistant in Minimum Essential Medium (MEM), all supplemented with 10% penicillin-streptomycin (Invitrogen) and 10% fetal calf serum (Invitrogen), in a humidified atmosphere with 5% CO_2. In the case of EMT6/AR10r DOX resistant cell lines, 1 µg/mL of DOX was added in the culture medium once a week.

4.7. Cell Proliferation

MTT (3-(4,5-Dimethylthiazol-2-yl)-2,5diphenyltetrazolium bromide; Sigma-Aldrich, St. Louis, MA, USA) analysis was performed in 96-well plates. Briefly, 1000–2000 cells/well were seeded in 100 µL of complete medium and the day after they were treated with DOX or BNS-DOX (10^{-5}–10^{-9} M) for 72 h. Subsequently, cells were supplemented with 5 mg/mL thiazolyl blue tetrazolium bromide (M2128; Sigma-Aldrich) for 2 h. Thereafter, the medium was removed and cells were lysed with 100 µL of DMSO. Absorbance was recorded at 570 nm by a 96-well-plate reader (PerkinElmer, Waltham, MA, USA). Controls were normalized to 100%, and the readings from treated cells were expressed as % of viability inhibition. Eight replicates were used to determine each data point, and five different experiments were performed.

4.8. Colony-Forming Assay

Cells (800/well) were seeded into six well plates and treated with the compounds. The medium was changed after 3 h and cells were cultured for additional 10 days. Subsequently, cells were fixed and stained with a solution of 80% crystal violet and 20% methanol. Colonies were then photographed and counted with a Gel Doc equipment (Bio-Rad Laboratories, Hercules, CA, USA). Then, cells were washed and 30% acetic acid were added to induce a complete dissolution of the crystal violet. Absorbance was recorded at 595 nm by a 96-well-plate ELISA reader. Controls were normalized to 100%, and the readings from treated cells were expressed as % of viability inhibition. Five different experiments were performed.

4.9. Cell Cycle Analysis

Treated and untreated cells were harvested 72 h after the treatment with DOX or BNS-DOX at different concentrations. Cells were washed with 1× PBS, fixed in 70% cold ethanol, resuspended in a buffer containing 0.02 mg/mL RNase A (Sigma-Aldrich), 0.05 mg/mL propidium iodide (Sigma-Aldrich), 0.2% v/v Nonidet P-40 (Sigma-Aldrich), 0.1% w/v sodium citrate (Sigma-Aldrich), and analyzed by a FACS Calibur cytometer (Becton Dickinson, Franklin Lakes, NJ, USA).

4.10. Cell Death

Treated and untreated cells were harvested 72 h after the treatment with different concentration of DOX or BNS-DOX, washed with 1× PBS, and subsequently resuspended in Annexin-V binding buffer (Life Technologies, Carlsbad, CA, USA) supplemented with 1:100 APC-conjugated Annexin-V (Immunotools, Friesoythe, Germany). Cells were analyzed by a FACS Calibur cytometer (Becton Dickinson, Franklin Lakes, NJ, USA). The analysis of apoptosis was performed by measuring the caspase 3 activity in cell lysates using a fluorimetric assay (BioVision, Milpitas, CA, USA) following the manufacture' instructions.

4.11. Cell Uptake Studies

EMT6 cells (4×10^4 cells per well) were seeded on Corning® cover glasses (Sigma-Aldrich) in a 24-well plate. The day after, the cells were incubated with BNS-DOX and DOX (30 µM) for 1 and 3 h.

Then, the cells were washed with PBS, fixed with 4% paraformaldehyde at room temperature for 15 min, and stained with 4′,6-diamidine-2-phenylindole (DAPI). Finally, coverslips were mounted and the image acquisition was performed with a Leica SPE Confocal microscope (Leica, Wetzlar, Germany), with 63X oil-immersion objective. The mean fluorescence intensity of Dox was quantified by ImageJ software (ImageJ, U.S. National Institutes of Health, Bethesda, MD, USA).

4.12. In Vivo Experiments

Transgenic (BALB-neuT) female mice, which over-express the rat HER2 (neu) oncogene under the mouse mammary tumor virus (MMTV) promoter [51] and wild type mice (BALB), 16–18 weeks old, were used. BALB-neuT and BALB mice were treated every week with intravenous injections (i.v.) of 2 mg/kg of DOX, BNS-DOX, empty nanoparticles (BNS), or PBS as control. Mice were bred under pathogen-free conditions in the animal facility of the Università del Piemonte Orientale, and treated in accordance with the Bioethics Committee of University of Turin, protocol NO. 479 of 1 November 2016. Body weight of the animals was monitored over time. Mice were sacrificed 7 weeks after the beginning of treatment and tumors were harvested and weighed. Immediately after dissection, tumor samples were embedded in OCT compound, snap-frozen and stored at −80 °C until use.

The biodistribution of DOX and BNS-DOX was evaluated after the mice sacrifice. The different tissues (liver, spleen, brain, heart, lungs, and kidneys) were collected, washed with saline solution, weighed, and frozen at −80 °C until analysis. Tissue extracts were prepared by adding 200 μL of methanol and 400 μL of TRIS buffer (1 M, pH 8.5) to the tissue and then homogenizing the mixtures.

The tissue homogenates were kept in ice for 15 min before adding 1.4 mL of acetonitrile. Then, the samples were vortex and centrifuged for 5 min at 15,000 rpm to separate the precipitated proteins.

After centrifugation clear supernatants (100 μL) were analyzed by HPLC analysis, to quantify the amount of DOX in the tissue extracts.

4.13. Immunofluorescence

Tumor tissues were cut with a cryostat (thickness 5–6 μm) and treated with 4% paraformaldehyde (Sigma-Aldrich) diluted in PBS for 5 min at room temperature to fix the sample on the glass slides. The samples were then blocked with 5% normal goat serum (NGS) in PBS for 1 h, in order to block aspecific sites to which the primary antibody could bind. To detect CD31 and LYVE-1 expression, slides were incubated with the primary rabbit antibody anti-CD31 or anti-LYVE-1 (dilution 1:100 and 1:200, respectively; Abcam, Cambridge, UK) overnight at 4 °C. The secondary antibody used was an anti-rabbit Ig Alexa fluor 488-conjugated (Invitrogen), diluted 1: 400. Then the sections were stained with 0.5 mg/mL of the fluorescent dye 4,6-diamidino-2-phenylindole-dihydrochloride (DAPI, Sigma-Aldrich) for 5 min, to stain the cell nuclei, and then mounted using Prolong anti-fade mounting medium (Light AntiFADE Kit, Molecular Probes Invitrogen). The sections were then observed by a fluorescence inverted Axiovert 40 CFL microscope (Carl Zeiss, Oberkochen, Germany), photographed with a Retiga 200R digital camera (QImaging, Surrey, BC, Canada), and analyzed with the Image Pro Plus Software for micro-imaging 5.0 (Media Cybernetics, version 5.0, Bethesda, MD, USA).

4.14. Histopathological Examination

Transverse midsections of hearts were fixed in 10% buffered formalin, embedded in paraffin, cut into 5 μm sections, and processed for hematoxylin and eosin (H&E) staining to determine the level of inflammation. Stained sections were analyzed by light microscope (DM 2500 Leica) connected to a digital camera (DFC 320, Leica, Milan, Italy). The sections were morphologically examined to evaluate the inflammatory infiltration levels.

4.15. Data Analysis

Data are shown as mean ± SEM. The statistical analyses were performed with GraphPad Prism 3.0 software (San Diego, CA, USA) using the one-way ANOVA and Dunnett test. IC_{50} was investigated using the two tailed unpaired *t*-test with Welch correction. The significance cut-off was *p* below 0.05.

5. Conclusions

BNS-DOX proved to be a promising effective nanoformulation in the treatment of breast cancer. The increased effectiveness, compared to DOX, may be due to a higher accumulation into the tumor mass and the neoplastic cells. Moreover, the reduced biodistribution in the heart tissue suggests a reduced cardiotoxicity of BNS-DOX. Therefore, this nanoformulation, which increases DOX efficacy and decreases its severe side effects, might be an attractive tool for improving the clinical management of breast cancer.

Author Contributions: M.A., B.F., C.L.G., N.C. and E.B. performed experiments and data analyses, and wrote the manuscript. F.B. carried out confocal microscopy analysis. F.T., S.P. and G.B. helped the design of experiments and wrote the manuscript. R.B. helped with the interpretation of results. R.C., U.D. and C.D. conceived the research, helped the design of experiments, data analyses, and wrote the manuscript. All authors have read and agreed to the published version of the manuscript.

Funding: This research has been supported by Associazione Italiana Ricerca sul Cancro (IG 20714, AIRC, Milano), Fondazione Cariplo (2017-0535), Fondazione Amici di Jean (Turin) and Progetti di Ricerca di Ateneo San Paolo 2016-2018.

Conflicts of Interest: No potential conflicts of interest were disclosed.

Abbreviations

DOX	doxorubicin
BNS-DOX	β-Cyclodextrins Nanosponges containing doxorubicin
EPR	enhanced permeability and retention effect
CD	cyclodextrin
BNS	β-cyclodextrin nanosponges
TBNC	Triple negative cell-lines
P-gp	P-glycoprotein
PLGA	poly (lactic-co-glycolic acid)
EGFR	epidermal growth factor receptors
MTT	(3-(4,5-Dimethylthiazol-2-yl)-2,5diphenyltetrazolium bromide
MMTV	mouse mammary tumor virus
NGS	normal goat serum
H&E	hematoxylin and eosin

References

1. Humber, C.E.; Tierney, J.F.; Symonds, R.P.; Collingwood, M.; Kirwan, J.; Williams, C.; Green, J.A. Chemotherapy for advanced, recurrent or metastatic endometrial cancer: A systematic review of Cochrane collaboration. *Ann. Oncol.* **2007**, *18*, 409–420. [CrossRef] [PubMed]
2. Prasad, P.; Shuhendler, A.; Cai, P.; Rauth, A.M.; Wu, X.Y. Doxorubicin and mitomycin C-loaded polymer-lipid hybrid nanoparticles inhibit growth of sensitive and multidrug resistant human mammary tumor xenografts. *Cancer Lett.* **2013**, *334*, 263–273. [CrossRef] [PubMed]
3. Jeong, Y.I.; Chung, K.D.; Choi, K.C. Doxorubicin release from self-assembled nanoparticles of deoxycholic acid-conjugated dextran. *Arch. Pharm. Res.* **2011**, *34*, 159–167. [CrossRef] [PubMed]
4. Hobbs, S.K.; Monsky, W.L.; Yuan, F.; Roberts, W.G.; Griffith, L.; Torchilin, V.P.; Jain, R.K. Regulation of transport pathways in tumor vessels: Role of tumor type and microenvironment. *Proc. Natl. Acad. Sci. USA* **1998**, *95*, 4607–4612. [CrossRef] [PubMed]
5. Laza-Knoerr, A.L.; Gref, R.; Couvreur, P. Cyclodextrins for drug delivery. *J. Drug Targets* **2010**, *18*, 645–656. [CrossRef] [PubMed]

6. Gigliotti, C.L.; Minelli, R.; Cavalli, R.; Occhipinti, S.; Barrera, G.; Pizzimenti, S.; Cappellano, G.; Boggio, E.; Conti, L.; Fantozzi, R.; et al. In Vitro and In Vivo therapeutic evaluation of camptothecin-encapsulated β-cyclodextrin nanosponges in prostate cancer. *J. Biomed. Nanotechnol.* **2016**, *12*, 14–27. [CrossRef]
7. Argenziano, M.; Lombardi, C.; Ferrara, B.; Trotta, F.; Caldera, F.; Blangetti, M.; Koltai, H.; Kapulnik, Y.; Yarden, R.; Gigliotti, L.; et al. Glutathione/pH-responsive nanosponges enhance strigolactone delivery to prostate cancer cells. *Oncotarget* **2018**, *9*, 35813–35829. [CrossRef]
8. Duchene, D.; Cavalli, R.; Gref, R. Cyclodextrin-based polymeric nanoparticles as efficient carriers for anticancer drugs. *Curr. Pharm. Biotechnol.* **2016**, *17*, 248–255. [CrossRef]
9. Swaminathan, S.; Pastero, L.; Serpe, L.; Trotta, F.; Vavia, P.; Aquilano, D.; Trotta, M.; Zara, G.; Cavalli, R. Cyclodextrin-based nanosponges encapsulating camptothecin: Physicochemical characterization, stability and cytotoxicity. *Eur. J. Pharm. Biopharm.* **2010**, *74*, 193–201. [CrossRef]
10. Swaminathan, S.; Vavia, P.R.; Trotta, F.; Cavalli, R.; Tumbiolo, S.; Bertinetti, L.; Coluccia, S. Structural evidence of differential forms of nanosponges of betacyclodextrin and its effect on solubilization of a model drug. *J. Incl. Phenom. Macrocycl. Chem.* **2013**, *76*, 201–211. [CrossRef]
11. Trotta, F.; Zanetti, M.; Cavalli, R. Cyclodextrin-based nanosponges as drug carriers. *Beilstein J. Org. Chem.* **2012**, *8*, 2091–2099. [CrossRef] [PubMed]
12. Swaminathan, S.; Cavalli, R.; Trotta, F. Cyclodextrin-based nanosponges: A versatile platform for cancer nanotherapeutics development. *Wiley Interdiscip. Rev. Nanomed. Nanobiotechnol.* **2016**, *8*, 579–601. [CrossRef] [PubMed]
13. Conti, L.; Ruiu, R.; Barutello, G.; Macagno, M.; Bandini, S.; Cavallo, F.; Lanzardo, S. Microenvironment, oncoantigens, and antitumor vaccination: Lessons learned from BALB-neuT mice. *Biomed. Res. Int.* **2014**, *2014*, 534969. [CrossRef]
14. Jänicke, R.U. MCF-7 breast carcinoma cells do not express caspase-3. *Breast Cancer Res. Treat.* **2009**, *117*, 219–221. [CrossRef] [PubMed]
15. Kagawa, S.; Gu, J.; Honda, T.; McDonnell, T.J.; Swisher, S.G.; Roth, J.A.; Fang, B. Deficiency of caspase-3 in MCF7 cells blocks Bax-mediated nuclear fragmentation but not cell death. *Clin. Cancer Res.* **2001**, *7*, 1474–1480. [PubMed]
16. Calogero, R.A.; Cordero, F.; Forni, G.; Cavallo, F. Inflammation and breast cancer. Inflammatory component of mammary carcinogenesis in ErbB2 transgenic mice. *Breast Cancer Res.* **2007**, *9*, e211. [CrossRef]
17. Di Carlo, E.; Diodoro, M.G.; Boggio, K.; Modesti, A.; Modesti, M.; Nanni, P.; Forni, G.; Musiani, P. Analysis of mammary carcinoma onset and progression in HER-2/neu oncogene transgenic mice reveals a lobular origin. *Lab. Investig.* **1999**, *79*, 1261–1269.
18. Iezzi, M.; Calogero, R.A.; Spadaro, M.; Musiani, P.; Forni, G.; Cavallo, F. BALB-neuT female mice as a dynamic model of mammary cancer. *Bentham Sci. Publ. Transl. Anim. Models Drug Discov. Dev.* **2012**, *28*, 136–166.
19. Rovero, S.; Amici, A.; Di Carlo, E.; Bei, R.; Nanni, P.; Quaglino, E.; Porcedda, P.; Boggio, K.; Smorlesi, A.; Lollini, P.L.; et al. DNA vaccination against rat her-2/Neu p185 more effectively inhibits carcinogenesis than transplantable carcinomas in transgenic BALB/c mice. *J. Immunol.* **2000**, *165*, 5133–5142. [CrossRef]
20. McClendon, A.K.; Osheroff, N. DNA topoisomerase II, genotoxicity, and cancer. *Mutat. Res.* **2007**, *623*, 83–97. [CrossRef]
21. Tewey, K.M.; Rowe, T.C.; Yang, L.; Halligan, B.D.; Liu, L.F. Adriamycin-induced DNA damage mediated by mammalian DNA topoisomerase II. *Science* **1984**, *226*, 466–468. [CrossRef] [PubMed]
22. Minotti, G.; Menna, P.; Salvatorelli, E.; Cairo, G.; Gianni, L. Anthracyclines: Molecular advances and pharmacologic developments in antitumor activity and cardiotoxicity. *Pharmacol. Rev.* **2004**, *56*, 185–229. [CrossRef] [PubMed]
23. Chang, G. Multidrug resistance ABC transporters. *FEBS Lett.* **2003**, *555*, 102–105. [CrossRef]
24. Shafei, A.; El-Bakly, W.; Sobhy, A.; Wagdy, O.; Reda, A.; Aboelenin, O.; Marzouk, A.; El Habak, K.; Mostafa, R.; Ali, M.A.; et al. A review on the efficacy and toxicity of different doxorubicin nanoparticles for targeted therapy in metastatic breast cancer. *Biomed. Pharmacother.* **2017**, *95*, 1209–1218. [CrossRef]
25. Kim, T.H.; Shin, Y.J.; Won, A.J.; Lee, B.M.; Choi, W.S.; Jung, J.H.; Chung, H.Y.; Kim, H.S. Resveratrol enhances chemosensitivity of doxorubicin in multidrug-resistant human breast cancer cells via increased cellular influx of doxorubicin. *Biochim. Biophys. Acta* **2014**, *1840*, 615–625. [CrossRef]

26. Ruiz de Almodóvar, C.; Ruiz-Ruiz, C.; Muñoz-Pinedo, C.; Robledo, G.; López-Rivas, A. The differential sensitivity of Bcl-2-overexpressing human breast tumor cells to TRAIL or doxorubicin-induced apoptosis is dependent on Bcl-2 protein levels. *Oncogene* **2001**, *20*, 7128–7133. [CrossRef]
27. Barenholz, Y. Doxil®—The first FDA-approved nano-drug: Lessons learned. *J. Control. Release* **2012**, *160*, 117–134. [CrossRef]
28. O'Brien, M.E.; Wigler, N.; Inbar, M.; Rosso, R.; Grischke, E.; Santoro, A.; Catane, R.; Kieback, D.G.; Tomczak, P.; Ackland, S.P.; et al. Reduced cardiotoxicity and comparable efficacy in a phase III trial of pegylated liposomal doxorubicin HCl (CAELYX/Doxil) versus conventional doxorubicin for first-line treatment of metastatic breast cancer. *Ann. Oncol.* **2004**, *3*, 440–449. [CrossRef]
29. Adair, J.H.; Parette, M.P.; Altınoğlu, E.I.; Kester, M. Nanoparticulate alternatives for drug delivery. *ACS Nano* **2010**, *4*, 4967–4970. [CrossRef]
30. Moosavian, S.A.; Abnous, K.; Badiee, A.; Jaafari, M.R. Improvement in the drug delivery and anti-tumor efficacy of PEGylated liposomal doxorubicin by targeting RNA aptamers in mice bearing breast tumor model. *Colloids Surf. B Biointerfaces* **2016**, *139*, 228–236. [CrossRef]
31. Gonçalves, M.; Mignani, S.; Rodrigues, J.; Tomás, H. A glance over doxorubicin based-nanotherapeutics: From proof-of-concept studies to solutions in the market. *J. Control. Release* **2020**, *317*, 347–374. [CrossRef] [PubMed]
32. Acharya, S.; Sahoo, S.K. PLGA nanoparticles containing various anticancer agents and tumour delivery by EPR effect. *Adv. Drug Deliv. Rev.* **2011**, *63*, 170–183. [CrossRef] [PubMed]
33. Fundarò, A.; Cavalli, R.; Bargoni, A.; Vighetto, D.; Zara, G.P.; Gasco, M.R. Non-stealth and stealth solid lipid nanoparticles (SLN) carrying doxorubicin: Pharmacokinetics and tissue distribution after iv administration to rats. *Pharmacol. Res.* **2000**, *42*, 337–343. [CrossRef] [PubMed]
34. Trotta, F.; Dianzani, C.; Caldera, F.; Mognetti, B.; Cavalli, R. The application of nanosponges to cancer drug delivery. *Expert Opin. Drug Deliv.* **2014**, *11*, 931–941. [CrossRef]
35. Cavalli, R.; Trotta, F.; Tumiatti, W. Cyclodextrin-based nanosponges for drug delivery. *J. Incl. Phenom. Macrocycl. Chem.* **2006**, *56*, 209–213. [CrossRef]
36. Caldera, F.; Argenziano, M.; Trotta, F.; Dianzani, C.; Gigliotti, L.; Tannous, M.; Pastero, L.; Aquilano, D.; Nishimoto, T.; Higashiyama, T.; et al. Cyclic nigerosyl-1, 6-nigerose-based nanosponges: An innovative pH and time-controlled nanocarrier for improving cancer treatment. *Carbohydr. Polym.* **2018**, *194*, 111–121. [CrossRef]
37. Daga, M.; Ullio, C.; Argenziano, M.; Dianzani, C.; Cavalli, R.; Trotta, F.; Ferretti, C.; Zara, G.P.; Gigliotti, C.L.; Ciamporcero, E.S.; et al. GSH-targeted nanosponges increase doxorubicin-induced toxicity "in vitro" and "in vivo" in cancer cells with high antioxidant defenses. *Free Radic. Biol. Med.* **2016**, *97*, 24–37. [CrossRef]
38. Scomparin, A.; Salmaso, S.; Eldar-Boock, A.; Ben-Shushan, D.; Ferber, S.; Tiram, G.; Shmeeda, H.; Landa-Rouben, N.; Leor, J.; Caliceti, P.; et al. A comparative study of folate receptor-targeted doxorubicin delivery systems: Dosing regimens and therapeutic index. *J. Control. Release* **2015**, *208*, 106–120. [CrossRef]
39. Sun, H.; Guo, X.; Zeng, S.; Wang, Y.; Hou, J.; Yang, D.; Zhou, S. A multifunctional liposomal nanoplatform co-delivering hydrophobic and hydrophilic doxorubicin for complete eradication of xenografted tumors. *Nanoscale* **2019**, *11*, 17759–17772. [CrossRef]
40. Wang, H.; Zheng, M.; Gao, J.; Wang, J.; Zhang, Q.; Fawcett, J.P.; He, Y.; Gu, J. Uptake and release profiles of PEGylated liposomal doxorubicin nanoparticles: A comprehensive picture based on separate determination of encapsulated and total drug concentrations in tissues of tumor-bearing mice. *Talanta* **2020**, *208*, e120358. [CrossRef]
41. Marano, F.; Argenziano, M.; Frairia, R.; Adamini, A.; Bosco, O.; Rinella, L.; Fortunati, N.; Cavalli, R.; Catalano, M.G. Doxorubicin-loaded nanobubbles combined with extracorporeal shock waves: Basis for a new drug delivery tool in anaplastic thyroid cancer. *Thyroid* **2016**, *26*, 705–716. [CrossRef] [PubMed]
42. Yang, Y.; Yang, Y.; Xie, X.; Cai, X.; Zhang, H.; Gong, W.; Wang, Z.; Mei, X. PEGylated liposomes with NGR ligand and heat-activable cell-penetrating peptide-doxorubicin conjugate for tumor-specific therapy. *Biomaterials* **2014**, *35*, 4368–4381. [CrossRef] [PubMed]
43. De, U.; Chun, P.; Choi, W.S.; Lee, B.M.; Kim, N.D.; Moon, H.R.; Jung, J.H.; Kim, H.S. A novel anthracene derivative, MHY412, induces apoptosis in doxorubicin-resistant MCF-7/Adr human breast cancer cells through cell cycle arrest and downregulation of P-glycoprotein expression. *Int. J. Oncol.* **2014**, *44*, 167–176. [CrossRef] [PubMed]

44. Kapse-Mistry, S.; Govender, T.; Srivastava, R.; Yergeri, M. Nanodrug delivery in reversing multidrug resistance in cancer cells. *Front. Pharmacol.* **2014**, *5*, e159.
45. Rosenbaum, A.I.; Zhang, G.; Warren, J.D.; Maxfield, F.R. Endocytosis of beta-cyclodextrins is responsible for cholesterol reduction in Niemann-Pick type C mutant cells. *Proc. Natl. Acad. Sci. USA* **2010**, *107*, 5477–5482. [CrossRef] [PubMed]
46. Guy, C.T.; Webster, M.A.; Schaller, M.; Parsons, T.J.; Cardiff, R.D.; Muller, W.J. Expression of the neu protooncogene in the mammary epithelium of transgenic mice induces metastatic disease. *Proc. Natl. Acad. Sci. USA* **1992**, *89*, 10578–10582. [CrossRef]
47. Mitri, Z.; Constantine, T.; O'Regan, R. The HER2 receptor in breast cancer: Pathophysiology, clinical use, and new advances in therapy. *Chemother. Res. Pract.* **2012**, *2012*, e743193. [CrossRef]
48. Clemente, N.; Argenziano, M.; Gigliotti, C.L.; Ferrara, B.; Boggio, E.; Chiocchetti, A.; Caldera, F.; Trotta, F.; Benetti, E.; Annaratone, L.; et al. Paclitaxel-loaded nanosponges inhibit growth and angiogenesis in melanoma cell models. *Front. Pharmacol.* **2019**, *10*, e776. [CrossRef]
49. DeJong, W.H.; Hagens, W.I.; Krystek, P.; Burger, M.C.; Sips, A.J.; Geertsma, R.E. Particle size-dependent organ distribution of gold nanoparticles after intravenous administration. *Biomaterials* **2008**, *29*, 1912–1919. [CrossRef]
50. Clemente, N.; Boggio, E.; Gigliotti, C.L.; Raineri, D.; Ferrara, B.; Miglio, G.; Argenziano, M.; Chiocchetti, A.; Cappellano, G.; Trotta, F.; et al. Immunotherapy of experimental melanoma with ICOS-Fc loaded in biocompatible and biodegradable nanoparticles. *J. Control. Release* **2019**, *11*, 48.
51. Quaglino, E.; Mastini, C.; Forni, G.; Cavallo, F. ErbB2 transgenic mice: A tool for investigation of the immune prevention and treatment of mammary carcinomas. *Curr. Protoc. Immunol.* **2008**, *82*, 20.9.1–20.9.10.

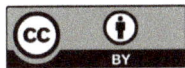

© 2020 by the authors. Licensee MDPI, Basel, Switzerland. This article is an open access article distributed under the terms and conditions of the Creative Commons Attribution (CC BY) license (http://creativecommons.org/licenses/by/4.0/).

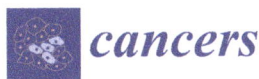

Article

Nanoformulated Zoledronic Acid Boosts the Vδ2 T Cell Immunotherapeutic Potential in Colorectal Cancer

Daniele Di Mascolo [1,†], **Serena Varesano** [2,†], **Roberto Benelli** [3], **Hilaria Mollica** [1], **Annalisa Salis** [4], **Maria Raffaella Zocchi** [5], **Paolo Decuzzi** [1,‡] and **Alessandro Poggi** [2,*,‡]

1. Laboratory of Nanotechnology for Precision Medicine, Fondazione Istituto Italiano di Tecnologia, 16163 Genoa, Italy; daniele.dimascolo@iit.it (D.D.M.); hilaria.mollica@iit.it (H.M.); Paolo.Decuzzi@iit.it (P.D.)
2. Molecular Oncology and Angiogenesis Unit, IRCCS Policlinico San Martino, 16132 Genoa, Italy; sere_varesano@hotmail.it
3. Immunology Unit, Ospedale Policlinico San Martino, University of Genoa, 16132 Genoa, Italy; roberto.benelli@hsanmartino.it
4. CEBR, University of Genoa, 16132 Genoa, Italy; annalisa.salis@unige.it
5. Division of Immunology, Transplants and Infectious Diseases, IRCCS San Raffaele Scientific Institute, 20132 Milan, Italy; zocchi.maria@hsr.it
* Correspondence: alessandro.poggi@hsanmartino.it
† These authors contributed equally to this work.
‡ P.D. and A.P. share the senior authorship.

Received: 20 November 2019; Accepted: 29 December 2019; Published: 31 December 2019

Abstract: Aminobisphosphonates, such as zoledronic acid (ZA), have shown potential in the treatment of different malignancies, including colorectal carcinoma (CRC). Yet, their clinical exploitation is limited by their high bone affinity and modest bioavailability. Here, ZA is encapsulated into the aqueous core of spherical polymeric nanoparticles (SPNs), whose size and architecture resemble that of biological vesicles. On Vδ2 T cells, derived from the peripheral blood of healthy donors and CRC patients, ZA-SPNs induce proliferation and trigger activation up to three orders of magnitude more efficiently than soluble ZA. These activated Vδ2 T cells kill CRC cells and tumor spheroids, and are able to migrate toward CRC cells in a microfluidic system. Notably, ZA-SPNs can also stimulate the proliferation of Vδ2 T cells from the tumor-infiltrating lymphocytes of CRC patients and boost their cytotoxic activity against patients' autologous tumor organoids. These data represent a first step toward the use of nanoformulated ZA for immunotherapy in CRC patients.

Keywords: Vδ2 T cells; zoledronic acid; polymeric nanoconstruct; anti-tumor immunity; colorectal carcinoma

---

1. Introduction

It is well established that the immune system is involved in controlling the growth and expansion of solid tumors, including colorectal carcinomas (CRCs) [1,2]. Tumor-infiltrating lymphocytes (TIL) comprise multiple cell subsets that can either kill tumor cells (effector anti-tumor lymphocytes) or modulate this response (regulatory T cells, Treg) [3,4]. A recent analysis of the overall survival of CRC patients revealed that the presence of intratumoral γδ T cells highly correlates with a significant favorable prognosis [3,4]. These cells are resident in the mucosal-associated lymphoid tissue of the gut epithelium and play a major role in controlling the integrity of the intestinal barrier when facing bacterial infections and pathogenic injuries [5–9]. Γδ T lymphocytes can be activated upon recognition of unprocessed non-peptide small molecules, including phosphoantigens (PA), derived from the mevalonate pathway in tumor cells [10–12]. Different drugs can be used to enhance γδ T cell activation, such as synthetic pyrophosphate-containing compounds [13,14]. Among these, aminobisphosphonates (N-BPs) are known to induce the activation and proliferation of the Vδ2 γδ T cell subset, thus increasing their blood concentration and anti-tumor activity [15–18]. For instance, the N-BP zoledronic acid (ZA) is a chemically stable analogue of inorganic pyrophosphate that inhibits the farnesyl pyrophosphate synthase (FPPS) of the mevalonate pathway and up-regulates isopentenyl pyrophosphate (IPP) accumulation, promoting the preferential growth of anti-tumor Vδ2 T cells in vitro and in vivo [19–21]. This immunostimulating property, together with the direct anti-tumor effects, have paved the way for clinical trials of different N-BPs [22–26]. We have recently reported that epithelial and mesenchymal cells from CRC specimens, upon exposure to ZA, stimulate the expansion of Vδ2 T cells with anti-tumor activity [21]. However, one of the main limitations in using free ZA for the treatment of CRC is its bone tropism. Indeed, N-BPs are used in the therapy of osteoporosis for their ability to reach the bone and activate the osteo-matrix deposition [16,17]. This property is a clear advantage when treating bone metastases of carcinomas or bone marrow tumors like multiple myeloma [16–19]. Nevertheless, the strong N-BPs' concentration in the bone limits the distribution in other districts, such as a neoplastic mass developing in the colon. Furthermore, as with most small molecules, ZA has a rapid blood clearance that also limits its effective use in γδ T cell stimulation [27,28]. Therefore, novel delivery strategies are needed to capitalize on the multifaceted therapeutic properties of ZA. To improve the biodistribution and bioavailability of N-BPs, prodrugs have been proposed [29]. Although these have been shown to trigger the expansion of Vδ2 T cells more efficiently than the corresponding soluble form, these formulations do not warrant a significant reduction in bone tropism.

On the other hand, nanomedicine [30] could represent an ideal tool to enhance the circulation half-life and intra-tumor accumulation of ZA, while preserving its pharmacological features. Moreover, the effective use of nanoparticles for stimulating the immune system response against tumors has been recently demonstrated [31,32].

Nanoparticles (smaller than 200 nm) can exploit the presence of large fenestrations in the tumor vessels, the so-called enhanced permeation and retention effect (EPR), to increase drug accumulation in the neoplastic tissue compared to free drugs [33,34]. Moreover, as the molecules are loaded inside the nanoparticle, drug solubility and stability could be notably improved, preventing degradation by serum proteins. Finally, it is possible to control the release of the drug, hindering early leakage, and its natural accumulation in bone tissue [35–37].

In this work, ZA was reformulated into spherical polymeric nanoparticles (ZA-SPNs) with an aqueous core containing the active molecule, enclosed in a thin polymer matrix and a lipid monolayer. This architecture confers to ZA-SPNs an appearance similar to biological vesicles. These ZA-SPNs enhance the efficiency of ZA in the stimulation of CRC patients' Vδ2 T cells that, in turn, kill autologous tumor organoids, supporting the proposal to use this drug formulation against CRC.

2. Results

2.1. Synthesis and Characterization of ZA-SPNs

In order to enhance tumor accumulation for future in vivo use, ZA was reformulated into nanoparticles. Briefly, spherical polymeric nanoparticles loaded with ZA (ZA-SPNs) were obtained via a double emulsion–evaporation process, modifying the single emulsion protocol that was previously described by Lee et al. [38]. This formulation comprised an aqueous core, entrapping the hydrophilic ZA molecule, confined within a polymer shell and an external lipid monolayer. A schematic representation of a ZA-SPN's architecture is given in Figure 1A. Note that some of the lipids were conjugated with 2 kDa polyethylene glicole (PEG) chains, which limit unspecific absorption of blood proteins and extend the half-life of SPNs in circulation [35]. The ZA-SPNs were spherical in shape (Figure 1B), exhibited a hydrodynamic diameter of ≈170 nm and a polydispersity index (PDI) lower than 0.2, indicating a monodisperse particle population, and a negative ζ-potential of approximately −40 mV, similar to that of biological vesicles (Figure 1C). The nanoparticles were found to be stable at 37 °C for more than

2 weeks, preserving both the size and the monodispersity index (Figure 1D). This should be ascribed to the negative surface ζ-potential that prevented particle aggregation over time. Indeed, the ζ-potential was also stable over the same period of observation (Figure S1A). Note that the geometry and shell core structure of ZA-SPNs make them similar to biological vesicles. The pharmacological properties of ZA-SPNs were analyzed in terms of ZA loading and release. Different input amounts of ZA were considered in formulating the nanoparticles, namely 50, 100, 300, and 800 μg. The best formulation was obtained for an initial input of 300 μg, which resulted in a final ZA concentration of ≈100 μM per batch (Figure 1E) and an encapsulation efficiency, defined as the weight percentage of the encapsulated ZA amount at the end of the process over the initial amount, of ≈10% (Figure S1B). This was identified as the best configuration in that it maximized the ZA loading per batch, thus minimizing the mass of nanoparticles needed to deliver a given amount of ZA. The release of ZA from SPNs is given in Figure 1F, documenting a modest initial burst, corresponding to ≈25% ZA released after 4 h, followed by a sustained release, with more than 60% of ZA still entrapped in the SPNs after 2 days (50 h). Only after about 7 days (150 h) had all loaded ZA been released out of SPNs, as evaluated using high pressure liquid chromatography. This assured that the effects observed further in the experiments were not due to the early release of ZA, but to the one entrapped within the nanoparticles, and were working only after they were internalized.

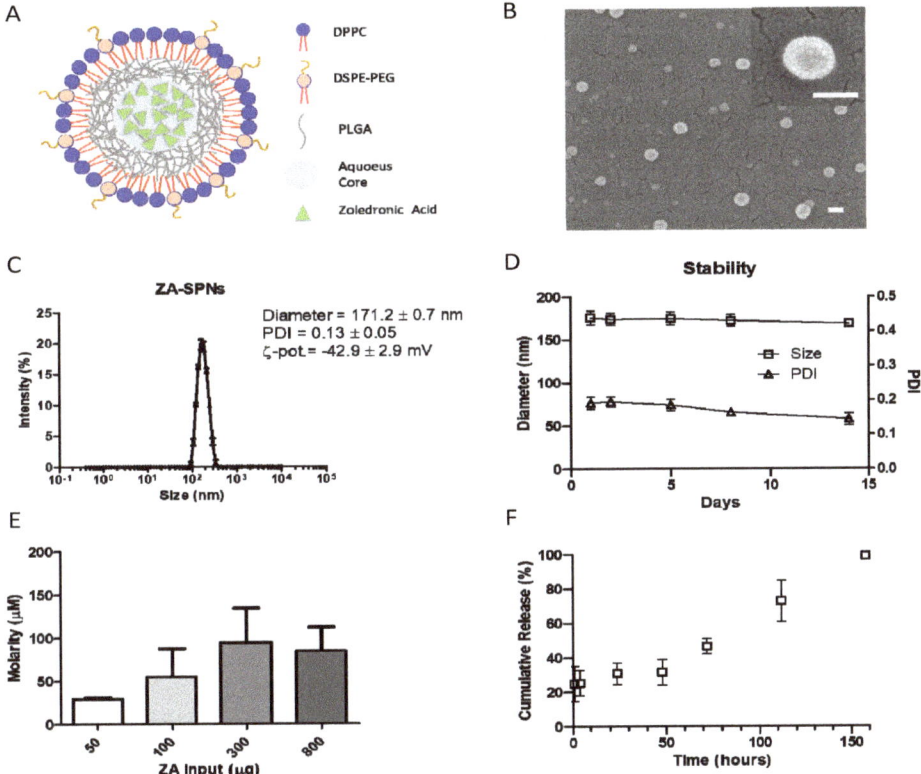

Figure 1. Zoledronic acid–spherical polymeric nanoparticles' (ZA-SPNs) physico-chemical properties. (**A**) Schematic of a ZA-SPN. DPPC: 1,2-dipalmitoyl-sn-glycero-3-phosphocholine; DSPE-PEG: 1,2-distearoyl-sn-glycero-3-phosphoethanolamine-N-[succinyl(polyethylene glycol)-2000]; PLGA: Poly(D,L-lactide-co-glycolic) acid. (**B**) SEM images of ZA-SPNs, showing their spherical shape and dimension (enlargement in the upper-right corner). Scale bar: 100 nm. (**C**) Size distribution of ZA-SPNs;

polydispersity index (PDI) and ζ-potential values are also shown. (**D**) Size and PDI stability over time of ZA-SPNs. (**E**) ZA-SPNs batch average molarity (μM) obtained for different input amounts of ZA in the synthesis process, showing 300 μg as the best input condition. (**F**) Release profile of ZA from ZA-SPNs, showing the minimal ZA loss within the first 48 h. Panels C–F: mean values ± SD.

2.2. ZA-SPNs Induce the Proliferation and Activation of Vδ2 T Lymphocytes

To test the ability of ZA-SPNs to trigger the expansion of Vδ2 T lymphocytes, peripheral blood mononuclear cells (PBMCs) of healthy donors were incubated with decreasing amounts of ZA-SPNs for 24 h. Then, cell cultures were supplemented with exogenous interleukin-2 (IL-2) and replaced with fresh IL-2 every three days. The amount of Vδ2 T cells was evaluated using immunofluorescence with an antibody specific for the Vδ2 chain of the T cell receptor (TCR), followed by florescence activated cell sorter (FACS) analysis, on days 0, 7, 14, and 21. The expansion rate of Vδ2 T lymphocytes were calculated by dividing the number of Vδ2 positive T cells at a given time point by their initial number. At the beginning, the amount of Vδ2 T cells present in the PBMCs was very low (2.5 ± 1.2% n = 10). As documented in Figure 2A (showing one representative experiment out of 10), both ZA-SPNs and soluble ZA were able to induce Vδ2 T cell proliferation, with a maximal expansion on day 21, although the effect of ZA-SPNs was more rapid than that of ZA. The second striking difference was the dose of ZA needed. Indeed, the maximum increase in the percentage of Vδ2 T cells (>90% of the whole cell culture) was reached in 21 days of culture with 0.05 μM of nanoformulated ZA (ZA-SPNs) against 1.0–5.0 μM of soluble ZA, depending on the PBMC donor (Figure 2B, mean ± SD of 10 donors). Specifically, the EC_{50} of ZA-SPNs was 1.355×10^{-3} μM, while that of ZA was 3.685×10^{-1} μM (Table 1). In other words, an almost 300 times higher soluble ZA dose was needed to obtain the same effect as ZA-SPNs. The expansion of Vδ2 T cells in response to ZA-SPNs was remarkable: the number of Vδ2 T cells rose from the initial value of 10^3 to 23×10^6 after 21 days, with a 23,000 fold increase (EC_{50} in Table 1); a similar effect was achieved with soluble ZA, only at two orders of magnitude higher concentrations (Figure 2B).

Due to the remarkable efficiency of ZA-SPNs, we further analyzed whether nanoformulated ZA, at the concentration of 0.05 μM (5×10^{-2} μM reported in Figure 1B), could trigger the proliferation of Vδ2 T cells, even without the addition of exogenous IL-2. Thus, PBMCs were labelled with carboxyfluorescein succinimidyl ester (CFSE), and on day 7 of the culture, proliferating Vδ2 T lymphocytes were identified using a double immunofluorescence assay, as cells with decreasing levels of CFSE content (green fluorescence intensity is inversely proportional to cell division rate) and reactivity with the anti-Vδ2 specific mAb. As shown in Figure 2C, a significant decrease of CFSE content in Vδ2 T cells was detected in ZA-SPNs cultures; in addition, an estimation of cell generations on day 7 showed that Vδ2 T cells incubated with ZA-SPNs had divided six to eight times, whereas cells treated with soluble ZA divided only one to two times (Figure 2D, ModFit LT analysis). At this time point, the percentage of Vδ2 T cells proliferating in ZA-SPN-stimulated cultures ranged from 20 to 35% in four out of five donors (Figure 2E); in contrast, no significant proliferation was detected with soluble ZA (Figure 2C–E) or empty SPNs (Figure 2E). This finding prompted the evaluation of whether ZA-SPNs could trigger the activation of Vδ2 T cells. It is well known that the neo-expression of activation antigens, such as cluster differentiation (CD) 25 and CD69, on T lymphocytes is a marker of cell triggering. Indeed, CD69 can function as a metabolic gatekeeper increasing glucose uptake [39], while CD25 is the α chain of the IL-2 receptor (IL2R) that increases the affinity for IL-2 of the βγ dimers of IL-2R [40]. Both these markers are involved in the growth of T lymphocytes [37,38]. CD25 expression on Vδ2 T cells, upon stimulation with ZA-SPNs, was detectable at 48 h, whereas no induction of CD25 was observed using soluble ZA or empty SPNs (Figure 2F). Neo-expression of the CD69 molecule on Vδ2 T cells was faster (detectable after 24 h) and stronger when PBMCs were incubated with ZA-SPNs compared to soluble ZA (Figure 2G,H). On the other hand, empty SPNs did not induce the expression of CD69 (not shown). Of note, the one donor whose Vδ2 T cells did not respond for proliferation (Figure 2E, light blue circle) also failed to express CD25 upon ZA-SPNs stimulation (Figure 2F, light blue circle). These data indicate that ZA carried by

SPNs can deliver a strong activation signal to Vδ2 T cells, leading to the neo-expression of activation antigens and expansion in the absence of exogenous growth factors.

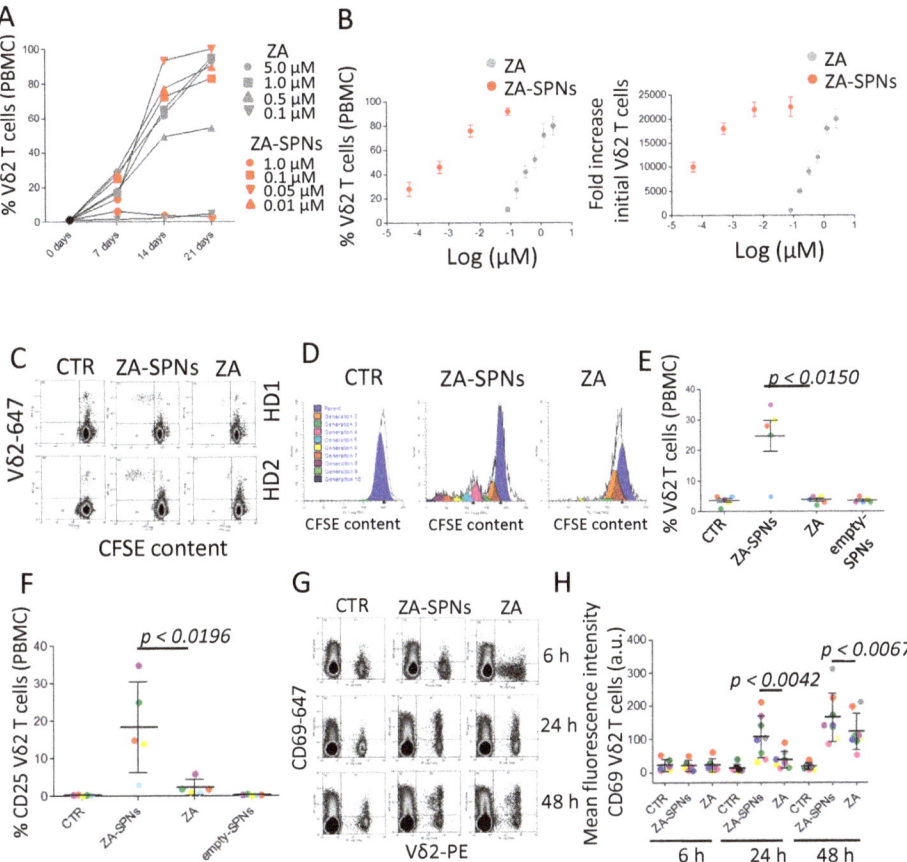

Figure 2. ZA-SPNs stimulated the expansion and activation of Vδ2 T lymphocytes. (**A**) PBMCs were incubated with ZA-SPNs (red) or soluble ZA (gray) at the indicated concentrations (μM) for 24 h before the addition of interleukin (IL)-2. The percentage of Vδ2 T lymphocytes was evaluated at different time points (7, 14, and 21 days) using fluorescence activated cell sorter FACS analysis. One representative experiment out of 10 is shown. (**B**) Left graph: PBMCs were incubated with ZA-SPNs (red) or soluble ZA (gray) (Log μM) for 24 h before the addition of IL-2. The percentage of Vδ2 T lymphocytes (2.5 ± 1.2% in the starting PBMCs) was evaluated on day 21 using FACS analysis. Mean ± SD of 10 healthy PBMCs. Right graph: Results of the left graph expressed as a fold increase of Vδ2 T lymphocytes/mL at the end of the culture compared to the initial number. Mean ± SD of 10 PBMCs. (**C**) Carboxyfluorescein succinimidyl ester (CFSE)-labeled PBMC from two representative donors (HD1, HD2) were cultured without (CTR) or with ZA-SPNs (0.05 μM) or soluble ZA (1 μM), without the addition of exogenous IL-2, and the decrease of CFSE intensity (green) was evaluated on day 7. Vδ2 T cells were identified with the specific mAb (red). (**D**) Vδ2 T cell proliferation, elicited as in (**C**), evaluated using the CFSE decrease in gated Vδ2 T cells with the ModFit LT5.4 software. CTR: CFSE content in cells with the medium alone. Experimental representative of five replicates performed. (**E**) Vδ2 T cell proliferation to ZA-SPNs or ZA or empty SPNs (same nanoparticle amounts as for the ZA-SPNs) elicited as in (**C**) in five donors; mean ± SD also shown. CTR: medium alone. (**F**) Expression of the IL-2Rα chain (CD25) at

48 h using FACS analysis on Vδ2 T lymphocytes in the indicated experimental conditions (CTR: medium alone; ZA-SPNs: 0.05 µM; ZA: 1.0 µM; empty SPNs). Results are expressed as a percentage of CD25$^+$ cells in gated Vδ2 T lymphocytes. (**G,H**) PBMCs cultured as in (C) for 6 h, 24 h, or 48 h were stained with the anti-Vδ2 and anti-CD69 mAbs and analyzed using FACS. Quadrants: lower-left—CD69$^-$Vδ2$^-$ cells; upper-left—CD69$^+$ cells; upper-right—CD69$^+$Vδ2$^+$ cells; lower-left—Vδ2$^+$ cells. In (H), PBMCs stained as in (G) and evaluated as the mean fluorescence intensity (MFI, a.u.) of CD69 expression on Vδ2 T cells at 6 h, 24 h, and 48 h. Mean ± SD from eight donors' PBMCs. CTR: medium alone.

Table 1. In vitro effect (EC$_{50}$) of ZA-SPNs and soluble ZA on Vδ2 T lymphocyte expansion.

Compound	Vδ2 Expansion [a]	Vδ2 Fold Increase [b]	Vδ2 Expansion from T + Mo [c]
ZA-SPNs	1.355×10^{-3}	2.067×10^{-4}	7.096×10^{-4}
Soluble ZA	3.685×10^{-1}	4.2×10^{-1}	5.449×10^{-1}

[a] EC$_{50}$ value expressed as the µM concentration needed to reach 50% of the maximal percentage of Vδ2 T cells grown in culture starting from PBMCs. [b] EC$_{50}$ value expressed as the µM concentration needed to reach 50% of maximal fold increase in Vδ2 T cell absolute number versus the initial Vδ2 T cell number. [c] EC$_{50}$ value expressed as the µM concentration needed to reach 50% of the maximal percentage of Vδ2 T cells grown in culture starting from 10^5 purified T lymphocytes with 10^3 monocytes (Mo) added (T:Mo ratio 1:100). Results are the average of three replicates with a standard deviation of <10%.

2.3. ZA-SPNs Mediated Vδ2 T Cell Expansion Is Associated with Isopentenyl-Pyrophosphate (IPP) Production

It is well established that monocytes (Mo) are the main peripheral blood cell population responsible for the N-BP-mediated triggering of Vδ2 T cells [6,20,21]. This is due to a monocyte's ability to efficiently accumulate IPP when exposed to N-BPs, including ZA [6,20]. As such, we examined whether ZA-SPNs could stimulate Vδ2 T cell expansion from highly purified T lymphocytes co-cultured with Mo and analyzed after 21 days. Different T cell to monocyte (T:Mo) ratios were considered, ranging from 10:1 to 1000:1. ZA-SPNs triggered the optimal proliferation of Vδ2 T cells at the T:Mo ratio of 10:1–100:1 (10^5 T vs. 10^3–10^4 Mo) (Figure 3A). Notably, the EC$_{50}$ for ZA-SPNs was 5.644×10^{-4} µM and 3.527×10^{-1} µM for ZA using 10^4 Mo, which was more than 600-fold higher compared to ZA-SPNs (Figure 3A vs. Figure 3B). With 10^3 Mo, EC$_{50}$ became 7.096×10^{-4} µM and 5.449×10^{-1} µM for ZA-SPNs and ZA, respectively; in this case, the difference was larger than 700 times in favor of ZA-SPNs (Table 1 and Figure 3A vs. Figure 3B). This demonstrated that ZA-SPNs efficiently stimulated Vδ2 T cell proliferation in the presence of very few Mo, with a strong gain in EC$_{50}$. Furthermore, it was assessed whether ZA-SPNs could stimulate the production of IPP, which is considered the product responsible for ZA-mediated effects [10–12,21]. Toward this aim, highly purified peripheral Mo were incubated with either ZA-SPNs (0.5 µM for 10^6 cells needed for IPP evaluation) or soluble ZA (0.5 µM for comparison with ZA-SPNs at the same concentration) for 24 h. The IPP concentration was determined using high performance liquid chromatography/time of flight-mass spectrometry (HPLC/TOF-MS). ZA-SPNs induced a twofold higher IPP production than soluble ZA, with a mean value of 3 pM for ZA-SPNs against 1.5 pM for ZA in three out of four Mo donors (Figure 3C). Then, we tested whether IPP could also be produced by CRC cell lines in response to ZA-SPNs. Indeed, this event is needed to trigger Vδ2-T-cell-mediated recognition and killing [10–12]. For this experiment, LS180 and SW620 were chosen, since we reported that the two cell lines produce high or low amounts, respectively, of IPP when stimulated with soluble ZA [21]. LS180 produced about 30% more IPP in response to 0.5 µM ZA-SPNs compared to soluble ZA (14.12 pM vs. 9.92 pM), while SW620 IPP production to 0.5 µM ZA-SPNs was superimposable (≈3 pM) with that obtained with soluble ZA at the same dose (Figure 3D,E). A small but detectable IPP production was also observed in LS180 using ZA-SPNs at a 0.05 µM concentration (5 pM). Empty SPNs did not evoke the production of IPP (<1 pM, Figure 3D,E).

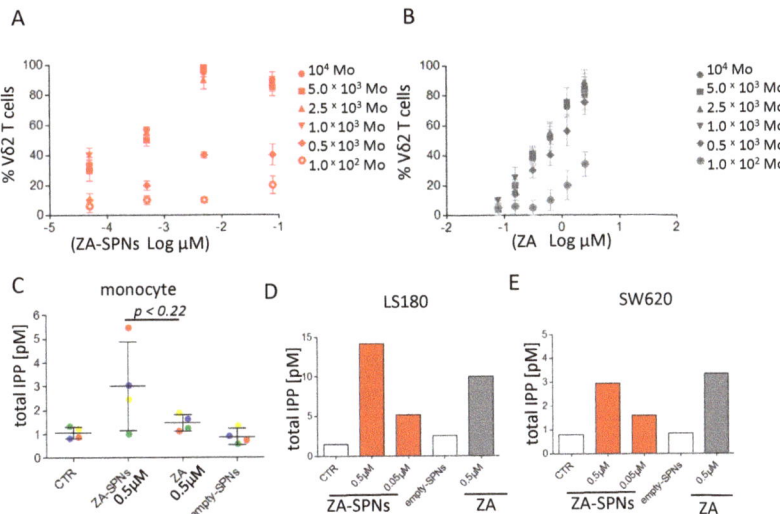

Figure 3. Monocyte requirement for Vδ2 T cell expansion and isopentenyl pyrophosphate (IPP) production in response to ZA-SPNs or ZA. (**A,B**) A total of 10^5 purified T lymphocytes were cultured with different amounts of autologous purified monocytes (Mo), as indicated, in the presence of ZA-SPNs (A) or soluble ZA (B) at different concentrations for 21 days. The percentage of Vδ2 T cells present in culture was evaluated using indirect immunofluorescence and FACS analysis; results are the mean ± SD of T cell populations from six healthy donors. (**C**) A total of 10^6 Mo were incubated for 24 h without (CTR) or with 0.5 μM ZA-SPNs or with 0.5 μM soluble ZA or with empty SPNs, and the amount of IPP produced (pM) was evaluated using high performance liquid chromatography/time of flight-mass spectrometry HPLC/TOF-MS. Colors indicate the four Mo donors. The mean ± SD for each condition is also shown. (**D,E**) A total of 5×10^5 LS180 or SW620 CRC cells were incubated for 24 h with 0.05 or 0.5 μM ZA-SPNs or 0.5 μM soluble ZA, and IPP production was evaluated as in panel (C). Results are shown as pmol of IPP extracted by acetonitrile/total protein content in each cell lysate analyzed using HPLC/TOF-MS. One representative experiment of two performed is shown.

2.4. CRC Cell Death Induced by Vδ2 T Lymphocytes Stimulated with ZA-SPNs

At first, the interaction of Vδ2 T lymphocytes with tumor cells challenged with ZA-SPNs was qualitatively analyzed through confocal microscopy and SEM imaging. SW620 CRC cells were incubated with Cy5-labeled ZA-SPNs to prove that nanoparticles could be internalized by tumor cells. Figure 4A shows that Cy5-ZA-SPNs (orange, arrows) accumulated in CRC cells, evidenced with the anti-epithelial cell adhesion molecule (EPCAM) mAb (red), in agreement with the notion that nanoparticles of this size are rapidly (by 4 h) engulfed by any cell, even if not professional phagocytes [41–43]. Then, Vδ2 T cells were added to CRCs engulfed with ZA-SPNs for a short incubation time (further 4 h), and their ability to interact with CRC cells was evaluated. Figure 4B shows an intimate contact between Vδ2 T cells, identified using the specific anti-Vδ2 mAb (green) and CRC (red); arrows indicate the engulfed Cy5-ZA-SPNs. Moreover, Vδ2 T cells also appeared clustered on CRCs, as it can be better appreciated in the representative SEM image (Figure 4C) where several Vδ2 T cells, false-colored in pink, surround and make contact with a much larger cancer cell.

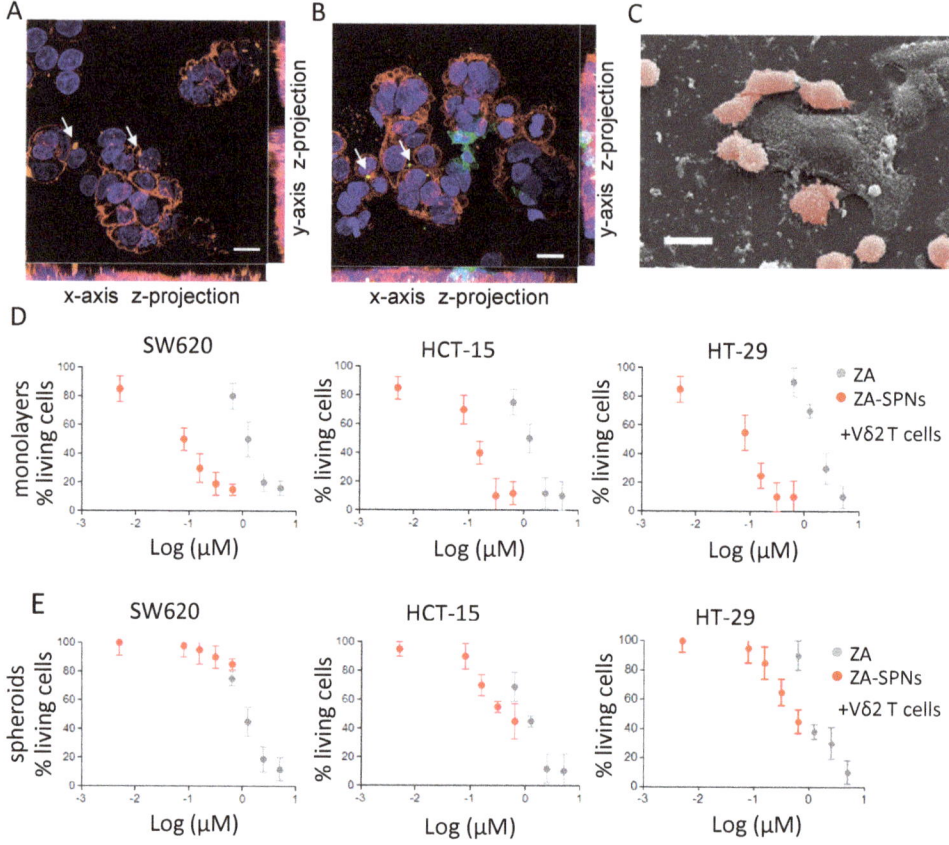

Figure 4. ZA-SPNs triggered the cytotoxicity of colorectal carcinoma (CRC) cell lines and spheroids using Vδ2 T cells. (**A**) Representative confocal microscopy image showing Cy5-conjugated ZA-SPNs' (orange, arrows) internalization in CRC cells, identified using the anti-EPCAM mAb and Alexafluor555 isotype-specific goat antimouse (GAM) (red). Blue: nuclei diamidino phenylindole (DAPI) staining. Scale bar: 10 μm. (**B**) Vδ2 T cells identified using the specific anti-Vδ2 mAb and Alexafluor488-anti-isotype GAM (green) interacting with CRC (EPCAM followed by Alexafluor555 GAM, red) previously exposed (24 h) to ZA-SPNs (white arrows). Blue: DAPI nuclear staining. Scale bar: 10 μm. (**C**) SEM images of a similar experiment in which Vδ2 T cells (pink) had surrounded a CRC (gray). Scale bar: 20 μm. (**D**) The CRC cell lines SW620, HCT-15, and HT-29 were cultured adherent in flat bottomed plates with ZA-SPNs (red) or with soluble ZA (gray) at different concentrations and challenged with activated Vδ2 T cells from healthy donors at the effector:target (E:T) ratio of 3:1 for 48 h. Then, viability was assessed using a crystal violet assay. Data is expressed as a percentage of living cells as compared to cells cultured in medium alone, are the mean ± SD of three independent experiments of six different replicates for each condition. (**E**) Spheroids of the CRC cell lines SW620, HCT-15, and HT-29 at day 5 were incubated with activated Vδ2 T cells at the E:T ratio of 3:1 and either ZA-SPNs (red) or soluble ZA (gray) at the indicated concentrations for 48 h. Spheroid cell viability was assessed using crystal violet assay modified as described in Varesano et al. [45]. Data are the mean ± SD of three independent experiments of six replicates for each condition.

Having shown that ZA-SPNs can be metabolized by CRC cells, and that Vδ2 T lymphocytes bind to ZA-SPN-treated CRC, we further analyzed whether these events resulted in an anti-tumor effect. Toward this aim, Vδ2 T lymphocytes were added to CRC cell lines exposed to ZA-SPNs at an effector:target (E:T) ratio of 3:1 to for allow the detection of the effect elicited by the nanoformulated ZA. Indeed, at this E:T ratio, the cytotoxic activity of Vδ2 T cells to the three CRC cell lines tested (SW620, HCT-15, and HT-29), evaluated as a reduction of living cells by the crystal violet assay, was almost negligible (less than 10%; see the cell viability ranging from 90 to 100% with the lowest ZA-SPNs concentrations in Figure 4D). The percentage of living CRC cells was strongly reduced in the presence of Vδ2 T cells when serial dilutions of ZA-SPNs were added to the lymphocyte–CRC cell co-cultures (Figure 4D). The ZA-SPNs' EC_{50} of cytotoxic activity was again lower (by 10 to 50 times) than that found for soluble ZA (Table 2). Both ZA-SPNs and ZA, in the absence of Vδ2 T cells, reduced the percentage of living adherent SW620 and HT-29 cells to some extent; this effect was more evident on HCT-15 (Figure S2A), but was always lower than that detected in the presence of Vδ2 T lymphocytes (EC_{50} 0.5 μM in Figure S2A vs. 0.1 μM depicted in Figure 4A and reported in Table 2).

Table 2. In vitro effect (EC_{50}) of ZA-SPNs and soluble ZA on the Vδ2-mediated cytotoxicity of CRC cells and spheroids.

Compound	SW620		HCT-15		HT-29	
	Adh [a]	Sph [b]	Adh	Sph	Adh	Sph
ZA-SPNs	8×10^{-2}	$>6 \times 10^{-1}$	1×10^{-1}	5×10^{-1}	1×10^{-1}	5×10^{-1}
ZA	1.2	1.0	1.0	1.1	1.7	1.0

[a] The indicated CRC cell lines were cultured adherent to plates and used as targets (Adh). [b] CRC cell lines were used as spheroid targets (Sph) in ultra-low attachment plates. The EC_{50} value is expressed as the micromolar concentration needed to reach 50% of the maximal cytotoxic effect evaluated calculating the percentage of non-living cells. Results are the average of three determinations with a standard deviation of <10%.

Since tumor cells grow in vivo as tridimensional (3D) structures, tumor spheroids have been used to mimic the initial stage of neoplastic growth in vitro [44,45]. Thus, we assessed whether Vδ2-T-cell-mediated killing of such structures could be stimulated by ZA-SPNs. We analyzed the tumor spheroids obtained after culturing the representative three CRC cells lines SW620, HCT-15, and HT-29 in ultra-low attachment plates, as described in Varesano et al. [45]. In these experimental conditions, spheroids from 50 to 250 μm in diameter can be obtained [45]. CRC tumor spheroids were able to engulf ZA-SPNs within 24 h of exposure (Figure S3A) and were killed by Vδ2 T cells; the ZA-SPNs EC_{50} was superimposable or lower than that of ZA for HCT-15 and HT-29 cell lines, while for SW620, the EC_{50} of ZA-SPNs was higher (Figure 4E and Table 2). A possible explanation for the discordant effect of ZA-SPNs and soluble ZA on SW620 as adherent cells or spheroids could be related to the different nanoparticle processing and/or mevalonate metabolism that follows the ZA-SPNs' entry, despite the detectable engulfment. The direct effect of ZA-SPNs on CRC cells growing adherent in conventional experimental conditions or cultured as spheroids was also evaluated using a crystal violet assay. Both ZA-SPNs and soluble ZA reduced the number of living cells by 30% when used on SW620 and HT-29 CRC cell monolayers, while the HCT-15 cell line was more sensitive (Figure S2A). On the other hand, SW620 and HT-29 spheroids were not directly affected by ZA-SPNs nor by soluble ZA at the concentrations used, while the effect on HCT-15 spheroids was detected only with ZA (Figure S2B). These findings were confirmed even after 96 h of incubation (not shown).

2.5. ZA-SPNs Elicited Vδ2 T Cell Proliferation from CRC Patients and the Killing of Autologous Tumor Organoids

To plan a potential therapeutic use of nanoformulated ZA, it is essential to prove that ZA-SPNs are actually able to trigger Vδ2 T cells from CRC patients' samples. Toward this aim, first, the ability of ZA-SPNs to expand Vδ2 T cells, either from peripheral blood or from tumor biopsies of CRC patients, was assessed; then, the cytotoxic potential of these cells from patients' PBMCs was quantified against CRC tumor cell lines or autologous tumor cells growing in vitro as colon mucosa organoids. A ZA-SPNs dose of 0.05 μM was chosen since it was the most effective on healthy donors' PBMCs (see Figure 1A,B). Figure 5A shows that expansion of Vδ2 T cells from the PBMCs of CRC patients was obtained with

0.05 µM ZA-SPNs. This expansion occurred in all samples from CRC patients (n = 20), and in 14 out of 20 samples reached ≈90% after 14 days; however, a 20-fold higher concentration (1.0 µM) of soluble ZA relative to the ZA-SPN concentration was needed to achieve this effect (Figure 5A). The absolute Vδ2 T cell numbers are reported in Figure S4. Of note, ZA-SPNs were able to expand tumor-infiltrating Vδ2 T cells (Table S1 reports the pathological features of these patients) when added to mononuclear cells isolated from the tumor (Figure 5B); the percentage of Vδ2 T cells obtained ranged from 10 to 90% in 5 out of 10 cases. This result was quite remarkable since in the bioptic cell suspensions, the starting amount of Vδ2 T cells was mostly lower than 0.1% and the $CD45^+$ leukocytes, containing infiltrating lymphocytes, were always less than 35% of the total cells (range 3–32% n = 10), as we reported elsewhere [21,44,45]. In addition, the presence of monocytes in these cell suspensions was almost negligible (range 0.02–0.5%, not shown) [21,46]. To define whether ZA-SPN-stimulated Vδ2 T cells from patients' PBMCs belonged to a population of effector cells, we analyzed the expression of CD27 and CD45RA that was reported to define different lymphocyte subsets. In particular, naïve (N) T cells bear CD27 and CD45RA molecules, as well as central memory (CM) T lymphocytes; express only CD27; effector memory (EM) T cells are double negative; and terminal differentiated memory cells (TEMRA) are surface CD45RA positive [45,47]. We reported that ZA can drive the expansion of Vδ2 T cells, showing the characteristics of effector memory (EM) T lymphocytes (i.e., absence of CD27 and CD45RA) [48]. As shown in Figure S5, also ZA-SPNs-stimulated Vδ2 T lymphocytes displayed an EM/TEMRA ($CD27^-CD45RA^-/CD27^-CD45RA^+$) phenotype.

Thus, Vδ2 T effector cells obtained upon ZA-SPNs stimulation from the PBMCs of three CRC patients were tested for their anti-tumor cytotoxic activity against the CRC cell lines HCT-15 and HT-29, either as adherent monolayers (Figure 5C) or as spheroids (Figure 5D), exposed to ZA-SPNs. The E:T ratio chosen was again 3:1 to emphasize the effect due to the nanoformulated ZA taken up by tumor cells. Indeed, at this E:T ratio, the percentage of living tumor cells upon incubation with Vδ2 T cells was still more than 80% for HCT-15 and ≈70% for HT-29 (Figure 5C,D). When the target tumor cells or spheroids were challenged with 0.05 µM ZA-SPNs, the cytotoxic effect of Vδ2 T effector cells was much more evident, as living tumor cells were less than 50% in all instances, decreasing by up to 20% for adherent HT-29 or HCT-15 spheroids (Figure 5C,D).

To test whether ZA-SPNs-expanded Vδ2 effector T lymphocytes could kill tumor cells in an autologous setting, organoids were derived from specimens of five CRC patients (listed in Table S1) in serum-free controlled culture conditions. Figure S6A shows these organoids, with variable sizes (perimeters and areas in Figure S6B), and expressing the epithelial marker EPCAM (Figure S6C). In particular, OMCR18-006TK organoids display a morphology typical of mucinous tumors, according to the histopathological diagnosis (Table S1). We first demonstrated the ability of organoids to engulf ZA-SPNs within 24 h of exposure (Figure S3B). Then, organoids, labeled with the green fluorescent probe calcein-acetoxy methyl ester (AM) and seeded in Geltrex domes, were exposed to ZA-SPNs (0.05, 0.1, 0.5 µM) and cultured with the corresponding autologous ZA-SPN-expanded Vδ2 T lymphocytes for 6 days to allow the effector cells to enter the domes and reach the organoids. Figure 5E shows a representative co-culture with Vδ2 T cells invading some organoids, where one is evident in subpanel a, and one appears almost destroyed in b; this is also shown with Z-stack images in Figure S7. The cytotoxic effect of Vδ2 T cells was evaluated by measuring the decrease in green fluorescence, as previously reported by Chung et al. [49]. Autologous ZA-expanded Vδ2 T cells decreased the vitality of tumor organoids by 10–30%; this cytotoxic effect was further increased when ZA-SPNs were added during the cytolytic assay. Indeed, in the presence of 0.05 µM ZA-SPNs, Vδ2 T cells could reduce the organoid viability by 50% (Figure 5F). In turn, 10- to 50-fold higher concentrations of soluble ZA were needed to obtain superimposable effects with soluble ZA (Figure 5F). Altogether, these results are the experimental proof that ZA-SPNs can efficiently trigger the growth and function of Vδ2 anti-tumor effector T cells from CRC patients.

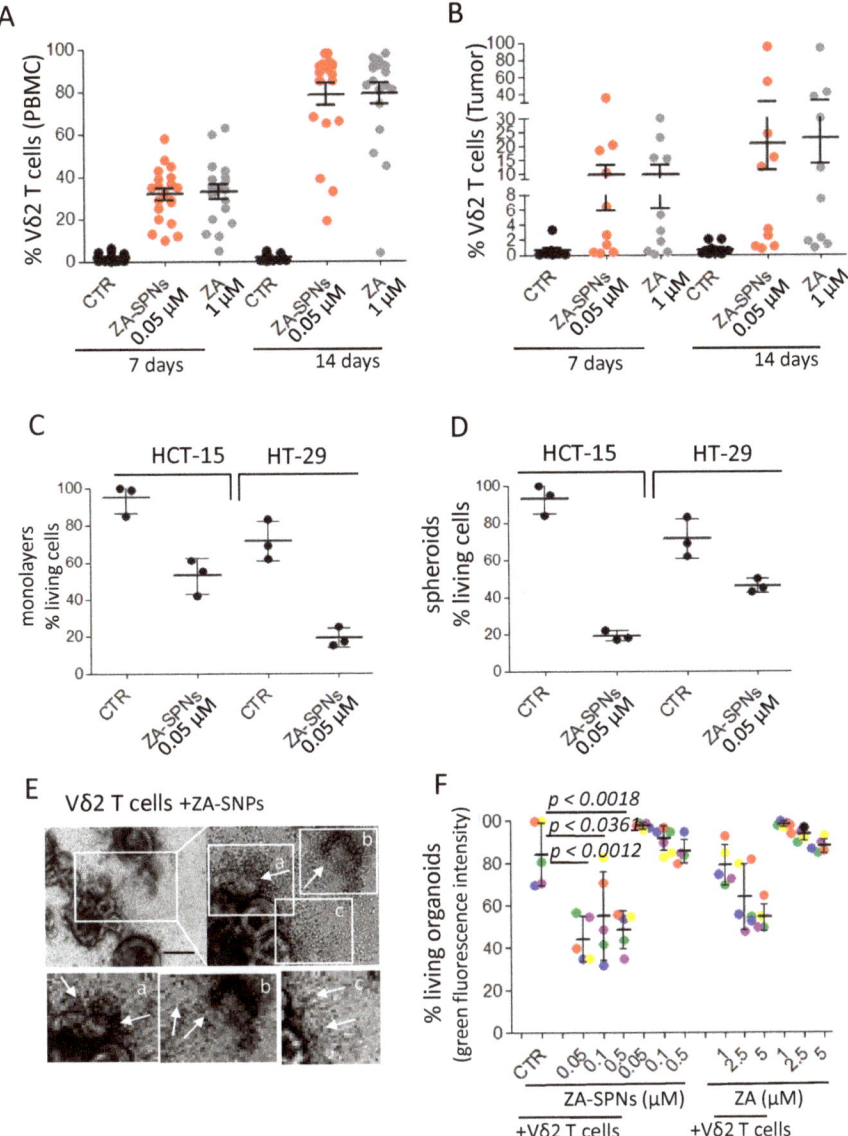

Figure 5. ZA-SPNs triggered the expansion of CRC patients' Vδ2 T lymphocytes to be able to kill CRC spheroids and autologous organoids. (**A**) PBMC from CRC patients were cultured with ZA-SPNs (0.05 µM) or soluble ZA (1.0 µM) and 10 ng/mL (30 IU/mL) IL-2. The percentage of Vδ2 T lymphocytes was evaluated using FACS analysis on days 7 and 14. Vδ2 T cells in the starting PBMCs: 1.4 ± 1.6%, mean ± SD of 20 patients. (**B**) Tumor cell suspensions were cultured as in (A), and Vδ2 T lymphocyte expansion was determined on days 7 and 14. Results are expressed as percentages of Vδ2 T lymphocytes as mean ± SD of 10 patients' specimens. Vδ2 T cells in the starting tumor-derived populations: 0.04 ± 0.05% (mean ± SD of 10 patients). (**C,D**) HCT-15 or HT-29 as adherent cells (C) or spheroids (D) were incubated with ZA-SPN-expanded Vδ2 T cells obtained from the PBMCs of three

CRC patients. ZA-SPNs (0.05 µM) were further added or not (CTR) at the onset of the 48 h assay. E:T ratio was 3:1. Data expressed as a percentage of living CRC cells (crystal violet staining) as mean ± SD of six replicates/condition in three independent experiments. (**E**) Representative co-cultures of ZA-SPN-expanded Vδ2 effector T cells and the autologous OMCR-016TK organoids exposed to ZA-SPN. Upper-left image: 100×. Scale bar: 100 µm. Upper-right image: 200×. Lower panels: enlargements of quadrants a, b, and c in the upper-right panel. Asterisks in each panel: organoids. Arrows in each panel: Vδ2 T cells invading organoids (c, one almost destroyed in b) or in their neighborhood (c). (**F**) Organoids from five patients (OMCR18-006TK, green; OMCR18-006TK, red; OMCR19-006TK, blue; OMCR19-009TK, yellow; OMCR19-016TK, purple) were labeled with calcein-acteoxy methyl ester (AM) and challenged with autologous ZA-SPN-expanded Vδ2 T cells for 6 days without ZA-SPNs (CTR) or in the presence of ZA-SPNs or soluble ZA at the indicated concentrations. E:T ratio was 3:1. Fluorescence of each culture well was quantified using spectrofluorometry and compared to that of organoid cultures considered to be 100%. Data expressed as a percentage of green fluorescence as mean ± SD of three independent experiments with six replicates/condition. The *p*-values of ZA-SPNs versus CTR are shown.

2.6. ZA-SPNs-Vδ2 T Lymphocytes Transendothelial Migration Toward CRC Tumor Cells in a Microfluidic System

To test the ability of ZA-SPN-expanded Vδ2 T cells (i.e., Vδ2 T lymphocytes obtained from PBMCs upon stimulation with ZA-SPNs and further culture for 21 days) to extravasate and reach CRC cells, a double-channel microfluidic chip was used [50]. This device comprised a vascular compartment (VC), uniformly coated with human umbilical vascular endothelial cells (HUVECs), and an extravascular compartment (EC), hosting a Matrigel matrix with CRC cells. The two compartments were separated by an array of micropillars, equally spaced by 3 µm (Figure 6A). HUVECs were seeded and also grew on the micropillars area, realizing an authentic vascular bed (Figure 6A,B showing the 3D reconstruction). By using this microfluidic system, the dynamics of ZA-SPN-expanded Vδ2 T cells infused into the VC was monitored over time. In the time-lapse experiments, these Vδ2 T cells fluxed into the VC (visible in blue due to the nuclear staining) and were able to cross HUVEC monolayer (red, CM-Dil membrane staining), and through the array of pillars, infiltrate the Matrigel matrix and reach the tumor cells (green, GFP$^+$) (Figure 6C).

The fluorescence intensity of the Vδ2 T cell nuclear staining was measured after 12 and 24 h in the VC and EC using the Image J software, quantifying the percentage increase over time in different regions of interest (ROIs) set for each channel (Figure 6D). Extravascular Vδ2 T cell accumulation was detectable within 24 h, with a fluorescence increase of about 300% in EC (Figure 6D, black histograms). While transported by the flow into the VC, the fluorescence increased up to 140 and 190% within the first 12 and 24 h of observation, respectively, documenting the interaction of Vδ2 T cells with endothelial cells (HUVECs) during the migration process (Figure 6D, white histograms). This interaction was also visible in confocal images of a separate experiment, in which Vδ2 T cells (CM-Dil stained, red) appeared in part in contact with HUVEC (green, phalloidin staining F-actin) in the VC and in part adherent to the CRC in the EC (green, phalloidin staining F-actin); notably, CRC cells interacting with Vδ2 T lymphocytes displayed a dim fluorescence and an altered actin distribution (Figure 6E). In conclusion, Vδ2 T cells grown upon a ZA-SPN stimulation, and tested in the microfluidic system, displayed the ability to extravasate and interact with tumor cells in the EC.

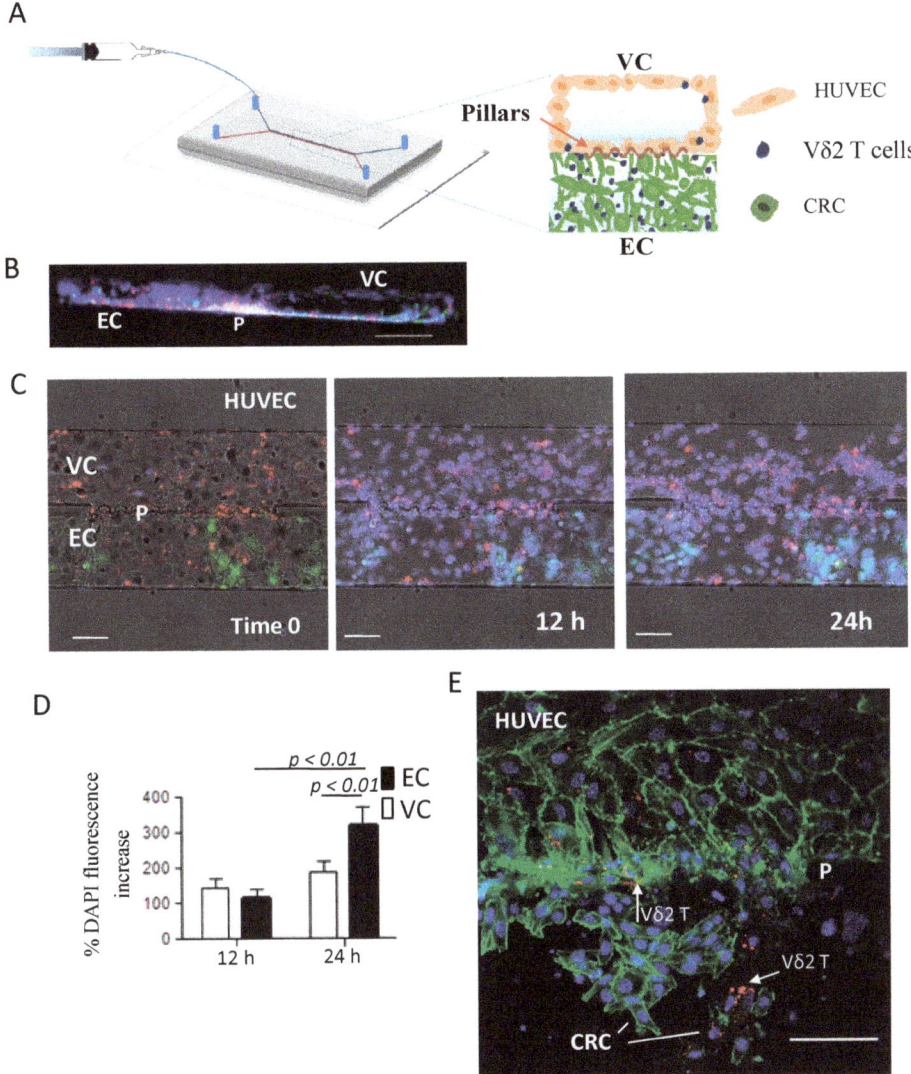

Figure 6. Transendothelial migration of ZA-SPN-expanded Vδ2 T lymphocytes toward CRC cells in a microfluidic system. (**A**) Double-chamber microfluidic chip [50] composed of a vascular compartment (VC), uniformly coated with human umbilical vascular endothelial cells (HUVECs), and an extravascular compartment (EC), hosting a Matrigel matrix with CRC cells. The two compartments were separated by an array of micropillars, equally spaced by 3 µm. ZA-SPN-expanded Vδ2 T cells were infused through the inlet into the VC, and their extravasation was mainly analyzed around the pillar area. (**B**) 3D reconstruction (lateral view) of the double channel microfluidic chip, showing on the right the HUVECs covering all of the channel (green/blue, phalloidin/DAPI) to mimic a complete vessel (VC); on the left, tumor cells (CRC, nuclear blue staining) in the EC. P: micropillar zone. Some Vδ2 T cells stained with CM-Dil (red) were visible in both compartments. Scale bar: 100 µm. (**C**) Time-lapse images following the localization of ZA-SPN-activated Vδ2 T lymphocytes before (time 0) and after (12 h, 24 h) injection into the VC. HUVEC membranes were stained using CM-Dil (red) and Vδ2 T cell

nuclei were stained by DAPI (blue). EC: extravascular channel populated with GFP⁺ SW480 CRC cells (green). P: micropillars. Scale bar: 100 μm. (**D**) Quantification (Image J software) of DAPI fluorescence intensity increase measured at 12 h and 24 h compared to time 0 (addition of Vδ2 T cells) in the VC (white columns) or the EC (black columns). Data expressed as a percentage of fluorescence increase, compared to time 0; mean ± SE. The *p*-values are shown. (**E**) Representative confocal image (top view) showing Vδ2 T cells (red, CM-Dil, white arrows), close to HUVECs in the VC, and surrounding CRC cells in the EC. Phalloidin (green) stained the F-actin filaments to show the organization of HUVECs; actin filaments were also visible in the CRC. DAPI (blue) stained both the HUVEC and CRC nuclei. P: micropillar zone. Scale bar: 100 μm.

3. Discussion

A major challenge in the hypothetical use of N-BPs as stimulators of anti-tumor Vδ2 T lymphocytes in solid cancers is related to the bone tropism of these compounds [16,17]. The encapsulation of ZA into spherical polymeric nanoparticles (ZA-SPNs), with a characteristic size of ≈200 nm, appears to be an effective solution to this hindrance. Indeed, nanoparticles up to a few hundreds of nanometers in diameter tend to passively accumulate in tumor tissues, following the so-called enhanced permeability and retention (EPR) effect [30,33,34]. This effect warrants the release of the drug into the tumor, preventing its early leakage and its natural accumulation in bone tissue.

In this work, we have demonstrated that SPNs can efficiently load ZA in such a way that large-scale production for clinical translation could be possible and that the payload was stably retained within its aqueous core for up to approximately one week. The architecture of ZA-SPNs, with an aqueous core confined within a lipid monolayer, resemble that of natural vesicles, likely favoring their penetration into cells. This would cause a progressive release of ZA inside tumor cells, leading to prompt activation of the mevalonate pathway responsible for IPP production [10], which eventually induces the activation and proliferation of Vδ2 T lymphocytes with anti-cancer functions.

Interestingly, not only do ZA-SPNs stimulate Vδ2 T cells at a concentration about 300-fold lower compared to soluble ZA, but can also, and unexpectedly, trigger their proliferation without exogenous IL-2, which is usually needed for T cells expansion. Possibly, ZA-SPNs induce a stronger signal than soluble ZA onto Vδ2 T cells, and in this way, promote the expression of activation molecules, such as the metabolic gatekeeper CD69 and the α-chain of the IL-2 receptor (CD25). Indeed, although not shown, a small fraction (≈17%) of Vδ2 T lymphocytes could actually express intracytoplasmic IL-2 upon stimulation with ZA-SPNs. Thus, ZA-SPNs could sensitize Vδ2 T cells to cytokines and growth factors present in the extracellular milieu. Yet, the underlying mechanism would have to be more precisely characterized in further studies.

Of note, ZA-SPNs were able to enhance the proliferation of Vδ2 T lymphocytes derived from the peripheral blood or tumor specimens of CRC patients. Based on the EC_{50}, the efficiency of ZA-SPNs to expand Vδ2 T lymphocytes was 2 to 3 orders of magnitude higher than that of soluble ZA. These Vδ2 T lymphocytes behaved as effector cells, exerting a strong cytolytic activity against CRC tumor cells exposed to ZA-SPNs. This was tested in two different 3D models, namely tumor spheroids and patient-derived organoids, to mimic cancer cell growth in vivo more closely. Indeed, there is increasing evidence that both tumor development and response to therapy in humans are not always predictable in animals [51,52]. Recently, zoledronic-acid-containing nanoparticles have been reported to localize into extra-skeletal tumors in a murine model, thus avoiding bone sequestration of such drug formulation [53]. This would also reinforce the proposal to use ZA-SPNs in therapeutic schemes aimed to activate an anti-cancer immune response, mainly through the activation of γδ T lymphocytes. Regrettably, murine cancer models present several limitations, considering that the two major γδ T cell subsets do not have orthologues in mice [54,55], and that even syngeneic mice would not be adequate as the response to N-BPs of γδ T cells is different in rodents than in humans [6,8]. On the other hand, 3D culture systems, including spheroids and organoids, have been validated as preclinical models to overcome these inconveniences by the present authors and others [44,45,56,57].

In a first set of 3D experiments, spheroids with diameters ranging from 50 to 250 μm were considered to mimic tumors at early stages. In this case, ZA-SPNs could trigger Vδ2 T lymphocyte-mediated cytotoxicity with different efficiencies depending on the used cell line. It is of note that this difference among the used CRC cell lines was not evident on the cell monolayers. This may have been due to the spatial heterogeneity in the IPP production by CRC cells because of the diverse depths of penetration of the drug within the 3D cell aggregates. The cell line SW620 generates compact spheroids that, although capable of ZA-SPNs engulfment, may limit drug penetration compared to HCT-15 and HT-29 spheroids [45]. Another explanation is based on the different mevalonate metabolism and IPP production that follows ZA-SPNs' entry; these features might be constitutive of each cell line or vary depending on the 3D structure acquired during tumor growth. Interestingly, the cytotoxic efficiency of ZA-SPNs was remarkable when patients' organoids were exposed to autologous Vδ2 T cells that had expanded upon stimulation with ZA-SPNs. This demonstrated the potential therapeutic relevance of ZA-SPNs in CRC patients, suggesting that 3D culture systems may have specific features influencing the treatment outcome. Although validated using reliable pre-clinical models [44,56,57], both spheroids and organoids have some limitations, including the lack of different cellular components of the tumor microenvironment. It should be recalled that effector lymphocytes must exert their anti-tumor activities in a microenvironment populated by suppressive cells, such as mesenchymal stromal cells (MSC), regulatory T lymphocytes (Treg), and myeloid derived suppressor cells (MDSC) [46,58].

Nevertheless, the present authors and others have previously reported that microenvironment immunosuppression can be reverted using ZA or phosphoantigens, resulting in Vδ2 T cell activation [48,59]. It is still to be established whether ZA-SPNs can affect the regulatory functions of Treg and MDSC. However, it is likely that ZA-SPNs could influence the function of leukocytes since a remarkable Vδ2 T cell stimulation was observed in the presence of a few monocytes. This should most likely be ascribed to the enhancement of IPP production by these cells.

Another property of ZA-SPN stimulation was that of enhancing the ability of Vδ2 T cells to sense tumor cells. Specifically, in a microfluidic chip, ZA-SPN-expanded Vδ2 T cells were able to extravasate and migrate toward tumor cells, overcoming the vascular barrier and the extracellular matrix. These findings indicate that Vδ2 T cells, after being activated by ZA-SPNs, could reach tumor cells and recirculate, even if triggered away from the tumor site.

4. Materials and Methods

4.1. Reagents

Zoledronic acid (ZA) was purchased from Selleckchem (Aurogene, Rome, Italy). Poly(D,L-lactide-co-glycolic) acid (PLGA, 50:50, CarboxyTerminated, molecular weight ≈ 60 kDa) was purchased from Sigma-Aldrich (St. Louis, MO, USA). 1,2-dipalmitoyl-sn-glycero-3-phosphocholine (DPPC), 1,2-distearoyl-sn-glycero-3-phosphoethanolamine-N-[succinyl(polyethylene glycol)-2000] (DSPE-PEG), and 1,2-distearoyl-sn-glycero-3-phosphoethanolamine (DSPE) were obtained from AvantiPolar Lipids (Alabaster, AL, USA). Analytical grade dimethyl sulfoxide (DMSO), acetonitrile, chloroform, absolute ethanol, dipotassium hydrogen phosphate anhydrous, and tetra butyl ammonium Bi-sulphateand 5(6) carboxyfluoresceindiacetate N-succinimidylester (CFSE) were purchased from Sigma-Aldrich (Milan, Italy). RPMI-1640 and FBS (One Shot™ Fetal Bovine Serum) were obtained from Gibco (Thermo Fisher Scientific, Monza, Italy). DMEM-F12,L-Glutamine, and penicillin/streptomycin (BioWhittaker® Reagents) were purchased from Lonza (Basel, Switzerland). Epidermal growth factor (EGF) was purchased from Peprotech Europe (London, UK) while IL-2 was purchased from Miltenyi (Miltenyi Biotec Italia, Bologna).

4.2. Zoledronic Acid-Loaded Spherical Polymeric Nanoparticles (ZA-SPNs) Synthesis

Spherical polymeric nanoparticles (SPNs) were obtained using a double emulsion–evaporation procedure, modifying the single emulsion protocol previously described by Lee et al. [38]. Briefly, ZA, dissolved in the aqueous phase, was slowly added under probe sonication to an organic phase containing 10 mg of PLGA and DPPC dissolved in chloroform. This first emulsion was added dropwise to a 4% ethanol solution containing DSPE-PEG under probe sonication. The molar ratio of DPPC:DSPE-PEG was 7.5:2.5, while both the lipids were at 20% w/w of the polymer. Empty SPNs were prepared following the same procedure, but without ZA in the aqueous phase. Fluorescent ZA-SPNs were prepared by substituting a small fraction of DPPC (10% of the total amount) with DSPE-Cy5. After the evaporation of all the organic solvent in a reduced pressure environment, SPNs were purified and collected through sequential centrifugation steps. The first centrifugation was performed at 1200 rpm for 2 min to remove large debris from the synthesis process. The supernatant was then centrifuged at 12,000 rpm for 15 min, and the remaining pellet was centrifuged at the same speed several times in order to remove the ZA not incorporated into the SPNs. Finally, the resulting SPNs were resuspended in 1 mL aqueous solution before their use in all the subsequent experiments.

4.3. ZA-SPNs Physico-Chemical and Pharmacological Characterization

The nanoparticle size distribution and PDI were measured at 37 °C using dynamic light scattering (DLS) with the Zetasizer Nano ZS (Malvern, UK). By using proper zeta-cells, the nanoparticles' ζ-potential was also measured. For the stability study, both the size and PDI were measured over time for a period of 2 weeks while maintaining nanoparticles at 37 °C in deionized (DI) water. Also, ζ-potential was measured and monitored for the same time period. To study the nanoparticle morphology, SPN samples were dropped on a silicon wafer and dried. Samples were then gold sputtered and analyzed using a JSM-7500FA (JEOL, Milan, Italy) analytical field-emission scanning electron microscope (SEM) at 15 keV. The amount of ZA entrapped in the nanoparticles (n = 3 for each experimental condition) were measured using HPLC (1260 Infinity, Agilent Technology, Milano, Italy), using a reverse phase C-18 column (Zorbax Eclipse plus, Agilent Technology, Milano, Italy). Samples were eluted in isocratic conditions using a mixture of methanol (5%), acetonitrile (12%), and a buffer made out of 4.5 g of dipotassium hydrogen phosphate anhydrous plus 2 g of tetra butyl ammonium bi-sulphate in 1 L of DI water. The provided molarity refers to the molarity of one batch of ZA-SPNs resuspended in 1 mL of solution. To evaluate the release profile of ZA from the nanoparticles, a known amount of ZA-SPNs was loaded into Slide-A-Lyzer MINI dialysis microtubes with a molecular cut-off of 10 kDa (Thermo Fisher Scientific, Waltham, MA, USA), and placed in 4 L of PBS in order to simulate the infinite sink condition. At predetermined time points (namely 1, 4, 24, 48, 72, 112, and 158 h), three samples were collected and the amount of ZA was measured using high pressure liquid chromatography (HPLC).

4.4. Patients

Twenty-six CRC patients suffering from CRC were studied (institutional informed consent signed at the time of donation and EC approval PR163REG201 renewed in 2017). The localization of tumors was determined by the surgery staff of the Oncological Surgery Unit of the Istituto di Ricerca e Cura a Carattere Scientifico (IRCCS) Ospedale Policlinico San Martino. The tumor stage was determined according to the Union for International Cancer Control (UICC) and Dukes classification modified by Aster and Coller [60], and the microsatellite status was analyzed by the Pathology Unit. The PBMCs were isolated from all patients and used for measuring Vδ2 T lymphocyte proliferation and cytotoxic activity in an allogenic or autologous setting. Tumor specimens from 14 patients were analyzed (Table S1): 10 for the isolation of cell suspensions, used in experiments aimed to determine the ability of ZA-SNPs to trigger the expansion of Vδ2 T cells, and 5 for the generation of organoids and used, within the fourth passage of culture, as targets to evaluate the cytotoxic activity of Vδ2 T cells from autologous PBMCs.

4.5. Ex Vivo Expansion of Vδ2 T Cells

ZA was solubilized in DMSO, following the manufacturer's instructions. The amount of soluble ZA to trigger Vδ2 T cell proliferation or activation of Vδ2-T-cell-mediated tumor cell lysis ranged from 0.5 μM to 5 μM, in keeping with our previous data [21,45,48]. At these concentrations, the dilution of DMSO in culture was less than $1:10^3$ (between $1:2 \times 10^3$ and $1:2 \times 10^4$). Neither DMSO at $1:10^3$ nor ZA at concentrations up to 1 μM induced toxic effects, as evaluated using a crystal violet assay and propidium iodide (PI, Sigma-Aldrich) staining, on the cells used in this study, nor did they influence the proliferation or cytotoxicity of Vδ2 T lymphocytes [45]. Using ZA at a 5-μM concentration, about 20% of dead cells were detected among the Vδ2 T cells after 14 days of culture. The amount of ZA-SPNs to be used for triggering the expansion of Vδ2 T cells was determined in preliminary experiments by adding decreasing amounts of SPNs to cell cultures (namely 0.5, 0.25, 0.12, 0.05, 5×10^{-3}, 5×10^{-4}, 5×10^{-5} μM). Notably, in all the in vitro experiments, the maximum concentration used of ZA-SPNs was 0.5 μM and the optimum was 0.05 μM, the latter being more than a thousand times lower than the batch concentration and free of direct toxic effect on T lymphocytes. Similarly, this protocol was used also to estimate the non-toxic amount of nanoparticles for PBMCs (not shown). As a control, empty nanoparticles were used, with the same polymer amounts used for the ZA-SPNs. A concentration of 0.5 μM for 10^5 cells, the highest concentration tested, was not toxic for either lymphocytes nor monocytes. A concentration of 50 nM of ZA-SPNs (from now on 0.05 μM for easier comparison with soluble ZA) was experimentally found to be adequate to follow the expansion of Vδ2 T cells in in vitro cultures.

PBMCs were obtained from both healthy adult donor's buffy coats (institutional informed consent signed at the time of donation) and venous blood samples of CRC patients using density gradient centrifugation with Lymphocyte Separating Medium (Pancoll human, density: 1.077 g/mL, PAN-Biotech, Munich, Germany), as described in Zocchi et al. [21]. To obtain Vδ2 T lymphocyte populations, PBMCs were cultured in 96-well U-bottomed plates in 200 μL of RPMI-1640 medium supplemented with 10% FBS, penicillin/streptomycin, and L-glutamine, and with serial dilutions of either free ZA or ZA-SPNs, in a 37 °C humidified cell incubator with 5% CO_2.

After 24 h, and on days 5 and 7, 100 μL of culture supernatant were discarded and substituted with 100 μL of fresh medium containing recombinant human IL-2 (30 UI/10 ng/mL final concentration, Miltenyi Biotec Italia, Bologna). On day 10, cells were split in the medium supplemented with IL-2 and this was repeated every three days. The percentage of Vδ2 T lymphocytes was determined at different time points (days 0, 7, 14, 21) using indirect immunofluorescence and cytofluorimetric analysis, which was always performed by gating viable cells using the anti-Vδ2 TCR specific monoclonal antibody (mAb) γδ123R3, as described in Musso et al. [48]. Lymphocyte populations were used as effector cells in co-culture experiments with tumor cells or tumor cell spheroids after day 21 when the percentage of Vδ2 lymphocytes were more than 96% of the total cells. In some experiments, T lymphocytes and monocytes (Mo) were isolated from PBMC using specific negative selection kits (Stemcells Biotecnologies, Voden, Italy). The purity of the selected T lymphocyte and Mo populations was always more than 97% and 95%, respectively; this was determined using immunofluorescence with specific anti-CD3 (to identify T cells) or anti-CD14 (to stain Mo) mAbs and FACS analysis (see below). Then, T cells and Mo were co-cultured in the presence of soluble ZA or ZA-SPNs at different T:Mo ratios (10:1, 20:1, 40:1, 100:1, 200:1, 1000:1) and the percentage of Vδ2 cells was analyzed using immunofluorescence with the specific anti-Vδ2 mAb.

4.6. Immunofluorescence Assay and Analysis of Lymphocyte Proliferation

The immunofluorescence assay was performed as described in Musso et al. [48] with anti-Vδ2 mAb (γδ123R3, IgG1) or anti-CD3 mAb (289/10/F11, IgG2a) or anti-CD69 (31C4, IgG2a) or anti-CD25

(4E3, IgG2b, Miltenyi Biotec) or anti-CD45RA (T60, IgG2a) or anti-CD27 (MT271, IgG1, Miltenyi Biotec), anti-EPCAM (15806, IgG2b, R and D System, Minneapolis, MN) or anti-CD14 (TUK4, IgG2a, Thermo Fisher Scientific) mAbs, followed by Alexafluor 647 or PE-anti-isotype specific goat anti-mouse antiserum (GAM) (Life Technologies, Milan, Italy). At least 10^4 cells/sample were run on a CyAn ADP cytofluorimeter (Beckman-Coulter Italia, Milan, Italy), and results were analyzed with the Summit 4.3 software (Beckman-Coulter) and expressed as percentage of fluorescent cells or mean fluorescence intensity arbitrary units (MFI a.u.).

To measure the proliferation of Vδ2 T lymphocytes, the PBMCs were labelled with CFSE as described in Musso et al. [61]. Briefly, 10^6 cells were incubated for 30 min at 37 °C in a water bath in complete medium with 100 nM CFSE. Then, cells were extensively washed and put in culture at 10^5 cells/microwell in 96-well U-bottomed plates. ZA (1 µM) or ZA-SPNs (0.05 µM) were added and the proliferation was analyzed at 7 days after labelling cells with anti-Vδ2-specific mAb, followed by Alexafluor 647 GAM. Samples were analyzed on a CyAn ADP cytofluorimeter and proliferation was indicated by the reduction of CFSE in the cell generations compared to the content of CFSE in the parental component. The different cell generations were defined using the software ModFit LT 5.4 (Verity Software House, Topsham, ME, USA) with different colors.

4.7. CRC Cell Cultures and Spheroid Generation

The human CRC cell lines SW620, HCT-15, HT-29, LS180, SW-48, and SW480, provided and certified as mycoplasma-free by the cell bank of the IRCCS Ospedale Policlinico San Martino (Blood Transfusion Centre, B. Parodi, Genoa, Italy), were cultured in RPMI-1640 medium supplemented with 10% FBS, penicillin/streptomycin, and L-glutamine in adherent culture plates in a humidified incubator at 37 °C with 5% CO_2. Experimental conditions for the generation of tumor cell spheroids were selected starting with decreasing numbers of each tumor cell line (2×10^4 to 1×10^4 to 5×10^3 per well) in flat-bottom 96-well plates (Ultra-Low attachment multiwell plates, Corning®Costar®, New York City, NY, USA), with DMEM-F12 serum free medium supplemented with EGF (Peprotech Europe, London, UK) at a 10 ng/mL final concentration ($\geq 1 \times 10^6$ IU/mg). EGF was selected, among other natural ligands of epidermal growth factor receptor (EGFR), due to reasons previously described in detail in Varesano et al. [45]. When plating, 10^4 cells of SW620, HCT-15, or HT-29 tumor cell spheroids were obtained in 5–6 days after changing the culture medium every two days [45].

On day 5, CRC spheroids with a maximum diameter of about 250 µm were composed of living cells, as assessed by culturing a sample under adherent conventional conditions for 24 h and the subsequent identification of living cells with propidium iodide (PI, Sigma-Aldrich) staining and a crystal violet assay (data not shown) as described in Varesano et al. [45]. Spheroid dimensions were measured using images taken with the Olympus IX70 bright field inverted microscope equipped with a CCD camera (ORCA-ER, C4742-80-12AG, Hamamatsu, Japan) via the analysis of regions of interest after defining each spheroid with the CellSens software (version 1.12, Olympus, Tokyo, Japan) [43].

4.8. CRC Cell Viability and Cytotoxicity Assay

The CRC cell viability was determined using the Crystal Violet Cell Cytotoxicity Assay Kit (Biovision, Milpitas, CA, USA) either upon exposure to serial dilution of ZA-SPNs from 0.5 to 0.005 µM or ZA from 5 µM to 0.5 µM, and/or following co-culture with Vδ2 T cells. In conventional adherent cultures, CRC cells were incubated with ZA-SPNs or free ZA at the above-mentioned concentrations with Vδ2 T cells for 48 h, while finding the minimum time point to detect cytotoxicity with this system [45]. The optimal amount of Vδ2 T cells to detect the cytotoxic effect elicited by the drugs added, as determined in preliminary experiments, was 7.5×10^4 Vδ2 T cells/2.5×10^4 CRC cells, corresponding to a 3:1 effector to target (E:T) ratio. Similarly, CRC spheroids were exposed to ZA-SPNs or ZA, as above, and co-cultured for 48 h with Vδ2 T cells at the E:T ratio of 3:1 calculated as described in Varesano et al. [45]. Then, spheroids were transferred in conventional adherent plates and incubated for an additional 24 h to allow for plastic attachment. The CRC cells were then washed four times with

PBS and the adherent cells were stained with crystal violet following the manufacturer's instructions. The amount of crystal violet, proportional to the amount of adherent/living cells, was measured with the Victor X5 multilabel plate reader (Perkin Elmer Italia SPA, Milan, Italy) at 595 nm [45]. Results are expressed as a percentage of living cells calculated as follows: (OD_{595} CRC/OD_{595} CRC plus drug and/or Vδ2 T cells) × 100%.

4.9. CRC Organoid Generation and Vδ2 T Cell Cytotoxicity Elicited Using ZA-SPNs

Primary CRC organoid cultures were obtained following published guidelines [62,63]. Tissue samples, obtained after patient informed consent (PR163REG2014 renewed in 2017) and collected by a trained pathologist, were enzymatically digested by collagenases type I and II in Leibovitz L15 medium (Gibco-Thermo Scientific Italia, Milan, Italy) without serum. The digested tissue was passed through a 100-μm strainer to completely eliminate the residual matrix and mucus. Cripts were washed several times in fresh L15 medium to eliminate cell debris, mixed with Geltrex (LDEV-free, hESC-qualified, reduced growth factor; Gibco-Thermo Scientific), and plated in a 24-well plate. After polymerization at 37 °C, Geltrex domes were covered with 500 μL of medium per well (DMEM-F12 plus B27 plus 10 ng/mL of EGF, ≥10^6 IU/mg) supplemented with antibiotics. Different cocktails of inhibitors were tested on different wells [61] to identify the best culture condition for each CRC tumor sample. This culture method naturally selects pure colorectal epithelial cells within a few in vitro passages, while not allowing for the expansion of other contaminating populations [64]. The absence of wnt3a and R-spondin in the culture medium excluded the contamination of normal epithelial cells from mucosa. In this study, we tested five organoid cultures (OMCR18-006TK, OMCR18-006TK, OMCR19-006TK, OMCR19-009TK, and OMCR19-016TK), as detailed in Table S1, which were photographed using a Leica DM-LB2 microscope (Leica Biosystems, Milan, Italy), equipped with a GX-CamU3-18 camera (GT-Vision, Stansfield, UK) and depicted in Figure S6.

Organoids in Geltrex domes (3 μL) were labeled with calcein-AM (Sigma-Aldrich, 500 nM), washed with culture medium, seeded in 96-well flat-bottomed plates (1 dome/well), and challenged with autologous Vδ2 T cells, previously expanded with ZA-SPNs, at the E:T ratio of 3:1. The number of tumor cells in the 3-μL dome was evaluated via counting with the Miltenyi MACS Quant Cytofluorometer (Miltenyi Biotec srl, Bologna, Italy). The E:T co-culture was performed in the presence of ZA-SPNs (0.5, 0.1, 0.05 μM) and prolonged for 6 days to allow for the penetration of lymphocytes into the domes (3–4 days, as evaluated using conventional microscopy in preliminary experiments, not shown), followed by effector cell function. Then, fluorescence of each culture well was quantified using spectrofluorometry (Ex:488 nm, Em: 530 nm, Victor X5, Perkin Elmer) and compared to the fluorescence of organoid cultures without Vδ2 T cells, which was considered to be 100%. Data are expressed as a percentage of green fluorescence.

4.10. Cell Preparation for Confocal and SEM Imaging

SW-48 cells were seeded on circular glass slides previously coated with fibronectin (1 mg/mL, Sigma-Aldrich). After 24 h at 37 °C, to allow for cell attachment on the slide, samples were incubated with 0.05 μM Cy5-conjugated ZA-SPNs for 4 h. Vδ2 T cells were then added for an additional 4 h. For confocal imaging, cells were washed three times with PBS, fixed with 4% paraformaldehyde, and stained with DAPI and anti-EPCAM mAb, followed by Alexafluor555 GAM for CRC cells and with the anti-Vδ2 specific mAb or Vδ2 followed by Alexafluor488 GAM. Images were taken with a spinning disc confocal microscopy system (Eclipse Ti with Revolution XDi acquisition System, Nikon Instruments, Firenze, Italy) in sequence mode to avoid overlapping among the different fluorochromes. In some experiments, SW620 spheroids, the OMCR18-016TK organoids, or Vδ2 T cells obtained from the PBMCs were exposed to 0.05 μM Cy5-ZA-SPNs for 24 h. Spheroids and T cells were also stained with 20 nM Syto16 (Life Technologies, Thermo Fisher Scientific, Milan, Italy) to identify nuclei (blue pseudocolor). Spheroids or Vδ2 T cells were seeded onto glass slides, while organoids were analyzed in Geltrex domes seeded into 96-well black plates with a clear bottom (Costar, Corning.

Inc., Minneapolis, MN, USA). In another series of experiments, ZA-SPN-expanded Vδ2 T cells were labeled with CFSE and incubated with the OMCR18-016TK organoids for 48 h and then analyzed using confocal microscopy. Samples were run under a FV500 confocal microscope (Olympus Italia srl, Milan, Italy with a PlanApo 20× objective or 40× NA1.00 oil objective, and data was analyzed with FluoView 4.3b software (Olympus Italia srl, Milan, Italy). Images were taken in sequence mode and shown in pseudocolor. For SEM, samples were washed with PBS and fixed with glutaraldehyde 2% in a sodium cacodylate buffer 0.1 M at pH 7.4; then, samples were post-fixed with osmium tetroxide 1% solution, dehydrated with a series of alcohol at 4 °C, and infiltrated with hexamethyldisilazane. After an overnight drying, they were sputter-coated with a thin (10 nm) layer of gold to protect them and make their surface conductive. Imaging was performed with an analytical low-vacuum SEM JSM 6490 (JEOL (Italia), Milan, Italy), at 15 kV.

4.11. Microfluidic Chip Fabrication

The double-channel microfluidic chip was realized following the same protocols of the present authors' recent paper [50]. Briefly, by using a direct laser writing machine (DWL 66+, Heidelberg Instruments, Heidelberg, Germany), optical masks were obtained and then used in sequential photolithographic processes to impress the two channels and the raw pillars, which separated them on the resist spun on a silicon wafer. After the resists development, the entire 2D geometry was made tridimensional through the inductively coupled plasma – reactive ion etching (ICP-RIE) that, using a Bosh process, dug the pattern into the silicon. This entire design was then transferred to polydimethylsiloxane (PDMS), the final material of the chip, by casting the latter onto the silicon and baking it at 60 °C overnight. Finally, the PDMS was treated with an oxygen plasma (20 W for 20 s) and bonded to a glass coverslip to produce a closed hollow structure. A biopsy punch was used to create the inlets and outlets. The final microfluidic chip presented two channels, which were 210 μm wide and 50 μm high. The region of contact of the two channels (500 μm in length) was constituted by an array of pillars, separated by a 3-μm gap.

4.12. Microfluidic Experiments

Before the seeding of the cells in the channels, the chip was autoclaved at 120 °C. A solution of Matrigel (8–12 mg/mL, Sigma-Aldrich) was half diluted with a suspension of the CRC cell lines SW-48 or SW-480 GFP+ (kindly provided by Dr. N.Ferrari, 15×10^6 cells/mL) and inserted in the extravascular channel. For the gelation of Matrigel, the chip was kept in an incubator for 5 min at 37 °C. Then, fibronectin (20 μg/mL, Sigma-Aldrich) was pipetted into the vascular channel, and after 15 min, HUVECs (6×10^6 cells/mL, PromoCell GmbH, Heidelberg, Germany) were inserted into the same channel. Experiments were then performed after overnight incubation in order to get an endothelial vessel in the vascular channel and to allow tumor cells to attach and adapt to the extravascular channel environment. Vδ2 T cells, previously stained with DAPI or CM-(Invitrogen Thermo Fisher Scientific, Milan, Italy) were injected into the vascular channel through a syringe pump (Harvard Pump 11 Elite, Harvard Apparatus, Holliston,, MA, USA) at a flow rate of 50 nL/min and at a E:T (Vδ2:CRC) ratio of 3:1. A Spinning disc confocal microscopy system (Nikon EclipseTi with Revolution XDi acquisition System) acquired images at predefined time intervals (4 min) for 24 h. Images were analyzed using the ImageJ software (1.52n, NIH, USA), quantifying the percentage increase in fluorescence intensity (i.e., DAPI for Vδ2 T cells) in different regions of interest (ROIs, 500 μm in length and 215 μm in height), close to the pillar area. Data represent the percentage increase of such fluorescence, compared to time 0, and are expressed as mean ± SE. For the confocal images, F-actin cytoskeleton filaments were stained in green using phalloidin (Alexa Fluor phalloidin, Life Technologies, Thermo Fisher Scientific, Milan, Italy), nuclei with DAPI and Vδ2 T cells with CM-Dil. Images were acquired using a confocal microscope (Nikon A1).

4.13. HPLC Negative-Ion Electrospray Ionization TOF-MS

The production of IPP by monocytes or LS180 or SW620CRC cells, after treatment with different amounts of 0.5 or 0.05 µM ZA-SPNs or 0.5 µM soluble ZA for 24 h, was evaluated on cell extracts, dissolved via vortex mixing in 80 µL MilliQ water and 250 µL Na_3VO_4, and cleared using centrifugation in an Eppendorf Minifuge (Eppendorf srl, Milan, Italy) (13,000 rpm, 3 min) using HPLC negative-ion electrospray ionization time of flight mass spectrometry (HPLC/TOF-MS) according to the method described by Jauhiainen et al. [65] with some modifications reported in detail in Zocchi et al. [21]. Calibration curves for IPP were generated with standards diluted in MilliQ water/0.25 mM Na_3VO_4 in the range 0.1–15 µM. The IPP content was determined using HPLC/TOF-MS, operating in reflection negative ion mode, using an Agilent 1200 series chromatographic system, equipped with G1379B degasser, G1376A capillary pump, and G1377A autosampler. Negative full-scan mass spectra were recorded using the Agilent's Mass Hunter software version n. B.05.00 in the mass range of m/z 60–500. The full scan data were processed using the Agilent Mass Hunter Qualitative Analysis, ver. B.02.00 software. The amount of IPP was measured using the extracted ion current (EIC) peak area (EIC m/z 244.99 $[M-H]^-$). Results are shown as pmol of IPP extracted using acetonitrile/total protein content in each cell lysate. The chromatographic method used could not separate the isomers IPP and 3,3-dimethylallyl pyrophosphate (DMAPP). The identity of the parent ion present in our cell extracts was confirmed by verifying the formation of fragment ions (m/z 79, m/z 159, m/z 177, and m/z 227), generating negative MS/MS spectra with a mass spectrometer Agilent 1100 series LC/MSD Trap, equipped with an orthogonal geometry electrospray source and ion trap analyzer (not shown) [21].

4.14. Statistical Analysis

Statistical analysis was performed using a two-tailed unpaired Student's *t*-test. For the time-lapse confocal studies, at first for assessing the homogeneity of variances, the equal-variance assumption was tested using the Brown–Forsy test. ANOVA was performed to evaluate the differences between groups, followed by the Tukey-HSD post-hoc test. The *p*-values are shown in the text or in the figure legends. Results are shown as mean ± SEM or mean ± SD.

4.15. Human Subjects

All human studies described in this manuscript have been approved by the appropriate institutional review board(s) as indicated in the Ethic Committee approval PR163REG2014 renewed in 2017. The written informed consent was received from participants prior to inclusion in the study and it is stored in the Molecular Oncology and Angiogenesis Unit.

5. Conclusions

In conclusion, this study demonstrates, for the first time to the present authors' knowledge, that the encapsulation of ZA into spherical polymeric nanoparticles can lead to the stimulation of Vδ2 T cell expansion and activation of anti-tumor activity far more effectively than soluble ZA. Moreover, the awareness that both peripheral-blood and tumor-infiltrating Vδ2 T cells can respond to ZA-SPNs and efficiently induce tumor cell death in patients' organoids in an autologous setting, would further support the use of this ZA nanoformulation in CRC. The eventual therapeutic plan may be preceded by testing the IPP production and Vδ2 T cell activation in the patient-specific 3D model of tumor organoids in order to pursue a personalized therapy. These results are a step toward the use of ZA-SPNs to trigger anti-tumor immunity in CRC and their possible translation in clinical practice.

Supplementary Materials: The following are available online at http://www.mdpi.com/2072-6694/12/1/104/s1. Figure S1: ZA-SPNs ζ-potential over time and encapsulation efficiency, Figure S2: Effect of ZA-SPNs and ZA on CRC viability, Figure S3: ZA-SPNs were internalized by CRC spheroids and organoids, Figure S4: ZA-SPNs triggered the expansion of CRC patients' Vδ2 T lymphocytes, Figure S5: Expression of CD45RA and CD27 in Vδ2 T lymphocytes after stimulation with ZA-SPNs, Figure S6: Colon organoid characterization, Figure S7:

ZA-SPN-expanded Vδ2 T cells can infiltrate colon organoids, Table S1: Pathology features of CRC patients from which tumor cell suspensions and/or organoids were derived.

Author Contributions: D.D.M. and S.V. performed the experiments and wrote and revised the paper, R.B. prepared the CRC tumor organoids; H.M. performed the microfluidic chip experiments, A.S. performed the IPP analysis, M.R.Z. planned some experiments and wrote and revised the paper, P.D. planned some experiments and wrote and revised the paper, and A.P. planned and performed some experiments and wrote and revised the paper. A.P. takes, together with D.D.M., S.V., and P.D., the major responsibility for the assembling of figures and the main message of the paper. All authors have read and agreed to the published version of the manuscript.

Acknowledgments: The authors thank N. Ferrari for the GFP + SW480 CRC cell line; C. Malfatto for separating PBMCs from CRC patients; D. La Torre for providing us venous blood samples of CRC patients; S. Scabini, E. Romairone, L. Mastracci, and F. Grillo for providing us the tumor specimens of CRC patients; F. Tosetti and A. Profumo for help in preparation and evaluation of for IPP content. A.P. acknowledges the partial support by the Italian Association for Cancer Research (AIRC) IG 21648, 5xmille 2014, 5xmille2015 from Ministero della Salute and Ricerca Corrente 2018–2021. P.D. acknowledges the partial support by the Italian Association for Cancer Research AIRC IG 17664; the Fondazione San Paolo project "Ligurian Alliance for Nanomedicine against cancer", and the European Union's Seventh Framework Programme (FP7/2007-2013) ERC 616695.

Conflicts of Interest: The authors declare no conflict of interest.

References

1. Fridman, W.H.; Pagès, F.; Sautès-Fridman, C.; Galon, J. The immune contexture in human tumours: Impact on clinical outcome. *Nat. Rev. Cancer* **2012**, *12*, 298–306. [CrossRef]
2. Church, S.E.; Galon, J. Tumor Microenvironment and immunotherapy: The whole picture is better than a glimpse. *Immunity* **2015**, *43*, 631–633. [CrossRef]
3. Gentles, A.J.; Newman, A.M.; Liu, C.L.; Bratman, S.V.; Feng, W.; Kim, D.; Nair, V.S.; Xu, Y.; Khuong, A.; Hoang, C.D.; et al. The prognostic landscape of genes and infiltrating immune cells across human cancers. *Nat. Med.* **2015**, *21*, 938–945. [CrossRef]
4. Meraviglia, S.; Lo Presti, E.; Tosolini, M.; La Mendola, C.; Orlando, V.; Todaro, M.; Catalano, V.; Stassi, G.; Cicero, G.; Vieni, S.; et al. Distinctive features of tumor-infiltrating γδ T lymphocytes in human colorectal cancer. *Oncoimmunology* **2017**, *6*, e1347742. [CrossRef]
5. Hayday, A.C. Gammadelta T cells and the lymphoid stress-surveillance response. *Immunity* **2009**, *31*, 184–196. [CrossRef] [PubMed]
6. Bonneville, M.; O'Brien, R.L.; Born, W.K. Gammadelta T cell effector functions: A blend of innate programming and acquired plasticity. *Nat. Rev. Immunol.* **2010**, *10*, 467–478. [CrossRef] [PubMed]
7. Corvaisier, M.; Moreau-Aubry, A.; Diez, E.; Bennouna, J.; Scotet, E.; Bonneville, M.; Jotereau, F. Vgamma9 Vdelta2 T cell response to colon carcinoma cells. *J. Immunol.* **2005**, *175*, 5481–5488. [CrossRef] [PubMed]
8. Kabelitz, D.; Wesch, D.; He, W. Perspectives of gammadelta T lymphocytes in tumor immunology. *Cancer Res.* **2007**, *67*, 5–8. [CrossRef]
9. Todaro, M.; D'Asaro, M.; Caccamo, N.; Iovino, F.; Francipane, M.G.; Meraviglia, S.; Orlando, V.; La Mendola, C.; Gulotta, G.; Salerno, A.; et al. Efficient killing of human colon cancer stem cells by gammadelta T lymphocytes. *J. Immunol.* **2009**, *182*, 7287–7296. [CrossRef]
10. Gober, H.J.; Kistowska, M.; Angman, L.; Jenö, P.; Mori, L.; De Libero, G. Human T cell receptor gammadelta cells recognize endogenous mevalonate metabolites in tumor cells. *J. Exp. Med.* **2003**, *197*, 163–168. [CrossRef]
11. Wang, H.; Sarikonda, G.; Puan, K.J.; Tanaka, Y.; Feng, J.; Giner, J.L.; Cao, R.; Mönkkönen, J.; Oldfield, E.; Morita, C.T. Indirect stimulation of human Vγ2Vδ2 T cells through alterations in isoprenoid metabolism. *J. Immunol.* **2011**, *187*, 5099–5113. [CrossRef] [PubMed]
12. Vavassori, S.; Kumar, A.; Wan, G.S.; Ramanjaneyulu, G.S.; Cavallari, M.; El Daker, S.; Beddoe, T.; Theodossis, A.; Williams, N.K.; Gostick, E.; et al. Butyrophilin 3A1 binds phosphorylated antigens and stimulates human γδ T cells. *Nat. Immunol.* **2013**, *14*, 908–916. [CrossRef] [PubMed]
13. Burjanadzé, M.; Condomines, M.; Reme, T.; Quittet, P.; Latry, P.; Lugagne, C.; Romagne, F.; Morel, Y.; Rossi, J.F.; Klein, B.; et al. In vitro expansion of gammadelta T cells with anti-myeloma cells activity by Phosphostim and IL-2 in patients with multiple myeloma. *Br. J. Haematol.* **2007**, *139*, 206–216. [CrossRef] [PubMed]

14. Gertner-Dardenne, J.; Bonnafous, C.; Bezombes, C.; Capietto, A.H.; Scaglione, V.; Ingoure, S.; Cendron, D.; Gross, E.; Lepage, J.F.; Quillet-Mary, A.; et al. Bromohydrin pyrophosphate enhances antibody-dependent cell-mediated cytotoxicity induced by therapeutic antibodies. *Blood* **2009**, *113*, 4875–4884. [CrossRef]
15. Das, H.; Wang, L.; Kamath, A.; Bukowski, J.F. Vgamma2Vdelta2 T-cell receptor-mediated recognition of aminobisphosphonates. *Blood* **2001**, *98*, 1616–1618. [CrossRef]
16. Santini, D.; Vespasiani Gentilucci, U.; Vincenzi, B.; Picardi, A.; Vasaturo, F.; La Cesa, A.; Onori, N.; Scarpa, S.; Tonini, G. The antineoplastic role of bisphosphonates: From basic research to clinical evidence. *Ann. Oncol.* **2003**, *14*, 1468–1476. [CrossRef]
17. Clézardin, P.; Fournier, P.; Boissier, S.; Peyruchaud, O. In vitro and in vivo anti-tumor effects of bisphopshonates. *Curr. Med. Chem.* **2003**, *10*, 173–180. [CrossRef]
18. Santolaria, T.; Robard, M.; Léger, A.; Catros, V.; Bonneville, M.; Scotet, E. Repeated systemic administration of aminobisphosphonates and human Vγ9Vδ2 T cells efficiently control tumor development in vivo. *J. Immunol.* **2013**, *191*, 1993–2000. [CrossRef]
19. Kunzmann, V.; Bauer, E.; Feurle, J.; Weissinger, F.; Tony, H.P.; Wilhelm, M. Stimulation of gammadelta T cells by aminobisphosphonates and induction of anti plasmacell activity in multiple myeloma. *Blood* **2000**, *96*, 384–392. [CrossRef]
20. Fiore, F.; Castella, B.; Nuschak, B.; Bertieri, R.; Mariani, S.; Bruno, B.; Pantaleoni, F.; Foglietta, M.; Boccadoro, M.; Massaia, M. Enhanced ability of dendritic cells to stimulate innate and adaptive immunity on short-term incubation with zoledronic acid. *Blood* **2007**, *110*, 921–927. [CrossRef]
21. Zocchi, M.R.; Costa, D.; Venè, R.; Tosetti, F.; Ferrari, N.; Minghelli, S.; Benelli, R.; Scabini, S.; Romairone, E.; Catellani, S.; et al. Zoledronate can induce colorectal cancer microenvironment expressing BTN3A1 to stimulate effector γδ T cells with anti-tumor activity. *Oncoimmunology* **2017**, *6*, e1278099. [CrossRef] [PubMed]
22. Bennouna, J.; Levy, V.; Sicard, H.; Senellart, H.; Audrain, M.; Hiret, S.; Rolland, F.; Bruzzoni-Giovanelli, H.; Rimbert, M.; Galéa, C.; et al. Phase I study of bromohydrinpyrophosphate (BrHPP, IPH 1101) a Vgamma9 Vdelta2 T lymphocyte agonist in patients with solid tumors. *Cancer Immunol. Immunother.* **2010**, *59*, 1521–1530. [CrossRef] [PubMed]
23. Lang, J.M.; Kaikobad, M.R.; Wallace, M.; Staab, M.J.; Horvath, D.L.; Wilding, G.; Liu, G.; Eickhoff, J.C.; McNeel, D.G.; Malkovsky, M. Pilot trial of interleukin-2 and zoledronic acid to augment γδ T cells as treatment for patients with refractory renal cell carcinoma. *Cancer Immunol. Immunother.* **2011**, *60*, 1447–1460. [CrossRef] [PubMed]
24. Sakamoto, M.; Nakajima, J.; Murakawa, T.; Fukami, T.; Yoshida, Y.; Murayama, T.; Takamoto, S.; Matsushita, H.; Kakimi, K. Adoptive immunotherapy for advanced non-small cell lung cancer using zoledronate-expanded γδT cells: A phase I clinical study. *J. Immunother.* **2011**, *34*, 202–211. [CrossRef]
25. Meraviglia, S.; Eberl, M.; Vermijlen, D.; Todaro, M.; Buccheri, S.; Cicero, G.; La Mendola, C.; Guggino, G.; D'Asaro, M.; Orlando, V.; et al. In vivo manipulation of Vgamma9Vdelta2 T cells with zoledronate and low-dose interleukin-2 for immunotherapy of advanced breast cancer patients. *Clin. Exp. Immunol.* **2010**, *161*, 290–297. [CrossRef]
26. Dieli, F.; Vermijlen, D.; Fulfaro, F.; Caccamo, N.; Meraviglia, S.; Cicero, G.; Roberts, A.; Buccheri, S.; D'Asaro, M.; Gebbia, N.; et al. Targeting human gammadelta T cells with zoledronate and interleukin-2 for immunotherapy of hormone-refractory prostate cancer. *Cancer Res.* **2007**, *67*, 7450–7457. [CrossRef]
27. Lin, J.H. Bisphosphonates: A review of their pharmacokinetic properties. *Bone* **1996**, *18*, 75–85. [CrossRef]
28. Dhillon, S. Zoledronic Acid (Reclast®, Aclasta®): A Review in Osteoporosis. *Drugs* **2016**, *76*, 1683–1697. [CrossRef]
29. Tanaka, Y.; Iwasaki, M.; Murata-Hirai, K.; Matsumoto, K.; Hayashi, K.; Okamura, H.; Sugie, T.; Minato, N.; Morita, C.T.; Toi, M. Anti-tumor activity and immunotherapeutic potential of a bisphosphonate prodrug. *Sci. Rep.* **2017**, *7*, 5987. [CrossRef]
30. Xiong, Y.; Wang, Y.; Tiruthani, K. Tumor immune microenvironment and nano-immunotherapeutics in colorectal cancer. *Nanomedicine* **2019**, *21*, 102034. [CrossRef]
31. Zeng, B.; Middelberg, A.P.; Gemiarto, A.; MacDonald, K.; Baxter, A.G.; Talekar, M.; Moi, D.; Tullett, K.M.; Caminschi, I.; Lahoud, M.H.; et al. Self-adjuvanting nanoemulsion targeting dendritic cell receptor Clec9A enables antigen-specific immunotherapy. *J. Clin. Investig.* **2018**, *128*, 1971–1984. [CrossRef] [PubMed]

32. Muraoka, D.; Seo, N.; Hayashi, T.; Tahara, Y.; Fujii, K.; Tawara, I.; Miyahara, Y.; Okamori, K.; Yagita, H.; Imoto, S.; et al. Antigen delivery targeted to tumor-associated macrophages overcomes tumor immune resistance. *J. Clin. Investig.* **2019**, *129*, 1278–1294. [CrossRef] [PubMed]
33. Maeda, H.; Matsumura, Y. EPR effect based drug design and clinical outlook for enhanced cancer chemotherapy. *Adv. Drug Deliv. Rev.* **2011**, *63*, 129–130. [CrossRef] [PubMed]
34. Matsumura, Y.; Maeda, H. A new concept for macromolecular therapeutics in cancer chemotherapy: Mechanism of tumoritropic accumulation of proteins and the antitumor agent smancs. *Cancer Res.* **1986**, *46*, 6387–6392.
35. Papahadjopoulos, D.; Allen, T.M.; Gabizon, A.; Mayhew, E.; Matthay, K.; Huang, S.K.; Lee, K.D.; Woodle, M.C.; Lasic, D.D.; Redemann, C.; et al. Sterically stabilized liposomes: Improvements in pharmacokinetics and antitumor therapeutic efficacy. *Proc. Natl. Acad. Sci. USA* **1991**, *88*, 11460–11464. [CrossRef]
36. He, K.; Tang, M. Safety of novel liposomal drugs for cancer treatment: Advances and prospects. *Chem. Biol. Interact.* **2018**, *295*, 13–19. [CrossRef]
37. Zang, X.; Zhang, X.; Hu, H.; Qiao, M.; Zhao, X.; Deng, Y.; Chen, D. Targeted Delivery of Zoledronate to Tumor-Associated Macrophages for Cancer Immunotherapy. *Mol. Pharm.* **2019**, *16*, 2249–2258. [CrossRef]
38. Lee, A.; Di Mascolo, D.; Francardi, M.; Piccardi, F.; Bandiera, T.; Decuzzi, P. Spherical polymeric nanoconstructs for combined chemotherapeutic and anti-inflammatory therapies. *Nanomedicine* **2016**, *12*, 2139–2147. [CrossRef]
39. Cibrián, D.; Sánchez-Madrid, F. CD69: From activation marker to metabolic gatekeeper. *Eur. J. Immunol.* **2017**, *47*, 946–953. [CrossRef]
40. Abbas, A.K.; Trotta, E.R.; Simeonov, D.; Marson, A.; Bluestone, J.A. Revisiting IL-2: Biology and therapeutic prospects. *Sci. Immunol.* **2018**, *3*, eaat1482. [CrossRef]
41. Ameruoso, A.; Palomba, R.; Palange, A.L.; Cervadoro, A.; Lee, A.; Di Mascolo, D.; Decuzzi, P. Ameliorating amyloid-β fibrils triggered inflammation via curcumin-loaded polymeric nanoconstructs. *Front. Immunol.* **2017**, *8*, 1411. [CrossRef] [PubMed]
42. Di Mascolo, D.; Basnett, P.; Palange, A.L.; Francardi, M.; Roy, I.; Decuzzi, P. Tuning core hydrophobicity of spherical polymeric nanoconstructs for docetaxel delivery. *Polym. Int.* **2016**, *65*, 741–746. [CrossRef]
43. He, C.; Hu, Y.; Yin, L.; Tang, C.; Yin, C. Effects of particle size and surface charge on cellular uptake and biodistribution of polymeric nanoparticles. *Biomaterials* **2010**, *31*, 3657–3666. [CrossRef] [PubMed]
44. Zanoni, M.; Piccinini, F.; Arienti, C.; Zamagni, A.; Santi, S.; Polico, R.; Bevilacqua, A.; Tesei, A. 3D tumor spheroid models for in vitro therapeutic screening: A systematic approach to enhance the biological relevance of data obtained. *Sci. Rep.* **2016**, *6*, 19103. [CrossRef] [PubMed]
45. Varesano, S.; Zocchi, M.R.; Poggi, A. Zoledronate triggers Vδ2 T cells to destroy and kill spheroids of colon carcinoma: Quantitative image analysis of three-dimensional cultures. *Front. Immunol.* **2018**, *9*, 998. [CrossRef]
46. Costa, D.; Venè, R.; Benelli, R.; Romairone, E.; Scabini, S.; Catellani, S.; Rebesco, B.; Mastracci, L.; Grillo, F.; Minghelli, S.; et al. Mesenchymal stromal cell-mediated inhibition of natural killer cell function in colorectal cancer can be regulated by epidermal growth factor receptor targeting. *Front. Immunol.* **2018**, *9*, 1150. [CrossRef]
47. Dieli, F.; Poccia, F.; Lipp, M.; Sireci, G.; Caccamo, N.; Di Sano, C.; Salerno, A. Differentiation of effector/memory Vdelta2 T cells and migratory routes in lymph nodes or inflammatory sites. *J. Exp. Med.* **2003**, *198*, 391–397. [CrossRef]
48. Musso, A.; Catellani, S.; Canevali, P.; Tavella, S.; Venè, R.; Boero, S.; Pierri, I.; Gobbi, M.; Kunkl, A.; Ravetti, J.L.; et al. Aminobisphosphonates prevent the inhibitory effects exerted by lymph node stromal cells on anti-tumor Vδ2 T lymphocytes in non-Hodgkin lymphomas. *Haematologica* **2014**, *99*, 131–139. [CrossRef]
49. Chung, S.; Nguyen, V.; Lin, Y.L.; Kamen, L.; Song, A. Thaw-and-use target cells pre-labeled with calcein AM for antibody-dependent cell-mediated cytotoxicity assays. *J. Immunol. Methods* **2017**, *447*, 37–46. [CrossRef]
50. Mollica, H.; Palomba, R.; Primavera, R.; Decuzzi, P. Two-Channel Compartmentalized Microfluidic Chip for Real-Time Monitoring of the Metastatic Cascade. *ACS Biomater. Sci. Eng.* **2019**, *5*, 4834–4843. [CrossRef]
51. Ellis, L.M.; Fidler, I.J. Finding the tumor copycat. Therapy fails, patients don't. *Nat. Med.* **2010**, *16*, 974–975. [CrossRef] [PubMed]
52. Akhtar, A. The flaws and human harms of animal experimentation. *Camb. Q. Health Eth.* **2015**, *24*, 407–419. [CrossRef] [PubMed]

53. Li, X.; Valdes, S.A.; Alzhrani, R.F.; Hufnagel, S.; Hursting, S.D.; Cui, Z. Zoledronic Acid-containing Nanoparticles with Minimum Premature Release Show Enhanced Activity Against Extraskeletal Tumor. *ACS Appl. Mater. Interfaces* **2019**, *11*, 7311–7319. [CrossRef] [PubMed]
54. Silva Santos, B.; Serre, K.; Norell, H. γδT cells in cancer. *Nat. Rev. Immunol.* **2015**, *15*, 683–691. [CrossRef]
55. Adams, E.J.; Gu, S.; Luoma, A.M. Human gamma delta T cells: Evolution and ligand recognition. *Cell. Immunol.* **2015**, *296*, 31–40. [CrossRef]
56. Dijkstra, K.K.; Cattaneo, C.M.; Weeber, F.; Chalabi, M.; van de Haar, J.; Fanchi, L.F.; Slagter, M.; van der Velden, D.L.; Kaing, S.; Kelderman, S.; et al. Generation of Tumor-Reactive T Cells by Co-culture of Peripheral Blood Lymphocytes and Tumor Organoids. *Cell* **2018**, *174*, 1586–1598. [CrossRef]
57. Sato, T.; Stange, D.E.; Ferrante, M.; Vries, R.G.; Van Es, J.H.; Van den Brink, S.; Van Houdt, W.J.; Pronk, A.; Van Gorp, J.; Siersema, P.D.; et al. Long-term expansion of epithelial organoids from human colon, adenoma, adenocarcinoma, and Barrett's epithelium. *Gastroenterology* **2011**, *141*, 1762–1772. [CrossRef]
58. Wu, P.; Wu, D.; Ni, C.; Ye, J.; Chen, W.; Hu, G.; Wang, Z.; Wang, C.; Zhang, Z.; Xia, W.; et al. γδ T 17 cells promote the accumulation and expansion of myeloid-derived suppressor cells in human colorectal cancer. *Immunity* **2014**, *40*, 785–800. [CrossRef]
59. Capietto, A.H.; Martinet, L.; Cendron, D.; Fruchon, S.; Pont, F.; Fournié, J.J. Phophoantigens overcome human TCRVgamma9+ gammadelta T cell immunosuppression by TGF-beta: Relevance for cancer immunotherapy. *J. Immunol.* **2010**, *184*, 6680–6687. [CrossRef]
60. Astler, V.B.; Coller, F.A. The prognostic significance of direct extension of carcinoma of the colon and rectum. *Ann. Surg.* **1954**, *139*, 846–852. [CrossRef]
61. Musso, A.; Zocchi, M.R.; Poggi, A. Relevance of the mevalonate biosynthetic pathway in the regulation of bone marrow mesenchymal stromal cell-mediated effects on T-cell proliferation and B-cell survival. *Haematologica* **2011**, *96*, 16–23. [CrossRef] [PubMed]
62. Van De Wetering, M.; Francies, H.E.; Francis, J.M.; Bounova, G.; Iorio, F.; Pronk, A.; van Houdt, W.; van Gor, J.; Taylor-Weiner, A.; Kester, L.; et al. Prospective derivation of a living organoid biobank of colorectal cancer patients. *Cell* **2015**, *161*, 933–945. [CrossRef] [PubMed]
63. Fujii, M.; Shimokawa, M.; Date, S.; Takano, A.; Matano, M.; Nanki, K.; Ohta, Y.; Toshimitsu, K.; Nakazato, Y.; Kawasaki, K.; et al. A colorectal tumor organoid library demonstrates progressive loss of niche factor requirements during tumorigenesis. *Cell Stem Cell* **2016**, *18*, 827–838. [CrossRef] [PubMed]
64. Neal, J.T.; Li, X.; Zhu, J.; Giangarra, V.; Grzeskowiak, C.L.; Ju, J.; Liu, I.H.; Chiou, S.H.; Salahudeen, A.A.; Smith, A.R.; et al. Organoid Modeling of the Tumor Immune Microenvironment. *Cell* **2018**, *175*, 1972–1988. [CrossRef]
65. Jauhiainen, M.; Monkkonen, H.; Raikkonen, J.; Monkkonen, J.; Auriola, S. Analysis of endogenous ATP analogs and mevalonate pathway mebolites in cancer cell cultures using liquid chromatography-electrospray ionization mass spectrometry. *J. Chromatogr. B* **2009**, *877*, 2967–2975. [CrossRef]

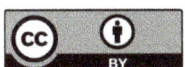

© 2019 by the authors. Licensee MDPI, Basel, Switzerland. This article is an open access article distributed under the terms and conditions of the Creative Commons Attribution (CC BY) license (http://creativecommons.org/licenses/by/4.0/).

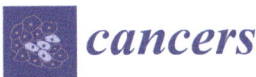

Article

Accuracy of Magnetometer-Guided Sentinel Lymphadenectomy after Intraprostatic Injection of Superparamagnetic Iron Oxide Nanoparticles in Prostate Cancer: The SentiMag Pro II Study

Alexander Winter [1,*,†], Svenja Engels [1,†], Philipp Goos [1], Marie-Christin Süykers [1], Stefan Gudenkauf [2], Rolf-Peter Henke [3] and Friedhelm Wawroschek [1]

[1] University Hospital for Urology, Klinikum Oldenburg, School of Medicine and Health Sciences, Carl von Ossietzky University Oldenburg, D-26111 Oldenburg, Germany; engels.svenja@klinikum-oldenburg.de (S.E.); philipp.goos@web.de (P.G.); marie_chr.sueykers@yahoo.de (M.-C.S.); wawroschek.friedhelm@klinikum-oldenburg.de (F.W.)

[2] Departments of Business Information Systems, University of Applied Sciences and Arts Hannover, D-30459 Hannover, Germany; stefan.gudenkauf@hs-hannover.de

[3] Institute of Pathology Oldenburg, D-26122 Oldenburg, Germany; r.p.henke@pathologie-oldenburg.de

* Correspondence: winter.alexander@klinikum-oldenburg.de; Tel.: +49-441-4032302

† These authors contributed equally to this work.

Received: 31 October 2019; Accepted: 17 December 2019; Published: 20 December 2019

Abstract: Radioisotope-guided sentinel lymph node dissection (sLND) has shown high diagnostic reliability in prostate (PCa) and other cancers. To overcome the limitations of the radioactive tracers, magnetometer-guided sLND using superparamagnetic iron oxide nanoparticles (SPIONs) has been successfully used in PCa. This prospective study (SentiMag Pro II, DRKS00007671) determined the diagnostic accuracy of magnetometer-guided sLND in intermediate- and high-risk PCa. Fifty intermediate- or high-risk PCa patients (prostate-specific antigen (PSA) ≥ 10 ng/mL and/or Gleason score ≥ 7; median PSA 10.8 ng/mL, IQR 7.4–19.2 ng/mL) were enrolled. After the intraprostatic SPIONs injection a day earlier, patients underwent magnetometer-guided sLND and extended lymph node dissection (eLND, followed by radical prostatectomy. SLNs were detected in vivo and in ex vivo samples. Diagnostic accuracy of sLND was assessed using eLND as the reference. SLNs were detected in all patients (detection rate 100%), with 447 sentinel lymph nodes SLNs (median 9, IQR 6–12) being identified and 966 LNs (median 18, IQR 15–23) being removed. Thirty-six percent (18/50) of patients had LN metastases (median 2, IQR 1–3). Magnetometer-guided sLND had 100% sensitivity, 97.0% specificity, 94.4% positive predictive value, 100% negative predictive value, 0.0% false negative rate, and 3.0% additional diagnostic value (LN metastases only in SLNs outside the eLND template). In vivo, one positive SLN/LN-positive patient was missed, resulting in a sensitivity of 94.4%. In conclusion, this new magnetic sentinel procedure has high accuracy for nodal staging in intermediate- and high-risk PCa. The reliability of intraoperative SLN detection using this magnetometer system requires verification in further multicentric studies.

Keywords: lymphadenectomy; magnetometer; prostate cancer; sentinel lymph node dissection; SPION; superparamagnetic iron oxide nanoparticles

1. Introduction

Histopathological examination or pelvic lymph node (LN) dissection (LND) is still the gold standard for LN staging in clinically localized prostate cancer (PCa). The number of removed LNs or the extent of LND directly influence the rate of detected LN-positive patients [1]. On the other hand, complications arise along with the number of LNs removed [2].

Because of relevant importance for further therapy and the complication rate of extended LND (eLND), as well as the low detection rate of limited LND methods, the concept of targeted radioisotope-guided sentinel LN (SLN) identification used in other tumor entities was implemented in PCa [3]. Conventionally, marking of SLNs with technetium-99m (^{99m}Tc) nanocolloid and a gamma probe for intraoperative SLN detection are used for the established radioisotope-guided SLN identification in PCa patients. The diagnostic accuracy of this radioactive sentinel LN dissection (sLND) approach was determined in a systematic literature review. Twenty-one studies including 2509 patients were analyzed [4]. The findings demonstrated that the diagnostic reliability of eLND and sLND were almost comparable. In sentinel cohorts, targeted sLND detected a higher rate of LN-positive patients than were expected from established nomograms [5–7].

Because of the ionizing radiation emitted by the radioactive tracer material, the benefits of the established SLN procedure are associated with certain limitations. The dependence on radioisotopes or nuclear medicine facilities imposes restrictions on patient planning and hospital logistics. In principle, the application of this procedure is thus limited to small parts of the developed world. Moreover, surgical staff and patients are exposed to ionizing radiation.

Superparamagnetic iron oxide nanoparticles (SPIONs) have received much attention in bioscientific research since the first report in the 1980s and have increasingly been used clinically in recent years. Biocompatible SPIONs with a suitable surface architecture have triggered research efforts for both cellular imaging and drug-delivery applications. One of the main features of SPIONs is the ability to show magnetization only in an applied magnetic field. SPIONs have the ability to form stable colloidal suspensions, which is crucial for in vivo biomedical applications [8]. SPIONs enhance both T1 and T2/T2* relaxation. In consequence, the uptake of SPION contrast agents results in a drop of signal intensity ('negative contrast') on T2* (susceptibility)-weighted magnetic resonance imaging (MRI) sequences [9]. In conjunction with a particle size optimized for filtration and retention by SLNs, these characteristics enable preoperative visualization of SLNs using MRI before intraoperative detection by handheld magnetometers [10,11]. The natural dark brown color can help to further identify SLNs intraoperatively and eliminates the need for separate (carbon or blue) dye injections in sentinel-guided surgery.

Based on these advantageous properties, SPIONs have been successfully applied for marking and intraoperative detection of SLNs in breast cancer to overcome the drawbacks of the radioisotope-based sentinel procedure [12]. In a pilot study, we presented the first results on the intraoperative detection of SLNs in PCa patients using a handheld magnetometer system after intraprostatic injection of SPIONs and demonstrated the feasibility and safety of this magnetic SLN identification procedure in PCa [13].

In view of these findings, we hypothesized that magnetometer-guided sLND based on intraoperative identification of SPION-marked SLNs would have high reliability in the identification of LN-positive PCa patients, being comparable with the radioisotope-guided sentinel procedure.

To assess the diagnostic accuracy of magnetometer-guided sLND in PCa, this prospective single-center study analyzed intermediate- and high-risk PCa patients who underwent magnetometer-guided sLND and eLND, followed by radical retropubic prostatectomy. The diagnostic accuracy of magnetometer-guided sLND was determined using eLND as the reference standard.

2. Results

As planned, the study included 50 intermediate- or high-risk PCa patients who underwent radical retropubic prostatectomy with magnetometer-guided sLND after intraprostatic injection of SPIONs, with eLND being performed as the reference standard. Table 1 summarizes the patient characteristics.

Table 1. Patient characteristics.

Characteristics	Overall	Patients with Negative LNs	Patients with Positive LNs
	$n = 50$	$n = 32$ (64%)	$n = 18$ (36%)
Age, years (median)	69.5	68.5	71.5
IQR	64–73	64–73	64.5–73
Total PSA, ng/mL (median)	10.8	9.8	12.0
IQR	7.4–19.2	6.9–14.7	8.3–30.1
Number of LNs removed (median)	18	19	17.5
IQR	15–23	15–23	16–22
Number of SLNs removed (median)	9	9	10
IQR	6–12	5–11	7–12
Number of positive LNs (median)			2
IQR			1–3
Tumor stage (%)			
T1c	28 (56)	22 (68.8)	6 (33.3)
T2a	2 (4)	1 (3.1)	1 (5.6)
T2b	6 (12)	4 (12.5)	2 (11.1)
T2c	12 (24)	5 (15.6)	7 (38.9)
T3	2 (4)	0 (0)	2 (11.1)
Biopsy Gleason score (%)			
6 (3 + 3)	8 (16)	8 (25.0)	0 (0)
7 (3 + 4)	26 (52)	18 (56.3)	8 (44.4)
7 (4 + 3)	6 (12)	5 (15.6)	1 (5.6)
≥8	10 (20)	1 (3.1)	9 (50.0)
Postoperative Gleason score (%)			
6 (3 + 3)	2 (4)	2 (6.3)	0 (0)
7 (3 + 4)	23 (46)	19 (59.4)	4 (22.2)
7 (4 + 3)	14 (28)	8 (25.0)	6 (33.3)
≥8	11 (22)	3 (9.4)	8 (44.4)
Pathologic stage (%)			
pT2	24 (48)	22 (68.8)	2 (11.1)
pT3a	12 (24)	7 (21.9)	5 (27.8)
pT3b	12 (24)	3 (9.4)	9 (50.0)
pT4	2 (4)	0 (0)	2 (11.1)

IQR, Interquartile range; (S)LN, (sentinel) lymph node; PSA, prostate-specific antigen.

In all, 966 LNs (median 18 per patient, interquartile range (IQR) 15–23) were removed. At least one SLN was successfully detected by magnetometer-guided sLND in all patients (50/50), resulting in a detection rate of 100%. According to the ex vivo measurements of magnetic LN activity, a total of 447 SLNs were identified. The median number of detected SLNs was 9 (IQR 6–12).

SLNs were also localized outside the established eLND template (e.g., the periprostatic region: 3.6%; presacral region: 2.2%). Figure 1 shows the detailed distributions of all SLNs per anatomical region.

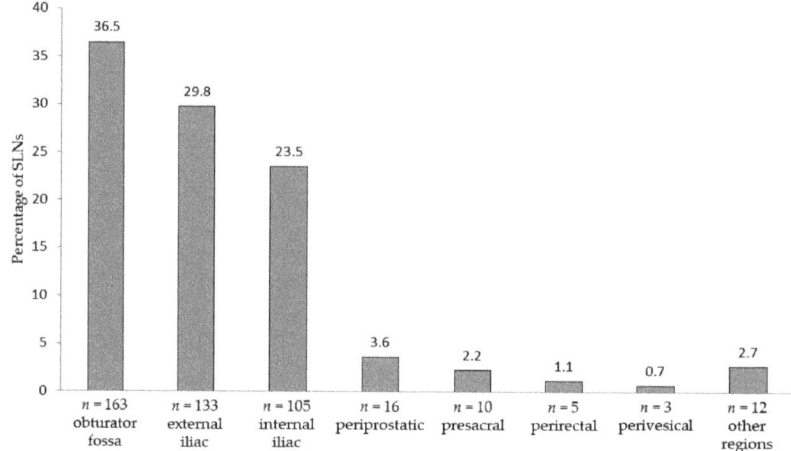

Figure 1. Areas and anatomical distribution of the 447 prostate sentinel lymph nodes from the 50 intermediate- or high-risk patients based on magnetometer-guided detection after intraprostatic injection of superparamagnetic iron oxide nanoparticles.

LN metastases were found in 36% (18/50) of patients. In total, 43 LNs were metastasis-positive, with the median number of positive nodes (when present) being 2 (IQR 1–3). Taking eLND as the reference standard, the sensitivity of the magnetic SLN procedure was 100%, i.e., all patients with LN metastases were correctly detected as LN-positive. The magnetometer-guided sLND results had a specificity of 97.0%, positive predictive value (PPV) of 94.4%, and negative predictive value (NPV) of 100%, resulting in a false negative rate of 0.0%. sLND was shown to be of additional diagnostic value in one of the 18 LN-positive patients. In this case, sLND resulted in the detection of one LN metastasis outside the eLND template (presacral), while eLND did not reveal any metastases (false positive rate 3%). Figure 2 shows the distribution of all detected LN metastases per anatomical region.

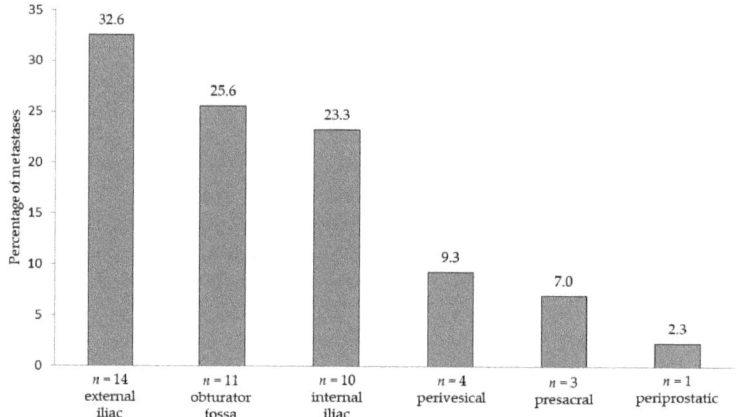

Figure 2. Areas and anatomical distribution of lymph node metastases ($n = 43$) detected by extended pelvic lymph node dissection and/or magnetometer-guided sentinel lymphadenectomy after intraprostatic injection of superparamagnetic iron oxide nanoparticles in 18 lymph node-positive patients with intermediate- or high-risk prostate cancer.

The percentage of LN-positive patients with metastases only in SLNs was 77.8% ($n = 14$).

Intraoperative measurement of magnetic activity or detection of SLNs using the handheld magnetometer missed one LN-positive patient, in whom one positive SLN was not detected, resulting in a sensitivity of 94.4% (17/18).

3. Discussion

After the successful application of the magnetometer-guided sentinel approach in breast cancer, the feasibility and safety of intraoperative detection of SPION-marked SLNs using a handheld magnetometer following intraprostatic SPIONs injection was demonstrated in PCa [13]. Currently, the use of this magnetic sentinel procedure is also being investigated in other tumor entities, for example, initial positive results have recently been shown for penile cancer [14].

On the basis of results comparable to the radioactive marking of SLNs in breast cancer and the promising first results presented in our PCa pilot study (SentiMag Pro I) [12,13,15], we hypothesized that magnetometer-guided sLND would also have high reliability in the identification of SLNs or LN-positive PCa patients, being comparable to the radioisotope-guided sentinel approach.

In the results presented for the SentiMag Pro II trial, which included PCa patients with an intermediate- or high-risk for the presence of lymphatic metastasis, SLNs were identified in all patients, resulting in a detection rate of 100%. This is better than in our pilot study, that included PCa patients with the same risk factors, where the magnetic technique successfully identified SLNs in only 89.5% of cases [13]. For radioisotope-guided sLND, a detection rate of 98.0% was reported in a study including over 2000 low-, intermediate-, and high-risk PCa patients [16]. One meta-analysis demonstrated a pooled detection rate of 93.8% for the radio-guided sentinel approach [17]. A systematic literature review considering 21 studies recruiting 2509 patients, found a median cumulative percentage detection rate of 95.9% (IQR 89.4–98.5%) [4]. However, in the SentiMag Pro II study, we adjusted the exclusion criteria according to some of the fundamental limitations of sLND already described by us and others (e.g., previous hormonal treatment or prostate surgery), which may have improved our detection rate [13].

In the ex vivo analysis using the handheld magnetometer to identify SLNs, all LN-positive patients were correctly detected in the SentiMag Pro II study. However, one metastatic SLN was not detected intracorporeally using the SentiMag probe, resulting in the missing of one LN-positive patient and a sensitivity of 94.4%. This patient had a high-risk tumor with large volume (Gleason score 4 + 5, pT3b (Union for International Cancer Control (UICC) tumor–node–metastasis (TNM) classification of malignant tumors, 7th Edition), PSA 44 ng/mL), which may have obstructed the outflow of the tracer. In vivo, only one SLN showing weakly magnetic activity (11 counts) could be identified using the SentiMag probe. In ex vivo measurement, magnetic activity was detected in five of the 35 LNs removed, which, like the metastasis-positive SLN overlooked intraoperatively (50 counts), had a comparatively low activity. The positive SLN, which was not detected intraoperatively, was located in the deep presacral area, so that the limitations of the intracorporeal detection of SPION-marked SLNs described in the next but one paragraph may have become noticeable, taking into account the weak activity.

In the systematic literature review mentioned above, the median cumulative percentage results for sLND showed a sensitivity of 95.2% (81.8–100%) and false negative rate of 4.8% (0–18.2%), taking into account in vivo SLN identification [4]. Accordingly, the SentiMag Pro II results can be considered comparable, and indicate that the use of intraprostatically injected SPIONs combined with intraoperative use of a handheld magnetometer forms a reliable replacement for the radioactive approach in PCa patients. In a meta-analysis of SLN biopsy in breast cancer using the same magnetic technique for SLN biopsy, pooled data could show that the magnetic technique was non-inferior to the standard technique ($z = 3.87$, $p < 0.001$), too. The mean detection rates for the technetium-based standard and magnetic techniques alone were 96.8% (94.2–99.0%) and 97.1% (94.4–98.0%), respectively. Mean false-negative rates were 10.9% (range 6–22%) for the standard technique and 8.4% (2–22%) for the magnetic technique. Using a random-effects model, the total number of LNs removed was significantly higher with the magnetic technique ($p = 0.003$) [18]. Similarly, in the SentiMag Pro II

Study, the number of SLNs removed (median 9, IQR 6–12) was higher than described in our own previous studies using the technetium-based procedure, in which 6 SLNs (median; IQR 4–8) were resected [5]. A possible cause for this could be the smaller size of SPION (60 nm; ^{99m}Tc nanocolloid: <80 nm) which could result in marking of secondary landing sites, too [19].

There are various possible causes limiting the effectiveness of intracorporal detection of SPION-marked SLNs using a magnetometer. One problem of intracorporeally detection is that adipose tissue surrounding SLNs can limit the proximity of the probe to the LN, resulting in insufficient exposure of the LN. An insufficient measurement of the magnetic signal can be the result. Moreover, the presence of tissue in the vicinity of the probe tip of the magnetometer and the LN reduces the in vivo magnetic signal because of the negative magnetic susceptibility of surrounding tissue [20]. The limited spatial resolution of the SentiMag® probe (~20 mm) could restrain the differentiation of SLN signals from the background signal from the injection site. In the near future, the higher resolution of novel probes using magnetic tunneling junction techniques (resolution ~4 mm) could lead to a sustainable improvement in intracorporeally SLN identification [20]. In addition, the now available possibility of preoperative localization of magnetically marked SLNs using magnetic resonance imaging (MRI) could further improve intraoperative detectability [10].

Other disadvantages of the magnetometer-guided procedure are the need for frequent balancing of the magnetic baseline level and the requirement for use of plastic or other non-magnetic retractors during surgery [18]. This circumstance also complicates the development of laparoscopic probes for magnetic SLN detection [21]. Another limitation of the magnetic technique is the maximum depth at which the magnetic signal can be detected. Currently available handheld magnetometers do not reach the same depth as a gamma probe (e.g., SentiMag: ~20 mm; TAKUMI® magnetic probe: 10 mm), which can have consequences for the identification of deeper nodes [22,23]. In the MELAMAG Trial, patients with melanoma who underwent SentiMag-guided SLN biopsy in the axillary basin had a lower SLN identification rate than those who required SLN biopsy in the groin basin, seemingly owing to SLNs being located deeper in the axilla compared with the groin [23]. In principle, it must be taken into account that unlike radioactive marking or the use of a gamma probe, contact of the magnetometer with the tissue is mandatory. This circumstance must be considered during intraoperative use of magnetometers and requires a certain adaptation to the radioactive approach.

Preoperative SLN identification offers the surgeon a roadmap with solid information on individual location of draining LNs. So far, lymphoscintigraphy cannot be undertaken without a radioisotope tracer. However, preoperative SLN visualization on MRI after intraprostatic SPION injection was demonstrated recently in PCa patients and could replace the conventional lymphoscintigraphic procedure [10]. MRI is highly sensitive to very small concentrations of SPION and very small SLNs could be visualized. The high spatial resolution of MRI allows the for differentiation of SLNs adjacent to each other, which appear as one hotspot in lymphoscintigraphy. In contrast, the spatial resolution of radioisotope-based lymphoscintigraphy is quite limited (~7–8 mm), which makes identification of smaller LNs, typical of pelvic LNs, difficult. The differentiation of SLNs, especially in the periprostatic, presacral, and perirectal region, is difficult because of high periprostatic activity and excreted radiotracer in the bladder [19].

Another important advantage for routine clinical use of the magnetic sentinel method is that this non-radioactive procedure does not require a radiation-controlled area or imaging facilities and can be safely implemented without facilities' restrictions in large parts of the world. For example, in Japan, currently, approximately 30% of the facilities do not have a radiation-controlled area [22]. Furthermore, SPION tracer is retained in LNs for a longer time, allowing for delayed sLND (up to 7 days for Sienna+ in breast cancer), which facilitates the patient planning. There is no dependence in radioactive isotope supply, which in recent years has been problematic because of cutbacks in production. Furthermore, the exposition of patients and surgical staff to ionizing radiation is avoided.

In the SentiMag Pro II study, in 22.2% ($n = 4$) of LN-positive cases, metastases were also found in non-SLNs. All four cases were patients with high aggressive PCa (PSA > 40 ng/mL, Gleason score ≥ 8), in accordance with previous reports showing poorer outcomes for sLND with highly aggressive tumors [24]. One fundamental problem of the SLN approach is that fully metastasized LNs or blocked lymph pathways can redirect the tracer, as has already been described for lymphatic spread, and LNs not detected by sLND might already be connected downstream [25]. However, magnetometer-guided sLND may detect LN metastases outside the established eLND template. For example, in the SentiMag Pro II study, 7% of positive nodes were detected in the presacral region. Others demonstrated that 7% of preoperatively SLNs were identified in the presacral region, and 8% of patients with LN metastasis would have been missed if an LND in the presacral region had not been performed [26]. Thus, if the goal is to remove as many positive LNs as possible and not just SLNs, sLND must be combined with eLND in high-risk PCa patients.

The limitations of this study include those inherent to the selection bias associated with surgical series from a single institution and a small sample size. In terms of limitations, it should be noted that the study center that conducted the SentiMag Pro II trial has a very high level of expertise in sLND approaches, which may have introduced bias. However, it remains to be emphasized that the staging reliability and rates of LN metastasis detected by magnetometer-guided sentinel lymphadenectomy in the monitored sample compare well with results from other sLND series [4]. To overcome these limitations, multicenter studies with a larger number of cases should be performed. In addition, a direct comparison of the new magnetic procedure with the radioisotope-guided approach, which can be accomplished by injecting both tracers, as performed by others in breast cancer patients, would be desirable [12,27]. However, our ethics committee did not allow us to perform this in the SentiMag Pro II study.

Initial studies on the magnetic sentinel method have also been carried out on several other tumor entities, which are to be continued in a comparable manner. Recently, the feasibility of intraoperative magnetic SLN identification using the SentiMag system in penile cancer patients could be shown in two pilot studies [14,28]. In addition, our working group was able to demonstrate the visualization of SLNs using MRI after peritumoral SPION injection in penile cancer [14]. Klimczak et al. compared the efficacy and safety of SLN detection in eight vulvar cancer patients using the SentiMag system with the standard radioactive tracer and reported a high detection rate (100%) and complete concordance to the standard procedure [29]. The magnetic sentinel technique is also feasible for SLN biopsy in melanoma with a high SLN identification rate [23]. However, comparing with the standard dual technique, the predefined non-inferiority margin was not reached in the MELAMAG Trial [23]. Furthermore, initial data on the use of magnetometer-guided SLN detection in lung cancer and colorectal cancer were reported [30,31].

In the future, non-invasive techniques could supplement surgical LN staging, including the sentinel procedure, or partially replace LND in longer term. Recent work highlights circulating tumor DNA (ctDNA) present in the blood as a supplemental, or perhaps an alternative, source of DNA to identify the clinically relevant cancer mutational landscape. This noninvasive approach may facilitate repeated monitoring of disease progression and treatment response. Potential applications of this noninvasive information in tumor staging, treatment, and disease prognosis are under discussion [32]. For example, Yang et al. propose the development of a staging system including analysis of ctDNA from liquid biopsy (B) (TNMB staging system) to enhance the current TNM cancer staging system. This model assumes that there is no LN metastasis in the case of undetectable ctDNA mutations in the blood [32]. A systematic metanalysis could demonstrate that cell-free DNA (cfDNA) levels detected by liquid biopsy can be predictive of axillary LN metastasis in patients with breast cancer [33]. Circulating epithelial tumor cells (CTCs) themselves can also provide noninvasive insights in the state of metastasis. However, CTCs are rare, comprising as few as 1–10 cells per 10⁹ hematological cells, and CTC shedding from a solid tumor into the bloodstream is a highly discontinuous process. Thus, the isolation of CTCs with high purity is still a very significant challenge [34]. To meet this challenge, Loeian et al. developed a nanotube-CTC-chip for isolation of tumor-derived epithelial cells (CTCs) from peripheral blood, with high purity, by exploiting the physical mechanisms of preferential adherence of CTCs on a nanotube surface [34]. In clinical studies they used this nanotube-CTC-chip to isolate CTCs with high purity from breast cancer patients. In this initial investigation, CTCs were captured in patients that were LN-positive and negative. However, an apparent increase in CTC counts between early stage (stage 1–3) and advanced disease (stage 4) using the nanotube-CTC-chip could be shown. In order to be able to use the chance, which these new non-invasive techniques offer also for the selection of LN-positive patients, their results should be correlated in further investigations also with the results of targeted sentinel lymphadenectomy showing a high reliability in the detection of patients with LN metastases.

4. Materials and Methods

4.1. Study Design and Patients

The prospective monocentric SentiMag Pro II study (German Clinical Trials Register: DRKS00007671) investigated the diagnostic accuracy of a novel technique for intraoperative SLN detection in PCa patients, using SPIONs and a handheld magnetometer.

Fifty patients with intermediate- or high-risk PCa (European Association of Urology risk group definitions) scheduled for open radical retropubic prostatectomy and pelvic LND between February and September 2015 were included in this study [35]. Inclusion criteria were a PSA level ≥10.0 ng/mL and/or a Gleason sore ≥7. Exclusion criteria included a known intolerance or hypersensitivity to iron or dextran compounds, iron overload disease, a pacemaker or other implantable device in the chest wall, hormonal treatment, and previous prostate surgery.

4.2. Magnetic Superparamagnetic Iron Oxide Nanoparticle (SPION) Tracer

The SPION tracer (Sienna+®) used in this study is a component of the SentiMag® system (Endomagnetics Ltd., Cambridge, UK). This system for marking and identifying SLNs comprises a handheld magnetometer, the SentiMag® unit, and the Sienna+® magnetic tracer. All are Conformité Européene (CE) certified as class IIa medical devices. The particles have a carboxydextran coating and a mean hydrodynamic diameter of 60 nm. Sienna+ has comparable functional properties to that of ^{99m}Tc nanocolloid, because upon interstitial injection the tracer flows through the lymph system and gets trapped in SLNs in the same manner as the radionuclide.

4.3. Tracer Injection

The sentinel technique in PCa differs from that in other tumor types. In breast cancer and malignant melanoma, a well-directed peritumoral injection is used to observe the lymphatic drainage of the tumor only. In PCa, which commonly occurs as a multifocal malignancy, it is not known with absolute certainty from which part of the organ the metastatic spread originated, or which lesion is the index lesion. Therefore, the aim of prostate lymph scintigraphy must be the imaging of all the primary draining LNs of the prostate, which must therefore include the SLN of the cancer.

In this study, one urologist injected 2 mL of SPION (Sienna+) into the prostate of patients using transrectal ultrasound guidance 24 h before surgery. Based on our examinations and those of others, the tracer was evenly spread as three deposits on both sides of the prostate in all cases, as described previously [13].

4.4. Magnetometer-Guided sLND, eLND, and Histopathological Examination

Patients underwent magnetometer (SentiMag)-guided sLND and eLND, followed by radical retropubic prostatectomy. All cases were performed by two high-volume surgeons, who applied the same anatomical template during eLND. The eLND template included the area along the external iliac vessels, with the distal limit being the femoral canal. Proximally, eLND was carried out to, and included, the bifurcation of the common iliac artery. All lymphatic fatty tissue along the internal iliac artery and within the obturator fossa and the area dorsal to the obturator nerve was removed, as described by Weingärtner et al. [36]. The lateral limit consisted of the pelvic sidewall, while the medial dissection limit was defined by the perivesical fat.

During sLND, all metal retractors were removed from the surgical field and polymer retractors (SUSI®, Aesculap®; B. Braun Melsungen AG, Melsungen, Germany) were used to avoid interference with the magnetometer when detecting SLNs with the SentiMag probe. All SLNs detected by the SentiMag were removed, with each magnetically active LN being considered as an SLN. In addition, the magnetic activity of all LNs was measured ex vivo. For surgical reasons, LNs other than SLNs directly adjoining and adhering to SLNs were also removed if in situ separation was not possible. In such cases, LNs were macroscopically detected (tactile and visually) ex vivo and the surgeon separated them from each other or from the containing fibro-fatty tissue. Thereafter, eLND was conducted to remove the remaining lymphatic fatty tissue from the above-named regions. Afterwards, LNs were macroscopically detected and separated from those containing fibro-fatty tissue by the surgeon.

Postoperatively, all LNs were detected and separated by the surgeon (SLNs and non-SLNs), cut into 3 mm transverse sections, and routinely processed and embedded in paraffin, while 4–5 µm-thick sections were further cut and stained with hematoxylin-eosin.

4.5. Outcome Measures of Magnetometer-Guided sLND

As established by our and other working groups, and in line with the results of an international sentinel consensus meeting, the diagnostic accuracy of sLND was assessed using conventional eLND in the same cohort as the reference standard [4,37]. Compliance with this standard ensures that our results can be compared with the results of other sentinel techniques.

The outcomes used to analyze the diagnostic test accuracy were detection rate (patients with at least one detected SLN/total number of patients operated on), sensitivity, specificity, PPV, NPV, false-positive, and false-negative rates, with all being measured at the patient level. False-negative cases were defined as patients with a histologically negative SLN, whilst cancer was found in other LNs. False-positive cases were defined as patients with SLNs containing metastases found outside the eLND template, while the eLND template did not reveal any metastases [4]. Thus, the false-positive rate provides a measure of the additional diagnostic value of sLND over and above eLND (false-negative on eLND).

A 2 × 2 table with sLND as the index test and eLND as the reference standard was used to calculate sensitivity, specificity, NPV, and PPV. Additionally, the anatomical distributions of detected LN metastases and identified SLNs were analyzed.

4.6. Ethical Approval

All subjects gave their informed consent for inclusion before they participated in the study. The protocol followed in this study was in accordance with the ethical standards of the 1964 Helsinki Declaration and its later amendments. The protocol was approved by the Medical Chamber of Lower Saxony, Germany (Bo/24/2014).

5. Conclusions

After interstitial injection, SPIONs are filtered and retained in SLNs allowing intraoperative identification of SLNs using handheld magnetometers. Based on these characteristics, SPIONs have been successfully applied for marking and intraoperative detection of SLNs in breast cancer to overcome the drawbacks of the radioisotope-based sentinel procedure. In several studies including breast cancer patients, the magnetic SentiMag technique for SLN biopsy was non-inferior to the standard method. The results of this prospective clinical trial suggest that the magnetometer-guided radiation-free sentinel procedure could be a reliable replacement for the established radioisotope-based approach in PCa patients who are at intermediate- or high-risk for LN involvement, too. With the aim of detecting all LN metastases in high-risk patients, sLND should be performed in addition to eLND, because of its additional diagnostic value and the detection of LN metastases outside the extended template.

The reliability of intraoperative SLN detection using the SentiMag system requires verification in further multicentric studies, including comparisons with other new magnetometer modalities (e.g., probes with permanent magnet and hall sensor or magnetic tunneling junction sensors), which were presented recently. In addition, the promising initial results in other tumor entities such as melanoma, vulvar, and penile cancer should also be pursued.

Author Contributions: Conceptualization, A.W., S.G. and F.W.; Data curation, S.E., P.G. and M.-C.S.; Formal analysis, A.W. and S.E.; Funding acquisition, A.W.; Investigation, A.W., S.E., P.G., M.-C.S., R.-P.H. and F.W.; Methodology, A.W. and F.W.; Project administration, S.E., P.G. and M.-C.S.; Software, S.G.; Supervision, F.W.; Validation, A.W. and S.E.; Writing—original draft, A.W. and S.E.; Writing—review and editing, S.G., R.-P.H. and F.W. All authors have read and agreed to the published version of the manuscript.

Funding: This study was funded by the Research Pool of the Carl von Ossietzky University Oldenburg, Oldenburg, Germany.

Acknowledgments: We thank Karl Embleton, from Edanz Group (www.edanzediting.com/ac) for editing a draft of this manuscript.

Conflicts of Interest: The authors declare no conflict of interest. The funder had no role in the design of the study, in the collection, analyses, or interpretation of data, in the writing of the manuscript, or in the decision to publish the results.

References

1. Heidenreich, A.; Ohlmann, C.H.; Polyakov, S. Anatomical extent of pelvic lymphadenectomy in patients undergoing radical prostatectomy. *Eur. Urol.* **2007**, *52*, 29–37. [CrossRef] [PubMed]
2. Briganti, A.; Chun, F.K.; Salonia, A.; Suardi, N.; Gallina, A.; Da Pozzo, L.F.; Roscigno, M.; Zanni, G.; Valiquette, L.; Rigatti, P.; et al. Complications and other surgical outcomes associated with extended pelvic lymphadenectomy in men with localized prostate cancer. *Eur. Urol.* **2006**, *50*, 1006–1013. [CrossRef] [PubMed]
3. Wawroschek, F.; Vogt, H.; Weckermann, D.; Wagner, T.; Harzmann, R. The sentinel lymph node concept in prostate cancer—first results of gamma probe-guided sentinel lymph node identification. *Eur. Urol.* **1999**, *36*, 595–600. [CrossRef] [PubMed]
4. Wit, E.M.K.; Acar, C.; Grivas, N.; Yuan, C.; Horenblas, S.; Liedberg, F.; Valdes Olmos, R.A.; van Leeuwen, F.W.B.; van den Berg, N.S.; Winter, A.; et al. Sentinel node procedure in prostate cancer: A systematic review to assess diagnostic accuracy. *Eur. Urol.* **2017**, *71*, 596–605. [CrossRef] [PubMed]
5. Winter, A.; Kneib, T.; Henke, R.P.; Wawroschek, F. Sentinel lymph node dissection in more than 1200 prostate cancer cases: Rate and prediction of lymph node involvement depending on preoperative tumor characteristics. *Int. J. Urol.* **2014**, *21*, 58–63. [CrossRef] [PubMed]
6. Winter, A.; Kneib, T.; Wasylow, C.; Reinhardt, L.; Henke, R.P.; Engels, S.; Gerullis, H.; Wawroschek, F. Updated nomogram incorporating percentage of positive cores to predict probability of lymph node invasion in prostate cancer patients undergoing sentinel lymph node dissection. *J. Cancer* **2017**, *8*, 2692–2698. [CrossRef]
7. Grivas, N.; Wit, E.; Tillier, C.; van Muilekom, E.; Pos, F.; Winter, A.; van der Poel, H. Validation and head-to-head comparison of three nomograms predicting probability of lymph node invasion of prostate cancer in patients undergoing extended and/or sentinel lymph node dissection. *Eur. J. Nucl. Med. Mol. Imaging* **2017**, *44*, 2213–2226. [CrossRef]
8. Wáng, Y.X.; Idée, J.M. A comprehensive literatures update of clinical researches of superparamagnetic resonance iron oxide nanoparticles for magnetic resonance imaging. *Quant. Imaging Med. Surg.* **2017**, *7*, 88–122.
9. Stark, D.D.; Weissleder, R.; Elizondo, G.; Hahn, P.F.; Saini, S.; Todd, L.E.; Wittenberg, J.; Ferrucci, J.T. Superparamagnetic iron oxide: Clinical application as a contrast agent for MR imaging of the liver. *Radiology* **1988**, *168*, 297–301. [CrossRef]
10. Winter, A.; Chavan, A.; Wawroschek, F. Magnetic resonance imaging of sentinel lymph nodes using intraprostatic injection of superparamagnetic iron oxide nanoparticles in prostate cancer patients: First-in-human results. *Eur. Urol.* **2018**, *73*, 813–814. [CrossRef]

11. Pouw, J.J.; Grootendorst, M.R.; Bezooijen, R.; Klazen, C.A.; De Bruin, W.I.; Klaase, J.M.; Hall-Craggs, M.A.; Douek, M.; Ten Haken, B. Pre-operative sentinel lymph node localization in breast cancer with superparamagnetic iron oxide MRI: The SentiMAG Multicentre Trial imaging subprotocol. *Br. J. Radiol.* **2015**, *88*, 20150634. [CrossRef] [PubMed]
12. Douek, M.; Klaase, J.; Monypenny, I.; Kothari, A.; Zechmeister, K.; Brown, D.; Wyld, L.; Drew, P.; Garmo, H.; Agbaje, O.; et al. Sentinel node biopsy using a magnetic tracer versus standard technique: The SentiMAG Multicentre Trial. *Ann. Surg. Oncol.* **2014**, *21*, 1237–1245. [CrossRef] [PubMed]
13. Winter, A.; Woenkhaus, J.; Wawroschek, F. A novel method for intraoperative sentinel lymph node detection in prostate cancer patients using superparamagnetic iron oxide nanoparticles and a handheld magnetometer: The initial clinical experience. *Ann. Surg. Oncol.* **2014**, *21*, 4390–4396. [CrossRef] [PubMed]
14. Winter, A.; Kowald, T.; Engels, S.; Wawroschek, F. Magnetic resonance sentinel lymph node imaging and magnetometer-guided intraoperative detection in penile cancer, using superparamagnetic iron oxide nanoparticles: First results. *Urol. Int.* **2019**, *29*, 1–4. [CrossRef] [PubMed]
15. Karakatsanis, A.; Daskalakis, K.; Stålberg, P.; Olofsson, H.; Andersson, Y.; Eriksson, S.; Bergkvist, L.; Wärnberg, F. Superparamagnetic iron oxide nanoparticles as the sole method for sentinel node biopsy detection in patients with breast cancer. *Br. J. Surg.* **2017**, *104*, 1675–1685. [CrossRef] [PubMed]
16. Holl, G.; Dorn, R.; Wengenmair, H.; Weckermann, D.; Sciuk, J. Validation of sentinel lymph node dissection in prostate cancer: Experience in more than 2000 patients. *Eur. J. Nucl. Med. Mol. Imaging* **2009**, *36*, 1377–1382. [CrossRef] [PubMed]
17. Sadeghi, R.; Tabasi, K.T.; Bazaz, S.M.; Kakhki, V.R.; Massoom, A.F.; Gholami, H.; Zakavi, S.R. Sentinel node mapping in the prostate cancer. Meta-analysis. *Nuklearmedizin* **2011**, *50*, 107–115. [PubMed]
18. Zada, A.; Peek, M.C.; Ahmed, M.; Anninga, B.; Baker, R.; Kusakabe, M.; Sekino, M.; Klaase, J.M.; Ten Haken, B.; Douek, M. Meta-analysis of sentinel lymph node biopsy in breast cancer using the magnetic technique. *Br. J. Surg.* **2016**, *103*, 1409–1419. [CrossRef]
19. Winter, A.; Kowald, T.; Paulo, T.S.; Goos, P.; Engels, S.; Gerullis, H.; Schiffmann, J.; Chavan, A.; Wawroschek, F. Magnetic resonance sentinel lymph node imaging and magnetometer-guided intraoperative detection in prostate cancer using superparamagnetic iron oxide nanoparticles. *Int. J. Nanomed.* **2018**, *13*, 6689–6698. [CrossRef]
20. Cousins, A.; Balalis, G.L.; Thompson, S.K.; Morales, D.F.; Mohtar, A.; Wedding, A.B.; Thierry, B. Novel handheld magnetometer probe based on magnetic tunnelling junction sensors for intraoperative sentinel lymph node identification. *Sci. Rep.* **2015**, *5*, 10842. [CrossRef]
21. Van de Loosdrecht, M.M.; Waanders, S.; Krooshoop, H.J.G.; ten Haken, B. Separation of excitation and detection coils for in vivo detection of superparamagnetic iron oxide nanoparticles. *J. Magn. Magn. Mater.* **2019**, *475*, 563–569. [CrossRef]
22. Taruno, K.; Kurita, T.; Kuwahata, A.; Yanagihara, K.; Enokido, K.; Katayose, Y.; Nakamura, S.; Takei, H.; Sekino, M.; Kusakabe, M. Multicenter clinical trial on sentinel lymph node biopsy using superparamagnetic iron oxide nanoparticles and a novel handheld magnetic probe. *J. Surg. Oncol.* **2019**, *120*, 1391–1396. [CrossRef] [PubMed]
23. Anninga, B.; White, S.H.; Moncrieff, M.; Dziewulski, P.; LC Geh, J.; Klaase, J.; Garmo, H.; Castro, F.; Pinder, S.; Pankhurst, Q.A.; et al. Magnetic technique for sentinel lymph node biopsy in melanoma: The MELAMAG trial. *Ann. Surg. Oncol.* **2016**, *23*, 2070–2078. [CrossRef] [PubMed]
24. Weckermann, D.; Dorn, R.; Holl, G.; Wagner, T.; Harzmann, R. Limitations of radioguided surgery in high-risk prostate cancer. *Eur. Urol.* **2007**, *51*, 1549–1556. [CrossRef]
25. Morgan-Parkes, J.H. Metastases: Mechanisms, pathways, and cascades. *AJR Am. J. Roentgenol.* **1995**, *164*, 1075–1082. [CrossRef]
26. Joniau, S.; Van den Bergh, L.; Lerut, E.; Deroose, C.M.; Haustermans, K.; Oyen, R.; Budiharto, T.; Ameye, F.; Bogaerts, K.; Van Poppel, H. Mapping of pelvic lymph node metastases in prostate cancer. *Eur. Urol.* **2013**, *63*, 450–458. [CrossRef]
27. Thill, M.; Kurylcio, A.; Welter, R.; van Haasteren, V.; Grosse, B.; Berclaz, G.; Polkowski, W.; Hauser, N. The Central-European SentiMag study: Sentinel lymph node biopsy with superparamagnetic iron oxide (SPIO) vs. radioisotope. *Breast* **2014**, *23*, 175–179. [CrossRef]

28. Cleaveland, P.; Lau, M.; Parnham, A.; Murby, B.; Ashworth, D.; Manohoran, P.; Taylor, B.; Bell, J.; Najran, P.; Oliveira, P.; et al. Testing the feasibility of sentimag/sienna+ for detecting inguinal sentinel nodes in penile cancer (SentiPen): An eUROGEN and national cancer research institute trial. *Eur. Urol.* **2019**, *76*, 874–875. [CrossRef]
29. Klimczak, P.; Kalus, M.; Kryszpin, M.; Manowiec, M.; Hirowska-Tracz, M.; Jedryka, M. A novel and promising technique of sentinel lymph nodes detection in vulvar cancer patients. *EJSO* **2019**, *45*, e151–e152. [CrossRef]
30. Pouw, J.J.; Grootendorst, M.R.; Klaase, J.M.; van Baarlen, J.; Ten Haken, B. Ex vivo sentinel lymph node mapping in colorectal cancer using a magnetic nanoparticle tracer to improve staging accuracy: A pilot study. *Colorectal Dis.* **2016**, *18*, 1147–1153. [CrossRef]
31. Imai, K.; Kawaharada, Y.; Ogawa, J.; Saito, H.; Kudo, S.; Takashima, S.; Saito, Y.; Atari, M.; Ito, A.; Terata, K.; et al. Development of a new magnetometer for sentinel lymph node mapping designed for video-assisted thoracic surgery in non-small cell lung cancer. *Surg. Innov.* **2015**, *22*, 401–405. [CrossRef] [PubMed]
32. Yang, M.; Forbes, M.E.; Bitting, R.L.; O'Neill, S.S.; Chou, P.C.; Topaloglu, U.; Miller, L.D.; Hawkins, G.A.; Grant, S.C.; DeYoung, B.R.; et al. Incorporating blood-based liquid biopsy information into cancer staging: Time for a TNMB system? *Ann. Oncol.* **2018**, *29*, 311–323. [CrossRef] [PubMed]
33. Lee, J.H.; Jeong, H.; Choi, J.W.; Oh, H.E.; Kim, Y.S. Liquid biopsy prediction of axillary lymph node metastasis, cancer recurrence, and patient survival in breast cancer: A meta-analysis. *Medicine* **2018**, *97*, e12862. [CrossRef] [PubMed]
34. Loeian, M.S.; Mehdi Aghaei, S.; Farhadi, F.; Rai, V.; Yang, H.W.; Johnson, M.D.; Aqil, F.; Mandadi, M.; Rai, S.N.; Panchapakesan, B. Liquid biopsy using the nanotube-CTC-chip: Capture of invasive CTCs with high purity using preferential adherence in breast cancer patients. *Lab. Chip.* **2019**, *19*, 1899–1915. [CrossRef]
35. Mottet, N.; Bellmunt, J.; Bolla, M.; Briers, E.; Cumberbatch, M.G.; De Santis, M.; Fossati, N.; Gross, T.; Henry, A.M.; Joniau, S.; et al. EAU-ESTRO-SIOG guidelines on prostate cancer. Part 1: Screening, diagnosis, and local treatment with curative intent. *Eur. Urol.* **2017**, *71*, 618–629. [CrossRef]
36. Weingärtner, K.; Ramaswamy, A.; Bittinger, A.; Gerharz, E.W.; Vöge, D.; Riedmiller, H. Anatomical basis for pelvic lymphadenectomy in prostate cancer: Results of an autopsy study and implications for the clinic. *J. Urol.* **1996**, *156*, 1969–1971. [CrossRef]
37. Van der Poel, H.G.; Wit, E.M.; Acar, C.; van den Berg, N.S.; van Leeuwen, F.W.B.; Valdes Olmos, R.A.; Winter, A.; Wawroschek, F.; Liedberg, F.; Maclennan, S.; et al. Sentinel node biopsy for prostate cancer: Report from a consensus panel meeting. *BJU Int.* **2017**, *120*, 204–211. [CrossRef]

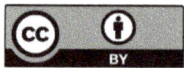

© 2019 by the authors. Licensee MDPI, Basel, Switzerland. This article is an open access article distributed under the terms and conditions of the Creative Commons Attribution (CC BY) license (http://creativecommons.org/licenses/by/4.0/).

Article

Magnetic Silica-Coated Iron Oxide Nanochains as Photothermal Agents, Disrupting the Extracellular Matrix, and Eradicating Cancer Cells

Jelena Kolosnjaj-Tabi [1,*], Slavko Kralj [2,3,*], Elena Griseti [1], Sebastjan Nemec [2,3], Claire Wilhelm [4], Anouchka Plan Sangnier [3], Elisabeth Bellard [1], Isabelle Fourquaux [5], Muriel Golzio [1] and Marie-Pierre Rols [1]

1. Institute of Pharmacology and Structural Biology, 205 Route de Narbonne, 31400 Toulouse, France; elena.griseti@ipbs.fr (E.G.); Elisabeth.Bellard@ipbs.fr (E.B.); muriel.golzio@ipbs.fr (M.G.); Marie-Pierre.Rols@ipbs.fr (M.-P.R.)
2. Department for Materials Synthesis, Jožef Stefan Institute, Jamova cesta 39, 1000 Ljubljana, Slovenia; sebastjan.nemec@ijs.si
3. Faculty of Pharmacy, University of Ljubljana, Askerceva cesta 7, 1000 Ljubljana, Slovenia; anouchka.plan@gmail.com
4. Laboratoire Matière et Systèmes Complexes (MSC), UMR 7057, Bâtiment Condorcet, Université Paris Diderot, 10 rue Alice Domon et Léonie Duquet, 75205 Paris, France; claire.wilhelm@univ-paris-diderot.fr
5. Centre de Microscopie Electronique Appliquée à la Biologie (CMEAB), Faculté de Médecine Rangueil, 133 Route de Narbonne, 31400 Toulouse, France; isabelle.fourquaux@univ-tlse3.fr
* Correspondence: jelena.kolosnjaj-tabi@ipbs.fr (J.K.-T.); slavko.kralj@ijs.si (S.K.)

Received: 30 October 2019; Accepted: 13 December 2019; Published: 17 December 2019

Abstract: Cancerous cells and the tumor microenvironment are among key elements involved in cancer development, progression, and resistance to treatment. In order to tackle the cells and the extracellular matrix, we herein propose the use of a class of silica-coated iron oxide nanochains, which have superior magnetic responsiveness and can act as efficient photothermal agents. When internalized by different cancer cell lines and normal (non-cancerous) cells, the nanochains are not toxic, as assessed on 2D and 3D cell culture models. Yet, upon irradiation with near infrared light, the nanochains become efficient cytotoxic photothermal agents. Besides, not only do they generate hyperthermia, which effectively eradicates tumor cells in vitro, but they also locally melt the collagen matrix, as we evidence in real-time, using engineered cell sheets with self-secreted extracellular matrix. By simultaneously acting as physical (magnetic and photothermal) effectors and chemical delivery systems, the nanochain-based platforms offer original multimodal possibilities for prospective cancer treatment, affecting both the cells and the extracellular matrix.

Keywords: magnetic silica-coated iron oxide nanochains; nanoparticles; photothermal treatment; hyperthermia; cancer; collagen; cellular microenvironment

1. Introduction

Iron oxide nanoparticles (IONPs) are among the most popular and most extensively studied inorganic nanoparticles, which have enabled a series of distinct therapeutic approaches in various biomedical domains [1].

Iron oxide nanoparticles were historically used as contrast agents for magnetic resonance imaging (MRI), mostly to detect liver metastases [2]. Subsequently, IONPs use evolved with the development of MRI-based technologies, enabling the in vivo tracking of single cells [3]. The magnetic responsiveness of IONPs [4] paved the way to magnetic cell manipulation approaches.

In order to be useful in biomedicine, nanoparticles should be superparamagnetic. Superparamagnetism is a form of magnetism where magnetization randomly flips at room temperature. In the absence of an external magnetic field, the overall magnetization of a group of superparamagnetic nanoparticles (smaller than 20 nm for iron oxides) is zero, because the magnetic moment of the nanoparticles is randomly distributed. The weakness of the attractive magnetic interactions among the superparamagnetic nanoparticles does not to allow them to magnetically aggregate. This magnetic behavior is crucial for the preparation of ferrofluids, which can therefore be applied to biological systems, because superparamagnetic nanoparticles remain well dispersed. Nevertheless, when an external magnet is applied, all magnetic moments align in the same direction, leading to a net magnetization. Nevertheless, individual superparamagnetic nanoparticles are too small for their effective translational movement even in the strongest magnetic fields. Therefore, in view of magnetic manipulation, iron oxides can be loaded in liposomes, confined within cell-derived vesicles or loaded within cells. When IONPs are loaded within the cells, the latter become magneto-responsive, and can thus migrate along a magnetic field gradient, allowing distal guidance of nanoparticle-loaded cells to the site of therapeutic interest [5].

Alternatively, to preserve superparamagnetism and achieve strong magnetic responsiveness, we here present a method by which we group a number of small superparamagnetic nanoparticles into larger and defined nanoparticle clusters. Such clusters are highly magnetically responsive and therefore form chain-like structures once exposed to magnetic field. In order to obtain permanent chain-like structures—the magnetic "nanochains"—we optimized the synthesis protocol. The nanochains are thus obtained when a suspension of superparamagnetic nanoparticle clusters is exposed to a defined magnetic field, while silica is added to fixate the clusters into permanent nanochains. Such nanochains are superparamagnetic, with superior magnetic responsiveness due to much larger magnetic moment (larger magnetic volume) than that of individual nanoparticle clusters.

In addition to magnetic targeting, other biomedical applications are applicable to IONPs. When magnetic nanoparticles are submitted to a high frequency alternating magnetic field (AMF) with suitable amplitude, the magnetic energy is transduced to nanoparticle heating, which dissipates into the surroundings. This phenomenon is exploited in magnetic hyperthermia [6], an experimental cancer treatment, where magnetic nanoparticles are locally injected and heated, in order to destroy unresectable tumors. Magnetic hyperthermia has an important advantage over other, more common hyperthermia treatments, such as the ones generated by microwaves, radiofrequency, or ultrasound. This advantage relies on the potential to heat solid tumors from the inside, preventing the heating of bystander tissues, located between the energy source and the target zone. Nevertheless, the main drawbacks for magnetic hyperthermia are: (1) the requirement of injecting high amounts of IONPs in order to obtain significant heating, thus requiring local (intra-tumoral) nanoparticles injections, and (2) the necessity to keep nanoparticles outside the cells, as intracellular processing dramatically decreases nanoparticle heating potential [7].

For a long time, magnetic hyperthermia was considered as the only nanoparticles-mediated thermal modality for cancer treatment. However, a few years ago, their remarkable conversion of light to heat in the near infrared window was demonstrated [8]. Photothermal therapy is a treatment that relies on the conversion of the energy of light into thermal energy. This phenomenon occurs because iron oxides are semiconductors, and have a small band gap between valence and conduction electrons. This band gap can be bridged by excitation, provided by the optical energy (the photons) of a laser beam. After excitation, valence electrons stay in the conduction band for a limited time, after which they fall back to the valence position. When this fall occurs, heat is emitted [9]. As light sources, such as lasers, can be accurately focused, the photothermal treatment can be limited only to the zone of therapeutic interest. The main advantage of photothermia over magnetic hyperthermia is that the treatment could be efficient even after cellular internalization of nanoparticles and at lower local nanoparticles concentrations [7].

Photothermia has been used in preclinical research, and mainly relies on heat generation mediated by gold [10], silver [11], and copper [12] nanoparticles or carbon nanotubes [13] and graphene [14]. These nanomaterials have a different mechanism for heat generation than IONPs. In metals, such as gold, silver, and copper, the light to heat conversion occurs when light interacts with conduction electrons on the surface of metallic nanoparticles [15]. In carbon-based nanoparticles, the delocalized electrons absorb light and the energy is converted to vibrations of the C-C reticule, which is released as heat when the vibrational states decay [15].

Photothermal therapy using gold nanoparticles already reached clinical trials (ClinicalTrials.gov Identifiers: NCT01270139 and NCT01436123), yet, as these materials might be extremely bio-persistent [16] and can potentially be toxic [17,18], we suggest alternative bio-compatible materials. Among them, iron oxides appear particularly attractive. The median lethal dose of intravenously applied citrate-coated IONPS (diameter 8.6 nm) to mice is very high, and was reportedly greater than 949 mg (17 mmol) Fe/kg body weight [19]. Indeed, once administered by the intravenous route, IONPs mainly accumulate in the liver. There they may induce oxidative stress, which results in an increased level of liver enzymes. Nevertheless, these changes are transient, and they do not lead to significant adverse reactions [20]. When synthetic nanoparticles degrade, the iron loads into ferritin proteins and integrates iron's physiological pathways of iron re-use or elimination [21]. Alternatively, the iron, released from synthetic nanoparticles, can be re-assembled in cells to form nanoparticles anew, and prevent the toxicity of ferrous iron [22].

While IONPs potential for MRI, magnetic targeting, and magnetic hyperthermia have been broadly documented in the literature, IONP-induced photothermia recently emerged [8,23].

With the aim to create bio-compatible, magnetically guidable, and photothermally responsive nanoparticles with long-term multimodal imaging properties, we intentionally prepared and optimized the functionalization protocol, as well as biologically tested magnetic silica-coated iron oxide nanochains [24]. The chains have an iron-oxide core and a silica shell, within which we covalently linked a fluorescent dye, allowing fluorescence imaging follow-up. The core conveys magnetic and photothermal properties, and the shell provides both (i) a large platform for nanoparticles surface functionalization and (ii) a porous compartment, which can covalently bind molecular components, such as dyes or drugs. The nanochains, which are presented in this study represent a promising and unique nanomaterial, possessing superparamagnetism, superior magnetic responsiveness, and good photothermal properties, which have been rarely combined in single nanostructures.

Cancerous cells and their microenvironment both play a pivotal role in cancer development, progression, and resistance to treatment [25]. In this regard, the nanochains, presented herein, which heat and thus simultaneously affect cellular and environmental components, could radically improve the therapeutic outcome. Moreover, one of the very important advantages of the magnetic nanochains is their superior magnetic responsiveness. The latter could be used for all applications where magnetic guidance is desired, such as magnetic drug delivery or magnetic targeting.

2. Results

2.1. Nanochains Characterization

Short, less than 1 μm long, anisotropic by shape, and superparamagnetic nanochains were synthesized by magnetic assembly of few (5 ± 1.4) nanoparticle clusters (Figure 1A, Scheme S1). The size of nanoparticle clusters coated with a 3-nm-thick silica shell was measured from TEM micrographs (>100 nanochains counted) and measured 90 ± 28 nm. The synthesis of nanoparticle clusters is based on self-assembly of 70 ± 14 superparamagnetic iron oxide (maghemite) nanoparticles within the size range of 10.4 ± 1.4 nm [24,26,27]. The core–shell nature of the nanochains, with the closely packed maghemite nanoparticles cluster cores and the amorphous silica shell, can be clearly distinguished in TEM micrographs (Figure 1A). Functionalized fluorescent nanochains showed superparamagnetic properties, excellent colloidal stability, and high magnetic responsiveness (Figure S1). When the suspension was placed on a magnet, the nanochains (Figure 1B left) readily assembled into slightly larger anisotropic nanochain bundles that could be detected by optical microscopy (Figure 1B right). These bundles are disaggregated as soon as the external magnet is removed. The nanochains' saturation magnetization Ms is ~37 Am^2kg^{-1} (Figure 1C). The efficiency of the functionalization was assessed using the Kaiser test, FTIR-ATR (Figure S2), and indirect methods such as the zeta-potential measurements of the fluorescent silica-coated nanochains (RB-nanochains), fluorescent amino-functionalized nanochains (RB-nanochains-NH_2), and fluorescent carboxyl functionalized nanochains (RB-nanochains-COOH) in aqueous suspensions (Figure 1D). The accessible primary amines on the surface of the RB-nanochains-NH_2 was quantified by Kaiser test. The spectroscopically determined mean value is 145 μmol per gram of the RB-nanochains-NH_2. A FTIR-ATR surface analysis method confirmed the transfer of surface amines of the RB-nanochains-NH_2 into carboxyl groups on the surface of the RB-nanochains-COOH (see Figure S2). The spectrum of the RB-nanochains-COOH shows the distinctive bands at wavenumbers 1703.1 cm^{-1}, 1442.9 cm^{-1}, and 1402.7 cm^{-1}, confirming the presence of carboxyl group and amide bond. However, the primary amines of the RB-nanochains-NH_2 are not clearly visible because they are overlapped with intensive silanol OH of silica at wavenumbers above 3000 cm^{-1}. The electrophoretic mobilities of the RB-nanochains, RB-nanochains-NH_2, and RB-nanochains-COOH were measured as the function of the operational pH. The silica surface shows a relatively acidic character, because its structure comprises negatively charged –OH groups at pH values above the isoelectric point (IEP) at ~ pH 3. The zeta-potential curve of pristine silica-coated nanochains reaches negative values of less than 15 mV at pH above 7. After amine functionalization, the zeta-potential of the RB-nanochains-NH_2 changed significantly and reached the value of ~ 6 mV at physiological pH 7.4. More pronouncedly, after carboxyl functionalization, the zeta potential significantly decreases to negative values, reaching negative values of less than ~ 40 mV at pH above 7. The high absolute values of the zeta-potential provide strong electrostatic repulsive forces between the nanochains, and result in a good colloidal stability of the suspension in neutral and alkaline conditions [28]. Therefore, the carboxyl-functionalized nanochains (nanochains-COOH and RB-nanochains-COOH) were chosen for further investigation. The heating efficiency was evaluated in nanochains suspensions up to [Fe] = 130 mM (7.3 g_{Fe}/L). The magnetic hyperthermia (MHT) yield after exposure to an alternating magnetic field was low even at the highest concentrations (130 mM): a 400 s exposure of the nanochains suspension led to a temperature increase of only 3.5 °C ± 0.2 °C. Heating potential can be evaluated using the mass-normalized specific absorption rate (SAR) parameter, expressed in W per gram of iron. Herein, the MHT SAR reached 25 ± 9 W/g_{Fe}. Conversely, the RB-nanochains-COOH suspension provided a high photothermal yield (Figure 1E) upon laser excitation at 808 nm and laser power density of 0.3 W/cm^2. A 400 s exposure of the same suspension led to a temperature increase of about 15.7 ± 2 °C (Figure 1E), and corresponded to a SAR of 202 ± 25 W/g_{Fe}. Indeed, the thermal yield is proportional to the laser power density, and reached a temperature increase of 30 ± 2 °C for the same suspension volume (100 μL) and iron concentration (130 mM), irradiated at λ = 808 nm at a laser power density of 1 W/cm^2.

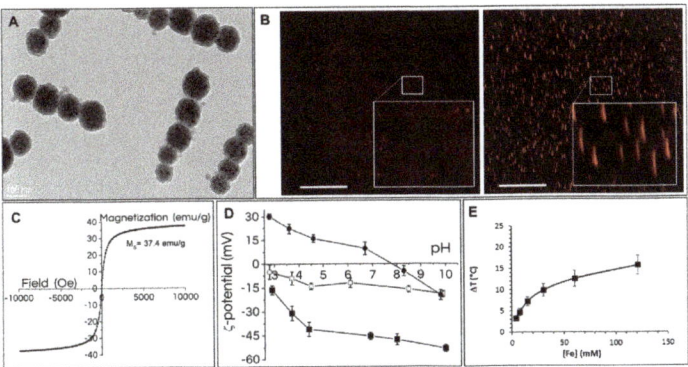

Figure 1. Structure and properties of RB-nanochains-COOH. (**A**) Transmission electron micrograph showing darker spherical nanoparticles cluster cores and less contrasted amorphous silica shell forming permanently sintered anisotropic nanochains, composed of ~5 clusters per nanochain. (**B**) Fluorescence micrographs of RB-nanochains-COOH dispersed in Dulbecco's Phosphate Buffered Saline (PBS) imaged (**left**) without the presence of a magnet and (**right**) with the magnet placed below the suspensions, showing the bundles of chains, which form well-defined, stable, transient super-assemblies, which align with the direction of magnetic field lines, and disassemble into individual nanochains as soon as the external magnet is removed. The inset shows a magnified view of the selected zone. Scale bar 100 μm (Mag. ×20). (**C**) Room-temperature measurements of the magnetization as a function of magnetic field strength (in emu/g of RB-nanochains-COOH). (**D**) The curves of the zeta-potential as a function of pH for RB-nanochains (white squares), for RB-nanochains-NH$_2$ (black spheres) and RB-nanochains-COOH (black squares). (**E**) Temperature elevation curve of RB-nanochains-COOH in 100 μL of aqueous suspension measured in an Eppendorf tube upon laser irradiation at λ = 808 nm and laser power density of 0.3 W/cm^2 at different iron concentrations expressed in millimoles (the bars represent the standard deviation (SD) obtained from 3 independent measurements).

2.2. Cell Loading

The cells were efficiently loaded with RB-nanochains-COOH, as shown in Figure 2A–D. RB-nanochains-COOH were internalized to the highest degree by the largest cells—the fibroblasts, while HCT-116 (wild type), HCT-116-GFP, and HeLa GFP-Rab7 internalized comparable quantities of chains, as assessed by average fluorescence intensity measurements. The mean red fluorescence intensity of internalized chains was 105 ± 6 for fibroblasts, 72 ± 1 for HeLa GFP-Rab7 cells, 74 ± 2 for HCT-116-GFP cells, and 71 ± 2 for HCT-116 wild type cells, respectively. Within the cells, the nanochains localized within endosomes, as evidenced in Figure 2E,F, showing HeLa cells expressing a green fluorescent rab7 protein, which is associated to early and late endosomes [25]. In HCT-116 wild type cells, which internalized the smallest amount of RB-nanochains-COOH, we quantified the iron load by single cell magnetophoresis, and determined an uptake of 17.3 ± 2.6 pg of iron per cell (Figure 2G). The mass of a single nanochain composed of 5 nanoparticle clusters is estimated to be 2.1×10^{-14} g. Since iron represents approximately 45% of nanochains, this equals 0.9×10^{-14} g of iron per chain. We thus estimate around 1800 ± 270 nanochains per cell in cancer cells. The uptake comparison among different cell types, used in this study, is shown in Figure 2H. While cancer cells internalized comparable amounts of RB-nanochains-COOH, the fibroblasts internalized about 30% more nanochains.

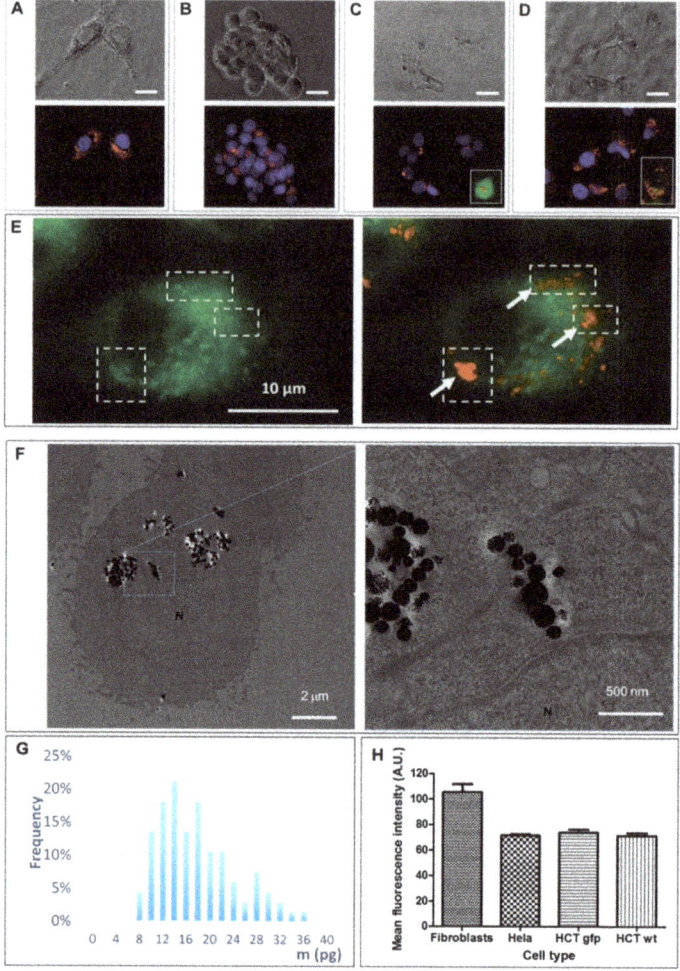

Figure 2. Cellular uptake of RB-nanochains-COOH obtained at an extracellular iron concentration of 5 mM within the RPMI medium. (**A–D**) Bright field (**top**) and fluorescence (**bottom**) micrographs showing RB-nanochain-COOH-loaded cells (**A**) Normal dermal fibroblasts, (**B**) HCT-116 wild type cells, (**C**) HCT-116 GFP cells, and (**D**) HeLa GFP-Rab7 cells (Scale bar 20 µm, Mag. ×40. Cell nuclei are stained in blue—Hoechst 33342 fluorescent stain. Insets in (**C,D**) show the intrinsic green fluorescence of GFP-expressing cells). (**E**) Left: Green fluorescence micrograph of a HeLa GFP-Rab7 cell, exhibiting characteristic green fluorescing endosomes, and right: green and red fluorescence micrographs overlay showing the co-localization of green fluorescing endosomes (white dashed line squares) with red fluorescing RB-nanochains-COOH clusters (squares and arrows) (Mag. ×100), (**F**) Representative transmission electron micrograph showing a loaded HCT-116 wild type cell (**left**) and the magnified view of internalized chains (**right**). N denotes the cell's nucleus. (**G**) Iron quantification in loaded HCT-116 wild type cells, as determined by single cell magnetophoresis. The graph shows the distribution of internalized iron (expressed in picograms of iron per cell) after cells incubation with 5 mM extracellular iron concentration. (**H**) RB-nanochains-COOH internalization in different cell types expressed as mean fluorescence intensity determined in a population of 500 cells. The error bars represent the SD of mean fluorescence intensities determined from 6 experiments per cell type.

2.3. Short and Long-Term Toxicity Assessment

Cell incubation with RB-nanochains-COOH (performed at 5 mM extracellular concentration of iron) did not alter cell viability of HCT116, HCT116-GFP, HeLa GFP-Rab7, and normal human dermal fibroblasts, as assessed with the Trypan Blue Exclusion Test, performed 24 h after cell loading. The viability of control and loaded cells was above 90%, respectively. In order to assess the long-term effect of RB-nanochains-COOH on cell survival and proliferation, we performed two distinct tests. The first approach involved a clonogenic test (Figure 3A,B). In the case of HCT-116, HCT-116-GFP, and HeLa-Rab7-GFP cells, the cells exhibited a colony-forming capacity of 83%, 90%, or 112%, respectively. In the case of normal dermal fibroblasts, the colony-forming capacity of loaded cells was of about 70% compared to control cells.

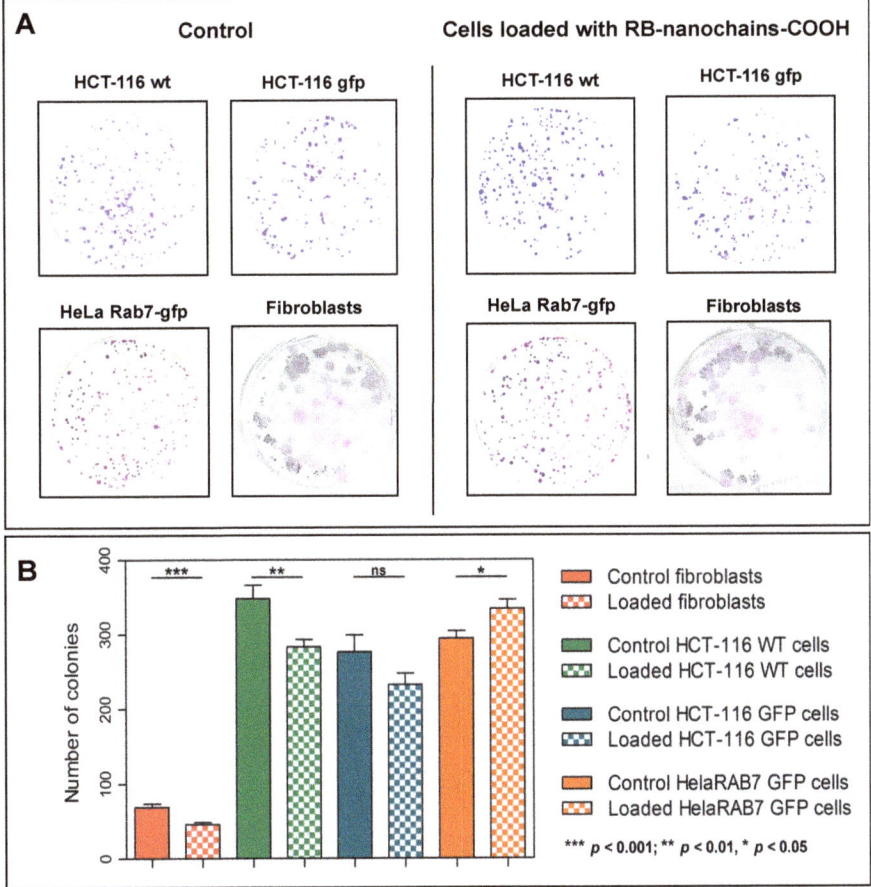

Figure 3. Colony-forming ability of control and RB-nanochain-COOH-loaded cells. (**A**) Images showing cell colonies after crystal violet staining. (**B**) Graph showing the number of colonies counted at D7 for cancer cell lines and at D 14 for normal dermal fibroblasts the term "loaded cells" refers to cells that internalized the RB-nanochains-COOH. The results (expressed as mean ± SEM) were obtained in three independent experiments made in triplicates. Differences between groups were assessed by an unpaired Student *t*-test and a *p*-value < 0.05 was considered significant.

The second approach involved the formation of cellular spheroids with unloaded (control) or loaded cells and the monitoring of spheroid growth over 9 days (Figure 4A). Unloaded- and loaded-cells' spheroids exhibited comparable growth (Figure 4B).

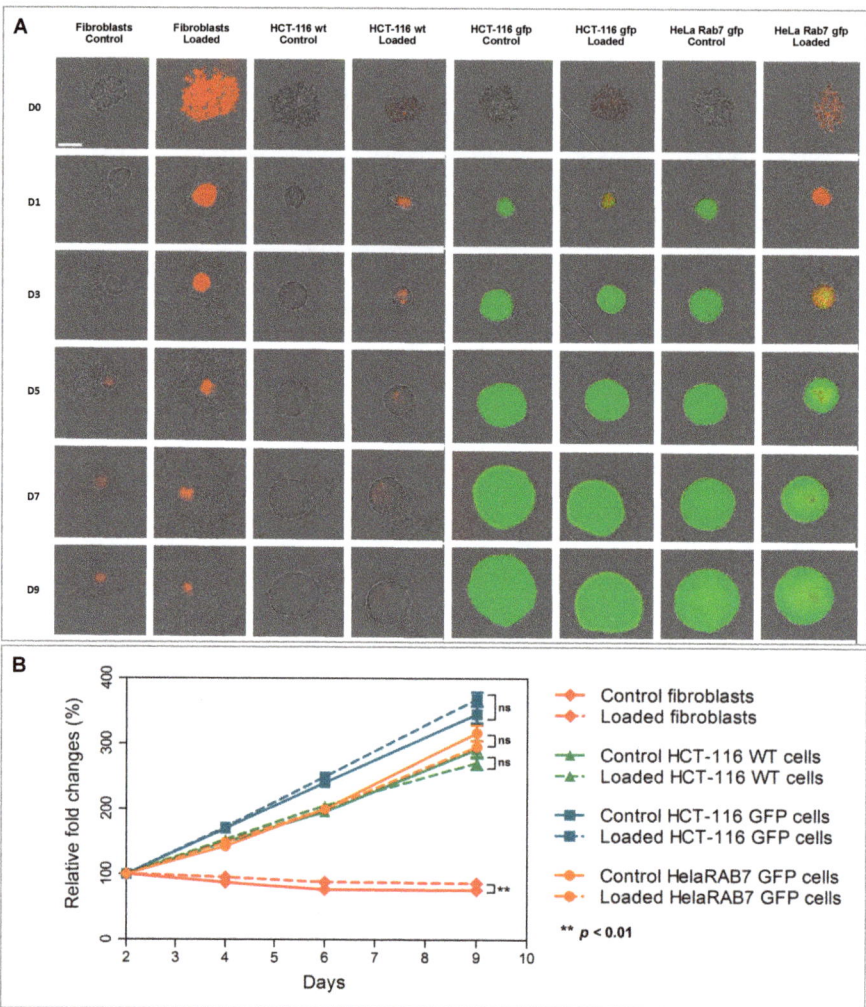

Figure 4. Control and RB-nanochain-COOH-containing cells (referred to as "loaded" in the figure), used to assess multicellular spheroids formation and growth. (**A**) Representative bright field and fluorescence micrographs overlays showing spheroids formation and growth over time. At the day of seeding (day 0—D0), the red fluorescence in cells, that internalized RB-nanochains-COOH, directly correlates with nanoparticle load. At D0 we see individual cells, which gradually agglomerate at day 1 after seeding (D1) and start forming cellular spheroids (D3 and onward). Scale bar 300 μm (mag. ×10). (**B**) Spheroid growth curve over time. Growth curves plotted from the area (mean ± standard error mean), $n = 3$ experiments, $n = 6$ spheroids per experiment per condition. Two-way ANOVA, p-value < 0.05 was considered significant.

2.4. Nanochain Distribution within Tumor Cells and Dermal Fibroblasts Spheroids

The distribution of RB-nanochains-COOH within the spheroids was assessed by a TEM investigation (Figure 5). In cellular spheroids composed of normal dermal fibroblasts, the nanochains are localized in endo-lysosomal compartments within the cells, and within the extracellular matrix, while in MCS made of cancer cells the nanochains are exclusively found in the endo-lysosomal compartments within cells.

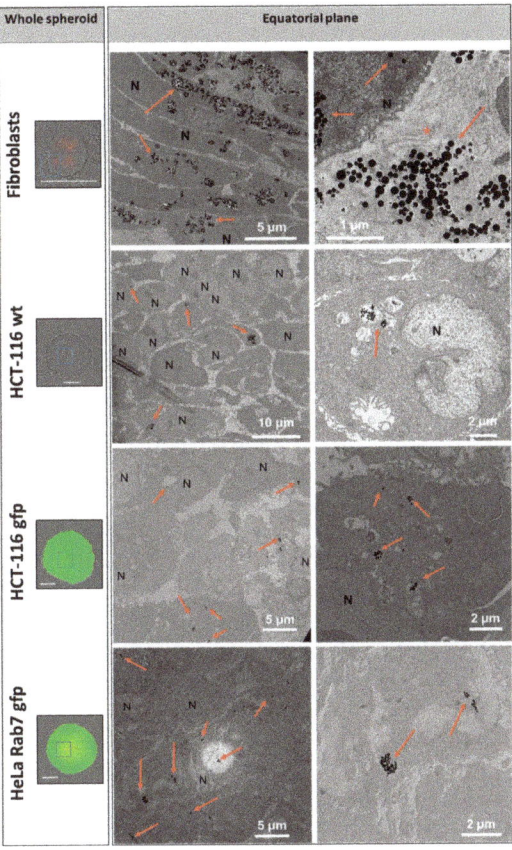

Figure 5. RB-nanochain-COOH distribution within multicellular spheroids. Left: Bright-field and fluorescence micrographs overlays of whole multicellular spheroids (scale bars 300 µm) fixed at day 11 and right: transmission electron microscopy (TEM) micrographs showing sections obtained at the equatorial plane of the spheroids. Nanochains are indicated with red arrows, N denotes cells' nuclei, * denotes the collagen fibers as evidenced within the extracellular matrix of the fibroblasts in the top right panel.

Within the extracellular matrix of spheroids, made of normal dermal fibroblasts, the RB-nanochains-COOH were found confined in the extracellular vesicles (Figure 6A) and non-confined, surrounded by fibrillary structures of the extracellular matrix (Figure 6B).

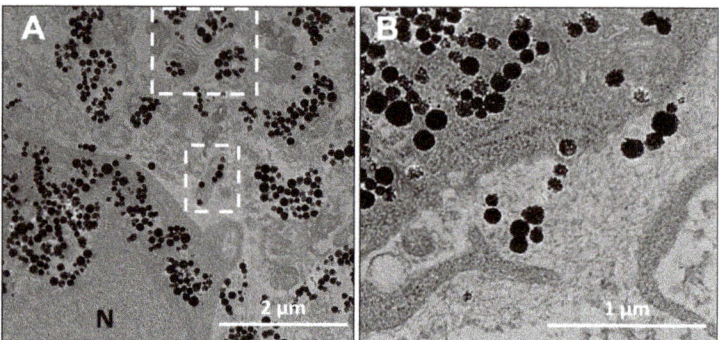

Figure 6. Comparison of extracellular locations of RB-nanochains-COOH within the extracellular matrix in multicellular spheroids. (**A**) Representative TEM micrograph showing RB-nanochains-COOH confined in extracellular vesicles (white dashed line squares) and (**B**) Non-confined RB-nanochains-COOH within fibroblast-secreted extracellular matrix.

2.5. Photothermia

After ascertaining that nanochains are well tolerated and not toxic to different cell types in vitro, we evaluated their potential for photothermal therapy. Plated cells, loaded with nanochains-COOH, or engineered cell sheets loaded with RB-nanochains-COOH, were exposed to the laser source operating within the multiphoton microscope. When loaded cells were exposed to the laser, all of them almost instantaneously underwent cell death. Figure 7A shows a characteristic example of loaded cells, which after nanochain-COOH heating underwent cell death, as evidenced by propidium iodide uptake (Figure 7B). Cell sheets, made of normal dermal fibroblasts, have a rich collagenous matrix. In the absence of RB-nanochains-COOH, the cells and their matrix were not altered after laser exposure under our experimental conditions (Figure 7C). When RB-nanochains-COOH were added to cell sheets (Figure 7D), they distributed transversally within the sheets and were found within both the cells and the collagen matrix (Figure 7E). While at low laser power (20 mW) the collagen remained unaltered, when the laser power was increased to 33 mW, the nanochains heated and melted the adjacent collagen fibers. The heating was well localized and was limited only to zones rich in nanochains and exposed to the higher laser power, as evidenced in Figure 7F. Zones where nanochains were not present and control cell sheets were not altered after 33 mW laser exposure.

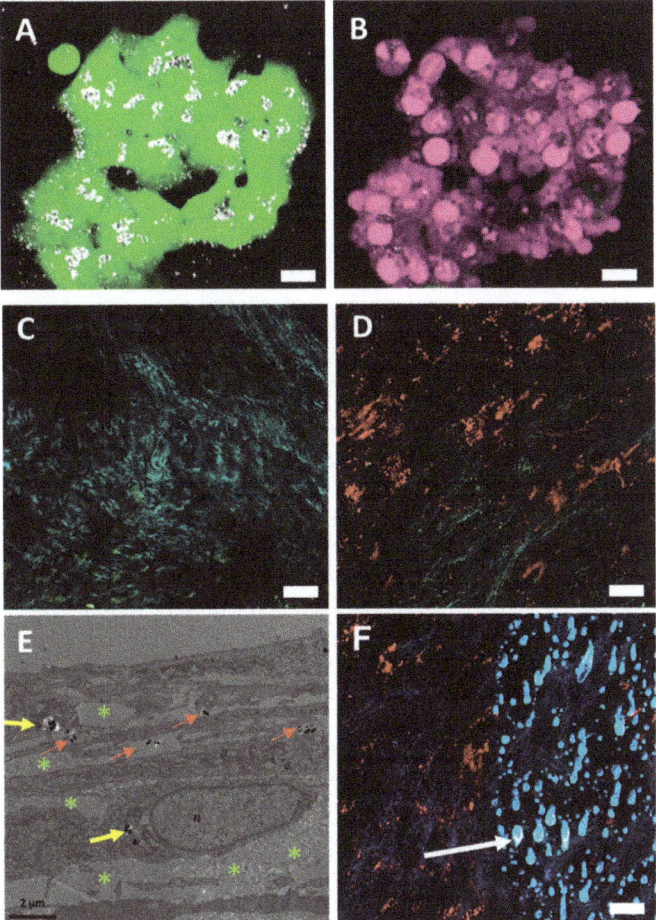

Figure 7. Nanochains as photothermal mediators affecting the cells and the extracellular matrix. (**A**) HCT-116-GFP cells (green) loaded with nanochains-COOH (white spots), exposed to the laser within the multiphoton microscope. (**B**) Nanochains-COOH-loaded HCT-116-GFP cells, which underwent cell death and thus internalized propidium iodide after laser exposure (the red fluorescence derived from cell-internalized propidium iodide is here represented by a magenta pseudo-color). (**C**) Representative micrograph of a control cell sheet exhibiting a rich collagenous matrix (turquoise) among auto-fluorescent (green) fibroblast cells (**D**) Representative micrograph of a cell sheet loaded with red-fluorescent RB-nanochains-COOH surrounded with collagen (turquoise) and fibroblasts (green). (**E**) TEM micrograph showing the distribution of RB-nanochains-COOH within the cell sheet. N denotes cell nucleus, yellow arrows point to intracellularly localized nanochains and red arrows point to extracellular nanochains. Green asterisks denote the collagen fibers in the extracellular matrix. (**F**) Representative micrograph of a cell sheet: exhibiting on the left side the intact collagen fibers (exposed to 20 mW laser power), and on the right side the melted collagen fibers (exposed to 33 mW laser power power). Scale bars in (**A**–**D**,**F**) equal 20 μm. White arrow in (**F**) points to a characteristic "drop" of melted collagen fibers.

3. Discussion

In this work we characterized a novel platform made of superparamagnetic iron oxide nanoparticle assemblies—silica-coated iron oxide nanochains [24]—that could have therapeutic potential once photoactivated.

Nanochains have high magnetic responsiveness, as we previously reported [24] and evidenced in Figure S2. Herein, we labeled the nanochains with rhodamine, which was covalently bound into the silica shell. This fluorescent labelling allows nanochains tracking by fluorescence imaging, while the surface of nanochains was functionalized with carboxyl groups (Figure 1), which are advantageous for cell-uptake, and allow endowing the cells with a high amount of nanoparticles (Figure 2). Presented nanostructures were characterized by different physico-chemical tests. Dynamic light scattering is frequently applied for determination of colloid hydrodynamic size, yet this analysis is designed for isotropic (spherical) particles. This method is therefore useless for characterization of nanochains due to their highly anisotropic shape. Alternatively, the behavior of colloidal stability in suspension could be estimated by monitoring the spontaneous sedimentation of the colloids over time. The RB-nanochains-COOH remained in suspension for at least three weeks (Figure S1A) and then only gradual could color change be seen, indicating a good stability for such relatively large "colloids". The RB-nanochains-COOH sediment completely due to gravity in two months, but they can be easily redispersed with a single gentle shake by hand. Another indirect method to determine the colloidal stability is the measurement of the RB-nanochains-COOH zeta potential, where high absolute values (over ± 30mV) at physiologically relevant pH 7.4 suggest good colloidal stability. In contrast, RB-nanochains are slightly negatively charged (−12 ± 3 mV) and RB-nanochains-NH$_2$ are slightly positively charged (6 ± 5 mV) at pH 7.4. These values are both inappropriate for achieving a suitable colloidal stability, but useful in biological settings. We therefore focused on carboxyl-functionalized nanochains (nanochains-COOH and RB-nanochains-COOH) for our in vitro studies.

Cell-loaded nanoparticles equaled a minimum of about 15 pg of iron per cell, as measured in HCT-116 cells (Figure 2), which were the smallest cells among the ones we used in this study and exhibited the lowest average red-fluorescence intensity. The quantity of iron per cell was determined by magnetophoresis. In the same way as for spherical nanoparticles, once internalized by cells, nanochains end up in large endo-lysosomal compartments [29], showing no shape anisotropy. Therefore, in the same way as for other nanoparticle-loaded cells, the translational movement of magnetic-nanochain-loaded cells derives from the overall load, which provides a global magnetic moment of the cell. Indeed, as the proportion of internalized material depends on cell size [29], fibroblasts internalized higher amounts of nanoparticles (Figure 4) and fluoresced about 30% more than cancerous cells.

In this study, the in vitro toxicity of nanochains was evaluated for the first time. The nanochains were not toxic to cancerous and non-cancerous cells (normal dermal fibroblasts, isolated from a skin biopsy), as assessed by three distinct approaches (trypan blue exclusion test, colony-forming ability, and RB-nanochain-COOH-loaded cells spheroid growth). While iron oxides are generally considered as safe and biocompatible, the toxicity assessment was indeed necessary because of the size and anisotropy of tested nanomaterials. In this regard, the toxicity was evaluated at different time points after cellular uptake of RB-nanochains-COOH. At first, we thus performed the toxicity assessment 24 h after cell loading. Cell viability (and thus short-term toxicity) is commonly evaluated using metabolic assays, which rely on read-out principles that include absorbance (colorimetry), fluorescence, or luminescence. Nevertheless, as iron oxides absorb light, colorimetric assays (such as MTT or MTS) or bio-luminescent tests (such as the ATP-based assays) might lead to false readouts, as studies reported [30]. Moreover, iron oxides can act as fluorescence quenchers [31–33], therefore redox-based viability tests, using fluorescent dyes, were also considered inappropriate for our study. We therefore assessed the viability with the trypan blue exclusion test [34]. This test relies on the capacity of viable cells to exclude the dye and the viability was assessed by direct visualization of cells and manual counting. As trypan blue exclusion only provides information about early events that occur after nanoparticles uptake, we used 2 additional tests, by which we evaluated the toxicity in the long term (7 days and beyond).

Our results indicate that nanochains are well tolerated by the cells. In the case of fibroblasts, we could observe a 30% decrease in colony-forming ability. This is probably due to two factors. Firstly, the fibroblasts have a surface that is relatively larger than the ones of cancerous cells, therefore they internalize more nanoparticles at the same extracellular nanoparticles concentration [35] (Figure 2H). Secondly, when cells divide, the nanoparticles load divides between daughter cells [36]. When cells have a short doubling time, which is the case of cancer cells, the iron load quickly splits and the burden of oxidative stress diminishes. The dermal fibroblasts which were used in this study had a doubling time of about 40 h, which was twice as much as the doubling time of cancer cells. Thus, fibroblasts were more exposed to the strain of oxidative stress, due to high, persistent, and prolonged iron presence. Moreover, studies show that gene expression of ferritin, the iron storage protein, and other proteins involved in iron homeostasis are upregulated after cell internalization of iron oxide nanoparticles [37], and this is even more emphasized in different cancers, as numerous studies suggest [38]. This explains why the colony-forming ability of cancer cells, used in this study, was less affected: cancer cells adapted easier than fibroblasts. In order to verify if nanoparticles could have a pro-proliferative effect, an additional test was made, and consisted in making cellular spheroids with cells, which were loaded with RB-nanochains-COOH. Spheroid growth was subsequently followed over 9 days (Figure 4). A modest but significant difference was only noted in the case of dermal fibroblasts, where spheroids made with particle-loaded cells were slightly larger than the spheroids made with unloaded cells. We assume that this difference is due to the overall volume of nanoparticles, internalized by cells, rather than to any potential cell growth stimulation, as the slopes of loaded and unloaded MCS growth curves are equivalent. As the volumes of cancer cell spheroids were much larger, the slight volume increase, which might be due to nanoparticles presence, affected the final volume to a much smaller extent, and the differences between loaded and non-loaded cells spheroids sizes were not significant. This result also allowed us to exclude a pro-proliferative effect induced by nanochains.

The distribution of nanochains was assessed on the ultrastructural level with transmission electron microscopy (TEM), by which we analyzed cells in 2D (at D1 post nanochains uptake—Figure 2) and 3D cultures (cellular spheroids—Figure 5, Figure 6 and Figure S3), as well as cell sheets (Figure 7). Nanochains are localized within cancer cells in multicellular spheroids, while in spheroids made of fibroblasts and in cell sheets the nanochains are distributed within cells and the extracellular matrix. On the ultrastructural level, the cells exhibited a normal morphology and we did not observe any signs of autophagy [28]. Nanochain load was much more prominent in spheroids made of fibroblasts, as these cells internalize more nanoparticles and have a smaller proliferation rate (as they exhibit contact inhibition when grown in 3D structures). This also explains why cell spheroids made of fibroblasts remain much smaller than the spheroids made of cancer cells and explains the auto-fluorescence of control fibroblasts spheroids, which started fluorescing (at λ_{Ex} = 560/40 nm and λ_{Em} = 630/75 nm) from day 5 onwards (Figure 4E first column). Dead cells have an increased autofluorescence, which is due to a decreased metabolic activity, and increased levels of denatured proteins [39,40]. Moreover, while cancerous cells divided their nanochain load and kept it within the cells, fibroblasts "expelled" nanochains into the matrix, (Figure 6), where chains were either contained within extracellular vesicles [41] or were not enclosed in membrane-derived structures. Based on this evidence, we stipulate that normal cells, which internalize more nanoparticles, have a smaller proliferation rate and a higher death rate (with respect to the overall number of cells constituting the spheroids), and generate more extracellular vesicles, which delocalize nanoparticles outside the cells into the extracellular matrix.

On the nanoparticle level, the nanochains did not undergo any major structural disintegration (Figure 6 and Figure S3). Their architecture at day 11 (when the spheroids were fixed and processed for TEM, as evidenced in multicellular spheroids in Figure 5, Figure 6 and Figure S3), remained comparable to their initial structure, which was observed in freshly loaded cells (Figure 2B) when the cells were seeded to form spheroids. Indeed, over time the chains are expected to degrade, as silica metabolizes to silicic acid [42], which is excreted in the urine [43]. On the other hand, the iron, stemming from iron oxides, is integrated into the metabolic pathway of endogenous iron [44].

Finally, our study demonstrates that presented nanochains have an excellent photothermal yield (Figure 1E), which can lead to both cell death (Figure 7B) and the melting of the extracellular matrix (Figure 7F). Most anticancer agents target cancerous cells. Nevertheless, the cellular matrix, which constitutes the tumor microenvironment, provides cancer cells with nutriments and structural support, as well as represents a substantial barrier to anticancer agent penetration. Moreover, the mechanical compression exerted by the tumor matrix was recognized to induce the metastatic phenotype in tumor cells [45].

Heat-induced cell death was previously reported for magnetic hyperthermia [6]. Nevertheless, magnetic heating can only occur when magnetic nanoparticles have enough freedom to rotate. When magnetic nanoparticles are submitted to an alternating magnetic field, they orient their magnetic moments. Magnetic energy is thus dissipated through nanoparticle movement, either by nanoparticle rotation due to Brownian relaxation or by the rotation of the magnetic moments within nanoparticles' cores due to Néel relaxation [7]. Therefore, if magnetic nanoparticles are confined, their magneto-thermal yield becomes much lower [7]. Nanoparticle confinement, for example, occurs within endo-lysosomes. In order to prevent such confinement after cellular internalization and in order to prevent nanoparticles dissemination throughout the body, the current therapeutic strategy (used by Magforce, the company that implemented the clinical use of magnetic hyperthermia) relies on the use of an aminosilane coating, which allows the formation of "stable deposits" within the tumoral tissue [46]. The nanochains, which are described in this study, are made of iron oxide nanoparticles confined within a silica shell. The low magnetic hyperthermia yield ($\Delta T = 3.5$ °C) was thus not surprising, and magnetic hyperthermia was not considered as a modality of choice. In contrast, the nanochains appeared to be excellent candidates for photothermia [7], exhibiting a high photothermal yield, even at low and physiologically useful laser power density ($\Delta T = 30$ °C at light wavelength of 808 nm and laser power density of 1 W/cm^2 and $\Delta T = 15.7$ °C at a laser power density of 0.3 W/cm^2). The photothermal functionality is particularly attractive, because the thermal yield does not decrease after endo-lysosomal internalization [7]. Nanochains can thus heat the surrounding environment when they are located outside and inside the cells (Figure 7).

Iron oxide nanoclusters, made of Fe$_3$O$_4$ nanocrystals interconnected by amorphous matrix bridges, were previously reported as efficient photothermal agents [23]. While this study was among the first to evidence that nanoclusters generate more heat than individual, non-clustered nanoparticles, the photothermal effect was obtained using a laser power density of 5 W/cm^2 [23]. Such laser power is high and detrimental to the tissue, and far exceeds the Maximum Permitted Exposure for the skin, as suggested by the American National Standards Institute Z136. In comparison, the nanochains could yield significant heat (more than 15 °C) at a much lower, and physiologically tolerable, laser power density of 0.3 W/cm^2.

The heating of nanochains was sufficient to induce cell death and to melt the collagen matrix, as evidenced in Figure 7. We have previously reported on collagen fibers slackening after tumor exposure to magnetic hyperthermia, generated by iron oxide cubic nanocrystals [47]. This slackening allowed a better permeation of doxorubicin, which was applied intravenously in a combined treatment with magnetic hyperthermia [47]. Collagen fiber slackening was assessed post mortem and was characterized by a larger spacing between collagen fibers, probably due to the phase transition of the collagen, in tissues that underwent hyperthermia [47]. Conversely, in the case of photothermia, performed in this study, we could observe how photothermia kills cancer cells, or disrupts (or melts) the extracellular matrix in a 3D micro-tissue model. These phenomena were observed in real time after cells (Video S1) or cell-sheets (Video S2) exposure to the laser within a multi-photon microscope.

Photothermal treatment could have an enormous potential for tackling highly desmoplastic tumors, which have an extremely poor therapeutic outcome. The tumor microenvironment, particularly the tightly woven collagen matrix, has a recognized capability to reduce the penetration of conventional (molecular) therapeutics and immune cells, therefore the nanochains, which could disrupt the collagen matrix, have a significant therapeutic perspective. In the future, such nanochain-based platforms could offer entirely new, synergistic, and multimodal possibilities. The latter would combine physical and chemical means in one individual nanostructure platform, allowing magnetic guiding, drug delivery, and cellular matrix destruction, as well as tumor cell eradication upon heat activation with a source of light.

4. Materials and Methods

4.1. Nanoparticles Synthesis, Functionalization, and Characterization

4.1.1. Raw Materials

The chemicals used for the synthesis of the superparamagnetic nanochains were of reagent grade quality and were obtained from commercial sources. Primary magnetic nanoparticle clusters were provided by Nanos SCI company (Ljubljana, Slovenia), and are commercially sold as iNANOvative™ (Nanos SCI, Ljubljana, Slovenia). Succinic anhydride (SA, 99%) and NH_4OH (28–30%) were supplied by Alfa Aesar (Lancashire, UK). Acetone (AppliChem GmbH, Darmstadt, Germany) and ethanol absolute (Carlo Erba, reagent—USP, Milano, Italy) were used without further processing. Hydroxy (polyethyleneoxy) propyl triethoxysilane (silane-PEG, 50% in ethanol) was supplied by Gelest Inc. (Morrisville, PA, USA). Tetraethoxysilane (TEOS; 98%), rhodamine B isothiocyanate (RB), (3-aminopropyl) triethoxysilane (APS; silane-NH2, 99%), dichloromethane (DCM), dimethylformamide (DMF), Keiser test kit, and polyvinyl pyrrolidone (PVP, 40 kDa) were obtained from Sigma Aldrich (St. Louis, MO, USA).

4.1.2. Syntheses of the Nanochains and Rhodamine-B-Labelled Nanochains

The commercial custom-made nanoparticle clusters with a ~3-nm-thick silica shell were provided by Nanos SCI company. The nanochain synthesis is based on dynamic magnetic assembly approach where parameters, such as (i) magnetic field strength, (ii) amount of TEOS added, (iii) duration of the exposure to the magnetic field, (iv) initial nanoparticle clusters concentration, and (v) nonmagnetic stirring rate, are precisely defined in order to control the nanochains length. The detailed syntheses procedures for the silica-coated nanoparticle clusters and nanochains have been published elsewhere [24,26,27,48]. Schematic demonstration of the crucial synthesis steps is presented in Supplementary Materials Scheme S1. Briefly, nanochains composed of approximately 5 nanoparticle clusters were prepared as follows. The suspension of commercial nanoparticle clusters was admixed with the polyvinyl pyrrolidone (PVP, molecular weight 40 kDa, pH 4.3 adjusted by 0.1M HCl) solution to reach final PVP concentration of 1.25×10^{-4} M and the final nanoparticle cluster concentration of 2.2×10^{-8} M. The reaction mixture (volume 90 mL) was stirred mechanically with glass propeller at 250 rpm for 8.5 h. The nanochain fabrication took place at a TEOS concentration of 45 mM, and an exposure to a magnetic field of 65 ± 15 mT. The whole amount of TEOS was admixed into the reaction mixture 10 min after the transfer of the nanoparticle clusters into the PVP solution. The silica was deposited on the chain-like nanostructures formed by a magnetic assembly of nanoparticle clusters after the pH was increased to a value 8.5 using NH_4OH. The pH was increased after 80 min of the TEOS addition. The nanochain synthesis with a ~15-nm-thick silica shell was completed in 3 h. The assemblies obtained by the mentioned procedure are denoted as "nanochains". For fluorescent labelling, rhodamine-B (RB) was covalently integrated into the matrix of the silica shell. The reaction between RB and APS was carried out first in the mixture of DCM/DMF = 4/1 overnight at room temperature. RB (0.00933 mmol) was dissolved in the solvent mixture (0.5 mL) and then APS (0.186 mmol) was added. Subsequently, the volatile solvent was removed using nitrogen flow and the product (RB-APS) was mixed with TEOS for the fluorescent silica coating. RB-labelled nanochains are denoted as "RB-nanochains". Finally, the synthesized nanochains and RB-nanochains were magnetically separated from the suspension and washed first with EtOH and then rinsed 3 times with distilled water.

4.1.3. Nanochains Functionalization

In order to improve the colloidal stability, the nanochain surface was modified by functionalization with carboxyl-carrying moieties. First, the amino-functionalized nanochains were prepared with the grafting of APS to the nanochains and RB-nanochains silica surface, as described elsewhere [35,49]. In brief, nanochains (150 mg, 15 mL distilled water) were diluted with 15 mL of ethanol to which 75 µL of APS and 250 µL of NH_4OH were added while the reaction mixture was stirred mechanically with glass propeller at 400 rpm for 5 h at 55 °C. The synthesized nanochains-NH_2 were magnetically separated from the suspension and washed first with ethanol and then rinsed 2 times with distilled water and transferred in DMF. For the preparation of carboxyl-functionalized nanochains (nanochains-COOH), the nanochains-NH_2 were further reacted with succinic anhydride (SA), applying a ring-opening elongation reaction. The nanochain-NH_2 suspension (50 mg in 35 mL DMF) was led to react with SA (10 mg in 15 mL DMF) solution, where a 0.5 mL aliquot of the solution of SA in DMF was added per minute into nanochain-NH_2 suspension, while being stirred mechanically with a glass propeller at 600 rpm overnight at room temperature. The produced nanochains-COOH formed a colloidal aqueous suspension. The same procedure of carboxyl functionalization was applied to RB-nanochains in order to produce RB-nanochains-COOH. Finally, both types of carboxyl-functionalized nanochains, nanochains-COOH and RB-nanochains-COOH, were thoroughly washed with acetone and ethanol, and dispersed in distilled water.

4.1.4. Nanochains Characterization

The RB-nanochain-COOH structure was assessed by transmission electron microscopy (TEM). A drop of RB-nanochains-COOH suspension was deposited on a copper grid coated with a perforated, transparent carbon foil. The suspension was dried prior to TEM observations performed with a transmission electron microscope (Jeol, JEM, 2100, Akishima, Japan), operating at 200 kV. Magnetic properties of the RB-nanochains-COOH were measured at room temperature by vibrational sample magnetometry (VSM) (Lake Shore 7307 VSM). The zeta-potential measurements as a function of the pH of the RB-nanochains, RB-nanochains-NH_2, and RB-nanochains-COOH suspensions (volume 15 mL) at final nanochains concentration of 0.2 mg/mL were monitored in an aqueous solution containing KCl (final concentration 10 mM). Zeta-potential measurements were performed on Zeta PALS, Brookhaven Instruments Corporation. FTIR-ATR analysis of the powders of the freeze-dried samples (RB-nanochains-NH_2, and RB-nanochains-COOH; 15–20 mg each) was performed on Perkin Elmer, Spectrum 400 Spectrometer. The quantitative analysis of primary amines of the RB-nanochains-NH_2 was determined by Keiser test, where accurately weighed 10 mg of the freeze-dried RB-nanochains-NH_2 was applied in the reaction with ninhydrin while following the manufacturer's protocol specified in the Kaiser kit.

4.2. Cell Culture and Loading of Cells with RB-Nanochains-COOH

The experiments were performed on four cell lines: the wild type human colorectal carcinoma cell line (HCT116) (ATCC® CCL-247TM), green fluorescent protein-expressing human colorectal carcinoma cell line (HCT116–GFP) [50], HeLa cells (ATCC® CCL-2TM) stably expressing GFP-RAB7 (HeLa GFP-Rab7) [51], and primary normal human dermal fibroblasts, isolated from a healthy skin biopsy [52]. Cells were grown the Dulbecco's Modified Eagle Medium (DMEM, Gibco-Invitrogen, Carlsbad, CA, USA) containing 4.5 g/L glucose, L-Glutamine and pyruvate, 1% of penicillin/streptomycin, and 10% of fetal bovine serum (the medium with additives is denoted as cDMEM). The cells were grown under standard cell-growing conditions (5% CO_2, 37 °C).

When the cells attained 60% confluence, they were rinsed with Dulbecco's Phosphate Buffered Saline with calcium chloride and magnesium chloride (Gibco-Invitrogen; PBS in the following text) and were incubated for 1 h with silica-coated iron oxide nanochains, dispersed in RPMI Medium 1640 (which was not supplemented with glutamine, serum, or antibiotics). Cells were either incubated with rhodamine-loaded functionalized silica-coated iron oxide nanochains (RB-nanochains-COOH) at iron concentrations of 5 mM; or 5 mM rhodamine-free carboxyl functionalized silica-coated iron oxide nanochains (Nanochains-COOH). The nanochain suspension dilutions used for cell loading were obtained after diluting a volume of the concentrated stock suspension of RB-nanochains-COOH or Nanochains-COOH (which had a known concentration of 62 mM of iron, as determined by chemical and magnetic measurements) in the RPMI Medium 1640. Cell loading was performed in T-25 flasks containing 2 mL of RPMI and the aliquot containing nanochain suspension, to obtain the final concentration of 5 mM of iron. Nanochains-COOH were favored in experiments involving multiphoton imaging, described in Section 4.8, last paragraph. During this imaging protocol, we intended to avoid red-fluorescence signal of RB-nanochains-COOH, in order to visualize propidium iodide uptake, which emits in the same spectrum and was used in this case as a cell viability probe during laser exposure under the multiphoton microscope.

After the one-hour incubation period with nanoparticle suspension in RPMI medium at 37 °C, the cells were gently rinsed with PBS and placed in cDMEM for an overnight chase. Particle-loaded cells were detached following the standard trypsin/EDTA-based cell detachment protocol and either fixed and processed for transmission electron microscopy (TEM) analyses, or re-plated for bright field, fluorescence, and multiphoton imaging (which included laser exposure and heating induction) or used to form multicellular spheroids (MCS) in toxicity/proliferation tests.

Cell sheets were made with primary normal human dermal fibroblasts, as previously described [53]. In summary, thirty thousand cells were plated in 24-well plates containing a round filter paper band (approximately 3 mm wide), where they grew for 6 weeks. During this period, the cells were supplied with cDMEM freshly supplemented with 50 µg/mL ascorbic acid (Sigma- Aldrich, St Quentin Fallavier, France), three times per week. Cell sheets were rinsed with PBS and co-incubated with RB-nanochains-COOH at iron concentrations of 0.25 mM in 500 µL RPMI during an incubation period of 1 h at 37 °C. The sheets were then rinsed with PBS and cDMEM was added for the overnight chase.

4.3. Bright Field and Fluorescence Microscopy and Image Analysis

Cells were imaged with a wide field Leica DM IRB microscope (Leica Microsystems, Wetzlar, Germany) coupled to a CoolSNAP HQ camera (Roper Scientific, Photometrics, Tucson, AZ, USA), using the following filter sets: for the GFP $\lambda_{Ex} = 480/40$ nm and $\lambda_{Em} = 527/30$ nm, for the RB-nanochains-COOH $\lambda_{Ex} = 560/40$ nm and $\lambda_{Em} = 630/75$ nm, and for Hoechst stain $\lambda_{Ex} = 360/40$ and $\lambda_{Em} > 425$ nm.

Cellular spheroids were monitored for 9 days using the IncuCyte Live Cell Analysis System Microscope (Essen BioScience IncuCyte™, Herts, Welwyn Garden City, UK) at a magnification × 10.

Images were analyzed with the ImageJ software (U.S. National Institute of Health, Bethesda, MD, USA). The software was used to determine the mean fluorescence intensity of loaded cells, and to measure spheroid growth. The average fluorescence intensity was measured on the first day after cellular uptake of RB-nanochains-COOH and comprised all cells that were seeded to form a spheroid. The mean average intensity was obtained by averaging 6 intensities of cells forming 6 different spheroids per cell type. Spheroid growth follow-up was obtained by measuring spheroid diameters (as the spheroids formed sphere-like structures). From the diameter of the whole spheroid, measured on daily basis, we calculated the equatorial area, which was used for growth comparison.

4.4. Transmission Electron Microscopy of Biological Matter

Cells, cellular spheroids, and engineered cell sheets were fixed (2% glutaraldehyde in 0.1 M sodium cacodylate buffer), post-fixed (1% osmium tetroxide), gradually dehydrated in ethanol, and embedded (Embed 812 resin, Electron Microscopy Sciences). Thin sections (70 nm thick) were observed with a HT 7700 Hitachi transmission electron microscope equipped with a CCD AMT XR41 camera.

4.5. Nanochains Acute and Long-Term Toxicity Assessment

4.5.1. Cell Viability Assessment by Trypan Blue Exclusion Test

Cell viability was determined 24 h after cellular uptake of RB-nanochains-COOH. The viability was assessed on the whole cell population: adherent cells and cells, which might have been floating in the culture medium. The media in which the cells were cultured and the tripsinized cells were pooled and centrifuged (5 min, 100× g). The supernatants were discarded and the pellets were re-suspended in PBS. Ten microliters of resulting cells suspensions were mixed with 10 µL of 0.4% Trypan Blue solution by gentle pipetting. Cells were manually counted using a Malassez hemocytometer within less than three minutes after preparation, and viability was calculated from the proportion of viable (undyed cells) in respect to the total number of cells (dyed and undyed). The counts were made in triplicates for each condition.

4.5.2. RB-Nanochain-Loaded Cells Survival and Proliferation Assessment

A clonogenic assay [54] was used to assess the impact of the RB-nanochains-COOH on cell long term survival. Five hundred unloaded (control) or loaded cancerous cells (prepared as described in Section 4.2.) or 250 unloaded or loaded normal dermal fibroblasts were seeded in 6-well plates. Seven or fourteen days after seeding (in case of cancer cells or fibroblasts, respectively), the colonies were rinsed with PBS, fixed with methanol, and stained with crystal violet (0.5% w/v) for 15 min under gentle stirring at room temperature, rinsed 3 times with PBS, and left to dry prior colony counting.

The impact of RB-nanochains-COOH on cell survival and proliferation was also determined in 3D cell cultures, where chain-loaded cells were used to make cellular spheroids. Multicellular cell spheroids (MCS) were made following the non-adherent technique, by seeding cells in Costar® Corning® Ultra-low attachment 96-well plates (Fisher Scientific, Illkirch, France). Approximately five hundred unloaded or loaded cancer cells (HCT116, HCT116-GFP, or HeLa GFP-Rab7) of five thousand unloaded or loaded fibroblasts were seeded per well in 250 µL of cDMEM. Plates were cultivated in 5% CO_2 humidified atmosphere at 37 °C. Single MCS were obtained in each well 24 h after seeding. The MCS growth was followed over a period of 9 days with video-microscopy, as described in Section 4.3. At the end of this period, the spheroids were fixed and processed for TEM, as described in Section 4.4.

4.6. Intracellular Iron Quantification by Single Cell Magnetophoresis

The iron load in loaded cells was determined by single cell magnetophoresis [55], which consists of measuring the velocity of cells loaded with magnetic nanoparticles, when loaded cells are submitted to a magnetic field gradient (B = 150 mT, gradB = 17 T/m). The migration of 100 cells was tracked by videomicroscopy for each cell-loading condition. Cell velocity and the average iron mass per cell were assessed as previously described [55].

4.7. Thermal Measurements

Thermal measurements were performed on nanoparticle aqueous suspensions. The measurements were made in 0.5 mL Eppendorf tubes containing 100 µL of RB-nanochains-COOH suspended in water, at an iron concentration of 130 mM. An alternating magnetic field generating device (DM3, NanoScale Biomagnetics, Zaragoza, Spain) operating at 471 kHz and 180 G was used to induce magnetic hyperthermia. Photothermal heating was obtained after NIR laser illumination operating at 808 nm at laser power densities of 0.3 and 1 W/cm^2. The temperature elevation was measured as a function of time using an infrared camera (FLIR SC7000) and imaging the sample from the side.

4.8. Second Harmonic Generation Imaging and Photothermal Treatment of Plated Cells and Cell Sheets

Second harmonic generation (SHG) imaging was performed with a 7 MP multiphoton laser scanning microscope (Carl Zeiss, Jena, Germany), equipped with a mag. 20 × objective (with a numerical aperture of 0.95), coupled to a Ti–sapphire femtosecond laser, Chameleon Ultra 2 (Coherent Inc., Santa Clara, CA, USA) tuned to 880 nm. In order to avoid nanochain heating and obtain the image of engineered cell sheets, we fixed the laser power to 18%, attaining an equivalent of the laser power of 20 mW, while non-descanned detectors collected emitted light from nanochains, SHG, and dermal fibroblasts through 565–610 nm, 435–485 nm, and 500–550 nm bandpass filters, respectively. The micrographs were acquired using a laser dwell time of 0.58 or 0.92 µs per pixel at an X, Y resolution of 0.15 µm, and the micrographs were obtained after averaging 4 frames. In experiments which involved nanochains heating, the laser power was fixed to 26%, attaining an equivalent a the laser power of 28 mW, and 30 images were acquired over a period of 8 min (4 s/image). In experiments involving the heating of nanochain-loaded green fluorescent protein (GFP) expressing plated HCT-116 cells, the laser power was fixed at 40%, attaining an equivalent of a laser power of 33 mW, while non-descanned detectors collected emitted light from permeabilized cells (propidium iodide positive) and GFP through 565–610 nm and 500–550 nm bandpass filters, respectively. Sixty images were acquired during 2 min using a laser dwell time of 0.79 µs per pixel, at a X, Y resolution of 0.415 µm.

4.9. Statistical Analysis

All biological tests were made in triplicates performed in three independent experiments, except for experiences where spheroid growth was monitored over time, where 6 spheroids were made per condition and three independent experiments were made. The results are expressed as mean ± SEM and the differences between groups were assessed by unpaired Student *t*-test or two-way ANOVA depending on data set. A p value < 0.05 was considered significant.

5. Conclusions

In the present study, we characterized and biologically tested nanochains, prepared by magnetic assembly of nanoparticle clusters, and coated with an additional layer of fluorescent silica. These nanochains have an extraordinary therapeutic potential and are not toxic to different cancerous and non-cancerous cells (human dermal fibroblasts). After irradiation with near infrared light, such nanochains eradicate tumor cells in vitro and have the capacity to melt the collagen matrix, as showed using engineered cell sheets made of cells secreting their own extracellular matrix. Further tests, namely tests on large cell populations and animal studies, will now be undertaken to go beyond the proof of principle described in this study, and to ascertain the practical therapeutic value of presented nanochains. The capacity of a therapeutic agent to act concomitantly on cancer cells and their environment could be a game changer in cancer treatment.

Supplementary Materials: The following are available online at http://www.mdpi.com/2072-6694/11/12/2040/s1, Video S1: Nanochain-loaded cell death induced by photothermal treatment, Video S2: Collagen melting after photothermal treatment of nanochains loaded cell-sheets, Scheme S1. Schematic representation of the main synthesis steps, Figure S1: Demonstration of magnetic responsiveness of the RB-nanochains-COOH, Figure S2: The FTIR-ATR spectra of the RB-nanochains, RB-nanochains-NH$_2$, and RB-nanochains-COOH, Figure S3: High-magnification TEM micrographs of RB-nanochains-COOH found within cancer cells

Author Contributions: Conceptualization, J.K.-T. and S.K.; Data curation, J.K.-T.; Formal analysis, E.G.; Funding acquisition, S.K. and M.-P.R.; Investigation, J.K.-T., S.K., E.G., S.N., C.W., A.P.S., E.B., I.F. and M.G.; Methodology, J.K.-T. and S.K.; Resources, S.K. and M.-P.R.; Supervision, M.G. and M.-P.R.; Validation, C.W., M.G. and M.-P.R.; Visualization, J.K.-T.; Writing—original draft, J.K.-T. and S.K.; Writing—review & editing, C.W., M.G. and M.-P.R.

Funding: This research was founded by an institutional grant of the ITMO Cancer AVIESAN (National Alliance for life sciences and Health) within the framework of the cancer Plan NUMEP (PC201615) and the Slovenian Research Agency (ARRS) for research core funding No. (P2-0089) No. (J1-7302 and J3-7494).

Acknowledgments: The authors thank Patricija Bostjancic Hribar for the assistance with FTIR-ATR measurements. The authors thank the "Toulouse Réseau Imagerie" core IPBS facility (Genotoul, Toulouse, France), the CMEAB (Toulouse, France) for electron microscopy and the CENN Nanocenter (Ljubljana, Slovenia) for the use of electron microscopy (TEM 2100) and magnetometry (VSM). The authors are grateful to Chantal Pichon from the Center for Molecular Biophysics, CNRS Orleans, who generously provided us with HeLa GFP-Rab7 cells. JKT, the Young Scientist Award Laureate of the FONROGA Foundation, kindly acknowledges Roland Garrigou and Georges Delsol for their initiative and their support of "Toulousain" scientists.

Conflicts of Interest: The authors declare no conflict of interest.

References

1. Silva, A.K.A.; Espinosa, A.; Kolosnjaj-Tabi, J.; Wilhelm, C.; Gazeau, F. Medical applications of iron oxide nanoparticles. *Iron Oxides Nat. Appl.* **2016**, 425–471. [CrossRef]
2. Marchal, G.; Van Hecke, P.; Demaerel, P.; Decrop, E.; Kennis, C.; Baert, A.; Van der Schueren, E. Detection of liver metastases with superparamagnetic iron oxide in 15 patients: Results of MR imaging at 1.5 T. *Am. J. Roentgenol.* **1989**, *152*, 771–775. [CrossRef]
3. Faraj, A.A.; Luciani, N.; Kolosnjaj-Tabi, J.; Mattar, E.; Clement, O.; Wilhelm, C.; Gazeau, F. Real-time high-resolution magnetic resonance tracking of macrophage subpopulations in a murine inflammation model: A pilot study with a commercially available cryogenic probe. *Contrast Media Mol. Imaging* **2013**, *8*, 193–203. [CrossRef]
4. Kralj, S.; Potrc, T.; Kocbek, P.; Marchesan, S.; Makovec, D. Design and fabrication of magnetically responsive nanocarriers for drug delivery. *Curr. Med. Chem.* **2017**, *24*, 454–469. [CrossRef]
5. Chaudeurge, A.; Wilhelm, C.; Chen-Tournoux, A.; Farahmand, P.; Bellamy, V.; Autret, G.; Ménager, C.; Hagège, A.; Larghéro, J.; Gazeau, F. Can magnetic targeting of magnetically labeled circulating cells optimize intramyocardial cell retention? *Cell Transplant.* **2012**, *21*, 679–691. [CrossRef]
6. Jordan, A.; Scholz, R.; Wust, P.; Fähling, H.; Felix, R. Magnetic fluid hyperthermia (MFH): Cancer treatment with AC magnetic field induced excitation of biocompatible superparamagnetic nanoparticles. *J. Magn. Magn. Mater.* **1999**, *201*, 413–419. [CrossRef]
7. Espinosa, A.; Kolosnjaj-Tabi, J.; Abou-Hassan, A.; Plan Sangnier, A.; Curcio, A.; Silva, A.K.; Di Corato, R.; Neveu, S.; Pellegrino, T.; Liz-Marzán, L.M. Magnetic (hyper) thermia or photothermia? Progressive comparison of iron oxide and gold nanoparticles heating in water, in cells, and in vivo. *Adv. Funct. Mater.* **2018**, *28*, 1803660. [CrossRef]
8. Chu, M.; Shao, Y.; Peng, J.; Dai, X.; Li, H.; Wu, Q.; Shi, D. Near-infrared laser light mediated cancer therapy by photothermal effect of Fe_3O_4 magnetic nanoparticles. *Biomaterials* **2013**, *34*, 4078–4088. [CrossRef] [PubMed]
9. Sattler, K.D. *Handbook of Nanophysics: Nanomedicine and Nanorobotics*; CRC press: Boca Raton, FL, USA, 2010.
10. Bardhan, R.; Lal, S.; Joshi, A.; Halas, N.J. Theranostic nanoshells: From probe design to imaging and treatment of cancer. *Acc. Chem. Res.* **2011**, *44*, 936–946. [CrossRef] [PubMed]
11. Boca, S.C.; Potara, M.; Gabudean, A.-M.; Juhem, A.; Baldeck, P.L.; Astilean, S. Chitosan-coated triangular silver nanoparticles as a novel class of biocompatible, highly effective photothermal transducers for in vitro cancer cell therapy. *Cancer Lett.* **2011**, *311*, 131–140. [CrossRef]
12. Zhou, M.; Zhang, R.; Huang, M.; Lu, W.; Song, S.; Melancon, M.P.; Tian, M.; Liang, D.; Li, C. A chelator-free multifunctional [^{64}Cu] CuS nanoparticle platform for simultaneous micro-PET/CT imaging and photothermal ablation therapy. *J. Am. Chem. Soc.* **2010**, *132*, 15351–15358. [CrossRef] [PubMed]
13. Murakami, T.; Nakatsuji, H.; Inada, M.; Matoba, Y.; Umeyama, T.; Tsujimoto, M.; Isoda, S.; Hashida, M.; Imahori, H. Photodynamic and photothermal effects of semiconducting and metallic-enriched single-walled carbon nanotubes. *J. Am. Chem. Soc.* **2012**, *134*, 17862–17865. [CrossRef]
14. Yang, K.; Zhang, S.; Zhang, G.; Sun, X.; Lee, S.-T.; Liu, Z. Graphene in mice: Ultrahigh in vivo tumor uptake and efficient photothermal therapy. *Nano Lett.* **2010**, *10*, 3318–3323. [CrossRef] [PubMed]
15. Sharma, S.; Shrivastava, N.; Rossi, F.; Thanh, N.T.K. Nanoparticles-based magnetic and photo induced hyperthermia for cancer treatment. *Nano Today* **2019**, 100795. [CrossRef]
16. Kolosnjaj-Tabi, J.; Javed, Y.; Lartigue, L.; Volatron, J.; Elgrabli, D.; Marangon, I.; Pugliese, G.; Caron, B.; Figuerola, A.; Luciani, N. The one year fate of iron oxide coated gold nanoparticles in mice. *ACS Nano* **2015**, *9*, 7925–7939. [CrossRef]
17. Chen, Z.; Meng, H.; Xing, G.; Chen, C.; Zhao, Y.; Jia, G.; Wang, T.; Yuan, H.; Ye, C.; Zhao, F. Acute toxicological effects of copper nanoparticles in vivo. *Toxicol. Lett.* **2006**, *163*, 109–120. [CrossRef]
18. Kolosnjaj-Tabi, J.; Szwarc, H.; Moussa, F. In vivo toxicity studies of pristine carbon nanotubes: A review. In *The Delivery of Nanoparticles*; IntechOpen: Rijeka, Croatia, 2012; ISBN 978-953-51-0615-9.
19. Wagner, S.; SCHNORR, J.; Pilgrimm, H.; Hamm, B.; Taupitz, M. Monomer-coated very small superparamagnetic iron oxide particles as contrast medium for magnetic resonance imaging: Preclinical in vivo characterization. *Investig. Radiol.* **2002**, *37*, 167–177. [CrossRef]

20. Jain, T.K.; Reddy, M.K.; Morales, M.A.; Leslie-Pelecky, D.L.; Labhasetwar, V. Biodistribution, clearance, and biocompatibility of iron oxide magnetic nanoparticles in rats. *Mol. Pharm.* **2008**, *5*, 316–327. [CrossRef]
21. Lartigue, L.; Alloyeau, D.; Kolosnjaj-Tabi, J.; Javed, Y.; Guardia, P.; Riedinger, A.; Péchoux, C.; Pellegrino, T.; Wilhelm, C.; Gazeau, F. Biodegradation of iron oxide nanocubes: High-resolution in situ monitoring. *ACS Nano* **2013**, *7*, 3939–3952. [CrossRef]
22. Van de Walle, A.; Sangnier, A.P.; Abou-Hassan, A.; Curcio, A.; Hémadi, M.; Menguy, N.; Lalatonne, Y.; Luciani, N.; Wilhelm, C. Biosynthesis of magnetic nanoparticles from nano-degradation products revealed in human stem cells. *Proc. Natl. Acad. Sci. USA* **2019**, *116*, 4044–4053. [CrossRef]
23. Shen, S.; Wang, S.; Zheng, R.; Zhu, X.; Jiang, X.; Fu, D.; Yang, W. Magnetic nanoparticle clusters for photothermal therapy with near-infrared irradiation. *Biomaterials* **2015**, *39*, 67–74. [CrossRef]
24. Kralj, S.; Makovec, D. Magnetic assembly of superparamagnetic iron oxide nanoparticle clusters into nanochains and nanobundles. *ACS Nano* **2015**, *9*, 9700–9707. [CrossRef]
25. Kolosnjaj-Tabi, J.; Marangon, I.; Nicolas-Boluda, A.; Silva, A.K.; Gazeau, F. Nanoparticle-based hyperthermia, a local treatment modulating the tumor extracellular matrix. *Pharmacol. Res.* **2017**, *126*, 123–137. [CrossRef]
26. Kopanja, L.; Kralj, S.; Zunic, D.; Loncar, B.; Tadic, M. Core–shell superparamagnetic iron oxide nanoparticle (SPION) clusters: TEM micrograph analysis, particle design and shape analysis. *Ceram. Int.* **2016**, *42*, 10976–10984. [CrossRef]
27. Masdeu, G.; Kralj, S.; Pajk, S.; López-Santín, J.; Makovec, D.; Álvaro, G. Hybrid chloroperoxidase-magnetic nanoparticle clusters: Effect of functionalization on biocatalyst performance. *J. Chem. Technol. Biotechnol.* **2018**, *93*, 233–245. [CrossRef]
28. Kralj, S.; Drofenik, M.; Makovec, D. Controlled surface functionalization of silica-coated magnetic nanoparticles with terminal amino and carboxyl groups. *J. Nanoparticle Res.* **2011**, *13*, 2829–2841. [CrossRef]
29. Wilhelm, C.; Gazeau, F. Universal cell labelling with anionic magnetic nanoparticles. *Biomaterials* **2008**, *29*, 3161–3174. [CrossRef]
30. Hoskins, C.; Wang, L.; Cheng, W.P.; Cuschieri, A. Dilemmas in the reliable estimation of the in-vitro cell viability in magnetic nanoparticle engineering: Which tests and what protocols? *Nanoscale Res. Lett.* **2012**, *7*, 77. [CrossRef]
31. Manciulea, A.; Baker, A.; Lead, J.R. A fluorescence quenching study of the interaction of Suwannee River fulvic acid with iron oxide nanoparticles. *Chemosphere* **2009**, *76*, 1023–1027. [CrossRef]
32. Al-Kady, A.S.; Gaber, M.; Hussein, M.M.; Ebeid, E.-Z.M. Structural and fluorescence quenching characterization of hematite nanoparticles. *Spectrochim. Acta Part A Mol. Biomol. Spectrosc.* **2011**, *83*, 398–405. [CrossRef]
33. Yu, C.-J.; Wu, S.-M.; Tseng, W.-L. Magnetite nanoparticle-induced fluorescence quenching of adenosine triphosphate–BODIPY conjugates: Application to adenosine triphosphate and pyrophosphate sensing. *Anal. Chem.* **2013**, *85*, 8559–8565. [CrossRef]
34. Strober, W. Trypan blue exclusion test of cell viability. *Curr. Protoc. Immunol.* **1997**, *21*, A–3B.
35. Kralj, S.; Rojnik, M.; Jagodič, M.; Kos, J.; Makovec, D. Effect of surface charge on the cellular uptake of fluorescent magnetic nanoparticles. *J. Nanoparticle Res.* **2012**, *14*, 1151. [CrossRef]
36. Kolosnjaj-Tabi, J.; Wilhelm, C.; Clément, O.; Gazeau, F. Cell labeling with magnetic nanoparticles: Opportunity for magnetic cell imaging and cell manipulation. *J. Nanobiotechnol.* **2013**, *11*, S7. [CrossRef]
37. Pawelczyk, E.; Arbab, A.S.; Pandit, S.; Hu, E.; Frank, J.A. Expression of transferrin receptor and ferritin following ferumoxides–protamine sulfate labeling of cells: Implications for cellular magnetic resonance imaging. *NMR Biomed. Int. J. Devoted Dev. Appl. Magn. Reson. Vivo* **2006**, *19*, 581–592. [CrossRef]
38. Petronek, M.S.; Spitz, D.R.; Buettner, G.R.; Allen, B.G. Linking cancer metabolic dysfunction and genetic instability through the lens of iron metabolism. *Cancers* **2019**, *11*, 1077. [CrossRef]
39. Majno, G.; Joris, I. Apoptosis, oncosis, and necrosis. An overview of cell death. *Am. J. Pathol.* **1995**, *146*, 3.
40. Majno, G.; La Gattuta, M.; Thompson, T. Cellular death and necrosis: Chemical, physical and morphologic changes in rat liver. *Virchows Arch. Pathol. Anat. Physiol. Klin. Med.* **1960**, *333*, 421–465. [CrossRef]
41. Yáñez-Mó, M.; Siljander, P.R.-M.; Andreu, Z.; Bedina Zavec, A.; Borràs, F.E.; Buzas, E.I.; Buzas, K.; Casal, E.; Cappello, F.; Carvalho, J. Biological properties of extracellular vesicles and their physiological functions. *J. Extracell. Vesicles* **2015**, *4*, 27066. [CrossRef]
42. Yang, S.-A.; Choi, S.; Jeon, S.M.; Yu, J. Silica nanoparticle stability in biological media revisited. *Sci. Rep.* **2018**, *8*, 185. [CrossRef]

43. Jurkić, L.M.; Cepanec, I.; Pavelić, S.K.; Pavelić, K. Biological and therapeutic effects of ortho-silicic acid and some ortho-silicic acid-releasing compounds: New perspectives for therapy. *Nutr. Metab.* **2013**, *10*, 2. [CrossRef]
44. Feliu, N.; Docter, D.; Heine, M.; del Pino, P.; Ashraf, S.; Kolosnjaj-Tabi, J.; Macchiarini, P.; Nielsen, P.; Alloyeau, D.; Gazeau, F. In vivo degeneration and the fate of inorganic nanoparticles. *Chem. Soc. Rev.* **2016**, *45*, 2440–2457. [CrossRef]
45. Janet, M.T.; Cheng, G.; Tyrrell, J.A.; Wilcox-Adelman, S.A.; Boucher, Y.; Jain, R.K.; Munn, L.L. Mechanical compression drives cancer cells toward invasive phenotype. *Proc. Natl. Acad. Sci. USA* **2012**, *109*, 911–916.
46. Jordan, A.; Scholz, R.; Maier-Hauff, K.; van Landeghem, F.K.; Waldoefner, N.; Teichgraeber, U.; Pinkernelle, J.; Bruhn, H.; Neumann, F.; Thiesen, B. The effect of thermotherapy using magnetic nanoparticles on rat malignant glioma. *J. Neuro Oncol.* **2006**, *78*, 7–14. [CrossRef]
47. Kolosnjaj-Tabi, J.; Di Corato, R.; Lartigue, L.; Marangon, I.; Guardia, P.; Silva, A.K.; Luciani, N.; Clément, O.; Flaud, P.; Singh, J.V. Heat-generating iron oxide nanocubes: Subtle destructurators of the tumoral microenvironment. *ACS Nano* **2014**, *8*, 4268–4283. [CrossRef]
48. Tadic, M.; Kralj, S.; Jagodic, M.; Hanzel, D.; Makovec, D. Magnetic properties of novel superparamagnetic iron oxide nanoclusters and their peculiarity under annealing treatment. *Appl. Surf. Sci.* **2014**, *322*, 255–264. [CrossRef]
49. Kralj, S.; Makovec, D. The chemically directed assembly of nanoparticle clusters from superparamagnetic iron-oxide nanoparticles. *RSC Adv.* **2014**, *4*, 13167–13171. [CrossRef]
50. Pelofy, S.; Teissié, J.; Golzio, M.; Chabot, S. Chemically modified oligonucleotide–increased stability negatively correlates with its efficacy despite efficient electrotransfer. *J. Membr. Biol.* **2012**, *245*, 565–571. [CrossRef]
51. Orio, J.; Bellard, E.; Baaziz, H.; Pichon, C.; Mouritzen, P.; Rols, M.-P.; Teissié, J.; Golzio, M.; Chabot, S. Sub-cellular temporal and spatial distribution of electrotransferred LNA/DNA oligomer. *J. RNAi Gene Silenc. Int. J. RNA Gene Target. Res.* **2013**, *9*, 479.
52. Gibot, L.; Galbraith, T.; Huot, J.; Auger, F.A. A preexisting microvascular network benefits in vivo revascularization of a microvascularized tissue-engineered skin substitute. *Tissue Eng. Part A* **2010**, *16*, 3199–3206. [CrossRef]
53. Pillet, F.; Gibot, L.; Madi, M.; Rols, M.-P.; Dague, E. Importance of endogenous extracellular matrix in biomechanical properties of human skin model. *Biofabrication* **2017**, *9*, 025017. [CrossRef]
54. Franken, N.A.; Rodermond, H.M.; Stap, J.; Haveman, J.; Van Bree, C. Clonogenic assay of cells in vitro. *Nat. Protoc.* **2006**, *1*, 2315. [CrossRef]
55. Wilhelm, C.; Gazeau, F.; Bacri, J.-C. Magnetophoresis and ferromagnetic resonance of magnetically labeled cells. *Eur. Biophys. J.* **2002**, *31*, 118–125. [CrossRef]

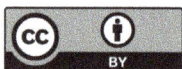

© 2019 by the authors. Licensee MDPI, Basel, Switzerland. This article is an open access article distributed under the terms and conditions of the Creative Commons Attribution (CC BY) license (http://creativecommons.org/licenses/by/4.0/).

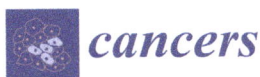

Article

An Effective Multi-Stage Liposomal DNA Origami Nanosystem for In Vivo Cancer Therapy

Stefano Palazzolo [1,2], Mohamad Hadla [2], Concetta Russo Spena [1], Isabella Caligiuri [1], Rossella Rotondo [1], Muhammad Adeel [1,3], Vinit Kumar [2,4], Giuseppe Corona [5], Vincenzo Canzonieri [1,6], Giuseppe Toffoli [2] and Flavio Rizzolio [1,3,*]

[1] Pathology unit, Centro di Riferimento Oncologico di Aviano (CRO) IRCCS, Aviano 33081, Italy; stpalazz85@gmail.com (S.P.); concettarussospena@gmail.com (C.R.S.); icaligiuri82@gmail.com (I.C.); rossellaross1988@gmail.com (R.R.); addistar60@yahoo.com (M.A.); vcanzonieri@cro.it (V.C.)
[2] Clinical and Experimental Pharmacology unit, Centro di Riferimento Oncologico di Aviano (CRO) IRCCS, Aviano 33081, Italy; m_hadla@hotmail.com (M.H.); vinitiitr@gmail.com (V.K.); gtoffoli@cro.it (G.T.)
[3] Department of Molecular Sciences and Nanosystems, Ca' Foscari University of Venice, Venice 30172, Italy
[4] Amity Institute of Molecular Medicine & Stem Cell Research, Amity University, Noida 201313, India
[5] Immunopathology and Cancer Biomarkers unit, Centro di Riferimento Oncologico di Aviano (CRO) IRCCS, Aviano 33081, Italy; giuseppe.corona@cro.it
[6] Department of Medical, Surgical and Health Science, University of Trieste, Trieste 34137, Italy
* Correspondence: flavio.rizzolio@unive.it; Tel.: +39-04-1234-8910; Fax: +39-04-1234-8594

Received: 30 October 2019; Accepted: 5 December 2019; Published: 12 December 2019

Abstract: DNA origami systems could be important candidates for clinical applications. Unfortunately, their intrinsic properties such as the activation of non-specific immune system responses leading to inflammation, instability in physiological solutions, and a short in vivo lifetime are the major challenges for real world applications. A compact short tube DNA origami (STDO) of 30 nm in length and 10 nm in width was designed to fit inside the core of a stealth liposome (LSTDO) of about 150 nm to remote load doxorubicin. Biocompatibility was tested in three-dimensional (3D) organoid cultures and in vivo. Efficacy was evaluated in different cell lines and in a xenograft breast cancer mouse model. As described in a previous work, LSTDO is highly stable and biocompatible, escaping the recognition of the immune system. Here we show that LSTDO have an increased toleration in mouse liver organoids used as an ex vivo model that recapitulate the tissue of origin. This innovative drug delivery system (DDS) improves the antitumoral efficacy and biodistribution of doxorubicin in tumor-bearing mice and decreases bone marrow toxicity. Our application is an attractive system for the remote loading of other drugs able to interact with DNA for the preparation of liposomal formulations.

Keywords: DNA origami; liposome; breast cancer; remote loading; doxorubicin; acute toxicity; organoids

1. Introduction

Cancer is the second major cause of death worldwide every year [1]. The standard methods to treat this deadly disease are surgery and chemotherapy with cytotoxic antitumor drugs [2]. Chemotherapeutic drugs possess unspecific targeting with a large biodistribution, leading to several side effects that make chemotherapy painful and even fail in some cases [3]. To overcome these limitations, the use of nanotechnologies marked important progressions in the development of a drug delivery system (DDS) able to improve the chemical, physical and pharmacological properties of drugs [4]. Ideally, the DDS to be applied in clinic should have the following properties: low toxicity, the ability to cross physiological barriers, high stability in body fluids (in particular in the blood stream), high loading efficiency and controlled drug release [5]. In order to meet the clinical requirements, nanotechnology plays a vital role in the development of smart delivery systems with excellent features such as size (around 100 nm), various functionalization and a high surface to volume ratio of nanomaterials. Recently, even though different nanomaterials like polymers and metal nanoparticles have been proposed for the development of nanostructures for smart DDS [6], the construction of biocompatible and stable vehicles for in vivo applications still remains the challenge for clinical therapy [7]. In the last decade, DNA technology received considerable attention for many attractive features such as easy synthesis in the predicted shape, precise nanopatterning, and mechanical rigidity, making DNA an interesting candidate for biomedical applications [8]. In the last three decades, scientists have developed different shapes of DNA nanostructures but, since 2000, the field was innovated with the advent of a folding technique called DNA origami [3]. DNA origami provides a platform for next generation DDS, becoming a potential candidate for clinics. In this regard, Hogberg et al. tested two different kinds of DNA origami structures for doxorubicin loading on three different breast cancer cell lines [5]. Ding et al. used self-assembled DNA origami as a carrier for doxorubicin that was able to circumvent drug resistance on multi-drug resistant breast cancer cells (MDR-MCF7) [6]. Yang et al. designed and synthesized triangular shaped DNA origami for the loading of doxorubicin to be used as a vehicle for in vivo cancer therapy [7]. Even though DNA nanostructures are an interesting DDS, they possess some limitations which prevent their in vivo application [9]. In particular, DNA nanovehicles, once in the blood stream, are rapidly recognized by circulating DNAses and by the immune system, inducing inflammatory responses. The possibility to encapsulate DNA nanostructures in double-layer membranes or in a protein coating could avoid DNAse degradation and immune system activation, improving pharmacokinetics, bioavailability and biodistribution [10–12].

Among the clinical-grade nanoparticle-based technologies, liposomal technology has become a very successful and rapidly developing area of preclinical and clinical research. With the advantages of biocompatibility, biodegradability, low toxicity, and aptitude to trap both hydrophilic and lipophilic drugs [13] as well as a desirable accumulation in tumor tissues [14], liposomes are very attractive and have been extensively investigated as a DDS. The size of liposomes makes them suitable to cross the fenestrations of blood vessels in the tumor site and to remain entrapped in the extracellular matrix. The long circulation time in the blood stream is obtained by adding polyethylene glycol (PEG) chains on the surface of the liposome, which allow it to escape the reticuloendothelial system (RES) and the immune system [15]. On this topic, Doxil represents one of the main examples of a liposomal formulation of doxorubicin. This anthracycline is loaded inside the liposome through a process called remote loading, by which doxorubicin precipitates inside the liposome, avoiding its release [16]. The net result is a high drug/lipid ratio that is essential for clinical application. Unfortunately, the liposomal system has certain limitations such as reaching an efficient drug loading only with weak base or acid molecules. Therefore, to overcome these limitations and improve the DNA nanostructure limitations (biodegradation and immune system activation), our group developed, for the first time, a robust bullet biomimetic system by making short tube DNA origami (STDO) of approximately 30 nm in length and 10 nm in width with high stability in physiological conditions for up to 48 h [17]. The compact size of STDO precisely fittted inside a stealthy liposome of about 150 nm and doxorubicin was efficiently remote loaded in liposomes (LSTDO). The LSTDO system had a controlled release at pH 7.4 with an increased release rate in acidic conditions (pH 5.5) typical of the tumor microenvironment. LSTDO also improved the biocompatibility of DNA origami injected into immunocompetent mice (FVB/N) [17]. Therefore, there was a need to test the system (LSTDO) in vivo in order to determine if it could be used in clinics for a better cancer therapy.

In this work, we studied the LSTDO remotely loaded with doxorubicin for in vivo applications. The combined properties of liposomes and DNA origami allowed for the introduction of a biocompatible innovative system for the delivery of doxorubicin, which improved tumor accumulation of the drug and efficiently inhibited tumor growth in mice (Figure 1).

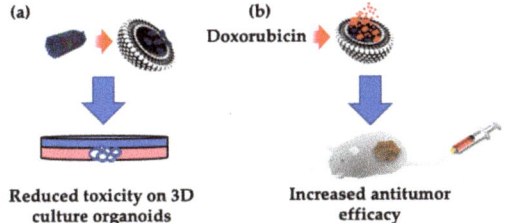

Figure 1. Schematic representation of the new liposomal/origami technology for the drug delivery of doxorubicin. (**a**) Liposomal short tube DNA origami (LSTDO) decreases the adverse effect of STDO on mouse liver derived organoids. (**b**) LSTDO-doxo increases the antitumor effect of doxorubicin on mice bearing breast cancer tumor cells.

2. Results

2.1. Synthesis and Characterization

The original data were published by our group in Palazzolo et al. [17]. Briefly, STDO was assembled in a one-step reaction. The expected dimensions were about 30 nm in length and 10 nm in width. After synthesis, STDO was purified by PEG precipitation as described by Stahl et al. [18]. The lipid composition used to create the liposomes to encapsulate the STDO was derived from Doxil. Liposomes were synthesized by applying the membrane extrusion method in a physiological buffer containing STDO (see Materials and Methods). After this process LSTDO were purified by removing excess of STDO with a cationic resin able to remove free DNA origami without interfering with liposomes. The DDS were analyzed by transmission electron microscopy (TEM) and dynamic light scattering (DLS). The calculated hydrodynamic radius of the STDO and of the LSTDO before and after purification from unencapsulated STDO were 37.6 ± 5.4 nm, 170.1 ± 67.0 nm and 163.9 ± 54.2 nm, respectively (Supplementary Materials Figure S1).

LSTDO was able to load doxo at about 50% (w/w) loading efficiency. The release of LSTDO was pH dependent and increased at pH 5.5, a typical condition of the tumor microenvironment. Other data, including STDO agarose gel electrophoresis, size distribution and stability in physiological conditions were described in Palazzolo et al. [17].

2.2. Liver Organoid Toxicity

Mouse liver organoids were isolated from eight weeks-old C57BL6 mice. Organoids were phenotypically characterized by histological and immunohistochemical (IHC) staining for the most common liver markers (Figure 2). In accordance with cyto-morphological evidence reported in the literature [19], microscopic examination of haematoxylin and eosin (H&E) staining showed that liver organoids had the typical features of hepatic progenitors and mature hepatocytes. Liver organoids retained their stemness and proliferative potential, confirmed respectively by the strong immunopositivity for CD133 and octamer-binding transcription factor 4 (OCT4) stem cell markers and Ki67 proliferation marker. Transcription factor SOX9 and cytokeratin 19 (KRT19)-immunopositive cells, typical markers of premature ductal hepatocytes, were observed in the single-layer epithelium (Figure 2a). Cells of the stratified epithelium differentiated into mature hepatocytes and resulted in albumin (ALB+) and HNF4α-positive (HNF4α+) cells (Figure 2a). Therefore, our results highlight that mouse liver organoids maintain their commitment to their tissue of origin.

On this note, a single-layer epithelium was composed of cuboidal cells positive for E-cadherin (E-Cad+) (Figure 2a), which surround a central lumen and alternated with pseudostratified epithelium in a structure that resembles a primordial hepatic diverticulum.

Since the liver is the organ which accumulates the majority of compounds administered intravenously and is the organ which detoxifies the blood from toxic substances, we decided to test if our DDS is biocompatible with liver organoids to predict in vivo biocompatibility. Organoids were plated and treated with STDO, LSTDO and liposomes at two different concentrations (100 µg/mL and 10 µg/mL). After 24 h, the caspase 3/7 assay was used to determine the activation of apoptotic enzymes (Figure 2b). The level of caspase 3/7 was increased significantly after treatment of liver organoids with 100 µg/mL of STDO compared with organoids treated with LSTDO or only liposomes. The quantity used is the same amount employed to treat mice.

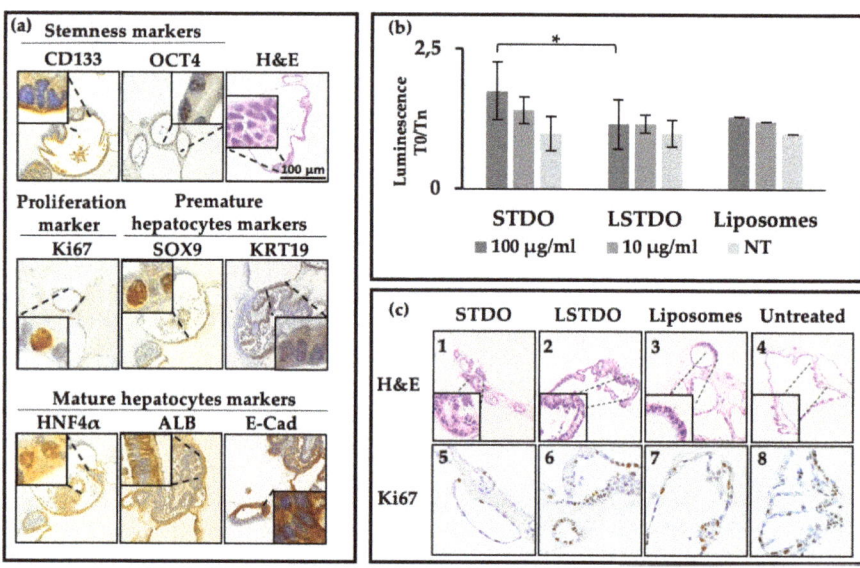

Figure 2. DNA origami-induced toxicity on mouse liver organoids. (**a**) Cytomorphological and immunohistochemical characterization of mouse liver organoids as a model to test the toxicity induced by origami. (**b**) Induced apoptosis (Cas 3/7 assay) as a toxicity marker of LSTDO and STDO. (**c**) Cytomorphological changes (H&E) induced by STDO (Panel 1) and LSTDO (Panel 2) compared with the control and liposomes (Panel 3 and 4, respectively). Ki67 expression in mouse liver organoids treated with STDO (Panel 5) and LSTDO (Panel 6) compared with the control and liposomes (Panel 7 and 8, respectively). Image magnification: 20×. (* p-value < 0.05).

Morphological examination of H&E staining revealed that organoids treated for 48 h with 100 µg/mL STDO exhibit cytostructural changes. Indeed, compared with the control, STDO induced a loss of epithelial cells and a loss of organoid structural complexity. Moreover, cellular atypia and nuclear karyorrhexis and karyolysis, accompanied by irregular clumping of chromatinic material, were detectable (Figure 2c, Panel 1). Treatment with 100 µg/mL of LSTDO did not affect the general structure of organoids, displaying unremarkable changes such as slight visible nuclear pyknosis and slight cellular atypia (Figure 2c, Panel 2). Untreated and liposome-treated mouse liver organoids appeared as similar glandular structures with active proliferations (Figure 2c, Panels 3 and 4).

In order to assess if STDO-induced cytotoxicity could affect organoid cell proliferation, immunohistochemical analysis of Ki67 was performed. The results showed a remarkable reduction of Ki67 staining in mouse liver organoids treated with 100 µg/mL STDO for 48 h (Figure 2c, Panel 5) compared with LSTDO- and liposome- treated and untreated organoids (Figure 2c, Panels 6, 7 and 8, respectively).

2.3. In Vitro Efficacy

After purification, STDO and LSTDO were loaded with doxorubicin (see Materials and Methods) [17]. The cytotoxic effects of STDO-doxo and LSTDO-doxo were tested on breast (MCF7 and MDA-MB-231) and colon (LoVo) cancer cell lines. The cell viability experiments showed no significant differences among the effects of free doxorubicin, STDO-doxo and LSTDO-doxo (Figure 3 and Supplementary Materials Figure S2). These results are in line with previous publications [5] and are supported by data obtained with liposomal doxorubicin which shown a benefit only in in vivo models [20]. Similarly, our group has previously demonstrated that doxorubicin encapsulated in exosomes, i.e., natural vesicles lined with a bilayer of phospholipids, was able to increase the therapeutic index of this drug only in vivo [21,22].

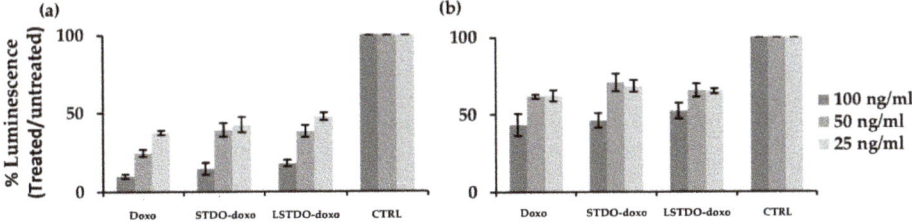

Figure 3. Cytotoxicity of LSTDO-doxo, STDO-doxo and doxo on (**a**) MCF7, (**b**) MDA-MB-231 breast cancer cell lines. Histograms represent the cell viability. Experiments were done in triplicate.

2.4. In Vivo Toxicity

To establish the toxic effect of LSTDO-doxo, STDO-doxo and doxorubicin, mice were intraperitoneally (i.p.) injected with a high dose of doxorubicin (15 mg/kg) and the acute toxicity was evaluated (Figure 4a). Body weight was monitored as a quantitative parameter describing animal health, with progressive weight loss indicating deteriorating health. Mice treated with STDO-doxo showed rapid weight loss over five days, after which they were sacrificed. On the other hand, the mice treated with LSTDO-doxo exhibited the same body weight decrease of those treated with free doxorubicin (Figure 4b).

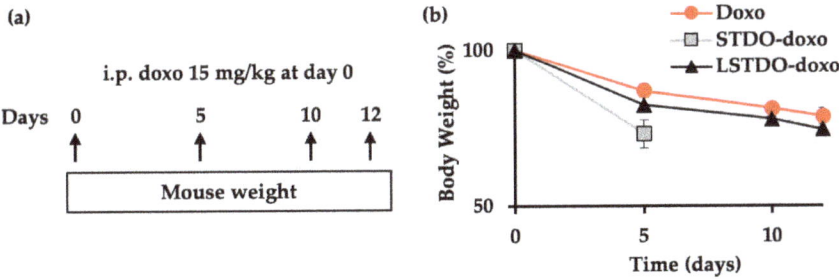

Figure 4. LSTDO-doxo is less toxic than STDO-doxo in vivo. (**a**) Schematic design of the study. Three mice per group were injected intraperitoneally (i.p.) with 15 mg/kg of doxo, STDO-doxo and LSTDO-doxo on day 0 and their body weight was measured at the indicated intervals. (**b**) Mice body weight was followed up for 12 days as an index of illness. Mice treated with LSTDO-doxo w comparable to mice treated with doxo. Mice treated with STDO-doxo had more rapid weight loss and were sacrificed earlier.

These results showed that LSTDO-doxo was safer than STDO-doxo. To explain the observed toxicity, the tissues of mice were analyzed by histopathology. Among the analyzed tissues (heart, liver, lung, kidney, intestine, spleen and skin; data not shown), we observed a reduced number of blasts in the bone marrow of STDO-doxo treated mice compared to doxo- or LSTDO-doxo-treated mice (Figure 5a,b), which could be a symptom of the observed toxicity.

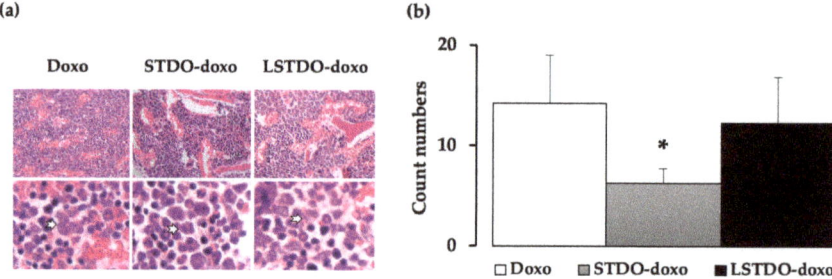

Figure 5. Bone marrow histological analysis of mice treated for acute toxicity. (**a**) The bone marrow was analyzed by histopathology. Representative H&E staining of the bone marrow at 40× magnification (upper panel). Lower panel shows examples of blasts (arrows). (**b**) The number of blast cells was less in STDO-doxo treated mice compared to the other treatments. (* p-value < 0.05).

2.5. LSTDO-Doxo is More Effective than Free Doxo In Vivo

To test the antitumor efficacy of LSTDO-doxo, the MDA-MB-231 cell line was orthotopically implanted into the breast of nude mice. After tumors reached >50 mm^3, mice were treated three times intravenously once per week with 3 mg/kg of doxo, STDO-doxo and LSTDO-doxo. Tumor volumes were followed up (Figure 6a). After 17 days, mice treated with LSTDO-doxo showed a reduced tumor burden compared to mice treated with STDO-doxo or free doxo (27%; p-value < 0.05) (Figure 6b). At the end of the experiment, the survival rate of doxo-treated mice was 0%, STDO-doxo was 12.5% and LSTDO-doxo was 33.3%. To support our data, the concentration of doxo was measured in the tumor. As demonstrated in Figure 6c, LSTDO-doxo accumulated in the tumor more than STDO-doxo and free doxo (1.39 fold; p-value < 0.05), confirming again that the new DDS presented in this work effectively delivered the drug at the target site, increasing its efficacy.

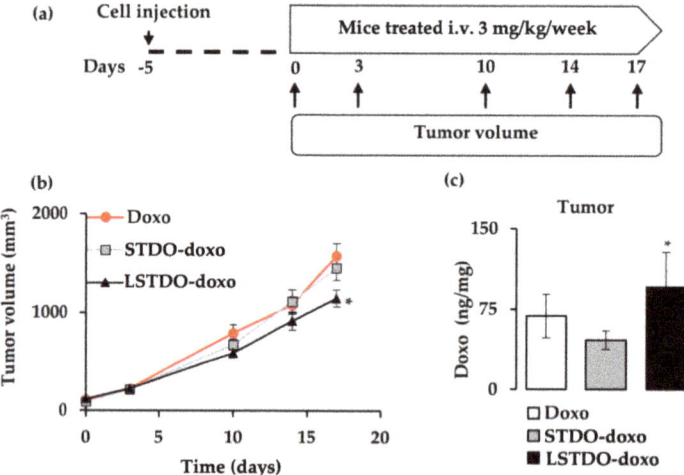

Figure 6. LSTDO-doxo increases the efficacy of doxo in vivo. (**a**) Schematic design of the tumor growth study. Mice were treated three times (3 mg/kg, once a week) and tumor volumes (n = 8) were followed up. (**b**) After 14 days, mice treated with LSTDO-doxo had a reduced tumor volume compared with mice treated with doxo and STDO-doxo (* p-value < 0.05). (**c**) After 72 h post-doxo injection, mice were sacrificed and tumors (n = 8) were collected to quantify the amount of doxo. (ng of doxo/mg of tissue; * p-value < 0.05).

Although the difference between LSTDO-doxo- and doxo-treated tumors are not impressive, we are proposing an alternative remote loading system based on DNA nanoparticles. Considering that DNA nanostructures have the ability to be functionalized with different chemical groups, we are able to customize the DNA origami accordingly with the drugs to loaded inside the liposomes.

3. Discussion

DNA nanotechnology is based on the properties of DNA to form structures through complementary base pair interactions such as robust self-assembly, which allows the design of DNA nanostructures with the required shape, geometry and additional functionalization sites. The modulation of size, shape and net charge of DNA nanostructures has been demonstrated to be important in order to overcome natural cell membrane barriers to deliver naked DNA or siRNA that otherwise would not enter the cells. Another advantageous feature of DNA origami could be the ability to exhibit controlled drug release. However, the in vivo application of DNA nanostructures also presents some limitations. In particular, the major limitation for low-density DNA nanostructures is represented by many circulating enzymes such as DNAses that (especially in tumour cells and the tumor microenvironment) are overrepresented and can degrade it quickly. A dense packaging of DNA helices within a DNA nanostructure is one of the strategies used to increase their stability against DNA-degrading enzymes. The encapsulation of DNA structures under a sheet of biocompatible materials like membranes could be another approach to protect them from recognition and degradation by non-specific immune activation [21,23]. From a therapeutic perspective (comparing the clearance half-life of most anticancer drugs), to obtain good in vivo results, we should develop DNA-based nanostructures with a half-life higher than 30 h to enable their clinical application in drug delivery. For instance, the terminal clearance half-life of doxo, which is among the most widely used chemotherapeutic agent, is around 30 h [24]. DNA nanostructures could be designed in order to create a nanodevice to control the activity of an external enzyme [25]. This additional feature could be exploited to actively release drugs through the modulation of the enzyme activity. This could be a key step for the development of a stealth DNA-based DDS to load drugs inside liposomes only by their interaction with DNA, independently of the pKa of the drugs themselves that could represent an important limitation. Furthermore, the possibility to modify oligonucleotides with functional groups could allow the loading of other drugs.

The present study highlights the excellent versatility of DNA nanotechnology for the development of innovative DDS with high biocompatibility, improved pharmacokinetic/biodistribution profiles and size/shape-dependent enhanced permeability and retention (EPR) effect [26]. Nonetheless, the cost for the synthesis and purification of this kind of DDS are still elevated, but there are many laboratories working to improve this new technology and some ameliorations were recently reached [25,27,28].

In our previous work, we addressed three key limitations in the bioapplication of DNA origami i.e., their short in vivo stability, non-specific immune system activation and poor cellular uptake, seeding the basis for a new drug remote loading concept. In the present work, we successfully applied the DDS in vivo, demonstrating that the system possesses very strong properties to be a candidate for future therapeutic applications. In particular, LSTDO-doxo was shown to improve the efficacy of doxo on mice bearing breast cancer-derived tumors, reducing tumor burden and decreasing the toxic effect of doxo on bone morrow. Toxicity tests on ex vivo three-dimensional (3D) cultures (mouse liver-derived organoids) that resembled the tissue of origin demonstrated that the LSTDO is less toxic than free DNA origami as evidenced by the caspase 3/7 assay and cytomorphological examination of organoids by H&E staining. Moreover, STDO could interfere with cellular proliferation as confirmed by Ki67 staining reduction compared to untreated and liposome-treated mouse liver organoids.

This work embodies strong and substantial innovations to the previously described DNA-based delivery approaches [7,29] for cancer therapy and enhances the translational prospects of DNA origami-based DDS. There are a lot of limitations for the loading of drugs inside liposomes. In some cases, the poor loading efficiency is a hurdle that prevents the use of liposomal drug formulations [30]. We strongly believe that the technology reported here could be applied to every drug able to interact with DNA, to build other biomimetic drug formulations and to obtain a more efficient and safe multistage system.

This work is a first step towards a new nanotechnology drug delivery era in which DNA nanostructures will play a key role. DNA nanotechnology is taking its first steps into the field of drug delivery and it is a necessary and remarkable step forward that could become the basis for the biomedical and pharmacological application of smart DNA nanodevices to translate this technology into clinics.

4. Materials and Methods

4.1. Materials and Reagents

MDA-MB-231, MCF7 (human breast cancer) and LoVo (human colorectal cancer) cell lines were grown as indicated by the suppliers. Nude and FVB/N mice were purchased from Harlan Laboratories (Udine, Italy). The experimental procedures were approved by the Italian Ministry of Health and performed in accordance with institutional guidelines. We utilized female mice of 6 weeks of age. Data were reported as mean and standard error of the mean. Oligonucleotides for DNA origami were purchased from IDT Technology (Coralville, IA, USA). M13mp18 single strand plasmids were purchased by Bayou Biolabs, LLC (Metairie, LA, USA).

4.2. Self-Assembly of DNA Origami

All DNA origami were assembled on ssDNA M13mp18 as a scaffold at a final concentration of 5 nM. Annealing and assembling of DNA origami were performed in 1× TAE-Mg^{2+} buffer (40 mM Tris-HCl; 20 mM acetic acid; 2 mM EDTA; 12.5 mM magnesium acetate; pH 8.0) in a thermocycler (Eppendorf Mastercycler®, Hamburg, Germany) by slowly cooling down from 90 °C to room temperature (RT) in 12 h. STDO was designed with CaDNAno software and assembled with the following protocol: 1× TE-Mg^{2+} buffer (10 mM Tris-HCl, 1 mM EDTA, 16 mM $MgCl_2$, pH 8) in a thermocycler by slowly cooling down from 65 °C to 4 °C in 19 h.

4.3. DNA Origami Purification

To obtain pure DNA origami structures, eliminating the excess of staple strands and scaffolds, we applied the protocol described by Stahl et al. based on PEG precipitation [18]. The DNA origami mixture was mixed 1:1 (v/v) with precipitation buffer containing 15% PEG 8000 (w/v), 5 mM Tris-HCl, 1 mM EDTA and 505 mM NaCl (all chemicals were purchased from Sigma-Aldrich Merck, Darmstadt, Germany). The solution was mixed by inversion and spun down at 10,000× g for 25 min at RT. The supernatant was discarded and the pellet was resuspended in physiological solution.

4.4. LSTDO Preparation and Purification

Lipid powders were resuspended in chloroform and dried overnight (ON) with a vacuum pump (EZ-2, SP scientific, Ipswich, UK) to form a lipid cake. The formulation of the lipid cake was: 1,2-distearoyl-sn-glycero-3-phosphocholine, 1,2-dihexadecanoyl-sn-glycero-3-phosphoethanolamine-PEG and cholesterol; 55:5:40). Lipid cake (2 mg) was rehydrated in a STDO solution (800 μg) and extruded ten times through 200 nm and 100 nm Millipore filters (Merck Millipore, Darmstadt, Germany). The excess of DNA origami was eliminated by a cationic resin (IONEX H, C.T.S., City, Italy) interaction. Resin (500 μg) was hydrated in 500 μL of mQ water, washed twice and resuspended in 1× PBS. This solution was mixed 1:1 with the LSTDO solution and incubated at RT in rotation for 1 h. After incubation, the solution was centrifuged at 0.2× g for 5 min in order to pellet the resin with free DNA origami and the supernatant containing the purified LSTDO was collected.

4.5. Doxorubicin Loading and Release

Doxorubicin-HCl was purchased from Accord (Accord Healthcare, Milan, Italy). LSTDO were incubated with a solution of 2 mg/mL doxorubicin 1:2 for 24 h at RT. The excess of unloaded drugs was eliminated by dialysis (1× PBS, pH 7.4, 15,000 MWCO semi-permeable membrane, 2 h at RT). Empty liposomes were treated with the same loading protocol for LSTDO to be used as a control. Intercalated doxorubicin was dosed by absorbance at 450 nm. The release of doxorubicin from liposomes and LSTDO (50 µg/500 µL) was evaluated with a dialysis membrane with a 15,000 MWCO dipped into 1 L of 1× PBS at pH 7.4 or pH 5.5.

4.6. Cell Viability Assay

Cells were seeded in 96-well plates (Becton Dickinson, Franklin Lake, NJ, USA) at a density of 1 × 10^3 cells/well and incubated for 24 h to allow for the attachment of cells. The cells were incubated with doxo, STDO-doxo and LSTDO-doxo at the same concentrations for 96 h. The cytotoxicity was correlated with the cell viability as evaluated by the CellTiter-Glo® Luminescence Assay (Promega, Madison, WI, USA) with an Infinite200 PRO instrument (Tecan, Männedorf, Switzerland).

4.7. Organoid Isolation

Mouse liver organoids were isolated from 8-week-old C57/BL6 mice following the protocol described by Stappenbeck [31]. In brief, a piece of liver was dissected and digested with 2 mg/mL collagenase II for 30 min. The digested tissue was transferred into a clean 15 mL tube with 10 mL of washing medium and centrifugated at 0.5× *g*. The supernatant was discarded and the pellet was resuspended in 10 µL of Cultrex® BME (Trevigen, Gaithersburg, MD, USA) and plated in a 24-well plate. After solidification of the matrix, 500 µL of medium was added to each well.

4.8. Toxicity Tests on Mouse Liver Organoids

To test the toxic effect of STDO and LSTDO, mouse liver organoids were plated in 96-well plates and treated with each compound at 100 µg/mL and 10 µg/mL. After 24 h, organoids were analyzed with Caspase-Glo® 3/7 (Promega, Madison, WI, USA). After 48 h, organoids were collected and embedded in paraffin for histopathological analysis.

4.9. Histopathology

The organs of mice were collected and fixed in phosphate-buffered 10% formalin, embedded in paraffin, sectioned at a thickness of 3 µm, and stained with hematoxylin and eosin (H&E). The tissues were analyzed with a light microscope using different magnifications. Morphological details were analyzed at 40× objective. Organoids, previously washed with pre-warmed PBS, were embedded using Bio-Agar (Bio-Optica, Milan, Italy) and the blocks were fixed overnight in 10% neutral buffered formalin. Subsequently, samples were processed for paraffin embedding. Sections were used for H&E staining using a Leica ST5020 multi-stainer. Immunohistochemistry (IHC) was performed with the UltraVision LP Detection System HRP DAB kit (Thermo Scientific, Waltham, MA, USA). Heat-induced antigen retrieval was performed using 10 mM citrate buffer, pH 6.0, and the slides were incubated with the following primary antibodies diluted in 0.5% BSA: rabbit anti-E-cadherin (E-cad, Genetex #GTX100443) diluted at 1:500, mouse anti-albumin (ALB (F-8), Santa Cruz #sc-374670) diluted at 1:100, rabbit anti-HNF4α (Abcam #ab181604) diluted at 1:200, rabbit anti-cytokeratin 19 (KRT19, Origene #TA313117) diluted at 1:50, rabbit anti-SOX9 (Millipore #AB5535) diluted at 1:250, rabbit anti-CD133 (Proteintech #18470-1-AP) diluted at 1:200, rabbit anti-OCT4 (Abcam, #18967) diluted at 1:100, and rabbit anti-Ki-67 (Invitrogen, #MA5-14520) diluted at 1:200.

4.10. Mouse Xenograft

MDA-MB-231 cells (3×10^6) were mixed with 30% Matrigel HC (BD Bioscience, Franklin Lake, NJ, USA) and implanted orthotopically into 6-week-old female nude mice. When tumors reached a measurable size (>50 mm^3), mice were treated i.v. with doxo, STDO-doxo and LSTDO-doxo once per week for a total of three treatments. Tumor volumes were measured with a caliper instrument and calculated using the following formula: (length × width^2)/2.

4.11. Biodistribution

Organs of mice were washed with 10 mL of cold PBS/heparin before collection, diluted in 500 µL of 4% PBS/BSA and homogenized with Qiagen Tissue Ruptor for 20 s at power 4 in ice. Samples were then stored at −80 °C. The concentrations of doxo were measured by liquid chromatography tandem mass spectrometry (LC-MS/MS) as described by Bayda et al. [32].

4.12. Statistical Analysis

The statistical significance was determined using a two-tailed *t*-test. A *p* value less than 0.05 was considered significant for all comparisons. Bars represent standard errors for tumor volume and body weight. All other bars are standard deviations.

5. Conclusions

In this work, we translate in vivo the system previously described in [17]. In particular, before starting the in vivo tests of LSTDO-doxo, we ensure its biocompatibility by performing toxicity tests on mouse liver-derived organoids. The internalization of DNA origami inside the liposomes favored and prevented the toxic effect of free DNA origami. In vivo tests highlighted both an improvement in tumor efficacy and a better drug accumulation in the tumor. We believe that the current work represents a strong and substantial step to translate DNA origami DDS into the clinic.

Supplementary Materials: The following are available online at http://www.mdpi.com/2072-6694/11/12/1997/s1, Figure S1: Characterization of liposomes, STDO and LSTDO. Figure S2: Efficacy of LSTDO-doxo on LoVo colorectal cancer (CRC) cell lines.

Author Contributions: Writing—original draft, S.P. and F.R.; writing—review, editing and investigation S.P., M.H., C.R.S., I.C., G.C., R.R., M.A., V.K. and V.C.; PhD mentor of S.P., G.T.; PhD mentor of S.P/supervision, F.R.

Funding: This research was funded by MyFirst AIRC No. 1569.

Acknowledgments: F.R. and S.P. are thankful to Associazione Italiana per la Ricerca sul Cancro (MyFirst AIRC No. 1569).

Conflicts of Interest: The authors declare no conflict of interest.

References

1. Li, J.; Fan, C.; Pei, H.; Shi, J.; Huang, Q. Smart drug delivery nanocarriers with self-assembled DNA nanostructures. *Adv. Mater.* **2013**, *25*, 4386–4396. [CrossRef] [PubMed]
2. Rothemund, P.W.K.; Ekani-Nkodo, A.; Papadakis, N.; Kumar, A.; Fygenson, D.K.; Winfree, E. Design and Characterization of Programmable DNA Nanotubes. *J. Am. Chem. Soc.* **2004**, *126*, 16344–16352. [CrossRef] [PubMed]
3. Tasciotti, E. Smart cancer therapy with DNA origami. *Nat. Biotechnol.* **2018**, *36*, 234–235. [CrossRef] [PubMed]
4. Palazzolo, S.; Bayda, S.; Hadla, M.; Caligiuri, I.; Corona, G.; Toffoli, G.; Rizzolio, F. The Clinical translation of Organic Nanomaterials for Cancer Therapy: A Focus on Polymeric Nanoparticles, Micelles, Liposomes and Exosomes. *Curr. Med. Chem.* **2018**, *25*, 4224–4268. [CrossRef] [PubMed]
5. Zhao, Y.X.; Shaw, A.; Zeng, X.; Benson, E.; Nyström, A.M.; Högberg, B. DNA origami delivery system for cancer therapy with tunable release properties. *ACS Nano* **2012**, *6*, 8684–8691. [CrossRef] [PubMed]

6. Jiang, Q.; Song, C.; Nangreave, J.; Liu, X.; Lin, L.; Qiu, D.; Wang, Z.G.; Zou, G.; Liang, X.; Yan, H.; et al. DNA origami as a carrier for circumvention of drug resistance. *J. Am. Chem. Soc.* **2012**, *134*, 13396–13403. [CrossRef]
7. Zhang, Q.; Jiang, Q.; Li, N.; Dai, L.; Liu, Q.; Song, L.; Wang, J.; Li, Y.; Tian, J.; Ding, B.; et al. DNA origami as an in vivo drug delivery vehicle for cancer therapy. *ACS Nano* **2014**, *8*, 6633–6643. [CrossRef]
8. Rothemund, P.W.K. Folding DNA to create nanoscale shapes and patterns. *Nature* **2006**, *440*, 297–302. [CrossRef]
9. Ponnuswamy, N.; Bastings, M.M.C.; Nathwani, B.; Ryu, J.H.; Chou, L.Y.T.; Vinther, M.; Li, W.A.; Anastassacos, F.M.; Mooney, D.J.; Shih, W.M. Oligolysine-based coating protects DNA nanostructures from low-salt denaturation and nuclease degradation. *Nat. Commun.* **2017**, *8*, 15654. [CrossRef]
10. Linko, V.; Mikkilä, J.; Kostiainen, M.A. Packaging DNA Origami into Viral Protein Cages. *Methods Mol. Biol.* **2018**, *1776*, 267–277.
11. Kiviaho, J.K.; Linko, V.; Ora, A.; Tiainen, T.; Järvihaavisto, E.; Mikkilä, J.; Tenhu, H.; Nonappa; Kostiainen, M.A. Cationic polymers for DNA origami coating—Examining their binding efficiency and tuning the enzymatic reaction rates. *Nanoscale* **2016**, *8*, 11674–11680. [CrossRef] [PubMed]
12. Perrault, S.D.; Shih, W.M. Virus-inspired membrane encapsulation of DNA nanostructures to achieve in vivo stability. *ACS Nano* **2014**, *8*, 5132–5140. [CrossRef] [PubMed]
13. Johnston, M.J.W.; Semple, S.C.; Klimuk, S.K.; Ansell, S.; Maurer, N.; Cullis, P.R. Characterization of the drug retention and pharmacokinetic properties of liposomal nanoparticles containing dihydrosphingomyelin. *Biochim. Biophys. Acta Biomembr.* **2007**, *1768*, 1121–1127. [CrossRef] [PubMed]
14. Hofheinz, R.D.; Gnad-Vogt, S.U.; Beyer, U.; Hochhaus, A. Liposomal encapsulated anti-cancer drugs. *Anticancer Drugs* **2005**, *16*, 691–707. [CrossRef]
15. Immordino, M.L.; Dosio, F.; Cattel, L. Stealth liposomes: Review of the basic science, rationale, and clinical applications, existing and potential. *Int. J. Nanomed.* **2006**, *1*, 297–315.
16. Barenholz, Y.C. Doxil®—The first FDA-approved nano-drug: Lessons learned. *J. Control. Release* **2012**, *160*, 117–134. [CrossRef]
17. Palazzolo, S.; Hadla, M.; Spena, C.R.; Bayda, S.; Kumar, V.; Lo Re, F.; Adeel, M.; Caligiuri, I.; Romano, F.; Corona, G.; et al. Proof-of-Concept Multistage Biomimetic Liposomal DNA Origami Nanosystem for the Remote Loading of Doxorubicin. *ACS Med. Chem. Lett.* **2019**, *10*, 517–521. [CrossRef]
18. Stahl, E.; Martin, T.G.; Praetorius, F.; Dietz, H. Facile and Scalable Preparation of Pure and Dense DNA Origami Solutions. *Angew. Chem. Int. Ed.* **2014**, *53*, 12735–12740. [CrossRef]
19. Bayda, S.; Hadla, M.; Palazzolo, S.; Kumar, V.; Caligiuri, I.; Ambrosi, E.; Pontoglio, E.; Agostini, M.; Tuccinardi, T.; Benedetti, A.; et al. Bottom-up synthesis of carbon nanoparticles with higher doxorubicin efficacy. *J. Control. Release* **2017**, *248*, 144–152. [CrossRef]
20. Garnier, D.; Li, R.; Delbos, F.; Fourrier, A.; Collet, C.; Guguen-Guillouzo, C.; Chesné, C.; Nguyen, T.H. Expansion of human primary hepatocytes in vitro through their amplification as liver progenitors in a 3D organoid system. *Sci. Rep.* **2018**, *8*, 8222. [CrossRef]
21. Min, Y.; Caster, J.M.; Eblan, M.J.; Wang, A.Z. Clinical Translation of Nanomedicine. *Chem. Rev.* **2015**, *115*, 11147–11190. [CrossRef] [PubMed]
22. Toffoli, G.; Hadla, M.; Corona, G.; Caligiuri, I.; Palazzolo, S.; Semeraro, S.; Gamini, A.; Canzonieri, V.; Rizzolio, F. Exosomal doxorubicin reduces the cardiac toxicity of doxorubicin. *Nanomedicine* **2015**, *10*, 2963–2971. [CrossRef] [PubMed]
23. Hadla, M.; Palazzolo, S.; Corona, G.; Caligiuri, I.; Canzonieri, V.; Toffoli, G.; Rizzolio, F. Exosomes increase the therapeutic index of doxorubicin in breast and ovarian cancer mouse models. *Nanomedicine* **2016**, *11*, 2431–2441. [CrossRef] [PubMed]
24. Perrault, S.D.; Shih, W.M. Lipid Membrane Encapsulation of a 3D DNA Nano Octahedron. *Methods Mol. Biol.* **2017**, *1500*, 165–184. [PubMed]
25. Greene, R.F.; Collins, J.M.; Jenkins, J.F.; Speyer, J.L.; Myers, C.E. Plasma pharmacokinetics of adriamycin and adriamycinol: Implications for the design of in vitro experiments and treatment protocols. *Cancer Res.* **1983**, *43*, 3417–3421.
26. Liu, M.; Fu, J.; Hejesen, C.; Yang, Y.; Woodbury, N.W.; Gothelf, K.; Liu, Y.; Yan, H. A DNA tweezer-actuated enzyme nanoreactor. *Nat. Commun.* **2013**, *4*, 2127. [CrossRef]

27. Kocabey, S.; Meinl, H.; MacPherson, I.S.; Cassinelli, V.; Manetto, A.; Rothenfusser, S.; Liedl, T.; Lichtenegger, F.S. Cellular Uptake of Tile-Assembled DNA Nanotubes. *Nanomaterials* **2014**, *5*, 47–60. [CrossRef]
28. Sobczak, J.P.J.; Martin, T.G.; Gerling, T.; Dietz, H. Rapid folding of DNA into nanoscale shapes at constant temperature. *Science* **2012**, *338*, 1458–1461. [CrossRef]
29. Fu, Y.; Zeng, D.; Chao, J.; Jin, Y.; Zhang, Z.; Liu, H.; Li, D.; Ma, H.; Huang, Q.; Gothelf, K.V.; et al. Single-step rapid assembly of DNA origami nanostructures for addressable nanoscale bioreactors. *J. Am. Chem. Soc.* **2013**, *135*, 696–702. [CrossRef]
30. Auvinen, H.; Zhang, H.; Kopilow, A.; Niemelä, E.H.; Nummelin, S.; Correia, A.; Santos, H.A.; Linko, V.; Kostiainen, M.A. Protein Coating of DNA Nanostructures for Enhanced Stability and Immunocompatibility. *Adv. Healthc. Mater.* **2017**, *6*, 1700692. [CrossRef]
31. Bandak, S.; Goren, D.; Horowitz, A.; Tzemach, D.; Gabizon, A. Pharmacological studies of cisplatin encapsulated in long-circulating liposomes in mouse tumor models. *Anticancer Drugs* **1999**, *10*, 911–920. [CrossRef] [PubMed]
32. Miyoshi, H.; Stappenbeck, T.S. In vitro expansion and genetic modification of gastrointestinal stem cells in spheroid culture. *Nat. Protoc.* **2013**, *8*, 2471–2482. [CrossRef] [PubMed]

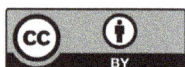

© 2019 by the authors. Licensee MDPI, Basel, Switzerland. This article is an open access article distributed under the terms and conditions of the Creative Commons Attribution (CC BY) license (http://creativecommons.org/licenses/by/4.0/).

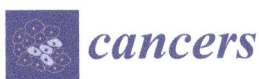

Article

A Triple Co-Delivery Liposomal Carrier That Enhances Apoptosis via an Intrinsic Pathway in Melanoma Cells

Nina Filipczak [1,*], Anna Jaromin [1], Adriana Piwoni [1], Mohamed Mahmud [1,2], Can Sarisozen [3], Vladimir Torchilin [3,4] and Jerzy Gubernator [1]

1. Department of Lipids and Liposomes, Faculty of Biotechnology, University of Wroclaw, 50-383 Wroclaw, Poland; anna.jaromin@uwr.edu.pl (A.J.); adriana.piwoni@gmail.com (A.P.); mohamedzwawi@yahoo.com (M.M.); jerzy.gubernator@uwr.edu.pl (J.G.)
2. Department of Food Science and Technology, Faculty of Agriculture, University of Misurata, Misurata 2478, Libya
3. Center for Pharmaceutical Biotechnology and Nanomedicine, Northeastern University, Boston, MA 02115, USA; cansarisozen@gmail.com (C.S.); v.torchilin@northeastern.edu (V.T.)
4. Department of Oncology, Radiotherapy and Plastic Surgery I.M. Sechenov First Moscow State Medical University (Sechenov University), 119991 Moscow, Russia
* Correspondence: nina.filipczak@uwr.edu.pl or nina.filipczak@gmail.com; Tel.: +48-713-756-318

Received: 1 November 2019; Accepted: 3 December 2019; Published: 9 December 2019

Abstract: The effectiveness of existing anti-cancer therapies is based mainly on the stimulation of apoptosis of cancer cells. Most of the existing therapies are somewhat toxic to normal cells. Therefore, the quest for nontoxic, cancer-specific therapies remains. We have demonstrated the ability of liposomes containing anacardic acid, mitoxantrone and ammonium ascorbate to induce the mitochondrial pathway of apoptosis via reactive oxygen species (ROS) production by the killing of cancer cells in monolayer culture and shown its specificity towards melanoma cells. Liposomes were prepared by a lipid hydration, freeze-and-thaw (FAT) procedure and extrusion through polycarbonate filters, a remote loading method was used for dug encapsulation. Following characterization, hemolytic activity, cytotoxicity and apoptosis inducing effects of loaded nanoparticles were investigated. To identify the anticancer activity mechanism of these liposomes, ROS level and caspase 9 activity were measured by fluorescence and by chemiluminescence respectively. We have demonstrated that the developed liposomal formulations produced a high ROS level, enhanced apoptosis and cell death in melanoma cells, but not in normal cells. The proposed mechanism of the cytotoxic action of these liposomes involved specific generation of free radicals by the iron ions mechanism.

Keywords: anacardic acid; mitoxantrone; targeted drug delivery; liposomes; melanoma; apoptosis; ascorbic acid

---

1. Introduction

Melanoma, one of the most aggressive types of cancer, arises from the transformation of normal melanocytes. This type of cancer is characterized by uncontrolled divisions, dysregulation of cell processes and the ability to invade and create metastases even at an early stage of development [1,2].

The basic method of treating melanoma is the surgical removal of the neoplastic lesions with a margin of healthy tissue. In addition, chemotherapy, radiotherapy and immunotherapy are also used. However, despite aggressive treatment, complete remission is often not observed. The prognosis depends on the depth of tumor cell infiltration and the clinical stage of the cancer. In early stages (infiltration depth up to 1 mm), a cure can be up to 90–100% and decreases as the cancer progresses.

Conventional chemotherapy with dacarbazine and temozolomide has few side effects, but it is not very effective. Interleukin-2 and other immunocytokines have been known to be effective in melanoma treatment, but their use is limited due to high systemic toxicity [3–5], which is why using this method of treatment is still problematic [6]. Another approach to melanoma treatment is to inhibit negative regulation by binding to CTLA-4. CTLA-4 blocking promotes stimulation of adaptive immunity and T cell activation. CTLA-4 blocking antibodies have shown efficacy in various mouse models of malignancy when administered alone or in combinations with vaccines, chemotherapy and radiation. Some of anti-CTLA-4 antibodies were recently developed, including ipilimumab and tremelimumab. Both of the letter antibodies have been extensively evaluated for melanoma; in particular, ipilimumab has recently been approved as second line monotherapy in the treatment of advanced melanoma. Tremelimumab is currently being evaluated in Phase II trials as monotherapy for melanoma [7,8], however standards of melanoma treatment are dacarbazine and temozolomide [8]. Other co-inhibitory pathway uses the programmed cell death receptor 1 (PD-1), which is an inhibitory receptor present on activated T cells. When PD-1 binds to its ligand (PD-L1), which is often expressed on activated cancer cells, the ability to T cells to produce an effective immune response is reduced. Antibodies directed against PD-1 (nivolumab, pembrolizumab) or PD-L1 may therefore help to restore or enhance the anti-tumor immune response and induce tumor remission in patients with advanced melanoma. Although this approach has a significant impact on survival, half of the patients do not respond well to treatment. Possible mechanisms of poor response to treatment are numerous and may include the following: (1) no preexisting anti-tumor immune response, (2) intratumoral development of immunosuppressive molecules such as indoleamine dioxygenase (3) and oncogenic pathways of melanoma, which activate immunosuppressive programs such as WNT/β-catenin. Therefore, more research is needed to enable appropriate selection of patients who are likely to benefit from this approach [9,10].

These results may be improved by using combination therapy. In this report, the main chemotherapeutic was mitoxantrone, used in combination with two additional active agents. Mitoxantrone (MIT) [11] has been used extensively in the treatment of cancers such as acute myeloid leukemia, non-Hodgkin's lymphoma, prostate cancer and breast cancer as well as in active forms of progressive multiple sclerosis [12,13]. The antitumor effect of MIT is based on its ability to interact with DNA, where it forms a covalent complex with topoisomerase II, which prevents the rejoining of the single DNA strand during replication, and consequently inhibits DNA replication and RNA transcription [14–16], and the cell cycle at various stages [17]. Despite its wide application, MIT can have many side effects including cardiotoxicity [18,19]. Recently, the use of natural dietary antioxidants has been considered for use, to minimize cytotoxicity and tissue damage with anti-cancer agents [20]. Some natural substances, such as ascorbic acid, improve anti-cancer activity of some chemotherapeutic drugs [21]. Ascorbic acid is a water-soluble antioxidant as well as an enzyme co-factor produced by plants and certain animals. It is a powerful reducing agent that effectively neutralizes potentially harmful free radicals generated as a result of metabolic processes [22–24]. In contrast to normal cells, ascorbic acid becomes more toxic towards cancer cells because of the increased uptake of its oxidized form, dehydroascorbate (DHA), via the GLUT1 glucose transporter. Release of iron ions from the cytoplasmic iron storage protein, ferritin (iron ions are much more abundant in cancer cells due to transferrin receptors overexpression), which become available for DHA, results in production of hydrogen peroxide and depletion of the reduced glutathione pool by a cyclic oxidation-reduction mechanism [25]. Several studies have shown a positive effect of ascorbic acid in the treatment of cancer and a significant reduction in chemotherapy-related adverse reactions in patients [26].

Iron can be released from ferritin by additional biological reductants including thiols and reduced flavins [27]. One of the anticancer activities of the anthracyclines and its derivatives is free radical formation by reaction with iron ions [28–30]. Therefore, it appeared reasonable to use the ammonium ascorbate ion gradient for the encapsulation of the anthracycline derivative, MIT, to maximize its anticancer potential. The iron-based free radical mechanism for MIT action is increased in cancer cells known to accumulate iron [31].

In this work, we tested liposomes for the ascorbic acid effect alone or combined with MIT or with anacardic acid (AA), which is another natural compound with potential anticancer activity. Anacardic acid inhibits histone acetyltransferases (HAT) activity of p300 and P300/CBP-associated factor (PCAF) in vitro [32]. Blocking the p300 protein inhibits the NF-κB pathway regulating cell proliferation, survival and inflammation [33]. Anacardic acid may also reduce VEGF-dependent angiogenesis, which can lead to inhibition of tumor growth [34]. Its activity has been demonstrated with melanoma cells [35], colon, breast, lung, cervical and renal cancers [36]. It may also affect the growth of hormone-dependent tumors by inhibiting the activity of androgen and estrogen receptors [37,38]. However, the exact mechanism of anticancer activity of anacardic acid is not fully understood. It is believed to be involved in the modulation of the expression of several genes involved in the cell cycle and apoptosis. The action of anacardic acid causes the arrest of the cell cycle in the S phase and the induction of apoptosis, most probably by reducing the expression of genes including Bcl-2 and Bax [39]. Remarkably, the hydrogenation of anacardic acid to form its saturated acid did not alter the inhibitory activity, thus eliminating the importance of saturation status in the mechanism of inhibition. [32]. Tested liposomal formulations containing 5 mol% of the AA with MTX encapsulated by means of an ammonium ascorbate gradient exhibited remarkably high toxicity toward both used melanoma cancer lines, but not to non-cancer NHDF cells, where the protective influence of ascorbate was observed. The main purpose of this research was to develop liposomes co-loaded with anacardic acid, mitoxantrone and ammonium ascorbate, and investigate the combined effects of these liposomal formulations on human melanoma cancer cells.

2. Results

2.1. Liposomes Preparation and Characterization

As shown in Table 1A, liposomes containing different amounts of anacardic acid had an average size around 110 nm with a narrow size distribution and slightly negative charge. Additionally, morphological analysis determined by TEM microscopy confirmed the presence of circular structures with uniform size in AA-containing liposome samples (Figure 1).

Table 1. Summary of size (Z-average), polydispersity index (PDI) and zeta potential of (**A**) all nano-preparations and (**B**) 5mol% anacardic acid nano-preparations before and after targeting with transferrin.

A				
Amount of Anacardic Acid in Liposome Membrane (mol%)	Diameter (nm)	Zeta Potential (mV)	PDI	Encapsulation Efficiency (%)
0	112 ± 1.2	0.87 ± 0.39	0.036	99.5
5	111 ± 1.5	−4.31 ± 0.49	0.042	99.6
10	115 ± 2.3	−5.42 ± 0.63	0.051	98.9
15	112 ± 0.8	−5.74 ± 1.1	0.046	99.2
20	105 ± 2.5	−4.12 ± 0.9	0.032	99.2
40	110 ± 2.1	−2.81 ± 0.5	0.06	98.6
B				
Liposomal Formulation	Diameter (nm)	Zeta Potential (mV)	PDI	Encapsulation Efficiency (%)
LipAA5 Vit. C	111 ± 1.5	−4.31 ± 0.49	0.042	99.0
LipAA5 Vit. C TF	119 ± 1.5	−3.71 ± 0.5	0.05	89.9

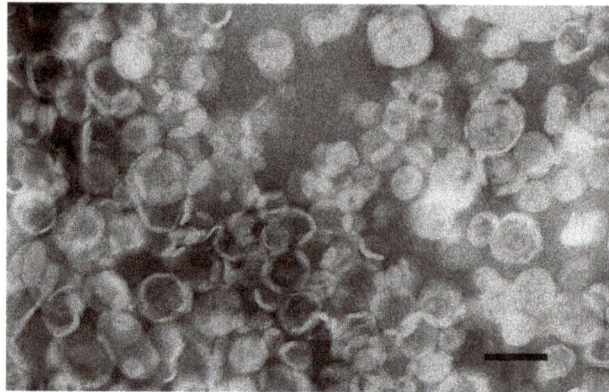

Figure 1. Transmission electron microscopy image of 5 mol% AA-incorporated liposomes. Scale bar = 100 nm.

In all cases MIT encapsulation was very efficient (above 98%). All of these parameters remained nearly the same (Table 1B) after targeting liposomes with transferrin.

2.2. Liposomes Demonstrate Selectivity toward Melanoma Cells and Low Cardio- and Hepatotoxicity and a Lower Hemolysis Ratio

The cytotoxicity of the free drug and liposomal formulations was tested on two human melanoma cell lines A375 and Hs294T. Mitoxantrone was entrapped in liposomes using two different gradients: ammonium ascorbate (Vit C) and ammonium sulphate (AS). Liposomes enriched with anacardic acid (AA) and liposomes without AA were investigated. Cell viability was measured by MTT assay after 48 or 72 hrs from the addition of free drug or liposomes and the cell survival curves were determined.

Both cell lines were sensitive to MIT in a dose-dependent manner. Empty AA liposomes with Vit. C showed only slight toxicity to melanoma cells, which was approximately the same in both cell lines. This toxicity was directly proportional to the amount of anacardic acid. This effect was much less visible for liposomes with ammonium sulphate. The presence of AA significantly increased the cytotoxicity of the liposomal MIT, both with liposomes containing ammonium ascorbate and for liposomes with ammonium sulphate. An additional significant cytotoxic effect of ascorbic acid was observed at higher concentration and after a longer incubation time (72 h), especially in the A375 cell line. The difference between Lip AA5 MIT Vit. C and Lip AA5 MIT AS was significant over the entire range of concentrations tested. The patterns observed after 48 hours of incubation remain practically unchanged when incubated for 72 hours.

The NHDF skin fibroblast cell line was used as a normal control for melanoma cells to check specificity of the action of anacardic acid and mitoxantrone, because the highly desirable feature of the drug carrier is its low toxicity against cells that are not cancerous.

A toxic effect of anacardic acid on normal cells, above 5 mol% concentration for formulations containing ammonium ascorbate was observed. However, a formulation containing 5 mol% of anacardic acid and ammonium ascorbate was not toxic to the normal skin cells.

Based on the survival curves for all formulations, the IC_{50} parameter was determined (Table 2). The plain liposomes were characterized by an IC_{50} concentration ranging from several to several hundred μM of total mol amount of lipids that form liposomes. In addition, anacardic acid in combination with ammonium ascorbate is more toxic to melanoma cells than in combination with ammonium sulfate (IC_{50} for Lip AA5 Vit. C. was 12.1 μM and for Lip AA5 AS was 35.8 μM for A375 after 48 h incubation). This tendency was evident for both melanoma cell lines and independent of incubation time. The reverse is true for the NHDF cell line, where the formulation with anacardic acid in combination with ammonium ascorbate is less toxic than the formulation of anacardic acid with a pH gradient generated by ammonium sulphate (IC_{50} value is more than three times higher for LipAA5 Vit.C for 48 h incubation and 138 times higher for 72 h).

Table 2. Comparison of IC_{50} values (µM) of mitoxantrone-free liposomes and mitoxantrone-containing liposomes for all cell lines. Values are averages of three independent measurements with standard deviation.

Liposomal Formulation	Cell Line					
	A375		Hs294T		NHDF	
	IC_{50} 48 h	IC_{50} 72 h	IC_{50} 48 h	IC_{50} 72 h	IC_{50} 48 h	IC_{50} 72 h
Lip Vit.C	286.5 ± 31	158.37 ± 35	74.92 ± 7.5	43.95 ± 0.3	174.3 ± 7.3	122.06 ± 9
LipAA5 Vit.C	15.4 ± 3	12.63 ± 5	30.43 ± 6.65	0.52 ± 0.03	188.5 ± 20.8	152.93 ± 11
Lip AA10 Vit.C	17 ± 0.3	58.71 ± 7.4	3.54 ± 0.5	1 ± 0.03	23.4 ± 1.5	20.01 ± 0.46
Lip AA15 Vit.C	14.8 ± 0.08	1.78 ± 0.5	1.93 ± 0.5	5.59 ± 1.34	19.57 ± 0.8	19.32 ± 0.93
Lip AA20 Vit.C	17.7 ± 2.1	2.71 ± 0.55	1.7 ± 0.4	0.6 ± 0.04	26.87 ± 3	12.12 ± 2.8
Lip AA40 Vit.C	1.35 ± 0.2	0.93 ± 0.09	1.26 ± 0.07	0.29 ± 0.06	20 ± 1.3	9.1 ± 0.84
Lip AS	240.5 ± 57	99.06 ± 14.2	123.15 ± 7	86.33 ± 6.8	44.5 ± 3.6	6 ± 1.1
Lip AA5 AS	36.1 ± 6	92.37 ± 18.9	109.43 ± 7.7	55.64 ± 9.4	58.36 ± 6.1	5.4 ± 1.3
Lip MIT Vit.C	50.44 ± 4.3	10.58 ± 3	19.52 ± 7.6	10.3 ± 2	41.25 ± 3.21	20.48 ± 4.25
Lip AA5 MIT Vit.C	0.4 ± 0.05	0.24 ± 0.1	1.69 ± 0.3	0.66 ± 0.13	84.04 ± 12.7	44.19 ± 5.7
Lip AA10 MIT Vit.C	0.47 ± 0.02	0.39 ± 0.02	1.88 ± 0.33	0.94 ± 0.04	4.7 ± 0.43	1. ± 0.04
Lip AA15 MIT Vit.C	0.37 ± 0.07	0.39 ± 0.01	0.77 ± 0.05	0.18 ± 0.005	1.5 ± 0.28	0.9 ± 0.006
Lip AA20 MIT Vit.C	0.46 ± 0.03	0.28 ± 0.002	0.18 ± 0.001	0.1 ± 0.007	0.84 ± 0.03	0.23 ± 0.009
Lip AA40 MIT Vit.C	0.04 ± 0.003	0.02 ± 0.002	0.12 ± 0.06	0.07 ± 0.006	0.3 ± 0.02	0.19 ± 0.004
Lip MIT AS	3.87 ± 1.34	32.5 ± 2.51	17.71 ± 1.22	7.11 ± 1.42	40.53 ± 6.2	1.03 ± 0.06
Lip AA5 MIT AS	19.88 ± 4.15	0.6 ± 0.2	16.6 ± 1.7	1.19 ± 0.26	35.92 ± 3.15	1 ± 0.28
MIT	0.22 ± 0.014	0.075 ± 0.001	0.165 ± 0.03	0.13 ± 0.02	0.43 ± 0.02	0.15 ± 0.02

For mitoxantrone-containing liposomes, IC_{50} values ranged from 0.02 to 75.05 µM (Table 2). There was also a protective effect of vitamin C in combination with anacardic acid for normal cell lines, as was the case with liposomes without a drug. Most current cancer therapies combine various therapeutic agents.

To determine the kind of interaction occurs between the anacardic acid and mitoxantrone, the CI was determined (Table 3). By comparing the combination index values, mitoxantrone and anacardic acid were clearly shown to act synergistically or additively on melanoma cells in the presence of ammonium sulphate or ammonium ascorbate. In the presence of vitamin c, AA and MIT acted antagonistically in normal cells by contrast to ammonium sulphate. These results suggest a different molecular mechanism of action in cancer cells and normal cells. The factor limiting the use of mitoxantrone in anticancer therapy is its high cardiotoxicity. In addition, this drug undergoes transformation in the liver, which leads to hepatotoxicity.

Table 3. Combination index (CI) values of liposomes containing mitoxantrone and anacardic acid in the presence of ammonium sulphate or ammonium ascorbate The CI values are at MIT concentration (50 µM).

Liposomal Formulation	Cell Line		
	A375	Hs294T	NHDF
Lip AA5 MIT AS	0.011	0.085	0.366
Lip AA5 MIT Vit.C	<0.01	0.194	57.064

The use of the lipid carrier was aimed to reduce of the side effects of mitoxantrone. The released LDH (Figure 2) and intracellular ATP (Figure 3) level were used to estimate hepatotoxicity and cardiotoxicity, respectively.

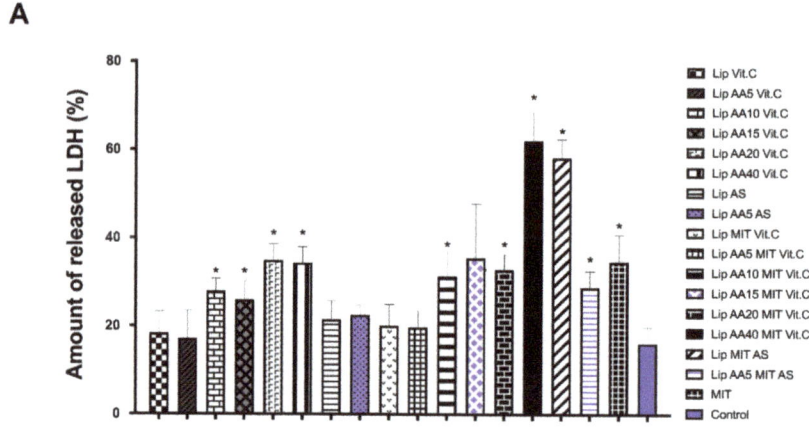

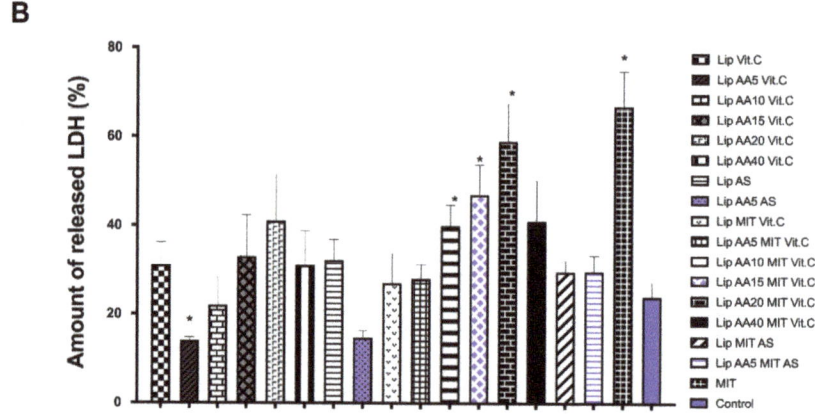

Figure 2. LDH released into the medium as a marker of cytotoxicity of liposomal formulation at a concentration of 10μM of MIT for line H9C2 (**A**), line H9C2 Hep-G2 (**B**). * the difference statistically significant to the control (T test) $p < 0.05$.

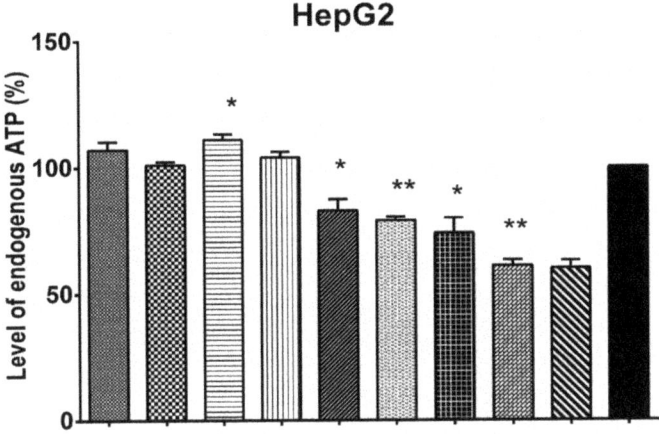

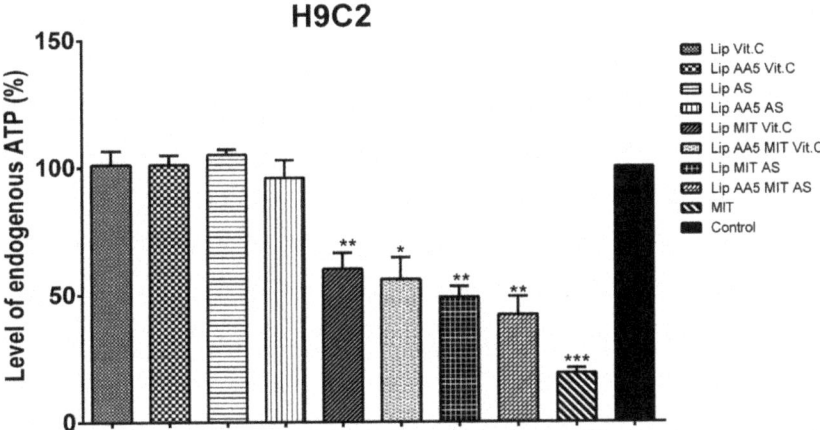

Figure 3. Intracellular ATP level in the Hep-G2 line (upper), line H9C2 (lower). * the difference statistically significant to the control (T test) $p < 0.05$; ** the difference statistically significant to the control (T test) $p < 0.01$; *** the difference statistically significant to the control (T test) $p < 0.001$.

The results obtained on the Hep-G2 liver cell line and H9C2 rat cardiomyocytes indicate a reduction in the toxicity of mitoxantrone in the liposomal form in relation to free drug for Hep-G2 cells. In addition, the formulation anacardic acid-enriched showed no increased toxicity to liver cells, even when combined with mitoxantrone. A similar effect was obtained for H9C2 myocardial cells, except for the formulation containing 40 mol% AA and MIT, and MIT formulations with AS, which were more toxic than free drug. The higher toxicity of the latter formulations suggests the involvement of vitamin C in the protection of cells against drug toxicity. The Lip MIT AS liposomes compared to Lip AA5 MIT AS liposomes showed a noticeable reduction in the toxicity in the presence of anacardic acid. The addition of anacardic acid to the liposome membrane did not change the level of intracellular ATP for either cell line (Figure 2B). Mitoxantrone significantly reduced ATP level (up to 60% for myocardial cells), but this effect is not observed in combination with anacardic acid and ammonium ascorbate.

MIT in the presence of AA and ammonium sulfate induced a much stronger cell response. In addition, MIT's influence on the level of ATP in liver cells is smaller than in the myocardial cells. This is opposite the effect in the case of LDH, which suggests that the toxicity of mitoxantrone in HeP-G2 cells is manifested by the release of LDH, while for H9C2 cells, by the reduction in ATP levels.

The hemolytic potential of free AA and AA-enriched liposomes without drug after incubation with human erythrocytes was observed (Figure 4). Formulations were characterized by their ability to induce the release of hemoglobin from red blood cells.

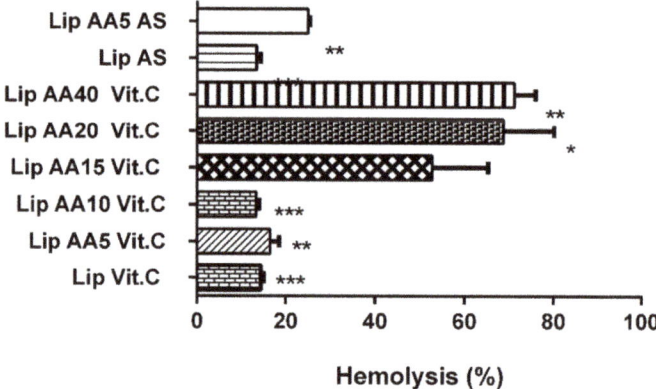

Figure 4. Hemolysis of human erythrocytes after incubation with liposome formulations (T test) * $p = 0.0176$; ** $p = 0.0058$; *** $p = 0.0008$.

Free AA at the concentration corresponding to 5 mol% caused 40.9% of hemolysis. Values obtained for Lip AA5 Vit. C and Lip AA5 AS 16.5 and 25%, respectively suggest a protective effect after its incorporation. It is worth noting that the free form of anacardic acid in concentrations equivalent to their content in liposomes 10 mol% or more is responsible for complete membrane damage under the conditions used. Therefore, the results obtained for Lip AA10 Vit. C are extremely interesting. The hemolysis determined was at the level of 13.4%, similar to the case of control compositions without AA (Lip Vit. C and Lip AS). This observation might indicate that AA located in the membrane probably has no direct contact with erythrocytes. Unfortunately, as the fraction of this compound increases in the remaining formulations (15, 20 and 40 mol%), the protective effect becomes weaker, probably due to presence of interactions with red blood cells. Summarizing, these results demonstrate that AA-incorporated liposomes are likely to cause less toxicity than free AA after intravenous administration and support the development of formulations for in vivo administration.

2.3. ROS Formation Induced by Liposome Formulations

A possible mechanism for caspase pathway activation is the excessive production of reactive oxygen species in response to cell treatment with liposomes. The highest increase in the level of reactive oxygen species was observed 4 h after addition of liposomes (Figure 5).

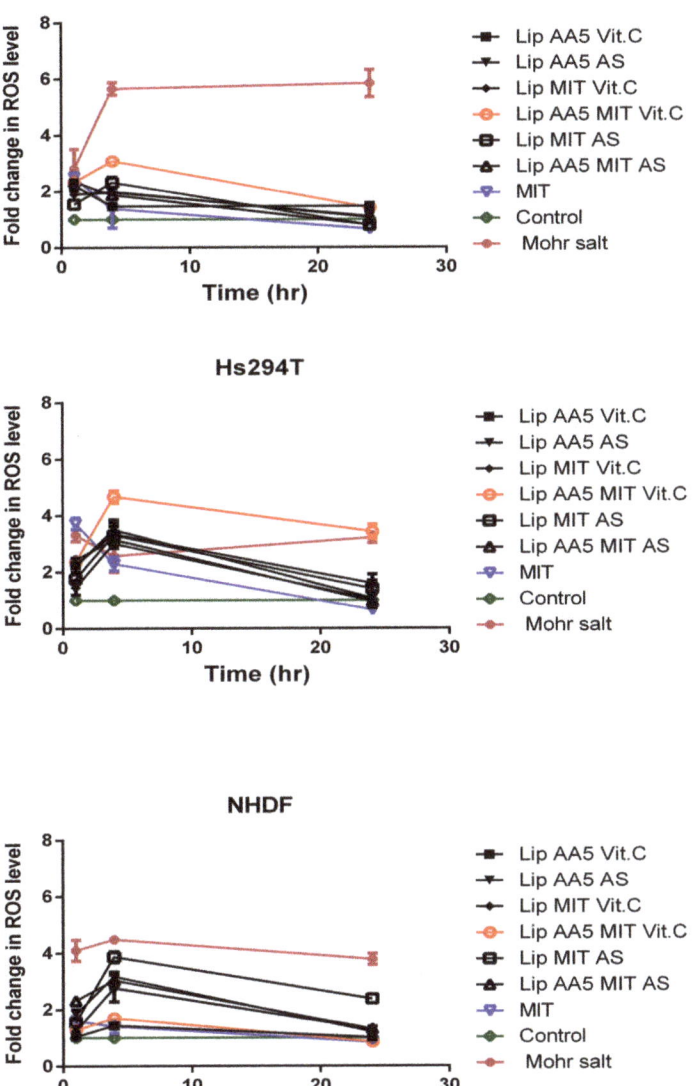

Figure 5. Reactive oxygen species levels in A375, Hs294T and NHDF cells after incubation with liposome formulations and free drug. The untreated cells (control) are considered as 100% of the endogenous ROS level. The Mohr salt was used as a positive control.

The formulation that most effectively raised the level of ROS in the cells of both melanoma lines was Lip AA5 MIT Vit. C, while the level of ROS induced by this formulation in NHDF cells was comparable to untreated cells. The time at which the level of ROS increase come before the increase in caspase activity, suggesting that increased ROS production was the cause of melanoma cell apoptosis.

2.4. Liposome Treatment Enhances the Apoptosis

Using flow cytometry, the progress of apoptosis in melanoma cells after 24 hours of incubation with liposomes and free drug at a dose corresponding to the IC_{50} (48 h) was analyzed. The controls were cells not treated with liposomes. After incubations, cells were labeled with Annexin V fluorescein-quenched and propidium iodide. In early apoptosis, phosphatidylserine dislocates from the inner side of the cell membrane to the exterior and can then bind to annexin V. Propidium iodide makes it possible to differentiate the population of cells with disturbances in the cell membrane integrity. Mitoxantrone in free form reduced the population of healthy cells in favor of a late-apoptotic form, regardless of the cellular model. For A375 melanoma cells (Figure 6), the liposomal form of mitoxantrone, anacardic acid and vitamin C worked in an almost identical manner (97% of cells were in the late stage of apoptosis or necrosis).

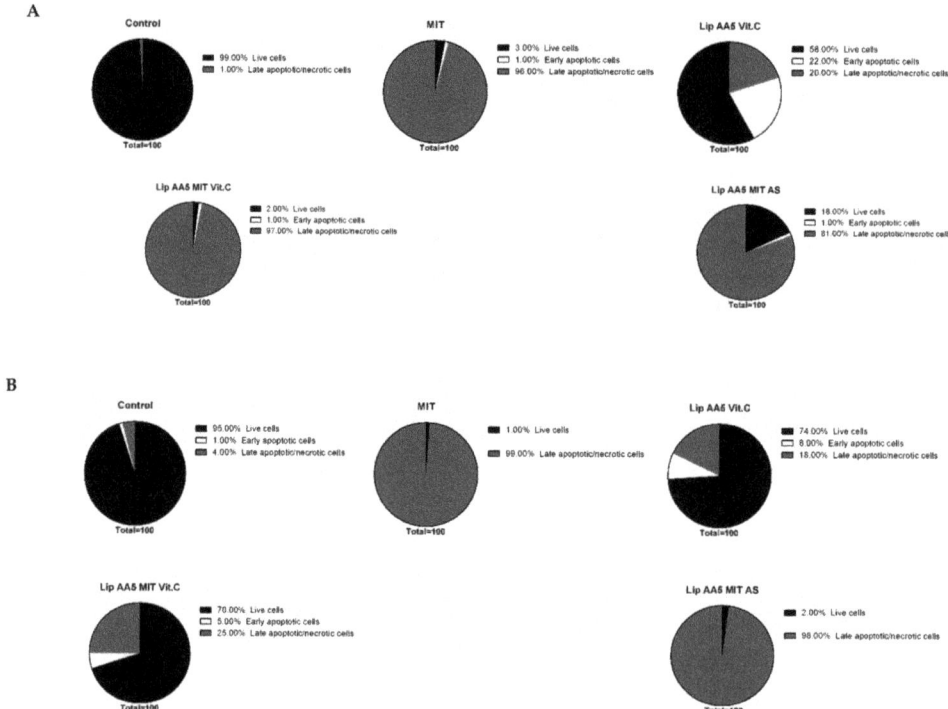

Figure 6. Percentage of the population of dead, living and early apoptotic (**A**) A375 and (**B**) NHDF cells after treatment with liposomes or free drug.

A similar effect was also observed with liposomal forms of anacardic acid, mitoxantrone and ammonium sulphate and formulations containing no anacardic acid. For the metastatic model of melanoma (Hs294T), the effect of free drug was comparable with Lip AA5 Vit C, while the change from vitamin C to ammonium sulfate no longer increased the population of late apoptotic or necrotic cells. This observation suggests the interaction of vitamin C, AA and mitoxantrone in the induction of melanoma cell death. It is noteworthy that the formulation of Lip AA5 Vit C was not toxic to normal skin cells (about 70% of cells remained intact).

This observation demonstrates the high efficacy and specificity of the developed formulation. The results indicate that cells treated with liposomes can die by apoptosis. The Caspase3/7 Glo® test was performed to check whether it was caspase-dependent apoptosis. A noticeable increase in caspase activity can be observed as early as the 6 h after treatment of cells with liposomal preparations (Figure 7).

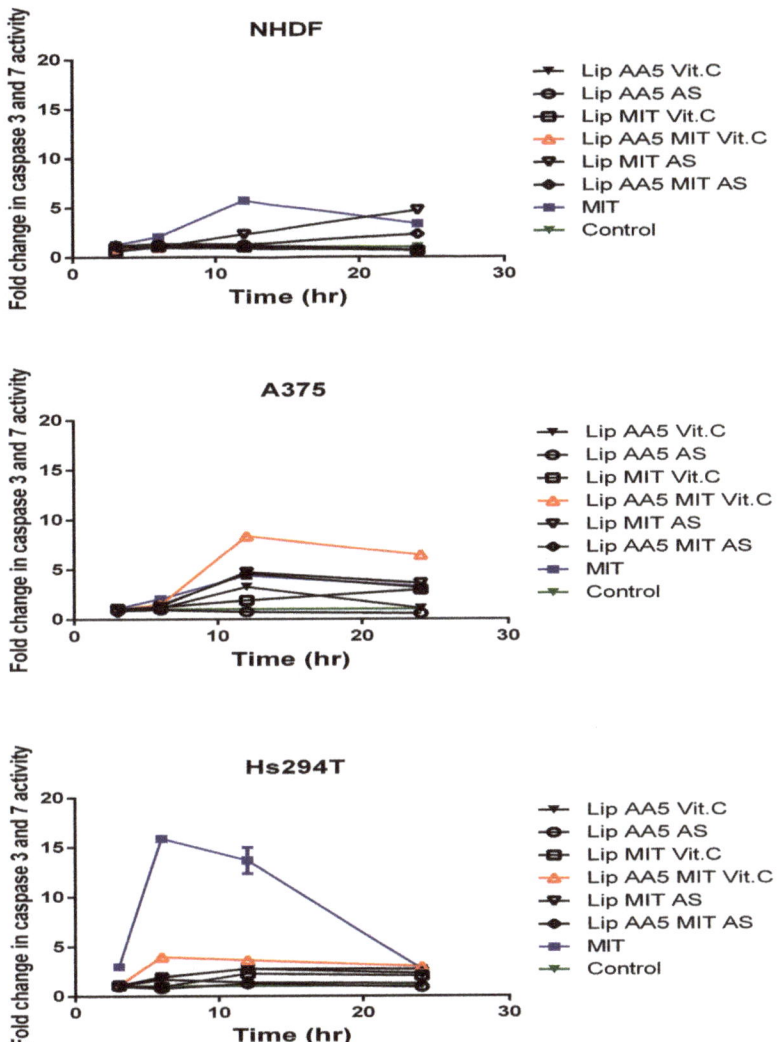

Figure 7. Activity of executive caspases within a 24-hour period after administration of liposomes or free drug. Caspase activity level was assumed to be 100% in cells not treated with liposomes.

The highest caspase activity was observed for the Hs294T line in response to the free drug and the Lip AA5 MIT Vit C. This formulation led to the highest increase in caspase activity (eight-fold) for A375 melanoma, but only 12 hr after administration of liposomes. Lip AA5 MIT Vit C did not elicit any response in NHDF normal cells, but the free drug and the ammonium sulfate-containing formulation caused an increase in caspase activity, after 24 hr of incubation. The results obtained indicate caspase-dependent apoptosis in response to treatment with liposome formulations, and that Lip AA5 MIT Vit C formulation selectively induced caspase-dependent apoptosis in melanoma cells. To check which apoptosis pathway is promoted cytochrome C released study was performed.

Cytochrome C appearance outside of mitochondria in treated with liposomes cells suggested activation of mitochondrial pathway of cell apoptosis (Figure 8).

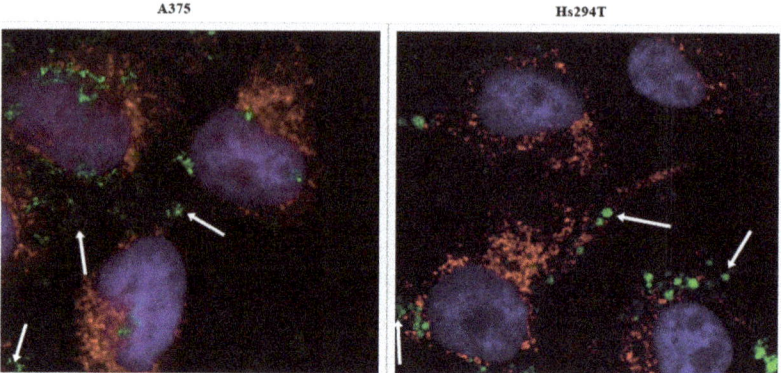

Figure 8. Microscopic photo of melanoma cells after treatment with liposomes (Lip AA5 MIT Vit.C). The cell nuclei are marked in blue, the red color indicates mitochondria, and the green color shows cytochrome c. The arrows indicate cytochrome c released from the mitochondria.

To check whether the release of cytochrome c from the mitochondria triggers Caspase 9 activation, the Caspase 9 Glo® test was used as in the case of caspase apoptosis (Figure 9). The results confirmed the hypothesis about the activation of the mitochondrial apoptosis pathway in response to the liposomal form of AA and MIT in the presence of vitamin C. The results show an increase in caspase 9 activity 6 hours after administration of liposomes in A375 cells. For the Hs294T line, this increase occurred after the fourth hour of incubation with the liposomes. The results indicate that the apoptosis occurs rapidly. No increase in the activity of this caspase was observed in normal cells, suggesting that another mechanism associated with caspases is responsible for their death.

2.5. Tf-Targeted Liposomes Demonstrate Efficient Melanoma Cell Killing

A 3D cell model was used to check how targeted liposomes interact with cells. Cells of melanoma line were plated on agarose plates in varying amounts and cultured for two weeks. As presented in Figure 10, the spheroids were fully mature on the seventh day of culture, as evidenced by the clear boundary of the spheroid. In the following days of the culture, the spheroids gradually changed their shape and the scattering of cells forming the spheroids was observed. Spheroids formed by approximately 13,000 cells on the seventh day of culture with diameter of approximately 500 μm for both cell lines were selected for further experiments.

Transferrin was selected for targeting liposomes. Liposomes were labeled with rhodamine. After incubation, rhodamine fluorescence in the cells was measured by flow cytometry (Figure 11A). Transferrin-targeted liposomes bound to the cells faster than non-targeted liposomes, regardless of the concentration of the liposomes administered. This effect was independent of the cell model.

The next step was an attempt to achieve greater association efficiency that translates into higher cytotoxicity of liposome formulation. ATP level measurements were performed as a toxicity indicator. The number of viable cells within spheroids, after treatment with liposomes (Figure 11B), indicated that targeting liposomes with transferrin increased the toxic effect of these liposomes. For the A375 cell line, the percent of viable cells that remained after administration of untargeted liposomes was approximately 50%, corresponding to a dose equivalent to the IC_{50}. The targeted formulation reduced cell viability by about 75%, so we have a significant increase in efficiency in the action of liposomes. For the second line of melanoma cells, this effect is slightly weaker, however, the difference between the targeted and non-targeted formulations remains statistically significant.

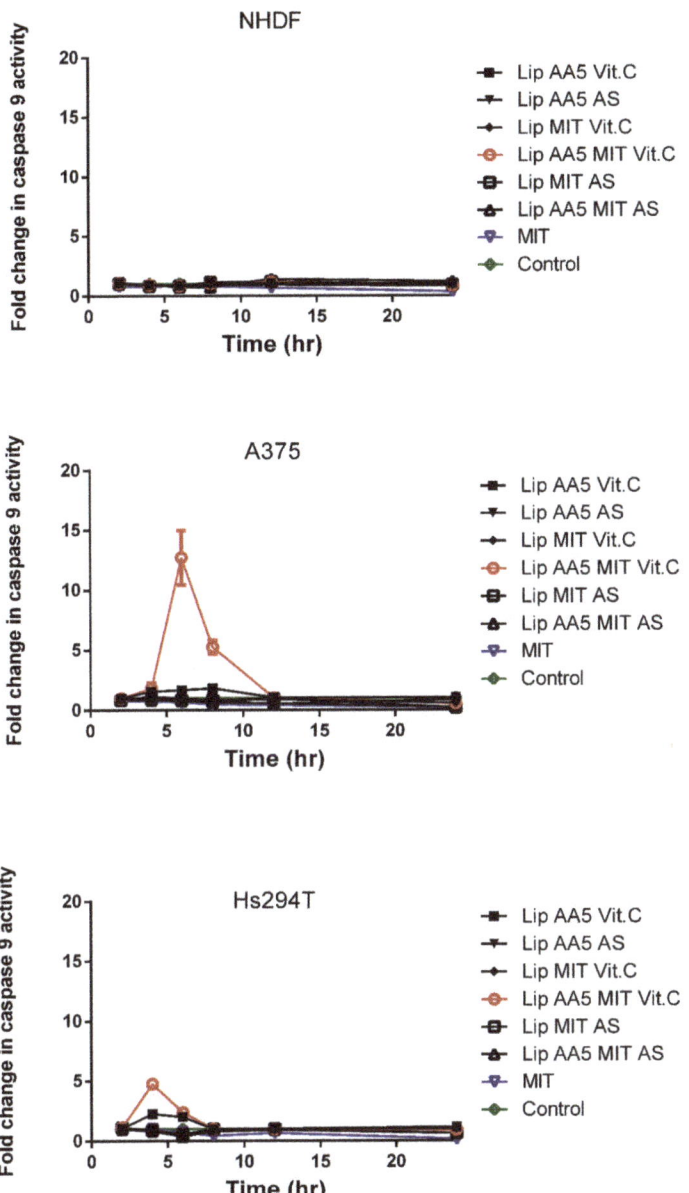

Figure 9. Caspase 9 activity in a 24-hour period after administration of liposomes and free drug. Cells untreated with any agent are marked as a control.

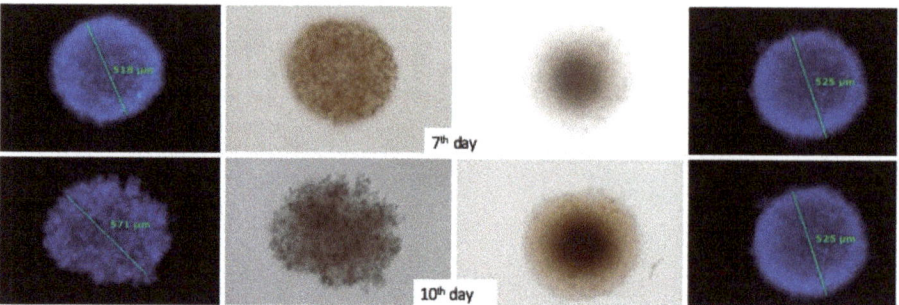

Figure 10. Microscopic image showing spheroids at various growth stages Cell nuclei were stained with Hoechst 33342.

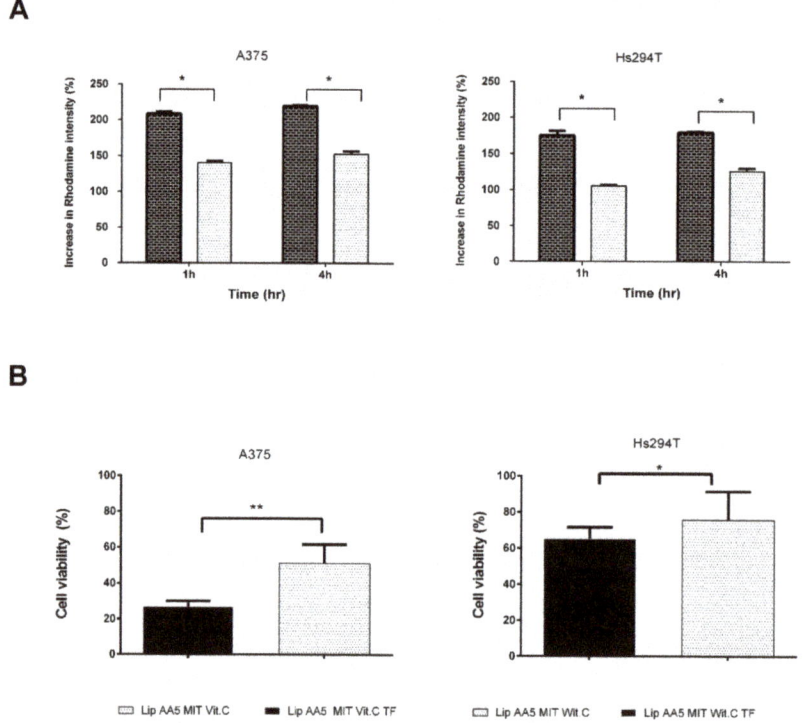

Figure 11. (**A**) Degree of association of liposomes with target A375 and Hs294T cells at 1 and 4 h. Autofluorescence of spheroid forming cells was taken as 100%. The results are the mean ± SD from three independent repetitions. (** two-way ANOVA $p < 0.01$). (**B**) Viability of melanoma cells forming spheroids 72 hours after administration of liposomes. Luminescence of untreated cells was accepted as 100% (control). The results are presented as mean ± SD from five independent repetitions. (test T * $p < 0.05$, ** $p < 0.01$).

3. Discussion

Current chemotherapy is usually insufficient to kill all cancer cells, even at maximum tolerated doses of the cytostatic. Even a relatively small increase in drug resistance in cancer cells may be enough to make a given agent completely ineffective. P-glycoprotein is a protein present on the surface of many types of tumors, and its overexpression is considered one of the main mechanisms by which cancer cells acquire resistance to chemotherapeutics. For this reason, it has been the target of many anticancer therapies. However, drugs such as verapamil and cyclosporine, which inhibit P-glycoprotein have many side effects and their use has become limited [40,41]. Therefore, additional compounds that may inhibit P-glycoprotein have been sought. The present study used a naturally occurring compound that inhibits the function of P-glycoprotein by blocking the NF-kB pathway to sensitize tumor cells to a known chemotherapeutic agent [42]. Anacardic acid is one of those compounds, which has been enriched in the liposomal membrane. The lipid carrier we developed was built from hydrogenated phosphatidylcholine, anacardic acid, dioleylphosphatidyl-ethanolamine, cholesterol, 1,2-distearoyl-sn-glycero-3-phosphatidylethanolamine-N-[amino(poly-ethylene glycol)-2000 and the *para*-nitrophenol derivative DOPE-PEG. In these liposomes mitoxantrone was actively entrapped using the pH gradient generated by ammonium sulfate or ammonium ascorbate.

However, it is known that for anti-cancer therapy to be fully effective, it is necessary to selectively target cancer while maintaining low toxicity towards normal cells. A breakthrough in the treatment of cancer was the transition from non-specific to strictly targeted therapy. The developed carrier represents this by targeting cells overexpressing the receptor for transferrin. The carrier is a targeted liposomal "cocktail" of three active substances with anticancer activity. The carrier of anti-cancer drugs is designed to not only improve its effectiveness, but to also reduce the side effects of the chemotherapeutic agent. In the case of mitoxantrone, its strongest side effects are cardiotoxicity and hepatotoxicity. As we managed to show, the carrier developed, allowed reduction of toxicity to the free drug for Hep-G2 cells. In addition, it was shown that anacardic acid, present in the formulation at 5–40 mole%, did not increase toxicity to liver cells, even in combination with mitoxantrone. A similar effect was obtained for H9C2 myocardial cells, with the exception of the formulation containing 40 mol% AA and MIT and the MIT formulation with AS, which proved to be more toxic than the free drug (Figures 2 and 3). The higher toxicity of the latter formulation suggests the involvement of vitamin c in the protection of cells against toxicity of the drug. The majority of the physiological and biochemical mechanisms of vitamin c's action result from the fact that it is an electron donor. Vitamin c is a powerful antioxidant due to the fact that, being such a donor, it protects other cellular components against oxidation [43]. Anacardic acid can also have a protective effect on myocardial cells. It allows for the differentiation of relevant stem cells towards cardiomyocytes, by affecting the change of chromatin structure and activation of the Castor 1 transcription factor necessary for the differentiation and maturation of these cells [44].

Next, how the liposomes developed interact with target cells was investigated. In vitro cytotoxicity measurements using melanoma cell lines A375 and Hs294T showed that anacardic acid significantly increases the activity of liposomal mitoxantrone at all concentrations tested, regardless of the gradient generator. One explanation may be the improvement of intracellular drug delivery. It should be noted that AA liposomes without MIT showed only a slight inhibition of melanoma cell line proliferation. As confirmed in these studies, mitoxantrone and anacardic acid act synergistically on melanoma cells in the presence of vitamin C or ammonium sulfate. The combination factor values indicate a very strong effect of this combination (Table 3). It may be more interesting that a combination of the antitumor factor with vitamin C usually causes the reverse effect [23] suggesting a key role for anacardic acid in this combination. Anacardic acid has antitumor activity that can induce apoptosis independent of caspase [45] and inhibit the NF-κB pathway [33]. It is also an epigenetic factor that inhibits the activity of histone acetyltransferases (HAT) involved in the regulation of gene expression. One of the HAT family members, Tip60, participates in cell responses to genotoxic events, such as plexus interruptions [46,47]. Inhibition of this enzyme causes weakening of DNA repair systems. Anacardic acid can sensitize cancer cells to genotoxic damage by inhibiting Tip60 [48]. It is known that one of the main mechanisms of action of mitoxantrone is promotion of DNA damage. Therefore, damage to the repair system by anacardic acid may contribute to the observed increase in toxicity.

An interesting observation is that the cytotoxicity of mitoxantrone and anacardic increased with ascorbic acid compared to liposomes with ammonium sulphate. Free vitamin c has previously been used to enhance the activity of several anthracyclines, in particular doxorubicin (DOX), which led to increased DNA damage caused by ROS [49]. Mitoxantrone and ammonium ascorbate cytotoxicity might be due to inhibition of COX expression [50] or activation of the p53 protein by vitamin c with induction of apoptosis, which has been demonstrated with the A375 melanoma cell line [51].

A different effect of this formulation seems very important with respect to normal skin cells, where the value of the combination factor calculated from the MIT survival curves indicates the antagonistic activity of anacardic acid and mitoxantrone in the presence of vitamin c, while in the presence of ammonium sulphate AA, maintains the synergistic effect of these factors. This is most likely due to the fact that ascorbic acid plays a role in protecting cells against genotoxic damage, but the exact protection mechanism is still unclear [52]. The main mechanism of the protective effect of ascorbic acid is its role in ROS removal [53]. However, most likely it is not the main factor that contributes to the protection of NHDF cells against mitoxantrone. Recent profile studies of gene expression in human skin cells treated with ascorbic acid have shown that this effect resulted in an increase in gene expression involved in cell proliferation and DNA repair [54]. Other studies have shown that vitamin c can stimulate chemical repair of DNA [55]. This may partly explain the ROS-independent protective mechanism of ascorbic acid in NHDF cells. It has turned out that liposomal formulations containing anacardic acid do not fully meet the objectives of this project, if the amount of anacardic acid exceeds 15 mol%. This observation is strongly supported by the human red blood hemolysis results. A study has been described previously by Stasiuk et al. the hemolytic activity of anacardic acid towards sheep erythrocytes [56]. As expected, the lytic potential of AA was decreased after its incorporation in liposomes. A similar phenomenon regarding the reduction of hemolytic activity after encapsulation in nanocarriers has already been reported [57,58]. Therefore, formulations containing only 5 mol% were used for the study, by meeting the criteria of stability. This particular formulation was chosen because, in addition to adequate stability, it was characterized by high toxicity to melanoma cells with little toxicity to normal cells. The toxic action of the designed carrier model involved the induction of cancer cells into the ROS-dependent apoptosis pathway. The results of in vitro analyses indicate that the developed lipid carrier effectively delivers the drug to cancer cells, translates into an enhanced production of reactive oxygen species (Figure 5), which then leads to the induction of the apoptosis shown by cytometric analyzes (Figure 6). The mechanism of this phenomenon is known to be dependent on the balance between the expression of pro-apoptotic and anti-apoptotic BCL2 proteins [59,60]. The increase in Bcl-2 levels in cancer cells blocks the release of cytochrome C from the mitochondria. Cytochrome C in the cytosol activates caspase 9 and then 3, leading to apoptosis.

The results suggest that the developed formulation causes the entry of tumor cells into the mitochondrial-dependent apoptosis pathway, as evidenced by the activity of caspase 9 (Figure 9). They also suggest a different mechanism of death for normal and cancerous cells. Based on the activity of caspases, a potential mechanism of action of the developed liposomes is proposed.

The proposed apoptosis model is based mainly on the lack of caspase 9 activation in NHDF cells and activation of executive caspases of apoptosis in all cellular models (Figure 7). The higher efficiency in introducing cells to the apoptosis pathway, and thus higher cytotoxicity, is dependent on the amount of drug delivered to the cells. The new mitoxantrone vehicle was designed so that the efficiency of active encapsulation was very high (over 95%) and the carrier was stable. However, it has been reported that even active encapsulation of the drug causes very rapid clearance of liposomes from the bloodstream (less than 5% of the drug remained in the bloodstream for more than two hours) [61]. In the case of sterically stabilized liposomes containing the PEG-lipid conjugate, over 80% of lipids and drug were present in the blood 4 hours after injection, and after 24 hours it remained more than 30%. Unfortunately, even prolonged circulation in the bloodstream does not necessarily lead to an increase in the effectiveness of the drug. It is believed that sterically stabilized liposomes containing mitoxantrone do not release the drug inside the cells. Instead there is a simple fusion of the liposome with the cell membrane and passive drug passage into the cell, or the drug is released as a result of carrier metabolism by macrophages present in tumor tissue [62,63]. One of the methods to reduce this effect is by targeting liposomes. In turn, longer persistence of liposomes in the blood enables better action on circulating cancer cells, which allows elimination of cells that metastasize to other organs [64]. In the case of melanoma, this is especially important because the primary way of treating skin cancers is surgical excision of the lesion and therapy preventing metastases. This argument supports the use of liposomes as a drug carrier in melanoma therapy.

As mentioned before, a desirable carrier feature for anti-cancer therapy is a high specificity that allows the drug to be introduced into the cells in a targeted and controlled manner. The developed liposomes with anacardic acid, containing ammonium ascorbate and mitoxantrone, may increase drug delivery to cells, by prolonging circulation time and targeting tumor tissue through the EPR effect, which is a known property of liposomes.

A very important step in the proposed project was to test the lipid carrier in the presence of transferrin. The addition of DOPE-PEG3400-pNP and the attachment of ligand to the surface of liposomes did not cause significant changes in the basic physicochemical properties of the preparation. The presence of DOPE in the coating promotes the fusion of liposomes with the endosomal membrane [65,66], which has been considered the most crucial step for the effective action of anticancer drugs [65]. In this case DOPE's main effect was to anchor the liposome of the long-chain PEG associated with the targeting factor. Using confocal microscopy and flow cytometry techniques, we observed clear differences in rhodamine-labelled Lip AA5 MIT Vit. C TF liposome effects with membrane of cells of different melanoma lines compared with Lip AA5 MIT Vit.C (Figure 11A). High specificity of interaction of the designed carrier with cells displaying the receptor for transferrin was also demonstrated. Furthermore, the results of cytotoxicity analysis (Figure 11B) indicate the relatively high specificity of TF immunoliposomes for target cells. The increased cytotoxicity of transferrin-targeted liposomes may be because these liposomes simultaneously delivered iron and vitamin c to cells. As a result, the iron pool available for the Fenton reaction doubles, since the vitamin c receives iron from ferritin, making them bioavailable [5,67].

High efficacy allows the potential use of this formulation in the therapy of other cancers, since transferrin receptor is overproduced in many types of cancer, especially those that show high growth rates [68–70]. The use of transferrin as a targeting agent is common, both for the management of anti-cancer drugs alone [71–73], for proteins with toxic effects [74–76] and for nucleic acids [77,78].

The targeting of the first type of transferrin receptor (TFR1) is made possible, by strategies that utilize its natural TF ligand, monoclonal antibodies or their fragments. Unfortunately, the blocking of the cytotoxicity of TF conjugates by native TF is a disadvantage. Therefore, its high concentrations circulating for long periods may disrupt the action of these conjugates, leading to a decrease in their therapeutic effectiveness. Because TF conjugates have the potential to interact with both TFR1 and TFR2 (which are predominantly present in the liver), they can be toxic to many normal cells. Targeting the TFR1 receptor carrier using monoclonal antibodies can help bypass these potential problems [79].

Hypoxia is a common feature of solid tumors and associated with tumor progression [80,81]. The expression of TFR in cells in an anaerobic microenvironment may be a more rational and effective use with targeted TFR molecules. The results of the tests conducted with the A375 cell line in hypoxia showed an increased expression of TFR in hypoxia at both the mRNA and protein level, which was confirmed by surface TFR analysis measured by flow cytometry [82]. The results of these tests confirm the validity of our use of transferrin as a driving factor, since its expression depends on the tumor environment. The developed liposomal formulation is a promising anticancer agent that may also be used as the basic platform for further modification.

In vitro studies have their limitations that make the interpretation of results difficult and do not always reflect the response of cancer cells growing in vivo. This is because most commercially available cancer lines have been derived by performing serial passages and selection of cells with desired traits, such as the expression of specific genes, morphological traits and functions. During their controlled growth, cancer cells acquire phenotypic traits that allow them to adapt to in vitro conditions [83]. In addition, in unilamellar cultures, the cells are provided with easy access to nutrients and oxygen, resulting in a homogeneous genotype and phenotypic cell population [84]. It should be emphasized that tumor cells cultured under such conditions lack the complexity of a tumor structure that grows in vivo [85]. Therefore, to evaluate the effectiveness of the developed anti-cancer drug carrier, spheroids (three-dimensional cultures)—aggregates of tumor cells that are grown in vitro were used. Multicellular tumor spheroids exhibit tumor traits that occur in vivo in the early phase of their growth and are therefore considered to be an intermediate form between cells from monolayer type cultures and spontaneously growing tumors [86–88].

4. Materials and Methods

4.1. Materials

Hydrogenated soy phosphatidylcholine (HSPC), 1,2-distearoyl-sn-glycero-phospho-ethanolamine-N-[poly(ethylene glycol)2000] (DSPE-PEG2000) were from Lipoid GmbH (Ludwigshafen, Germany). Cholesterol (CHOL) and 1,2-dioleoyl-sn-glycero-3-phosphoethanolamine (DOPE) were purchased from Northern Lipids, Inc. (Vancouver, BC, Canada). Nitrophenyl carbonate-PEG-nitrophenyl carbonate, MW 3400 (pNp-PEG-pNp) was purchased from Laysan Bio, Inc. (Arab, AL, USA). Natural cashew nutshell liquid (CNSL) was from Sandor Cashew (Delhi, India). AA was extracted from natural CNSL and subsequently hydrogenated using a method described by Legut et al. [89]. Sodium dihydrogen phosphate, disodium hydrogen phosphate, sodium chloride, dimethyl sulfoxide (DMSO), hydrogen peroxide, ascorbic acid and ammonium hydroxide were purchased from POCH (Gliwice, Poland). Sephadex G-50 Fine, Sepharose CL-4B, 3-(4,5-dimethylthiazol-2-yl)-2,5-diphenyltetrazolium bromide (MTT), rhodamine B, triethylamine (TEA), molybdenum blue spray solution, Dragendorff spray reagent, ninhydrin spray solution, transferrin, pyruvate, anti-cytochrome C antibody (N-terminal), paraformaldehyde (PFA), protease inhibitor cocktails and 4-Nonylphenyl-polyethylene glycol (Nonidet™ P40) where obtained from Sigma-Aldrich (St. Louis, MO, USA). Mitoxantrone hydrochloride (MIT) was a gift from the Pharmaceutical Research Institute (Warsaw, Poland). Cell culture media (DMEM, MEMα,), antibiotic-antimycotic solution and DPBS buffer were purchased from Lonza (Basel, Switzerland). Fetal Bovine Serum (FBS) was purchased from EuroClone (Pero, Italy). Nucleopore™, filters were obtained from WHATMAN® (Maidstone, UK). Hoechst 33342, GlutaMAX, 2′, 7′ DCFH-DA (2′, 7′-dichlorodihydrofluorescein diacetate); MitoTracker® Red CMXRos were purchased from Life Technologies (Carlsbad, CA, USA). Annexin V Apoptosis Detection Kit was obtained from BD Pharmingen™ (Franklin Lakes, NJ, USA). CellTiter-Glo® Luminescent Cell Viability Assay, Caspase-Glo® 3/7 Assay, Caspase-Glo® 9 Assay and GSH-Glo™ Glutathione Assay were purchased from Promega (Madison, WI, USA). All the other reagents were of analytical grade.

4.2. Preparation and Characterization OF Liposomes

Liposomes were prepared by a lipid hydration, freeze-and-thaw (FAT) procedure and extrusion through polycarbonate filters as described before [89]. In brief chloroform stock solutions of lipids (HSPC, CHOL, DSPE-PEG2000 and AA) were prepared and appropriate volumes were then used to obtain specific molar ratios of lipids presented in Table 4.

Table 4. The table presents a full list of the formulations developed and their lipid composition along with abbreviations. The last column contains the name of the factor used to generate the transmembrane pH gradient in liposomes.

Formulation Name/Abbreviation	HSPC	AA	DSPE-PEG2000	Cholesterol	Drug/Lipid Ratio	Ion Gradient Generator
Lip MIT Vit. C	55	0	5	40	0.2	Ammonium ascorbate
Lip AA5 MIT Vit. C	55	5	5	35	0.2	Ammonium ascorbate
Lip AA10 MIT Vit. C	55	10	5	30	0.2	Ammonium ascorbate
Lip AA15 MIT Vit. C	55	15	5	25	0.2	Ammonium ascorbate
Lip AA20 MIT Vit. C	55	20	5	20	0.2	Ammonium ascorbate
Lip AA40 MIT Vit. C	55	40	5	0	0.2	Ammonium ascorbate
Lip AA5 Vit. C	55	5	5	35	0	Ammonium ascorbate
Lip AA10 Vit. C	55	10	5	30	0	Ammonium ascorbate
Lip AA15 Vit. C	55	15	5	25	0	Ammonium ascorbate
Lip AA20 Vit. C	55	20	5	20	0	Ammonium ascorbate
Lip AA40 Vit. C	55	40	5	0	0	Ammonium ascorbate
Lip AS	55	0	5	40	0	Ammonium sulfate
Lip MIT AS	55	0	5	40	0.2	Ammonium sulfate
Lip AA5 AS	55	5	5	35	0	Ammonium sulfate
Lip AA5 MIT AS	55	5	5	35	0.2	Ammonium sulfate

AA—anacardic acid.

Chloroform solutions of the lipids were mixed, and chloroform was then evaporated using a nitrogen stream. Thin lipid films were dissolved in cyclohexane and the mixture subsequently frozen in liquid nitrogen and freeze-dried overnight at low pressure using a Savant Modulyo apparatus (Savant, Waltham, MA, USA).

Thin lipid films were hydrated with 300 mM ammonium ascorbate, pH = 4.0 or 300 mM ammonium sulfate, pH 5.5. The obtained multilamellar vesicles (MLVs) were freezed and thawed (FAT) ten times, followed by extrusion 10 times through polycarbonate filters with pore size of 100 nm on Thermobarrel Extruder (PPHU Marker, Wroclaw, Poland).

The ion and/or pH gradient was subsequently generated by exchanging the extravesicular liposomal solution on Sephadex G-50 Fine (1 × 20 cm) columns as described previously [89].

Afterwards liposome size, polydispersity index (PDI) and zeta potential were determined by the dynamic light scattering, Zetasizer Nano-ZS (Malvern Instruments Ltd., Malvern, UK). Phospholipid concentration was determined by ammonium ferrothiocyanate assay [90] on the Shimadzu UV 2401

PC spectrophotometer (Shimadzu, Kyoto, Japan). Methanolic solution of liposomes was used for mitoxantrone concentration measurement at $\lambda = 667$ nm.

After the remote loading, non-encapsulated drug was separated from MIT-containing liposomes on Sephadex G-50 Fine mini-columns (5.5 × 70 mm) and the MIT in collected fractions was determined. The encapsulation efficiency (EE) was calculated according to the formula: EE [%] = ((MIT[mM])/(lipid [mM]))/(initial D/(L)), where initial D/L is the drug-to-lipid ratio when drug was mixed with liposomes. The morphology of liposomes was determined by using a TESLA BS 540 transmission electron microscope. A drop of liposomes was placed on a copper grid and dried at room temperature. This step was followed by staining with 2% uranyl acetate and dried at room temperature.

4.3. Targeting of the Liposomes

4.3.1. Synthesis of pNP-PEG-PE

The pNP-PEG-PE synthesis reaction was carried out at room temperature by mixing pNP-PEG-pNP dissolved in chloroform and DOPE in the ratio of 4.8:1 as described [91]. The progress of the reaction was monitored by TLC chromatography. Dragendorff reagent was used to visualize PEG, molybdenum blue to visualize phosphate groups and ninhydrin to visualize primary amino groups. After completion of the reaction, the solvent was evaporated. The next step purified the product by gel filtration (Sepharsose CL-4B (2.5 × 50 cm). To identify the fractions containing the product, thin layer chromatography and visualization identical to that used during reaction monitoring were used. The fractions containing the product were frozen and lyophilized. The resulting and purified product was used for further modifications.

4.3.2. Attachment of Protein

The pNP-PEG-PE conjugate was used for the following reaction. A thin lipid film of the conjugate was hydrated with the transferrin saline solution (4 × molar excess to pNP-PEG-PE). The spontaneous hydrolysis of *para*-nitrophenol and the attachment of amino groups from peptide to terminal PEG chains were allowed for 12 hours at 4 °C. The excess of unbound transferrin was removed by dialysis into normal saline. The reaction efficiency was then checked by measuring protein with the BCA test. To obtain a targeted formulation, Tf-PEG-PE micelles were added to pre-prepared liposomes for post-insertion of PEG with attached targeting moieties. The insertion process was for 12 hours at 37 °C with gentle agitation.

4.4. Ex Vivo Red Blood Cell Hemolysis Assay

The study was approved by the Bioethics Commission at the Lower Silesian Medical Chamber (1/PNHAB/2018). Hemolysis was determined by measurement of hemoglobin release from human erythrocyte suspensions after incubation with a methanolic solution of AA or different liposomes formulations as previously described [92].

4.5. Cell Culture and Treatment

Human melanoma cell lines A375 (kindly provided by the Laboratory of Cell Pathology, Faculty of Biotechnology, University of Wroclaw, Poland) and Hs294T (kindly provided by Institute of Immunology and Experimental Therapy, Polish Academy of Sciences, Wroclaw, Poland) was cultured in DMEM medium supplemented with 2 mM glutamine and 5 or 10% fetal bovine serum. The human skin fibroblast cell line NHDF (CC-2511, Lonza) was cultured in MEM α medium supplemented with 2 mM glutamine and 10% fetal bovine serum. All the media contained 100 U/mL penicillin, 0.1 mg/mL streptomycin and 0.25 µg/mL amphotericin B. Ninety-six-well plates coated with 1.5% agarose were used to obtain the spheroids. 12,000 cells were plated on such prepared plates and the plates were centrifuged for 15 minutes at 10 °C at 3000 rpm. The cells were cultured at 37 °C in humid atmosphere saturated with 5% CO_2.

4.6. Cell Viability

4.6.1. MTT Assay

The cell viability was determined using a MTT assay by the method described by Mosmann [18]. Briefly, 10,000 cells/well were seeded onto 96-well plates and allowed to adhere for 24 hours. After treatment with liposomes and free drug cells were incubated in a solution of MTT in culture medium (0.5 mg/mL) for 4 hours. After incubation, the solution was removed and 0.05 mL of DMSO was added to each well, and plates were shaken gently for 5 min. Absorbance was measured at 550 nm with a reference wavelength of 630 nm on a UVM 340 microplate reader (Biogenet, Jozefow, Poland). The cell viability was estimated as the percentage of the control, which was cells untreated with any agents (100%). All experiments were performed a minimum of three times in triplicate.

4.6.2. ATP Measurement

A CellTiter-Glo® kit was used to measure cell viability. Cells were plated in a 96-well white plate at 10,000 cells/well and then incubated with the liposomes for a specified time. After incubation, the medium was replaced by fresh medium (100 µL). The plate was then left for 30 minutes at room temperature. An equal volume of CellTiter Glo reagent was added and incubated for 2 minutes with shaking to lyse the cells. Luminescence measurements were made using an EG & G Berthold luminometer (Wildbad, Germany).

4.7. Determination of the Association of Targeted Liposomes with Cells

After treatment with rhodamine-labeled liposomes (rhodamine-DOPE was added to the lipids at 1% mol ratio during preparation), spheroids were harvested at specified time intervals and rinsed twice with PBS and then trypsinized to break down the spheroid structure into a single cell suspension. The cells were centrifuged and rinsed again with PBS buffer. The cells were analyzed using a BD FACS Calibur™ (BD Biosciences, San Jose, CA, USA) flow cytometer based on 10,000 counts for each population tested. The fluorescence of rhodamine labeled cells was evaluated using a standard FL-2 filter, λ = 585 nm. The BD CellQuest™Pro software (version 5.2.1, BD Biosciences®) was used to analyze and visualize the results. Single samples were represented by 10 randomly selected spheroids from a given group.

4.8. Analysis of Apoptosis

Apoptosis and necrosis of treated cells was measured using flow cytometry using a FACSCalibur instrument (BD Biosciences) with a modified version of the protocol described previously [19]. Briefly, cells (500,000 cells/well) were grown on 6-well plates. Thirty minutes before the end of incubation, hydrogen peroxide (10% v/v) was added to the cells for a positive control of apoptosis. As a positive control for necrosis, 8 µL of Triton X-100 (0.1% v/v) was added to the cells and incubated for 5 min at room temperature. After incubation, cells were harvested by trypsinization and centrifuged (2000 rpm, 5 min, room temperature) and processed according to the manufacturer protocol. The results were analyzed using CellQuest™ Pro software (BD). The results from treated cells were compared to control, untreated cells. All experiments were performed a minimum of three times in triplicate

4.9. Lactate Dehydrogenase Leakage Assay

A lactate dehydrogenase (LDH) leakage assay was used to measure hepatotoxicity. Lactate dehydrogenase activity in the culture medium was used as an indicator of the integrity of the cell membrane. The LDH assay was performed as a modification of the method described previously [20]. Briefly, cells (50,000 cells/well) were grown on 48-well plates. Cells were treated with liposomes and free drug. After the incubation, the culture medium was collected, and the cells were washed twice with PBS. Then, the cells were lysed with 100 µL of lysis buffer Nonidet P-40 consisting of 1% Triton

X-100, 150 mM NaCl and 50 mM Tris HCl (pH 8.0) with a protease inhibitor cocktail for 10 min at 4 °C. Lysates were collected and centrifuged (10,000 rpm, 10 min, 4 °C), and the supernatant was collected and stored at 4°C. The activities of LDH in the medium (LDH_{out}) and in the cells (LDH_{in}) were measured according to the manufacturer's instructions (Biosystems Reagents & Instruments, Quezon City, Philippines). The enzyme activity was measured at 37 °C via quantification of NADH (1.55 mM) consumption using spectrophotometry (at λ = 340 nm) with pyruvate (2.75 mM) as the substrate in 100 mM Tris-HCl buffer (pH 7.2). The absorption was read directly (T_0) and after 3 min (T_3) using a UV-2401PC spectrophotometer (Shimadzu, Kyoto, Japan). The cytotoxicity = $LDH_{out}/(LDH_{out} + LDH_{in})$ expressed as a percentage of the control, untreated cells. All experiments were performed a minimum of three time in triplicate.

4.10. Measurement of Intracellular Reactive Oxygen Species

Fluorescence spectrophotometry was used to measure the intracellular levels of ROS with 2′,7′-dichlorodihydrofluorescein diacetate (H_2DCFDA) as the probe. The measurements were conducted by modifying the manufacturer protocol. Briefly 10,000 melanoma cells and control cells were grown in 96-well black plates and treated with liposomes at selected time intervals (at 1 to 24 hours). The cells were treated as described in the MTT assay. Ammonium iron (II) sulfate (Mohr's salt, 50 mM) was added to the cells as a positive control. After incubation, the culture medium was removed, cells were washed twice in PBS, and 100 µL of probe (10 µM in DPBS) was added to each well and incubated for 30 min at 37 °C in the dark. After incubation, the probe was removed, and the cells were washed twice in PBS. Then 200 µL of DPBS was added to each well and the intensity of fluorescence was read immediately on a Varian Cary Eclipse Fluorescence Spectrophotometer (Varian Ltd., Victoria, Australia) at λ = 498 nm for excitation and at λ = 525 nm for emission. Results were expressed as a percentage of arbitrary units of fluorescence compared to the control level, which was the cells untreated with any agents. All experiments were performed a minimum of three times, in triplicate.

4.11. Caspase 9 and 3/7 Assays

Harvested cells were seeded on white 96-well microplates with 10, 000 cells/well and allowed to adhere overnight and then treated with liposomes. After treatment, plates containing cells were removed from the incubator and allowed to equilibrate to room temperature. Caspase-Glo® 9 Reagent or Caspase-Glo® 3/7 Reagent was added to each well containing 100 µl of blank, negative control cells or treated cells in culture medium. Contents of plates were gently mixed using a plate shaker at 300–500 rpm for 2 minutes and incubated at room temperature for 30 minutes. Chemiluminescence measurement was done with an EG&G Berthold luminometer. The results are expressed as the percentage with respect to the control (stained cells).

4.12. Cytochrome C Staining

Harvested cells were seeded on cover glasses (50,000 cells), allowed to adhere overnight before treatment with liposomes. After treatment, cells were washed with PBS and then fixed and permeabilized. Primary anti-cytochrome C antibodies, secondary antibodies (FITC), Hoechst dye and MitoTracker® Red CMXRos dye were used for staining. Cells were incubated with primary antibodies (1: 100 dilution) for 12 hours at 4 °C, followed by incubation with secondary antibodies (1: 200 dilution) for two hours at room temperature. Incubation with MitoTracker Red® (250 nM) dye lasted 20 minutes at room temperature. For visualization Zeiss LSM 880 Airyscan confocal microscope (Zeiss, Jena, Germany) was used.

4.13. Statistical Analysis

Results were presented as mean values and standard deviations. Statistical significance analysis of data differences was performed using the GraphPad Prism software (software version 7.0 VA, GraphPad Software, San Diego, CA, USA). The IC_{50} value was also determined using that software.

Combination index values (CI) were calculated using CompuSyn software version 1.0 (freeware, The ComboSyn, Inc., Paramus, NJ, USA).

5. Conclusions

Here, we have prepared transferrin targeted liposomal formulations for co-delivery of mitoxantrone, anacardic acid and ammonium ascorbate to melanoma cells. We have demonstrated that one of developed liposomal formulations enhanced the level of apoptosis and cell death in melanoma cell lines but not in normal cells. The proposed mechanism of the cytotoxic action of liposomes involves specific generation of the free radicals by an iron ions mechanism and the induction of the apoptotic pathway in the melanoma cells. In summary we have successfully prepared a peptide-modified co-delivery system for chemotherapeutics and natural bioactive substances with an enhanced active tumor-targeting effect and therapeutic efficacy.

Author Contributions: Conceptualization, N.F., C.S. and J.G.; Methodology, N.F., A.J., A.P., M.M. and C.S.; Formal analysis, N.F., A.P. and M.M.; Investigation, N.F.; Resources, J.G. and V.T.; Writing—original draft preparation, N.F.; Writing—review and editing, A.J. and J.G.; Visualization, N.F., A.J. and J.G.; Supervision, J.G. and V.T.; Project administration, J.G.; Funding acquisition, J.G.

Funding: This study was supported by the National Science Center Foundation (grant number 2015/16/T/NZ3/00383; ETIUDA) and by a statutory activity of subsidy from the Polish Ministry of Science and Higher Education for the Faculty of Biotechnology of University of Wroclaw.

Acknowledgments: The authors thank William C. Hartner for helpful comments and English usage during the preparation of the manuscript.

Conflicts of Interest: The authors declare no conflict of interest.

References

1. Haass, N.K.; Smalley, K.S.M.; Herlyn, M. The role of altered cell-cell communication in melanoma progression. *J. Mol. Histol.* **2004**, *35*, 309–318. [CrossRef]
2. Pleshkan, V.V.; Zinov'eva, M.V.; Sverdlov, E.D. Melanoma: Surface markers as the first point of targeted delivery of therapeutic genes in multilevel gene therapy. *Mol. Biol.* **2011**, *45*, 416–433. [CrossRef]
3. Vultur, A.; Herlyn, M. SnapShot: Melanoma. *Cancer Cell* **2013**, *23*, 706. [CrossRef] [PubMed]
4. Eggermont, A.M.M.; Kirkwood, J.M. Re-evaluating the role of dacarbazine in metastatic melanoma: What have we learned in 30 years? *Eur. J. Cancer* **2004**, *40*, 1825–1836. [CrossRef] [PubMed]
5. Frinton, E.; Tong, D.; Tan, J.; Read, G.; Kumar, V.; Kennedy, S.; Lim, C.; Board, R.E. Metastatic melanoma: Prognostic factors and survival in patients with brain metastases. *J. Neurooncol.* **2017**, *135*, 507–512. [CrossRef]
6. Dickson, P.V.; Gershenwald, J.E. Staging and prognosis of cutaneous melanoma. *Surg. Oncol. Clin.* **2011**, *20*, 1–17. [CrossRef]
7. Grosso, J.F.; Jure-Kunkel, M.N. CTLA-4 blockade in tumor models: An overview of preclinical and translational research. *Cancer Immun. Arch.* **2013**, *13*, 5.
8. Mishra, H.; Mishra, P.K.; Ekielski, A.; Jaggi, M.; Iqbal, Z.; Talegaonkar, S. Melanoma treatment: From conventional to nanotechnology. *J. Cancer Res. Clin. Oncol.* **2018**, *144*, 2283–2302. [CrossRef]
9. Seremet, T.; Jansen, Y.; Planken, S.; Njimi, H.; Delaunoy, M.; El Housni, H.; Awada, G.; Schwarze, J.K.; Keyaerts, M.; Everaert, H.; et al. Undetectable circulating tumor DNA (ctDNA) levels correlate with favorable outcome in metastatic melanoma patients treated with anti-PD1 therapy. *J. Transl. Med.* **2019**, *17*, 303. [CrossRef]
10. Bhatia, S.; Thompson, J.A. PD-1 Blockade in Melanoma: A Promising Start, but a Long Way to Go. *JAMA* **2016**, *315*, 1573–1575. [CrossRef]
11. Brück, T.B.; Brück, D.W. Oxidative metabolism of the anti-cancer agent mitoxantrone by horseradish, lacto-and lignin peroxidase. *Biochimie* **2011**, *93*, 217–226. [CrossRef] [PubMed]
12. Seiter, K. Toxicity of the topoisomerase II inhibitors. *Expert Opin. Drug Saf.* **2005**, *4*, 219–234. [CrossRef] [PubMed]
13. Neuhaus, O.; Kieseier, B.C.; Hartung, H.-P. Therapeutic role of mitoxantrone in multiple sclerosis. *Pharmacol. Ther.* **2006**, *109*, 198–209. [CrossRef] [PubMed]

14. Seifrtová, M.; Havelek, R.; Chmelařová, M.; Cmielová, J.; Muthná, D.; Stoklasová, A.; Zemánková, S.; Rezáčová, M. The effect of ATM and ERK1/2 inhibition on mitoxantrone-induced cell death of leukaemic cells. *Folia Biol. (Praha)* **2011**, *57*, 74–81.
15. Fan, J.-T.; Kuang, B.; Zeng, G.-Z.; Zhao, S.-M.; Ji, C.-J.; Zhang, Y.-M.; Tan, N.-H. Biologically active arborinane-type triterpenoids and anthraquinones from Rubia yunnanensis. *J. Nat. Prod.* **2011**, *74*, 2069–2080. [CrossRef]
16. Wang, J.; Gao, R.; Li, Q.; Xie, S.; Zhao, J.; Wang, C. Synthesis, cytotoxicity, and cell death profile of polyaminoanthraquinones as antitumor agents. *Chem. Biol. Drug Des.* **2012**, *80*, 909–917. [CrossRef]
17. Khan, S.N.; Lal, S.K.; Kumar, P.; Khan, A.U. Effect of mitoxantrone on proliferation dynamics and cell-cycle progression. *Biosci. Rep.* **2010**, *30*, 375–381. [CrossRef]
18. Avasarala, J.R.; Cross, A.H.; Clifford, D.B.; Singer, B.A.; Siegel, B.A.; Abbey, E.E. Rapid onset mitoxantrone-induced cardiotoxicity in secondary progressive multiple sclerosis. *Mult. Scler.* **2003**, *9*, 59–62. [CrossRef]
19. Rossato, L.G.; Costa, V.M.; de Pinho, P.G.; Arbo, M.D.; de Freitas, V.; Vilain, L.; de Lourdes Bastos, M.; Palmeira, C.; Remião, F. The metabolic profile of mitoxantrone and its relation with mitoxantrone-induced cardiotoxicity. *Arch. Toxicol.* **2013**, *87*, 1809–1820. [CrossRef]
20. Krishnaja, A.P.; Sharma, N.K. Ascorbic acid potentiates mitomycin C-induced micronuclei and sister chromatid exchanges in human peripheral blood lymphocytes in vitro. *Teratog. Carcinog. Mutagen.* **2003**, *23*, 99–112. [CrossRef]
21. Kurbacher, C.M.; Wagner, U.; Kolster, B.; Andreotti, P.E.; Krebs, D.; Bruckner, H.W. Ascorbic acid (vitamin C) improves the antineoplastic activity of doxorubicin, cisplatin, and paclitaxel in human breast carcinoma cells in vitro. *Cancer Lett.* **1996**, *103*, 183–189. [CrossRef]
22. Sorice, A.; Guerriero, E.; Capone, F.; Colonna, G.; Castello, G.; Costantini, S. Ascorbic acid: Its role in immune system and chronic inflammation diseases. *Mini Rev. Med. Chem.* **2014**, *14*, 444–452. [CrossRef] [PubMed]
23. Heaney, M.L.; Gardner, J.R.; Karasavvas, N.; Golde, D.W.; Scheinberg, D.A.; Smith, E.A.; O'Connor, O.A. Vitamin C antagonizes the cytotoxic effects of antineoplastic drugs. *Cancer Res.* **2008**, *68*, 8031–8038. [CrossRef] [PubMed]
24. Verrax, J.; Calderon, P.B. The controversial place of vitamin C in cancer treatment. *Biochem. Pharmacol.* **2008**, *76*, 1644–1652. [CrossRef]
25. Yun, J.; Mullarky, E.; Lu, C.; Bosch, K.N.; Kavalier, A.; Rivera, K.; Roper, J.; Chio, I.I.C.; Giannopoulou, E.G.; Rago, C.; et al. Vitamin C selectively kills KRAS and BRAF mutant colorectal cancer cells by targeting GAPDH. *Science* **2015**, *350*, 1391–1396. [CrossRef]
26. Mamede, A.C.; Tavares, S.D.; Abrantes, A.M.; Trindade, J.; Maia, J.M.; Botelho, M.F. The role of vitamins in cancer: A review. *Nutr. Cancer* **2011**, *63*, 479–494. [CrossRef]
27. Sirivech, S.; Frieden, E.; Osaki, S. The release of iron from horse spleen ferritin by reduced flavins. *Biochem. J.* **1974**, *143*, 311–315. [CrossRef]
28. Eliot, H.; Gianni, L.; Myers, C. Oxidative destruction of DNA by the adriamycin-iron complex. *Biochemistry* **1984**, *23*, 928–936. [CrossRef]
29. Muindi, J.R.; Sinha, B.K.; Gianni, L.; Myers, C.E. Hydroxyl radical production and DNA damage induced by anthracycline-iron complex. *FEBS Lett.* **1984**, *172*, 226–230. [CrossRef]
30. Zweier, J.L. Reduction of O_2 by iron-adriamycin. *J. Biol. Chem.* **1984**, *259*, 6056–6058.
31. Du, J.; Cullen, J.J.; Buettner, G.R. Ascorbic acid: Chemistry, biology and the treatment of cancer. *Biochim. Biophys. Acta* **2012**, *1826*, 443–457. [CrossRef]
32. Balasubramanyam, K.; Swaminathan, V.; Ranganathan, A.; Kundu, T.K. Small molecule modulators of histone acetyltransferase p300. *J. Biol. Chem.* **2003**, *278*, 19134–19140. [CrossRef]
33. Sung, B.; Pandey, M.K.; Ahn, K.S.; Yi, T.; Chaturvedi, M.M.; Liu, M.; Aggarwal, B.B. Anacardic acid (6-nonadecyl salicylic acid), an inhibitor of histone acetyltransferase, suppresses expression of nuclear factor-kappaB-regulated gene products involved in cell survival, proliferation, invasion, and inflammation through inhibition of the inhibitory subunit of nuclear factor-kappaBalpha kinase, leading to potentiation of apoptosis. *Blood* **2008**, *111*, 4880–4891. [CrossRef] [PubMed]
34. Wu, Y.; He, L.; Zhang, L.; Chen, J.; Yi, Z.; Zhang, J.; Liu, M.; Pang, X. Anacardic acid (6-pentadecylsalicylic acid) inhibits tumor angiogenesis by targeting Src/FAK/Rho GTPases signaling pathway. *J. Pharmacol. Exp. Ther.* **2011**, *339*, 403–411. [CrossRef] [PubMed]

35. Tamura, S.; Nitoda, T.; Kubo, I. Effects of salicylic acid on mushroom tyrosinase and B16 melanoma cells. *Z. Naturforsch. C J. Biosci.* **2007**, *62*, 227–233. [CrossRef]
36. Park, W.J.; Ma, E. Inhibition of PCAF histone acetyltransferase, cytotoxicity and cell permeability of 2-acylamino-1-(3-or 4-carboxy-phenyl)benzamides. *Molecules* **2012**, *17*, 13116–13131. [CrossRef]
37. Schultz, D.J.; Wickramasinghe, N.S.; Ivanova, M.M.; Isaacs, S.M.; Dougherty, S.M.; Imbert-Fernandez, Y.; Cunningham, A.R.; Chen, C.; Klinge, C.M. Anacardic acid inhibits estrogen receptor alpha-DNA binding and reduces target gene transcription and breast cancer cell proliferation. *Mol. Cancer Ther.* **2010**, *9*, 594–605. [CrossRef]
38. Tan, J.; Chen, B.; He, L.; Tang, Y.; Jiang, Z.; Yin, G.; Wang, J.; Jiang, X. Anacardic acid (6-pentadecylsalicylic acid) induces apoptosis of prostate cancer cells through inhibition of androgen receptor and activation of p53 signaling. *Chin. J. Cancer Res.* **2012**, *24*, 275–283. [CrossRef]
39. Hsieh, C.-C.; Hernández-Ledesma, B.; de Lumen, B.O. Cell proliferation inhibitory and apoptosis-inducing properties of anacardic acid and lunasin in human breast cancer MDA-MB-231 cells. *Food Chem.* **2011**, *125*, 630–636. [CrossRef]
40. Ambudkar, S.V.; Dey, S.; Hrycyna, C.A.; Ramachandra, M.; Pastan, I.; Gottesman, M.M. Biochemical, cellular, and pharmacological aspects of the multidrug transporter. *Annu. Rev. Pharmacol. Toxicol.* **1999**, *39*, 361–398. [CrossRef]
41. Ueda, K. ABC proteins protect the human body and maintain optimal health. *Biosci. Biotechnol. Biochem.* **2011**, *75*, 401–409. [CrossRef] [PubMed]
42. Nabekura, T.; Hiroi, T.; Kawasaki, T.; Uwai, Y. Effects of natural nuclear factor-kappa B inhibitors on anticancer drug efflux transporter human P-glycoprotein. *Biomed. Pharmacother.* **2015**, *70*, 140–145. [CrossRef] [PubMed]
43. Padayatty, S.J.; Katz, A.; Wang, Y.; Eck, P.; Kwon, O.; Lee, J.-H.; Chen, S.; Corpe, C.; Dutta, A.; Dutta, S.K.; et al. Vitamin C as an antioxidant: Evaluation of its role in disease prevention. *J. Am. Coll. Nutr.* **2003**, *22*, 18–35. [CrossRef] [PubMed]
44. Re, A.; Nanni, S.; Aiello, A.; Granata, S.; Colussi, C.; Campostrini, G.; Spallotta, F.; Mattiussi, S.; Pantisano, V.; D'Angelo, C.; et al. Anacardic acid and thyroid hormone enhance cardiomyocytes production from undifferentiated mouse ES cells along functionally distinct pathways. *Endocrine* **2016**, *53*, 681–688. [CrossRef] [PubMed]
45. Seong, Y.-A.; Shin, P.-G.; Kim, G.-D. Anacardic acid induces mitochondrial-mediated apoptosis in the A549 human lung adenocarcinoma cells. *Int. J. Oncol.* **2013**, *42*, 1045–1051. [CrossRef] [PubMed]
46. Sun, Y.; Jiang, X.; Chen, S.; Fernandes, N.; Price, B.D. A role for the Tip60 histone acetyltransferase in the acetylation and activation of ATM. *Proc. Natl. Acad. Sci. USA* **2005**, *102*, 13182–13187. [CrossRef] [PubMed]
47. Jiang, Z.; Kamath, R.; Jin, S.; Balasubramani, M.; Pandita, T.K.; Rajasekaran, B. Tip60-mediated acetylation activates transcription independent apoptotic activity of Abl. *Mol. Cancer* **2011**, *10*, 88. [CrossRef]
48. Sun, Y.; Jiang, X.; Chen, S.; Price, B.D. Inhibition of histone acetyltransferase activity by anacardic acid sensitizes tumor cells to ionizing radiation. *FEBS Lett.* **2006**, *580*, 4353–4356. [CrossRef]
49. Ashino, H.; Shimamura, M.; Nakajima, H.; Dombou, M.; Kawanaka, S.; Oikawa, T.; Iwaguchi, T.; Kawashima, S. Novel function of ascorbic acid as an angiostatic factor. *Angiogenesis* **2003**, *6*, 259–269. [CrossRef]
50. Lee, S.K.; Kang, J.S.; Jung, D.J.; Hur, D.Y.; Kim, J.E.; Hahm, E.; Bae, S.; Kim, H.W.; Kim, D.; Cho, B.J.; et al. Vitamin C suppresses proliferation of the human melanoma cell SK-MEL-2 through the inhibition of cyclooxygenase-2 (COX-2) expression and the modulation of insulin-like growth factor II (IGF-II) production. *J. Cell Physiol.* **2008**, *216*, 180–188. [CrossRef]
51. Lin, S.-Y.; Lai, W.-W.; Chou, C.-C.; Kuo, H.-M.; Li, T.-M.; Chung, J.-G.; Yang, J.-H. Sodium ascorbate inhibits growth via the induction of cell cycle arrest and apoptosis in human malignant melanoma A375.S2 cells. *Melanoma Res.* **2006**, *16*, 509–519. [CrossRef] [PubMed]
52. Türkez, H.; Aydin, E. The protective role of ascorbic acid on imazalil-induced genetic damage assessed by the cytogenetic tests. *Toxicol. Ind. Health* **2012**, *28*, 648–654. [CrossRef] [PubMed]
53. Eguchi, M.; Miyazaki, T.; Masatsuji-Kato, E.; Tsuzuki, T.; Oribe, T.; Miwa, N. Cytoprotection against ischemia-induced DNA cleavages and cell injuries in the rat liver by pro-vitamin C via hydrolytic conversion into ascorbate. *Mol. Cell. Biochem.* **2003**, *252*, 17–23. [CrossRef] [PubMed]
54. Duarte, T.L.; Cooke, M.S.; Jones, G.D.D. Gene expression profiling reveals new protective roles for vitamin C in human skin cells. *Free Radic. Biol. Med.* **2009**, *46*, 78–87. [CrossRef] [PubMed]

55. Hata, K.; Urushibara, A.; Yamashita, S.; Shikazono, N.; Yokoya, A.; Katsumura, Y. Chemical repair of base lesions, AP-sites, and strand breaks on plasmid DNA in dilute aqueous solution by ascorbic acid. *Biochem. Biophys. Res. Commun.* **2013**, *434*, 341–345. [CrossRef]
56. Stasiuk, M.; Kozubek, A. Membrane perturbing properties of natural phenolic and resorcinolic lipids. *FEBS Lett.* **2008**, *582*, 3607–3613. [CrossRef]
57. Jaromin, A.; Zarnowski, R.; Kozubek, A. Emulsions of oil from Adenanthera pavonina L. seeds and their protective effect. *Cell Mol. Biol. Lett.* **2006**, *11*, 438–448. [CrossRef]
58. Jaromin, A.; Kozubek, A.; Suchoszek-Lukaniuk, K.; Malicka-Blaszkiewicz, M.; Peczynska-Czoch, W.; Kaczmarek, L. Liposomal formulation of DIMIQ, potential antitumor indolo[2,3-b]quinoline agent and its cytotoxicity on hepatoma Morris 5123 cells. *Drug Deliv.* **2008**, *15*, 49–56. [CrossRef]
59. Luo, X.; Budihardjo, I.; Zou, H.; Slaughter, C.; Wang, X. Bid, a Bcl2 interacting protein, mediates cytochrome c release from mitochondria in response to activation of cell surface death receptors. *Cell* **1998**, *94*, 481–490. [CrossRef]
60. Borner, C. The Bcl-2 protein family: Sensors and checkpoints for life-or-death decisions. *Mol. Immunol.* **2003**, *39*, 615–647. [CrossRef]
61. Allen, T.M. Long-circulating (sterically stabilized) liposomes for targeted drug delivery. *Trends Pharmacol. Sci.* **1994**, *15*, 215–220. [CrossRef]
62. Regev, R.; Yeheskely-Hayon, D.; Katzir, H.; Eytan, G.D. Transport of anthracyclines and mitoxantrone across membranes by a flip-flop mechanism. *Biochem. Pharmacol.* **2005**, *70*, 161–169. [CrossRef] [PubMed]
63. Mayer, L.D.; Cullis, P.R.; Bally, M.B. The Use of Transmembrane pH Gradient-Driven Drug Encapsulation in the Pharmacodynamic Evaluation of Liposomal Doxorubicin. *J. Liposome Res.* **1994**, *4*, 529–553. [CrossRef]
64. Reszka, R.; Beck, P.; Fichtner, I.; Hentschel, M.; Richter, J.; Kreuter, J. Body distribution of free, liposomal and nanoparticle-associated mitoxantrone in B16-melanoma-bearing mice. *J. Pharmacol. Exp. Ther.* **1997**, *280*, 232–237. [PubMed]
65. Bellosillo, B.; Villamor, N.; López-Guillermo, A.; Marcé, S.; Bosch, F.; Campo, E.; Montserrat, E.; Colomer, D. Spontaneous and drug-induced apoptosis is mediated by conformational changes of Bax and Bak in B-cell chronic lymphocytic leukemia. *Blood* **2002**, *100*, 1810–1816. [CrossRef]
66. Blagosklonny, M.V. Targeting cancer cells by exploiting their resistance. *Trends Mol. Med.* **2003**, *9*, 307–312. [CrossRef]
67. Weinberg, E.D. Iron and neoplasia. *Biol. Trace Elem. Res.* **1981**, *3*, 55–80. [CrossRef]
68. Daniels, T.R.; Delgado, T.; Helguera, G.; Penichet, M.L. The transferrin receptor part II: Targeted delivery of therapeutic agents into cancer cells. *Clin. Immunol.* **2006**, *121*, 159–176. [CrossRef]
69. O'Donnell, J.L.; Joyce, M.R.; Shannon, A.M.; Harmey, J.; Geraghty, J.; Bouchier-Hayes, D. Oncological implications of hypoxia inducible factor-1alpha (HIF-1alpha) expression. *Cancer Treat. Rev.* **2006**, *32*, 407–416. [CrossRef]
70. Qing, Y.; Shuo, W.; Zhihua, W.; Huifen, Z.; Ping, L.; Lijiang, L.; Xiaorong, Z.; Liming, C.; Daiwen, X.; Yu, H.; et al. The in vitro antitumor effect and in vivo tumor-specificity distribution of human-mouse chimeric antibody against transferrin receptor. *Cancer Immunol. Immunother.* **2006**, *55*, 1111–1121. [CrossRef]
71. Elliott, R.L.; Stjernholm, R.; Elliott, M.C. Preliminary evaluation of platinum transferrin (MPTC-63) as a potential nontoxic treatment for breast cancer. *Cancer Detect. Prev.* **1988**, *12*, 469–480. [PubMed]
72. Beyer, U.; Roth, T.; Schumacher, P.; Maier, G.; Unold, A.; Frahm, A.W.; Fiebig, H.H.; Unger, C.; Kratz, F. Synthesis and in vitro efficacy of transferrin conjugates of the anticancer drug chlorambucil. *J. Med. Chem.* **1998**, *41*, 2701–2708. [CrossRef] [PubMed]
73. Tanaka, T.; Shiramoto, S.; Miyashita, M.; Fujishima, Y.; Kaneo, Y. Tumor targeting based on the effect of enhanced permeability and retention (EPR) and the mechanism of receptor-mediated endocytosis (RME). *Int. J. Pharm.* **2004**, *277*, 39–61. [CrossRef] [PubMed]
74. Raso, V.; Basala, M. A highly cytotoxic human transferrin-ricin A chain conjugate used to select receptor-modified cells. *J. Biol. Chem.* **1984**, *259*, 1143–1149.
75. O'Keefe, D.O.; Draper, R.K. Characterization of a transferrin-diphtheria toxin conjugate. *J. Biol. Chem.* **1985**, *260*, 932–937.
76. Nakase, I.; Lai, H.; Singh, N.P.; Sasaki, T. Anticancer properties of artemisinin derivatives and their targeted delivery by transferrin conjugation. *Int. J. Pharm.* **2008**, *354*, 28–33. [CrossRef]

77. Ward, C.M.; Read, M.L.; Seymour, L.W. Systemic circulation of poly(L-lysine)/DNA vectors is influenced by polycation molecular weight and type of DNA: Differential circulation in mice and rats and the implications for human gene therapy. *Blood* **2001**, *97*, 2221–2229. [CrossRef]
78. Tang, M.X.; Szoka, F.C. The influence of polymer structure on the interactions of cationic polymers with DNA and morphology of the resulting complexes. *Gene Ther.* **1997**, *4*, 823–832. [CrossRef]
79. White, S.; Taetle, R.; Seligman, P.A.; Rutherford, M.; Trowbridge, I.S. Combinations of anti-transferrin receptor monoclonal antibodies inhibit human tumor cell growth in vitro and in vivo: Evidence for synergistic antiproliferative effects. *Cancer Res.* **1990**, *50*, 6295–6301.
80. Nagasawa, H.; Uto, Y.; Kirk, K.L.; Hori, H. Design of hypoxia-targeting drugs as new cancer chemotherapeutics. *Biol. Pharm. Bull.* **2006**, *29*, 2335–2342. [CrossRef]
81. Ang, S.O.; Chen, H.; Hirota, K.; Gordeuk, V.R.; Jelinek, J.; Guan, Y.; Liu, E.; Sergueeva, A.I.; Miasnikova, G.Y.; Mole, D.; et al. Disruption of oxygen homeostasis underlies congenital Chuvash polycythemia. *Nat. Genet.* **2002**, *32*, 614–621. [CrossRef] [PubMed]
82. Tao, J.; Liu, Y.; Li, Y.; Peng, J.; Li, L.; Liu, J.; Shen, X.; Shen, G.; Tu, Y. Hypoxia: Dual effect on the expression of transferrin receptor in human melanoma A375 cell line. *Exp. Dermatol.* **2007**, *16*, 899–904. [CrossRef] [PubMed]
83. Pinho, S.S.; Carvalho, S.; Cabral, J.; Reis, C.A.; Gärtner, F. Canine tumors: A spontaneous animal model of human carcinogenesis. *Transl. Res.* **2012**, *159*, 165–172. [CrossRef] [PubMed]
84. Zhang, X.; Wang, W.; Yu, W.; Xie, Y.; Zhang, X.; Zhang, Y.; Ma, X. Development of an in vitro multicellular tumor spheroid model using microencapsulation and its application in anticancer drug screening and testing. *Biotechnol. Prog.* **2005**, *21*, 1289–1296. [CrossRef] [PubMed]
85. Becher, O.J.; Holland, E.C. Genetically engineered models have advantages over xenografts for preclinical studies. *Cancer Res.* **2006**, *66*, 3355–3359. [CrossRef] [PubMed]
86. Madsen, S.J.; Sun, C.-H.; Tromberg, B.J.; Cristini, V.; De Magalhães, N.; Hirschberg, H. Multicell tumor spheroids in photodynamic therapy. *Lasers Surg. Med.* **2006**, *38*, 555–564. [CrossRef]
87. Santini, M.T.; Rainaldi, G.; Indovina, P.L. Apoptosis, cell adhesion and the extracellular matrix in the three-dimensional growth of multicellular tumor spheroids. *Crit. Rev. Oncol. Hematol.* **2000**, *36*, 75–87. [CrossRef]
88. Anada, T.; Masuda, T.; Honda, Y.; Fukuda, J.; Arai, F.; Fukuda, T.; Suzuki, O. Three-dimensional cell culture device utilizing thin membrane deformation by decompression. *Sens. Actuators B Chem.* **2010**, *147*, 376–379. [CrossRef]
89. Legut, M.; Lipka, D.; Filipczak, N.; Piwoni, A.; Kozubek, A.; Gubernator, J. Anacardic acid enhances the anticancer activity of liposomal mitoxantrone towards melanoma cell lines-in vitro studies. *Int. J. Nanomed.* **2014**, *9*, 653–668. [CrossRef]
90. Stewart, J.C. Colorimetric determination of phospholipids with ammonium ferrothiocyanate. *Anal. Biochem.* **1980**, *104*, 10–14. [CrossRef]
91. Biswas, S.; Deshpande, P.P.; Navarro, G.; Dodwadkar, N.S.; Torchilin, V.P. Lipid modified triblock PAMAM-based nanocarriers for siRNA drug co-delivery. *Biomaterials* **2013**, *34*, 1289–1301. [CrossRef] [PubMed]
92. Jaromin, A.; Korycińska, M.; Piętka-Ottlik, M.; Musiał, W.; Peczyńska-Czoch, W.; Kaczmarek, Ł.; Kozubek, A. Membrane perturbations induced by new analogs of neocryptolepine. *Biol. Pharm. Bull.* **2012**, *35*, 1432–1439. [CrossRef] [PubMed]

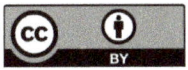

© 2019 by the authors. Licensee MDPI, Basel, Switzerland. This article is an open access article distributed under the terms and conditions of the Creative Commons Attribution (CC BY) license (http://creativecommons.org/licenses/by/4.0/).

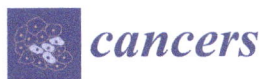

Article

Mangiferin-Loaded Polymeric Nanoparticles: Optical Characterization, Effect of Anti-topoisomerase I, and Cytotoxicity

Francisco Fabian Razura-Carmona [1], Alejandro Pérez-Larios [2,*], Napoleón González-Silva [2], Mayra Herrera-Martínez [3], Luis Medina-Torres [4], Sonia Guadalupe Sáyago-Ayerdi [1] and Jorge Alberto Sánchez-Burgos [1,*]

1. Tecnológico Nacional de México/I.T. Tepic, Laboratorio Integran de Investigación en Alimentos, Lagos del Country, Tepic CP 63175, Nayarit, Mexico; fabianrazura@gmail.com (F.F.R.-C.); sonia.sayago@gmail.com (S.G.S.-A.)
2. Division of Agricultural Sciences and Engineering, University Center of the Altos, University of Guadalajara, Tepatitlán de Morelos CP 47620, Jalisco, Mexico; napoleon.gonzalez@cualtos.udg.mx
3. Instituto de Farmacobiología, Universidad de la Cañada, Teotitlán de Flores Magón CP 68540, Oaxaca, Mexico; chimay_2002@hotmail.com
4. Facultad de Química, Universidad Nacional Autónoma de México, México D.F. CP 04510, Mexico; luismt@unam.mx

* Correspondence: alex.perez.larios@gmail.com (A.P.-L.); jorgealberto_sanchezburgos@yahoo.com.mx (J.A.S.-B.)

Received: 29 October 2019; Accepted: 2 December 2019; Published: 6 December 2019

Abstract: Mangiferin is an important xanthone compound presenting various biological activities. The objective of this study was to develop, characterize physicochemical properties, and evaluate the anti-topoisomerase activity of poly(lactic-co-glycolic acid) (PLGA) nanoparticles containing mangiferin. The nanoparticles were developed by the emulsion solvent evaporation method and the optimal formulation was obtained with a response surface methodology (RSM); this formulation showed a mean size of 176.7 ± 1.021 nm with a 0.153 polydispersibility index (PDI) value, and mangiferin encapsulation efficiency was about 55%. The optimal conditions (6000 rpm, 10 min, and 300 µg of mangiferin) obtained 77% and the highest entrapment efficiency (97%). The in vitro release profile demonstrated a gradual release of mangiferin from 15 to 180 min in acidic conditions (pH 1.5). The fingerprint showed a modification in the maximum absorption wavelength of both the polymer and the mangiferin. Results of anti-toposiomerase assay showed that the optimal formulation (MG4, 25 µg/mL) had antiproliferative activity. High concentrations (2500 µg/mL) of MG4 showed non-in vitro cytotoxic effect on BEAS 2B and HEPG2. Finally, this study showed an encapsulation process with in vitro gastric digestion resistance (1.5 h) and without interfering with the metabolism of healthy cells and their biological activity.

Keywords: nanoparticles; mangiferin; anti-topoisomerase activity; cytotoxicity

1. Introduction

Mangiferin (2-C-β-Dglucopyranosyl-1,3,6,7-tetra-hydroxyxanthone) is a xanthone C-glucoside, present in several plants [1]. It is considered as a bioactive compound (BC) that has been studied for its biosynthetic and medicinal properties. In *Mangifera indica* L. tree stem in an aqueous extract the mangiferin is the major BC [2]. Despite the potential broad applications, some chemical problems have limited its clinical use; for instance, its low solubility and poor intestinal permeability [3]. About 40 mangiferin metabolites can be biotransformed in processes like deglycosylation, dihydroxylation, methylation, glucuronidation, glycosylation, and sulfatation [4].

These metabolites are the basis to consider that mangiferin can have multiple applications, overcoming the chemical limitations for its clinical use, considering different physicochemical strategies that improve its permeability and solubility [5–7]—since several studies indicate the power of this compounds to prevent a TNF-α and nitric oxide (NO) production [8] and down-regulating COX-2 expression [9]. However, the use of pure BC is very limited due to fast release, low solubility, poor bioavailability, as well as easy deterioration [10,11]. Therefore, to preserve the quality of a BC or to enhance its applicability in food, nutraceutical, or biological formulations, a feasible alternative has been considered, namely, nanoencapsulation. Nanoencapsulation is an important technology for the protection of bioactive compounds (BCs) [12], recently, it has focused on increasing functionalities, such as high entrapment efficiency, bioavailability, mechanical stability, controlled release, and masking undesirable flavors [13,14]. Some of the applications in the food and pharmaceutical industry seek to encapsulate BCs, with the objective of forming protective barriers that increase the specialized application in the development of nutraceuticals [15].

Generate nanoparticles (NPs) of mangiferin, a BC that has shown biological activities such as antioxidant, antihypertensive, and anti-inflammatory, will allow to increase its resistance to acidic conditions, which is related to human digestion. These NPs are encapsulated with a biocompatible polymer such as poly(lactic-co-glycolic acid) (PLGA), which can resist this process and consequently have a controlled release [13]. Thereby, the aim of this study was to develop PLGA nanoparticles containing mangiferin and to evaluate their physicochemical properties, effect cytotoxic, and the anti-topoisomerase activity.

2. Results and Discussion

2.1. Encapsulation Efficiency (EE%) and Entrapment Efficiency (AE%)

In the NP preparation, it was observed that one of the critical steps was the previous solubilization of mangiferin (MG) in polyvinyl alcohol (PVA) solution; therefore, solubility tests were performed, obtaining the maximum concentration of MG in the formulations of 435 µg/mL of PVA solution. The EE% and AE% in each treatment were obtained for each NP formulation. EE% indicates the amount of compound that is inside the NPs, and that its behavior is reflected in a gradual release with respect to time, while the AE% is the one that is in the first layers of the nanoparticles added to the surface of the particles [14].

In Figure 1a, the EE% and EA% corresponding to the MG formulations are shown. The treatment that presented the highest encapsulation efficiency was MG4 (6000 rpm, 10 min, 300 µg) and MG14 (9000 rpm, 5 min, 435 µg) with EE% of 77 ± 3.02% and 76 ± 1.09%, respectively; while those of lower EE% were MG3 (6000 rpm, 5 min, 435 µg) and MG6 (7000 rpm, 3 min, 435 µg) with EE% values of 34 ± 1.22% and 36 ± 1.80%. Regarding the EA%, only MG4 presented significant difference with respect to the other treatments, presenting an AE% of 93 ± 4.95%, while the lowest corresponding to MG2 (6000 rpm, 5 min, 200 µg).

Treatment	Speed (RPM)	Time (min)	Concentration (µg)	%EE	%AE
MG1	6000	3	300	66±2.99[b]	78±3.51[b]
MG2	6000	5	200	37±1.63[f]	53±2.76[d]
MG3	6000	5	435	34±1.22[g]	48±1.75[e]
MG4	6000	10	300	77±3.02[a]	93±4.95[a]
MG5	7000	3	200	64±1.64[c]	79±4.32[b]
MG6	7000	3	435	36±1.80	46±1.54[e]
MG7	7000	5	300	60±2.11[d]	76±1.96[b]
MG8	7000	5	300	59±2.01[d]	75±1.43[b]
MG9	7000	5	300	61±2.79[c]	77±1.65[b]
MG10	7000	10	200	65±2.33[b]	75±3.21[b]
MG11	7000	10	435	49±1.34[e]	63±4.22[c]
MG12	9000	3	300	59±1.78[d]	76±2.01[b]
MG13	9000	5	200	65±3.37[b]	77±3.29[b]
MG14	9000	5	435	76±1.09[a]	68±2.52[c]
MG15	9000	10	300	57±1.94[d]	77±2.63[b]

Data is expressed as mean media ± deviation standard. Uppercase letters indicate significant difference between treatment ($p < 0.05$)

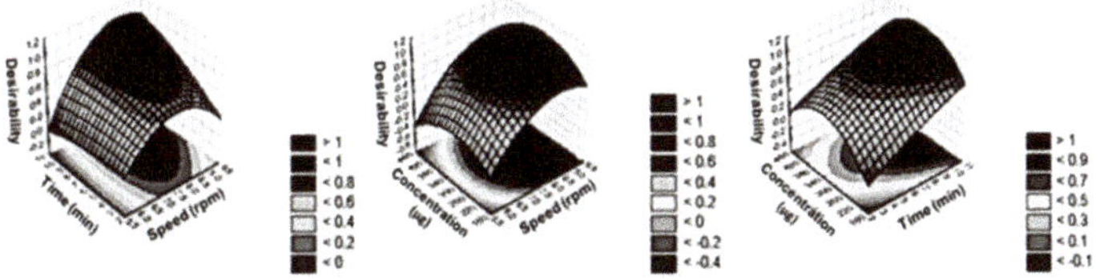

Figure 1. Optimization of mangiferin (MG) encapsulation. (**a**) Percentage of mangiferin encapsulation efficiency (EE%) and percentage of mangiferin entrapment efficiency (AE%) for each treatment. (**b**) Pareto chart of standardized effects; variable: Percentage of mangiferin encapsulation efficiency (EE%); (L) and (Q) describes the linear and quadratic interactions effects on the variable. (**c**) Desirability surface contours of percentage of mangiferin encapsulation efficiency; method: Spline.

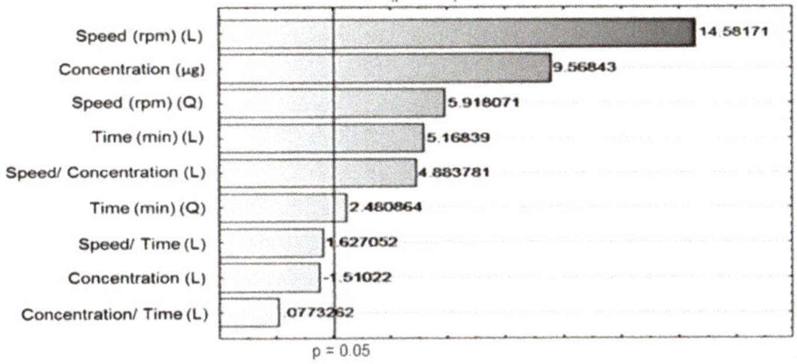

Some studies reported that different polymers have shown that the EE% of some compounds is a function of the charges present between the polymer and the compound [15–17]. The different charges between the molecules of mangiferin and PLGA promote the interactions between both, so when the mangiferin concentration increases, the EE% increases; however, some authors have described that this increase of encapsulating compounds promotes the saturation of the system, as is observed in the MG3 and MG6 treatments, which increased the concentration of mangiferin—however, the EE% was about 36% [18]. With high stirring speeds, EE% can be increased, since there is an increase in electrostatic charges but at short times [19]; this explains why MG14 presents EE% values close to the best MG4 treatment. However, low concentrations of the compound to be encapsulated are trapped on the surface of the particles, and this behavior is observed in MG13 and MG15. According to statistical analysis ($p < 0.5$), the factor that has the greatest effect on the EE% is the speed, followed by concentration ratio and the interaction between this variables, as shown in the Pareto chart (Figure 1b); MG4 showed the highest EE% with the lowest homogenization rate studied, unlike other treatments with the same concentration but at higher speeds (MG9 and MG15). Some studies have shown that the time in which the molecules are exposed to a certain speed can be decisive, so that a molecular interaction can be exerted [20]. Therefore, the treatment with the highest EE% was formulated with the following conditions: 6000 rpm, 10 min, and 300 µg of mangiferin according to the response surface obtained in the statistical analysis (Figure 1c), which is expressed in Equation (1).

$$Z = 283.56242804966 + 62.848482862581 \times x 4.3090184425532 \times x^2 2.7320158696753 \times y.36691981479872 \times y^2 + 1.1853803871635 \times x \times y + 0.012224096786592 \times 300 \times x + 0.00024480875382114 \times 300 \times y + 69.8885631 \quad (1)$$

where R-sqr = 0.90756, z describes EE%, x describes the homogenization speed, and y is the time at fixed concentration (300 µg).

An optimal condition was obtained when 317 µg of mangiferin was used in accordance to response surface, but this concentration can generate an increase in the size of the particles and in the polydispersity index. The size obtained in MG4 was 171 nm with a polydispersity index of 0.153 (Figure 2e).

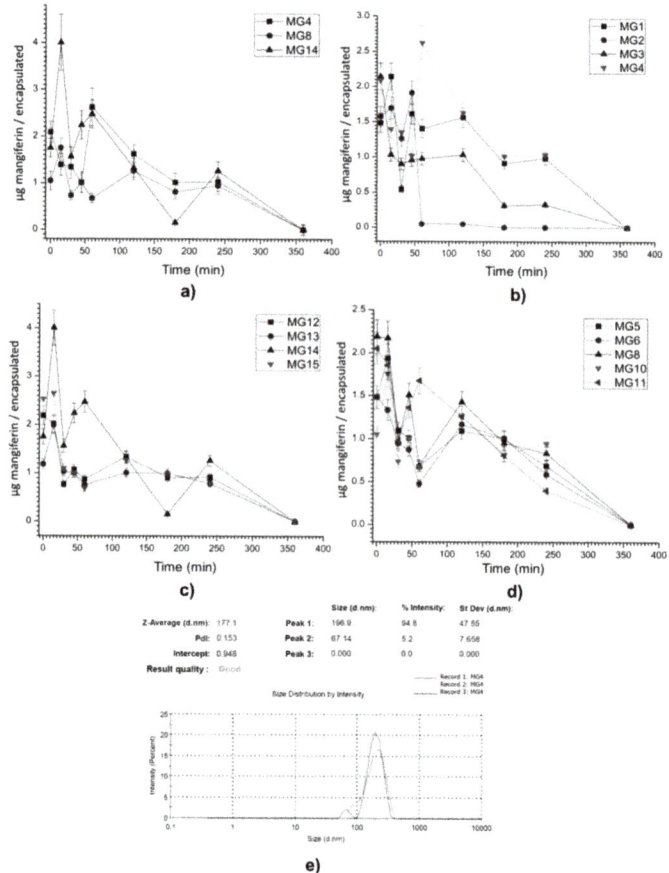

Figure 2. Mangiferin release profile and size distribution of best treatment; (**a**) best release profiles, (**b**) treatments at 6000 rpm, (**c**) treatments at 7000 rpm, and (**d**) treatments at 9000 rpm. (**e**) Size distribution on optimal condition (MG4).

2.2. Mangiferin Release Profile

The results of the kinetic release assay are described in Figure 2, where the release profiles of each encapsulated mangiferin formulation are shown (Figure 2a–d), includeing the polydispersibility index (PDI) and the average size of the resulting particle as an optimal treatment (Figure 2e). MG2 (Figure 2a) shows a rapid release, which coincides with the results of AE% for this treatment, since the highest concentration of mangiferin is found on the surface of the NPs; MG1 and MG3 (Figure 2a) show similar release profiles, since the release presents with variations without significant differences after 60 min. Figure 2c shows the treatments obtained at 7000 rpm, observing that there is no significant difference in the release after 60 min in the MG12, MG13, and MG15 treatments. Finally, in Figure 2d, it is observed that the differences between the release profiles are related to the concentrations of mangiferin used in the treatments (MG5, MG6, MG10, and MG11), observing that at long times of homogenization, EE% and EA% trend to be of the same values, which is reflected in a release of 50% before 60 min and then in three intervals (120, 180, and 240 min), with a release of 16.6% by interval.

Three fluctuations can be identified; the first occurs at 15 min, the second at 60 min, and the last after 2 h, almost in all the treatments. Nevertheless, some treatments such as MG4 (Figure 2a), MG14 (Figure 2c), and MG8 (Figure 2d) showed the highest mangiferin fluctuation after 1 h of exposure in an acid medium.

These treatments are shown in Figure 2b, which shows that MG14 presents its maximum release at 20 min and then presents a controlled release, while MG4 presents its maximum release at 60 min and subsequently shows a linear release until 180 min, without significant differences between 180 and 240 min. Studies carried out with the same phytochemical, but with a different polymer, showed a behavior like that shown in this study; this irregular behavior (ascending, descending, and ascending) was attributed mainly to the interactions between the present molecules (electrostatic interactions and hydrogen bridges) and the diffusivity of the nanoparticles [21,22]. Another result showed that when PLGA was used as an encapsulating agent, but under other encapsulation conditions, a similar diffusivity was observed [23]. During the first phase of release, agglomeration of nanoparticles occurs, and this strongly depends on the particle size, further affecting the release of the drug (amount and rate of release) from the nanoparticles.

The PLGA might have a higher tendency to agglomerate due to smaller sizes, and the release of the drug was also higher from these particles compared to other polymers. Among the factors that affect drug release, particle size is very important. We know that the particles with smaller sizes can degrade faster due to the increased surface area to volume ratio, and this might be a reason for the faster release of the mangiferin from PLGA particles in some treatments, but it is shown that at least three of the treatments (MG4, MG8, and MG14) show a controlled release in acidic conditions, maintaining the highest amount of MG and releasing it completely after 2 h of acidic exposure, which sets a pattern for the emulation of the gastrointestinal tract [24].

2.3. Scanning Electron Microscopy (SEM)

Figure 3 shows, scanning electron microscopy images of the optimal treatment (Figure 3a,b, MG4; Figure 3c, control). In the images related to MG4, agglomerations of nanoparticles can be seen, which were counted 100 particles independents, and Figure 3d shows the Pareto diagram of the size distribution of NPs. Previous studies show a similar behavior in agglomerated nanoparticles of the same polymer loaded with catechins larger than 500 nm; however, there is evidence that nanometer sizes are achieved with PLGA-loaded gold [25,26]. The results shown by SEM coincide with peak two of Figure 2e, which shows an average size of 67.14. It is possible that the dispersion of the particles is not adequate, and therefore, the distributions in that technique were greater, thus quantifying conglomerates of smaller particles.

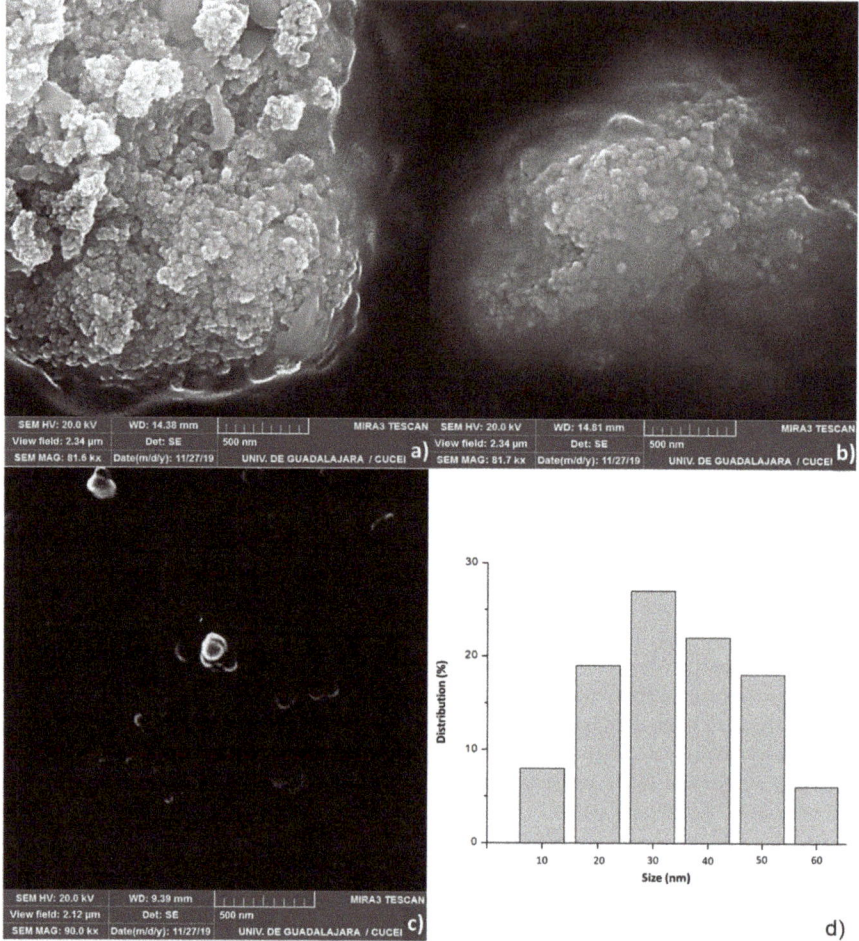

Figure 3. Scanning electron microscopy (SEM) of the mangiferin optimal nanoparticles (MG4); (**a**,**b**) images of optimal treatment; (**c**) control PLGA whitout mangiferin; (**d**) Pareto diagram of size distribution of optimal treatment.

Moreover, it has been described that the chemical structure of mangiferin creates a xanthone framework made up of four phenolic units and a glucose moiety [27]. Hence, it may be assumed that mangiferin might exhibit high affinity by PLGA and PVA forming a long structure that occurs for interaction of OH groups in the chemical composition [28]. In addition, the phenolic and glucose units present in mangiferin can efficiently stabilize the formed nanoparticle. Despite its bio-relevance and strong reducing capability, the use of mangiferin is not limited towards the preparation of nanoparticles [29].

2.4. UV-Visible Spectroscopy

The spectra obtained and reported in Figure 4 represents the optimal treatment (MG4) and only PLGA; this is related to the table that describes the same figure, in which the MG4 treatment is identified in two signals traveling to the infrared spectral region. The wavelength of greater absorption (λmax) in the PLGA-only was identified at 220 nm; this value was obtained for other authors [30]. The λmax for MG was 415 nm; according to this result, mangiferin slightly modified its orientation towards a different value UV signal. Atoms and molecules only absorb and emit radiation of certain frequencies, which implies the quantization of their energy levels. The electronic levels of a molecule are widely separated and usually only the absorption of a high energy photon can excite a molecule. UV spectroscopy studies the absorption of visible ultraviolet radiation by a molecule. By influencing UV-visible radiation of adequate energy, the molecules pass from the ground state to a state of higher energy (excited). If energy of the radiation matches the energy difference between the last occupied state and the first empty state, the transition from an electron to a higher energy state occurs. Therefore, a molecule absorbs the excitation of its busy orbital of higher energy (HOMO) to one occupied by a single electron (SOMO), according to the molecular orbital theory [31]. Some molecules have the ability to transfer between 1 to 3 electrons in this way, generating interactions and structural–energetic modifications which occur in the orbitals of each molecule; when this change take place is very likely that a molecule absorbs energy of certain wavelength modifying its spectral area [32–34]. Although it is not a specific method for identification of link vibration, it is possible to elucidate whether the formation of a new complex exists, or simply molecules are found. Contrary to the functionalized treatments where a modification of the spectral area of each component is shown, as there are interactions between polymeric matrix and phytochemicals, resistance of these occurs in an aqueous system.

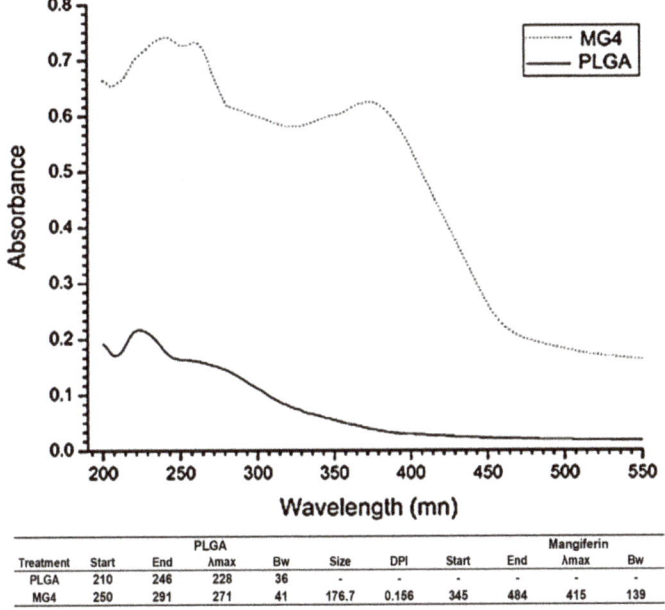

Treatment	PLGA						Mangiferin		
	Start	End	λmax	Bw	Size	DPI	Start	End	λmax	Bw
PLGA	210	246	228	36	-	-	-	-	-	-
MG4	250	291	271	41	176.7	0.156	345	484	415	139

Figure 4. Fingerprint UV-vis of mangiferin optimal nanoparticles (MG4) and poly (lactic-co-glycolic acid) (PLGA).

2.5. Powder X-ray Diffraction (XRD)

The powder X-ray diffraction patterns of MG and PLGA are illustrated in Figure 5. PLGA was in a crystalline form; however, in contrast, the XRD of the MG4 shows amplified signals corresponding to mangiferin between the θ 10–30 already described by other authors, indicating the change from a highly crystalline nature to an amorphous state of the complex mangiferin–PLGA [35,36]. However, these morphologies can also be attributed to the remnants of phosphate salts present in the formulation [36].

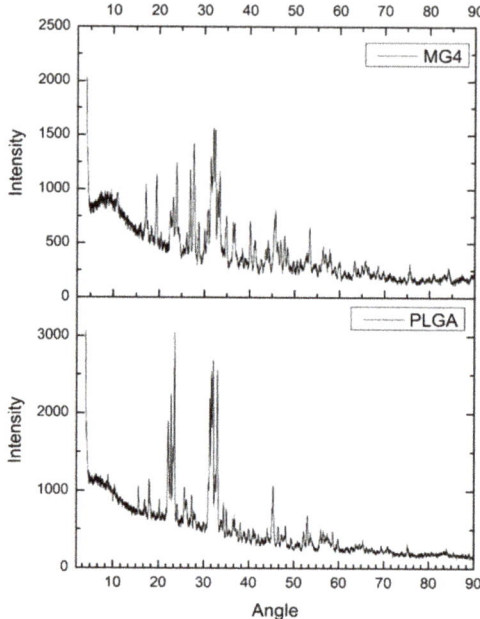

Figure 5. Powder X-ray diffraction patterns of mangiferin optimal nanoparticles (MG4) and poly (lactic-co-glycolic acid) (PLGA).

2.6. Anti-Topoisomerase Activity

It has been shown that during the development of a carcinoma, there is an increase in topoisomerases, because these enzymes are involved in cell replication [37]. Previous studies confirmed that mangiferin is capable of inhibiting the topoisomerase I enzyme (Topo I), involved in the splitting of DNA during cell division [38], Therefore, for this study, it was considered to evaluate its activity on Topo I in order to evaluate if there is loss of biological power or if it can be increased due to the controlled release of MG. Due to this, the used JN394 genetically modified strain (Matα ura3-52, leu2, trp1, his7, ade1-2, ISE2, rad52::LEU2) promotes a deficiency in the regeneration of DNA, greater permeability in the cell membrane y JN362a (Matα, ura3–52, leu2, trp1, his7, ade1–2, ISE2) resistant to DNA repair but sensitive to antimicrobial agents.

The concentration of extracts used in the assay was based on the solubility factor for each solid extract in dimethylsulfoxide (DMSO). As shown in Figure 6, the strain JN394 was hypersensitive to camptotecin (CPT) (69 ± 2.3% inhibition), which is a Topo I poison. MG4 showed 14.71 ± 1.2% inhibition (14.28 µg mangiferin/mg encapsulated) in this strain, while MG without encapsulation showed a percentage of inhibition of 28.5 ± 1.8% at the same concentration as CPT (50 µg/mL). The evaluated concentration of MG in MG4 is 5.71 times higher than that used in the camptothecin; so, to have a 69% inhibition, 66.98 µg of mangiferin (4.69 mg/mL of nanoparticles) is required.

JN394 is a strain that is DNA repair-deficient and drug-permeable (carry ise2 and rad52 mutations) [39]. These mutations increase the sensitivity of these cells to drugs [40]. The yeast JN362a, a DNA repair-proficient strain [35], was not affected by any NP treatment (+8 ± 0.43%) PLGA and (+5.3 ± 0.21%) MG4. These results mean that the MG4 has compounds with anti-topoisomerase activity against Topo I. Mangiferin has been identified as an inhibitor of the enzyme topoisomerase I by other authors [41].

The difference observed with respect to inhibition is related to the controlled release of MG4, since there is a time difference of 45 min, so that the total concentration of the encapsulated MG can be released in the media grown while CPT and MG come in contact with the yeasts from time 0 of growth. However, it has been shown that encapsulation can ensure that the amount of compound released can have a direct effect, without undergoing possible alterations during the process to reach the target cells. Mangiferin studies at a concentration of 50 µM have demonstrated an antiproliferative effect on cancer cells without affecting healthy cells; this is due to the activation of Nrf2–ARE signaling cascades [42], the controlled release of the phytochemical contributes to the inhibition of the topoisomerase enzyme, when mangiferin is expelled during the different phases of the cellular reproduction of the yeast, promoting cell death due to encapsulation [43]. A similar behavior was observed in the encapsulation of topotecan, which is a selective topoisomerase II inhibitor. A difference in cell viability between the encapsulated and non-encapsulated compound was observed—when the compound was encapsulated, the cytotoxicity remains constant after 24 h, whereas the non-encapsulated compound tended to decrease, confirming a controlled released on cell proliferation inhibition [44]. Modify strains from *Saccharomyces cerevisiae* have been used in cytotoxicity studies against topoisomerases, which were found in greater proportion in cancer cells, in addition to the modification in the gene that codes for topoisomerase [45], and these strains were like those used in the present study.

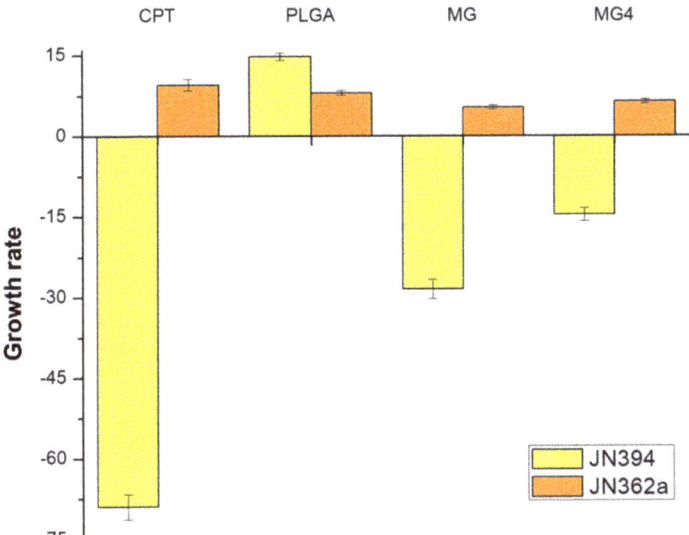

Figure 6. Growth rate of Camptotecin (CPT), poly (lactic-co-glycolic acid) (PLGA), mangiferin (MG), and mangiferin nanoparticles (MG4) in the proliferation of modified strains of *Saccharomyces cereviseae* JN362a and JN394.

2.7. Cell Viability

The NPs may have a high risk on human health, and to evaluate this, different types of cell cultures have been used as toxicity models under in vitro condition. HEPG2 derivate from hepatocellular carcinoma is a cell line well established and widely used as a model for drug metabolism and cytotoxicity studies, because these cells display many features of normal liver cells [46]. BEAS2B is an immortalized cell line isolated from normal human bronchial epithelium, and it has been employed to evaluate in vitro toxicity of some nanomaterials, because it is a non-cancerous epithelial cell type [47,48]. Thus, we selected HEPG2 and BEAS2B cells as a model system for studying the in vitro toxic effects of MG4.

HEPG2 and BEAS-2B cells were treated with varying concentrations of MG4. MTT is a tetrazolium salt that is converted to formazan salt (blue color) by mitochondrial dehydrogenase enzymes; thus, color can be measured, and it correlated with cell metabolic activity or live cells. Violet crystal dye stains cell proteins and DNA, and the cells that suffer cell death lose their adhesion; thus, adherent cells can be stained, and color can be quantified. Both methods showed that MG4 high concentrations (2500 µg/mL) were not able to decrease cell viability in BEAS-2B or HEPG2 cells (Figure 7). Furthermore, MG4 did not alter cell morphology in either cell line. Reports have shown that glycosylated bioactive compounds do not have an hepatotoxic effect on the in vitro model. Furthermore, the mangiferin conjugated with other similar compounds could have a positive role on hepatic glucose metabolism [44], as well as studies on encapsulation with PLGA showing that it does not appear to have an hepatotoxic effect on HEPG2, and therefore, it has been cataloged as a safe biopolymer [49].

Particularly, at 1250 mg/mL, an increase in the cell viability of HEPG2 is shown compared to the negative control. Other studies with this cell line have shown that some plant phenol extracts promote cell growth, but with isolated phenolic compounds, and the viability in healthy liver cells decreases at concentrations greater than 2 mg/mL [50,51]. Therefore, it is likely that this concentration allows the cellular replication of healthy cells; nevertheless, studies in cancer cells to corroborate this hypothesis are lacking.

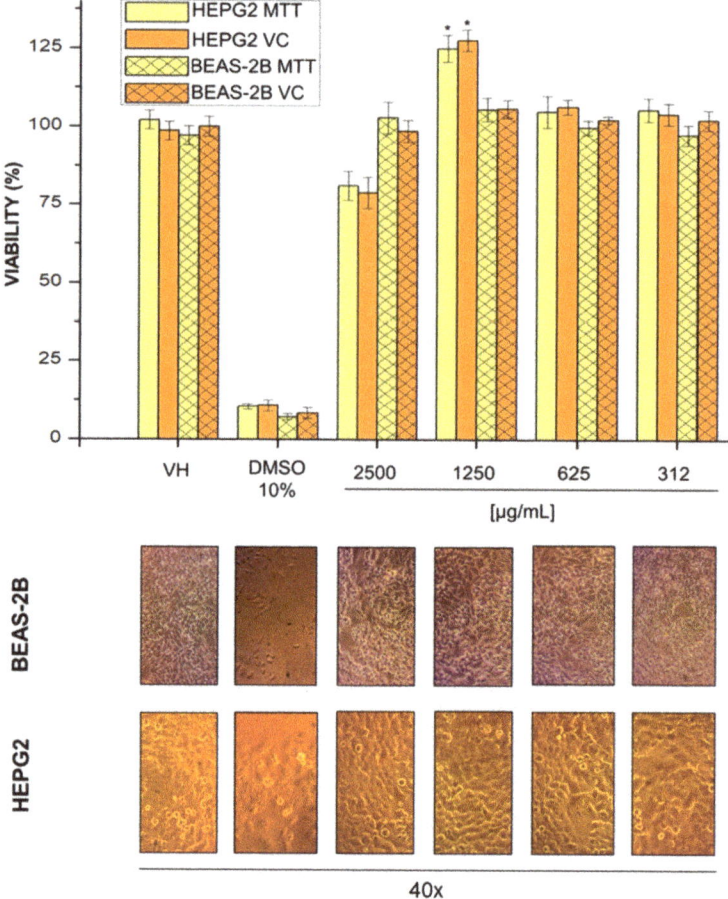

Figure 7. Cell viability of the various mangiferin nanoparticle concentrations for HepG2 and BEAS-2B cells using the violet crystal and MTT assay. * $p < 0.05$, statistical difference between treatment and control.

3. Materials and Methods

3.1. Reactives

Poly (lactic-co-glycolic acid) (PLGA), 75:25, Mw 25,000; polyvinyl alcohol (PVA) Mw 85,000–124,000, mangiferin, and dichloromethane (DCM) were obtained from Sigma-Aldrich (St. Louis, MO 63118, USA).

3.2. Preparation of Nanoparticles (NPs)

The NPs were developed following the method of solvent evaporation [52] using 15 mg of PLGA (75:25) and adding 500 µL of DCM in a flask. The aqueous phase composition was 5 mL of PVA solution (0.5%), and the quantity of mangiferin was added according to the amount required (Figure 1). The emulsion was sonicated for 5 min. Samples were homogenized by an Ultra-turrax® (IKA, T18; Germany) disperser and the organic phase was added drop-by-drop. Organic solvent was separated by rotoevaporation (Buchi, R-300; Essen, Germany). After, NPs were kept for 2 h at −80 °C and freeze-dried at −50 °C in a freeze-dryer (Labconco, FreeZone 6; Kansas, MO, USA). Finally, the lyophilized samples were stored in a desiccator and placed in the freezer (−20 °C) (Torrey, CHTC-255; Monterrey, Nuevo León, México). Loaded NPs were named MG1 to MG15, depending on the processing conditions. Unloaded NPs (PLGA) were also prepared and used as control.

3.3. Experimental Design

According to Box–Behnken design, a total number of 15 experiments, including 12 factorial points at the midpoints of the edges of the process space and three replicates at the center point for estimation of pure error sum of squares, were performed to choose the best model among the linear, two-factor interaction model and quadratic model due to the analysis of variance (ANOVA). An obtained p-value less than 0.05 was considered statistically significant. The selected independent variables were speed (A), time (B), and concentration (C) at three different levels as low (−1), medium (0), and high (+1). Dependent variables were encapsulation efficiency (EE%) and entrapment efficiency (AE%). The coded factors and responses of the variables are given in Figure 1.

3.4. Evaluation of Mangiferin Encapsulation Efficiency (EE%) and Entrapment Efficiency (AE%)

The samples were dissolved in phosphate-buffered solution (PBS) at pH of 7.0 solution and mangiferin AE% was determined indirectly [53]. An aliquot (200 µL) of sample was placed in a microplate reader (Biotek, Synergy HT; Winooski, VT, USA), the reading was recorded at 365 nm, and the concentration was obtained by a calibration curve of manguiferin (0.4, 0.8, 1.6, 3.2, and 6.4 µg/mL) using Equation (2).

$$AE\% = \left(\frac{A1 - AA}{A1}\right) \times 100 \qquad (2)$$

where $A1$ is the initial amount of mangiferin, and AA is the amount of free no-entrapped mangiferin determined by UV-vis [54].

EE% was determined later to expose the NPs under the conditions mentioned above; nevertheless, for this analysis, aliquots were taken at the time 0.15 min and 24 h. EE% was obtained using Equation (3).

$$EE\% = \left(\frac{E1 - E24}{E1}\right) \times 100 \qquad (3)$$

$E1$ is the difference in time concentration from t0 to 15 min, $E24$ is the total concentration released at 24 h. With this model it can wash the surface of the NPs with the objective of obtaining the concentration retained inside the particle.

Optimization of Data Using Response Surface Methodology (RSM)

Optimization by RSM was based on the highest possible value of EE% and AE% that we evaluated in terms of statistically significant coefficients and R^2 values. A Pareto chart was used for identification the quadratic and lineal effects from independent variables.

3.5. Mangiferin Release Profile in NPs

The in vitro release profile of mangiferin from NPs was evaluated suspending a 1.0 mg of NPs into 5 mL of PBS solution at different pH value (1.13 and 7.05) [55]. The suspension was maintained at 37 °C and 150 rpm (magnetic stirrers). The samples were read at 0, 15, 30, 45, 60, 120, 180, 240, and 360 min. The kinetic analyses of the release data were performed using various mathematical models [56–58]. From the optimum condition, particle size, size distribution, and the physicochemical properties were evaluated.

3.6. Optical Characterization

3.6.1. Size Distribution of Mangiferin NPs

The size distribution was determined in pure water at 18 °C using a particle size analyzer (Malvern, Mastersizer 2000; UK). For the measurements, 200 mL of the NP suspension was dispersed in 2 mL of filtered water. The analysis was performed at a scattering angle of 90°, refractive index of 1.590 (corresponding to PLGA), and 18 ± 3 °C.

3.6.2. Evaluation Morphology by Scanning Electron Microscopy (SEM)

The NPs were observed under scanning electron microscope (Tescan, MIRA3 LMU, London, UK). The samples were sputter-coated with gold before observation under SEM. Both low and high magnification images were obtained to confirm the uniformity of the particle sizes and to determine the exact size of the particle, respectively. The high magnification SEM images were interpreted by ImageJ software to determine the size of the particles.

3.6.3. UV-Visible Spectroscopy

UV–visible spectrums of NPs were recorded from 300 to 600 nm. Particle size distribution was carried out by a Dynamic Light Scattering (DLS) analyzer (Shimadzu, UV- 26000; Kyoto, Japan).

3.6.4. Surface Composition of the Np´s by X-ray Diffraction (XRD)

The XRD patterns were obtained using a Bruker D8 Advance equipment diffractometer (Tokyo, Japan) (k = 1.5460 Å, 40 KV, 30 mA), The diffraction intensity as a function of the diffraction angle (2θ) was measured between 10 and 90°, using a step of 0.02° and counting time of 0.25 s per step.

3.7. Biological Material

Mutant yeasts of *Saccharomyces cerevisiae*, JN362a and JN394 cells, were donated by Dr. John Nitiss of St. Jude Children's Research Hospital, Memphis, Tennessee. Cell lines were obtained of American Type Culture Collection: Primary and immortalized human bronchial epithelial cells, BEAS-2B (ATCC CRL-9609), and hepatocarcinoma adherent epithelial cell, HEPG2 (ATCC HB-8065).

3.8. Yeast Anti-Topoisomerase Assay

The anti-topoisomerase activity was evaluated using mutants *S. cerevisiae* JN362a and JN394 strains [59]. Briefly, yeast cells were grown in YPDA media at 30 °C for 18 h in a shaking incubator. The logarithmically growing cells were then counted using a hemocytometer and adjusted to a concentration of 2×10^6 cells/mL media. Yeast cells (6×10^6 cells) were incubated at 30 °C for 24 h in the shaking incubator (Thermo scientific, SHKE4450; Bedford, MA, USA) in the presence of the NPs, mangiferin, or CPT previously dissolved in 50 µL DMSO. DMSO (1.66%) was used as negative control, while CPT (50 µg/mL), a topoisomerase I inhibitor, was the positive control. Treated cells from each mixture were then duplicate plated to petri dishes containing 1.75% Agar bacto solidified YPDA media. Cells were incubated at growth temperature of 30 or 25 °C for 48 h. The anti-topoisomerase activity was determined as number of counted colonies in each plate by comparing to that of the negative control (DMSO).

3.9. Cell Line Culture

The cell lines BEAS-2B and HEPG2 were cultured in Dulbeco's Modified Eagle's Medium (Gibco 12320-032 and 12100-038, respectively; Gaithersburg, MD, USA) supplemented with 10% fetal bovine serum (JRScientific Inc., 43640-500; Woodland, CA, USA) and 1% streptomycin/penicillin (PAA, P11-002). Cultures were maintained at 37 °C in 5% CO_2.

3.10. Cell Viability Assay

Cell lines were seeded (1×10^4 cells/100 µL/well) in 96-well plates for 24 h in complete media [60]. Then, cells were treated with MG4 in concentrations of 2500, 1250, 625, and 312 µL/mL, medium volume was completed at 200 µL, and cells were incubated by 72 h at 37 °C in 5% CO_2. The DMSO (at the same volume that NPs, 1%) was used as a negative control and DMSO to high concentration (10%) was used as a positive control. Citotoxicity was evaluated by violet crystal and 3-(4,5-dimethylthiazol-2-yl)-2,5-diphenyl tetrazolium bromide (MTT), where all experiments were performed in triplicate in three independent experiments; thus, all data are reported as the mean value ± the standard error of the mean. The cells were observed with an inverted optical microscope (Olympus, CKX-41; Waltham, MA, USA.) and photographs were taken with the Microscope Eyepiece camera (AmScope, MU130; Irvine, CA, USA).

3.10.1. Staining with Violet Crystal

After 72 h of exposure to the NPs, cells were fixed with p-formaldehyde 4% (75 µL each well), and incubated at 37 °C for 1 h. Next, three washes were performed with PBS, and the plate was inverted and dried for 2 h in absorbent paper. Then, violet crystal 0.5% (50 µL to each well) was added and incubated at 37 °C for 20 min. Each well was washed three times with PBS, and subsequently, it was dried for 24 h. Finally, methanol (200 µL) was added to each well, and the plate was shaken and read at 570 nm in a BioRad microplate reader (iMark™ Microplate Absorbance Reader). The cell viability percentage was calculated as a ratio to the values obtained by the untreated cells. The results were analyzed with GraphPad Prism 5.0 software.

3.10.2. MTT Tetrazolium Assay

The cell cytotoxicity was evaluated using MTT stock solution (0.5 mg/mL); for that, MTT was dissolved in phosphate-buffered saline (PBS) (pH 7.4), and then it was filtered and stored at −20 °C in the absence of light. The assay was performed according to [61]; briefly, cells treated with NPs were washed once with PBS, then MTT (50 µL) and PBS (50 µL) were added to each well and incubated for 4 h at 37 °C in 5% CO_2. MTT solution was removed, and 100 µL DMSO was added to each well to dissolve the formazan crystals. Then, the plate was shaken and read at 570 nm in a BioRad microplate reader (iMark™ Microplate Absorbance Reader). The cell viability percentage was obtained by comparing the results with those of untreated cells. The results were analyzed with GraphPad Prism 5.0 software.

4. Conclusions

The nanoparticles made under the solvent emulsion and evaporation method with PLGA are potentially resistant to acidic conditions for up to 45 min; the best encapsulation and entrapment efficiency (77% and 93%) was achieved at a concentration of mangiferin of 300 µg. It was observed that the three factors studied (concentration, time, and speed of homogenization) affect the efficiency of encapsulation and modify the release profile of mangiferin. Interactions between the molecules in the formulation affected the fingerprint of the compounds when encapsulated; however, this formation of bonds does not produce a negative effect on the antipopoisomerase activity of mangiferin and does not present hepatotoxicity in vitro.

Author Contributions: Writing—original draft preparation, F.F.R.-C.; methodology, A.P.-L. and J.A.S.-B.; validation, M.H.-M., L.M.-T., and A.P.L.; formal analysis, N.G.-S.; investigation, F.F.R.-C.; writing—review and editing, J.A.S.-B. and A.P.-L.; supervision, J.A.S.-B. and S.G.S.-A.

Funding: Tecnológico Nacional de México (TecNM) with the project code 5857.16-P.

Acknowledgments: The authors gratefully acknowledge the financial support for the scholarship (787023) from CONACYT-Mexico, the Materials Lab (Technical Sergio Oliva and Martin Flores) for the use of the XRD and SEM equipment from the Centro Universitario de Ciencias Exactas e Ingenierias of the Universidad de Guadalajara, Jalisco, Mexico and to the Biopolymer's Lab (Gabriel Luna Barcenas) for the use of the Mastersizer equipment from the Cinvestav, Querétaro, México.

Conflicts of Interest: The authors declare no conflict of interest.

References

1. Vyas, A.; Syeda, K.; Ahmad, A.; Padhye, S.; Sarkar, F.H. Perspective on medical properties of mangiferin. *Mini Rev. Med. Chem.* **2012**, *12*, 412–425. [CrossRef] [PubMed]
2. Nunez Selles, A.J.; Velez Castro, H.T.; Aguero-Aguero, J.; Gonzalez-Gonzalez, J.; Naddeo, F.; De Simone, F.; Rastrelli, L. Isolation and quantitative analysis of phenolic antioxidants, free sugars, and polyols from mango (Mangifera indica L.) stem bark aqueous decoction used in Cuba as a nutritional supplement. *J. Agric. Food Chem.* **2002**, *50*, 762–766. [CrossRef] [PubMed]
3. Nunez Selles, A.J.; Daglia, M.; Rastrelli, L. The potential role of mangiferin in cancer treatment through its immunomodulatory, anti-angiogenic, apoptopic, and gene regulatory effects. *Biofactors* **2016**, *42*, 475–491. [CrossRef] [PubMed]
4. Liu, H.; Wang, K.; Tang, Y.; Sun, Z.; Jian, L.; Li, Z.; Wu, B.; Huang, C. Structure elucidation of in vivo and in vitro metabolites of mangiferin. *J. Pharm. Biomed. Anal.* **2011**, *55*, 1075–1082. [CrossRef] [PubMed]
5. Leiro, J.; Arranz, J.A.; Yanez, M.; Ubeira, F.M.; Sanmartin, M.L.; Orallo, F. Expression profiles of genes involved in the mouse nuclear factor-kappa B signal transduction pathway are modulated by mangiferin. *Int. Immunopharmacol.* **2004**, *4*, 763–778. [CrossRef]
6. Takeda, T.; Tsubaki, M.; Kino, T.; Yamagishi, M.; Iida, M.; Itoh, T.; Imano, M.; Tanabe, G.; Muraoka, O.; Satou, T.; et al. Mangiferin induces apoptosis in multiple myeloma cell lines by suppressing the activation of nuclear factor kappa B-inducing kinase. *Chem. Biol. Interact.* **2016**, *251*, 26–33. [CrossRef]
7. Takeda, T.; Tsubaki, M.; Sakamoto, K.; Ichimura, E.; Enomoto, A.; Suzuki, Y.; Itoh, T.; Imano, M.; Tanabe, G.; Muraoka, O.; et al. Mangiferin, a novel nuclear factor kappa B-inducing kinase inhibitor, suppresses metastasis and tumor growth in a mouse metastatic melanoma model. *Toxicol. Appl. Pharmacol.* **2016**, *306*, 105–112. [CrossRef]
8. Garrido, G.; Delgado, R.; Lemus, Y.; Rodriguez, J.; Garcia, D.; Nunez-Selles, A.J. Protection against septic shock and suppression of tumor necrosis factor alpha and nitric oxide production on macrophages and microglia by a standard aqueous extract of Mangifera indica L. (VIMANG). Role of mangiferin isolated from the extract. *Pharmacol. Res.* **2004**, *50*, 165–172. [CrossRef]
9. Bhatia, H.S.; Candelario-Jalil, E.; de Oliveira, A.C.; Olajide, O.A.; Martinez-Sanchez, G.; Fiebich, B.L. Mangiferin inhibits cyclooxygenase-2 expression and prostaglandin E2 production in activated rat microglial cells. *Arch. Biochem. Biophys.* **2008**, *477*, 253–258. [CrossRef]
10. Ariyarathna, I.R.; Karunaratne, D.N. Microencapsulation stabilizes curcumin for efficient delivery in food applications. *Food Packag. Shelf Life* **2016**, *10*, 79–86. [CrossRef]
11. Rodríguez, J.; Martín, M.J.; Ruiz, M.A.; Clares, B. Current encapsulation strategies for bioactive oils: From alimentary to pharmaceutical perspectives. *Food Res. Int.* **2016**, *83*, 41–59. [CrossRef]
12. Esfanjani, A.F.; Jafari, S.M. Biopolymer nano-particles and natural nanocarriers for nano-encapsulation of phenolic compounds. *Colloids Surf. B Biointerfaces* **2016**, *146*, 532–543. [CrossRef] [PubMed]

13. Liang, J.; Yan, H.; Puligundla, P.; Gao, X.; Zhou, Y.; Wan, X. Applications of chitosan nanoparticles to enhance absorption and bioavailability of tea polyphenols: A review. *Food Hydrocolloids* **2017**, *69*, 286–292. [CrossRef]
14. Anwer, M.K.; Mohammad, M.; Ezzeldin, E.; Fatima, F.; Alalaiwe, A.; Iqbal, M. Preparation of sustained release apremilast-loaded PLGA nanoparticles: In vitro characterization and in vivo pharmacokinetic study in rats. *Int. J. Nanomed.* **2019**, *14*, 1587. [CrossRef] [PubMed]
15. Benitez, S.; Benoit, J.P.; Puisioux, F.; Thies, C. Characterization of drug loaded poly (d,l-lactide) microespheres. *J. Pharmacol. Sci.* **1994**, *732*, 1721–1728.
16. Fernandez, D.M.; Gómez, M.; Núñez, L.; Ramos, D.; Moya, A.; Chang, A. Características físico-químicas de las microesferas obtenidas con diferentes polímeros y la liberación del principio activo. *Rev. Cuba. Farm.* **2005**, *37*, 5–9.
17. Busatto, C.A.; Helbling, I.; Casis, N.; Luna, N.; Estenoz, D.A. Microesferas biodegradables de PLGA para la liberación controlada de progesterona. In Proceedings of the 13st Congresso da Sociedade Latino Americana de Biomateriais, Orgãos Artificiais e Engenharia de Tecidos—SLABO, Foz do Iguaçu, Brazil, 24–27 August 2016.
18. Gracia, E.; García, M.T.; Rodríguez, J.F.; de Lucas, A.; Gracia, I. Improvement of PLGA loading and release of curcumin by supercritical technology. *J. Supercrit. Fluids* **2018**, *141*, 60–67. [CrossRef]
19. Varga, N.; Hornok, V.; Janovák, L.; Dékány, I.; Csapó, E. The effect of synthesis conditions and tunable hydrophilicity on the drug encapsulation capability of PLA and PLGA nanoparticles. *Colloids Surf. B Biointerfaces* **2019**, *176*, 212–218. [CrossRef]
20. Mahapatro, A.; Singh, D.K. Biodegradable nanoparticles are excellent vehicle for site directed in-vivo delivery of drugs and vaccines. *J. Nanobiotechnol.* **2011**, *9*, 2–11. [CrossRef]
21. Souza, J.R.; Feitosa, J.P.; De Carvalho, J.I.; Trevisan, M.T.; De Paula, H.C.; Nágila, M.P. Chitosan-coated pectin beads: Characterization and in vitro release of mangiferin. *Food Hydrocoll.* **2009**, *23*, 2278–2286. [CrossRef]
22. Owen, R.W. Spray-drying encapsulation of mangiferin using natural polymers. *Food Hydrocoll.* **2013**, *33*, 10–18.
23. Dhand, V.; Soumya, L.; Bharadwaj, S.; Chakra, S.; Bhatt, D.; Sreedhar, B. Green synthesis of silver nanoparticles using Coffea arabica seed extract and its antibacterial activity. *Mater. Sci. Eng. C* **2016**, *58*, 36–43. [CrossRef] [PubMed]
24. Venugopal, N.; Mitra, A. Influence of temperature dependent morphology on localized surface plasmon resonance in ultra-thin silver island films. *Appl. Surf. Sci.* **2013**, *85*, 357–372. [CrossRef]
25. Pool, H.; Quintanar, D.; Figueroa, J.D.; Mano, C.; Bechara, H.; Godínez, L.A.; Mendoza, S. Antioxidant effects of quercetin and catechin encapsulated into PLGA nanoparticles. *J. Nanomater.* **2012**, *2012*, 1–12. [CrossRef]
26. Patra, N.; Dehury, N.; Pal, A.; Behera, A.; Patra, S. Preparation and mechanistic aspect of natural xanthone functionalized gold nanoparticle. *Mater. Sci. Eng. C* **2018**, *90*, 439–445. [CrossRef]
27. Engelbrekt, C.; Sørensen, K.H.; Zhang, J.; Welinder, A.C.; Jensen, P.S.; Ulstrup, J. Green synthesis of gold nanoparticles with starch–glucose and application in bioelectrochemistry. *J. Mater. Chem.* **2009**, *42*, 7839–7847. [CrossRef]
28. Pereira, M.C.; Oliveira, D.A.; Hill, L.E.; Zambiazi, R.C.; Borges, C.D.; Vizzotto, M.; Mertens-Talcott, S.; Talcott, S.; Gomes, C.L. Effect of nanoencapsulation using PLGA on antioxidant and antimicrobial activities of guabiroba fruit phenolic extract. *Food Chem.* **2018**, *240*, 396–404. [CrossRef]
29. Kumawat, M.K.; Thakur, M.; Gurung, R.B.; Srivastava, R. Graphene Quantum Dots from Mangifera indica: Application in Near-Infrared Bioimaging and Intracellular Nanothermometry. *ACS Sustain. Chem. Eng.* **2017**, *5*, 1382–1391. [CrossRef]
30. Kim, K.; Luu, Y.K.; Chang, C.; Fang, D.; Hsiao, B.S.; Chu, B.; Hadjiargyrou, M. Incorporation and controlled release of a hydrophilicantibiotic using poly(lactide-co-glycolide)-based electrospun nanofibrous scaffolds. *J. Controll. Release* **2004**, *98*, 47–56. [CrossRef]
31. Chaitanya, K. Molecular structure, vibrational spectroscopic (FT-IR, FT-Raman), UV–vis spectra, first order hyperpolarizability, NBO analysis, HOMO and LUMO analysis, thermodynamic properties of benzophenone 2,4-dicarboxylic acid by ab initio HF and density functional method. *Spectrochim. Acta Part A Mol. Biomol. Spectrosc.* **2012**, *86*, 159–173.
32. Thomas, M. *Ultraviolet and Visible Spectroscopy*, 2nd ed.; John Wiley & Sons: New York, NY, USA, 1996; p. 172.
33. Pearson, R.G. Absolute electronegativity and hardness correlated with molecular orbital theory. *Proc. Natl. Acad. Sci. USA* **1986**, *83*, 8440–8441. [CrossRef] [PubMed]

34. Yang, X.; Zhao, Y.; Chen, Y.; Liao, X.; Gao, C.; Xiao, D.; Qin, Q.; Yi, D.; Yang, B. Host–guest inclusion system of mangiferin with β-cyclodextrin and its derivatives. *Mater. Sci. Eng. C* **2013**, *33*, 2386–2391. [CrossRef] [PubMed]
35. Liu, R.; Liu, Z.; Zhang, C.; Zhang, B. Nanostructured Lipid Carriers As Novel Ophthalmic Delivery System for Mangiferin: Improving In Vivo Ocular Bioavailability. *J. Pharm. Sci.* **2012**, *101*, 3833–3844. [CrossRef] [PubMed]
36. Sangeetha, G.; Rajeshwari, S.; Venckatesh, R. Green synthesis of zinc oxide nanoparticles by aloe barbadensis miller leaf extract: Structure and optical properties. *Mater. Res. Bull.* **2011**, *46*, 2560–2566. [CrossRef]
37. Pona, A.; Cline, A.; Kolli, S.S.; Taylor, S.L.; Feldman, S.R. Review of future insights of Dragon's Blood in dermatology. *Dermatol. Ther.* **2019**, *32*, 1–20. [CrossRef]
38. Arunkumar, J.; Rajarajan, S. A Study on the in vitro Cytotoxicity and Anti- HSV-2 Activity of Lyophilized Extracts of Terminalia Catappa Lin., Mangifera Indica Lin.and Phytochemical Compound Mangiferin. *Int. J. Med. Pharm. Virol.* **2015**, *2*, 22–26.
39. Nitiss, J.; Wang, J.C. DNA topoisomerase-targeting antitumor drugs can be studied in yeast. *Proc. Natl. Acad. Sci. USA* **1988**, *85*, 7501–7505. [CrossRef]
40. Ramírez-Mares, M.V.; Sánchez-Burgos, J.A.; Hernández-Carlos, B. Antioxidant, antimicrobial and antitopoisomerase screening of the stem bark extracts of Ardisia compressa. *Pak. J. Nutr.* **2010**, *9*, 307–313.
41. Qin, J.L.; Deng, S.P.; Zhang, Y.L.; Yuan, T.; Li, Y.B.; Han, H.H.; Chen, Z.F. Water soluble copper (II) and zinc (II) complexes of mangiferin: Synthesis, antitumour activity and DNA binding studies. *J. Chem. Res.* **2016**, *40*, 659–663. [CrossRef]
42. Zhang, B.P.; Zhao, J.; Li, S.S.; Yang, L.J.; Zeng, L.L.; Chen, Y.; Fang, J. Mangiferin activates Nrf2-antioxidant response element signaling without reducing the sensitivity to etoposide of human myeloid leukemia cells in vitro. *Acta Pharmacol. Sin.* **2014**, *35*, 257. [CrossRef]
43. Villamizar, G.; Parra-Monroy, M.L. Uso de Nanopartículas de plata en el control de microorganismos patógenos presentes en alimentos. *Nano Cienc. Tecnol.* **2015**, *13*, 54–59.
44. Broderick, L.; Yost, S.; Li, D.; McGeough, M.D.; Booshehri, L.M.; Guaderrama, M.; Hakonarson, H. Mutations in topoisomerase IIβ result in a B cell immunodeficiency. *Nat. Commun.* **2019**, *10*, 1–15. [CrossRef] [PubMed]
45. Souza, L.G.; Silva, E.J.; Martins, A.L.L.; Mota, M.F.; Braga, R.C.; Lima, E.M.; Marreto, R.N. Development of topotecan loaded lipid nanoparticles for chemical stabilization and prolonged release. *Eur. J. Pharm. Biopharm.* **2011**, *79*, 189–196. [CrossRef] [PubMed]
46. Bahadar, H.; Maqbool, F.; Niaz, K.; Abdollahi, M. Toxicity of Nanoparticles and an Overview of Current Experimental Models. *Iran. Biomed. J.* **2016**, *20*, 1–11.
47. Chatterjee, N.; Yang, J.; Kim, H.M.; Jo, E.; Kim, P.J.; Choi, K.; Choi, J. Potential toxicity of differential functionalized multiwalled carbon nanotubes (MWCNT) in human cell line (BEAS2B) and Caenorhabditis elegans. *J. Toxicol. Environ. Health Part A* **2014**, *77*, 1399–1408. [CrossRef]
48. Chatterjee, N.; Yang, J.S.; Park, K.; Oh, S.M.; Park, J.; Choi, J. Screening of toxic potential of graphene family nanomaterials using in vitro and alternative in vivo toxicity testing systems. *Environ. Health Toxicol.* **2015**, *15*, 1–7. [CrossRef]
49. Wang, C.; Jian-Dong, J.; Wei, W.; Wei-Jia, K. The Compound of Mangiferin-Berberine Salt Has Potent Activities in Modulating Lipid and Glucose Metabolisms in HepG2 Cell. *BioMed Res. Int.* **2016**, *2016*, 1–15. [CrossRef]
50. Ahmed, A.; Rabou, A.; Hanaa, H. CS-PEG decorated PLGA nano-prototype for delivery of bioactive compounds: A novel approach for induction of apoptosis in HepG2 cell line. *Adv. Med. Sci.* **2017**, *207*, 1–11.
51. Amararathana, M.; Johnston, M.R.; Vasantha-Rupasinghe, H.P. Plant Polyphenols as Chemopreventive Agents For Lung Cancer. *Int. J. Mol. Sci.* **2016**, *17*, 1352. [CrossRef]
52. Grauzdytė, D.; Raudoniutė, J.; Kulvinskienė, I.; Bagdonas, E.; Stasiulaitienė, I.; Martuzevicius, D.; Bironaite, D.; Aldonyte, R.; Venskutonis, P.R. Cytoprotective Effects of Mangiferin and Z-Ligustilide in PAH-Exposed Human Airway Epithelium in Vitro. *Nutrients* **2019**, *11*, 218. [CrossRef]
53. Venugopal, V.; Kumar, K.J.; Muralidharan, S.; Parasuraman, S.; Raj, P.V.; Kumar, K.V. Optimization and in-vivo evaluation of isradipine nanoparticles using Box-Behnken design surface response methodology. *OpenNano* **2016**, *1*, 1–15. [CrossRef]

54. Gomes, C.; Moreira, R.G.; Castell-Perez, E. Poly (DL-lactide-co-glycolide) (PLGA) nanoparticles with entrapped trans-cinnamaldehyde and eugenol for antimicrobial delivery applications. *J. Food Sci.* **2011**, *76*, N16–N24. [CrossRef] [PubMed]
55. Casa, D.M.; Moraes, T.C.M.; De Camargo, L.E.A.; Khalil, L.F.; Dalmolin, N.M.; Mainardes, R.M. Poly(L-lactide) nanoparticles reduce Amphotericin B cytotoxicity and maintain its in vitro antifungal activity. *J. Nanosci. Nanotechnol.* **2014**, *15*, 848–854. [CrossRef]
56. Alves, A.C.S.; Minardes, R.M.; Khalil, N.M. Nanoencapsulation of gallic acid and evaluation of its cytotoxicity and antioxidant activity. *Mater. Sci. Eng. C* **2016**, *60*, 126–134. [CrossRef] [PubMed]
57. Ritger, P.L.; Peppas, N.A. Simple equation for description of solute release II. Fickian and anomalous release from swellable devices. *J. Controll. Release* **1987**, *5*, 37–42. [CrossRef]
58. Siepmann, J.; Peppas, N.A. Modeling of drug release from delivery systems based on hydroxypropyl methylcellulose (HPMC). *Adv. Drug Deliv. Rev.* **2001**, *64*, 163–174. [CrossRef]
59. Nitiss, J.L.; Nitiss, K.C. Yeast systems for demonstrating the targets of antitopoisomerase II agents. *Methods Mol. Biol.* **2001**, *95*, 315–327.
60. Kizhedath, A.; Wilkinson, S.; Glassey, J. Assessment of hepatotoxicity and dermal toxicity of butyl paraben and methyl paraben using HepG2 and HDFn in vitro models. *Toxicol. Vitro* **2019**, *55*, 108–115. [CrossRef]
61. Kim, Y.J.; Haribalan, P.; Castro-Aceituno, V.; Kim, D.; Markus, J.; Lee, S.; Kim, S.; Liu, Y.; Chun-Yang, D. Photoluminescent And Self-Assembled Hyaluronic Acid-Zinc Oxide-Ginsenoside Rh2 Nanoparticles And Their Potential Caspase-9 Apoptotic Mechanism Towards Cancer Cell Lines. *Int. J. Nanomed.* **2019**, *14*, 8195–8208. [CrossRef]

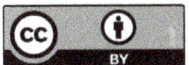

© 2019 by the authors. Licensee MDPI, Basel, Switzerland. This article is an open access article distributed under the terms and conditions of the Creative Commons Attribution (CC BY) license (http://creativecommons.org/licenses/by/4.0/).

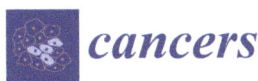

Article

Titanate Nanotubes Engineered with Gold Nanoparticles and Docetaxel to Enhance Radiotherapy on Xenografted Prostate Tumors

Alexis Loiseau [1], Julien Boudon [1,*], Alexandra Oudot [2], Mathieu Moreau [3], Romain Boidot [4], Rémi Chassagnon [1], Nasser Mohamed Saïd [5], Stéphane Roux [5], Céline Mirjolet [6,7,*] and Nadine Millot [1,*]

1. Laboratoire Interdisciplinaire Carnot de Bourgogne, UMR 6303, CNRS-Université Bourgogne Franche Comté, BP 47870, 21078 Dijon Cedex, France; alexis_loiseau@yahoo.fr (A.L.); remi.chassagnon@u-bourgogne.fr (R.C.)
2. Preclinical Imaging Platform, Nuclear Medicine Department, Georges-Francois Leclerc Cancer Center, 21079 Dijon Cedex, France; AOudot@cgfl.fr
3. Institut de Chimie Moléculaire de l'Université Bourgogne, UMR 6302, CNRS-Université Bourgogne Franche Comté, 21078 Dijon Cedex, France; mathieu.moreau@u-bourgogne.fr
4. Department of Biology and Pathology of Tumors, Georges-François Leclerc Cancer Center–UNICANCER, 21079 Dijon Cedex, France; RBoidot@cgfl.fr
5. Institut UTINAM, UMR 6213, CNRS-Université Bourgogne Franche-Comté, 25030 Besançon Cedex, France; said.nasser_mohamed@univ-fcomte.fr (N.M.S.); stephane.roux@univ-fcomte.fr (S.R.)
6. INSERM LNC UMR 1231, 21078 Dijon Cedex, France
7. Radiotherapy Department, Georges-Francois Leclerc Cancer Center, 21079 Dijon Cedex, France
* Correspondence: julien.boudon@u-bourgogne.fr (J.B.); CMirjolet@cgfl.fr (C.M.); Nadine.Millot@u-bourgogne.fr (N.M.)

Received: 23 October 2019; Accepted: 2 December 2019; Published: 6 December 2019

Abstract: Nanohybrids based on titanate nanotubes (TiONts) were developed to fight prostate cancer by intratumoral (IT) injection, and particular attention was paid to their step-by-step synthesis. TiONts were synthesized by a hydrothermal process. To develop the custom-engineered nanohybrids, the surface of TiONts was coated beforehand with a siloxane (APTES), and coupled with both dithiolated diethylenetriaminepentaacetic acid-modified gold nanoparticles (Au@DTDTPA NPs) and a heterobifunctional polymer (PEG$_{3000}$) to significantly improve suspension stability and biocompatibility of TiONts for targeted biomedical applications. The pre-functionalized surface of this scaffold had reactive sites to graft therapeutic agents, such as docetaxel (DTX). This novel combination, aimed at retaining the AuNPs inside the tumor via TiONts, was able to enhance the radiation effect. Nanohybrids have been extensively characterized and were detectable by SPECT/CT imaging through grafted Au@DTDTPA NPs, radiolabeled with ^{111}In. In vitro results showed that TiONts-AuNPs-PEG$_{3000}$-DTX had a substantial cytotoxic activity on human PC-3 prostate adenocarcinoma cells, unlike initial nanohybrids without DTX (Au@DTDTPA NPs and TiONts-AuNPs-PEG$_{3000}$). Biodistribution studies demonstrated that these novel nanocarriers, consisting of AuNP- and DTX-grafted TiONts, were retained within the tumor for at least 20 days on mice PC-3 xenografted tumors after IT injection, delaying tumor growth upon irradiation.

Keywords: titanate nanotubes; gold nanoparticles; vectorization; nanocarrier; colloidal stability; docetaxel; cytotoxicity; biodistribution; radiotherapy; prostate cancer

1. Introduction

Cancer remains one of the world's most devastating diseases with approximately 0.2% of people worldwide diagnosed with cancer at some point during their life [1]. However, even if mortality has a tendency to decrease, due to a better understanding of tumor biology and improvement of diagnostic tools and treatments, the prevalence of prostate cancer remains very high, especially in developed countries [2]. As an example, in 2019 in the United States, prostate cancer was the third-most diagnosed cancer, with close to 175,000 estimated new cases, corresponding to 1 prostate cancer over 10 detected cancers, being the second leading cause of cancer-related deaths in men with more than 31,000 estimated deaths [3]. In Europe, in 2018, the number of new prostate cancer cases was estimated at 450,000 [4].

Currently, anticancer chemotherapeutic agents such as docetaxel (DTX) are used to target tumor cells in prostate cancer treatment. DTX is an anti-mitotic chemotherapeutic agent, well known to decrease androgen receptor activation in castration-resistant prostate cancer cells [5,6]. It has been approved by Food and Drug Administration (FDA) in particular for the treatment of hormone-refractory prostate cancers [7]. Chemotherapy is often associated with radiotherapy (RT) to increase its efficiency during tumor treatment [8]. Nevertheless, injected drugs weakly reach tumor sites, and patients who undergo repeated treatments develop drug resistance within 24 months of initial exposure [6,9,10]. Thus, high doses, relative to the patient's needs, are administered, causing harmful side effects and excessive toxicities [11–13].

The development of nanotechnologies has offered a new strategy to incorporate and vectorize an active substance specifically to sick cells, increasing its efficacy while limiting systemic concentration. Theranostic nanohybrids have been considerably developed over the past decade as a new generation of nanocarriers for therapeutic and diagnosis purposes [14,15]. This emergent nanotechnology can be used to control injected doses, to perform medical diagnostic imaging based on nanohybrids monitoring inside the organism, and to improve the intracellular concentration of drugs and allow their accumulation within tumor site by enhanced permeability and retention (EPR) mechanisms while limiting toxicity in normal tissues [16–19]. Nevertheless, further increasing treatment efficacy is a relevant issue. Direct tumor administration through intratumoral (IT) injection might be a relevant approach. Accordingly, there is an interest to develop new nanocarriers for docetaxel to increase therapeutic efficiency and enhance radiation sensitization by maintaining radiosensitizing agents inside cancer cells. Among all nanovectors, carbon nanotubes (CNTs) have been widely investigated for drug delivery applications [20] as well as halloysite clay nanotubes (HNTs) [21]. CNTs are pioneer nanovectors, representing a novel set of nanomaterials available for cancer therapy [22]. Their unique physicochemical properties and their ability to cross cell membranes provide a higher capacity of drug loading when compared to conventional liposomes and dendrimer drug carriers [23]. In addition, CNTs may prolong circulation time and improve bioavailability of conjugated drug molecules [24]. However, these molecules are largely insoluble. To become biologically compatible, appropriate surface modifications leading to a better water solubility should be envisaged [25]. As for HNTs, considered as viable and inexpensive nanoscale containers for encapsulation of drugs [26,27], they also require surface modification for increased colloidal stability, and even though some coated HNTs are evaluated as being non-cytotoxic up to 75 $\mu g.mL^{-1}$ [27], some others appear to have toxic effects [28]. To overcome CNT and HNT drawbacks, titanate nanotubes (TiONts) have received particular attention as a new generation of nanovectors with adequate surface chemistry that are highly adaptable when compared to the relatively inert chemistry of CNTs. Similarly, TiONts are widely studied [29–31] in a broad range of applications since their discovery in the late 1990s [32]. Recently, TiONt applications have been developed in several fields of biomedicine [29,33], such as orthopedics and dental implants [34], dopamine detection [35], DNA transfection [36] and adsorption [37], bioimaging [38,39], safe nanocarrier [36,40,41], drug delivery (genistein and docetaxel) [42–44], and cancer cell radiosensitization [44,45]. These TiONt applications are possible due to the atypical morphology shared with CNTs and HNTs. However, they present a shorter length (about 100–300 nm), an opening at the extremities, and a wide versatility of surface chemistry compared with CNTs [29]. It has been shown that shape and functionalization of nanoparticles, used as carriers, affects biodistribution [19,46]. Moreover, our group demonstrated that TiONts can be internalized with no cytotoxicity induction and maintained inside cells for at least 10 days in vitro [36,45]. Finally, the exposure to TiONts combined with irradiation induced a radiosensitizing effect [45]. The functionalization of nanocarrier-TiONts is mandatory in order to have new or complementary functionalities such as stability and biocompatibility in physiological conditions for biomedical applications [19,40,43,47]. In addition, functionalization enables TiONts to carry therapeutic molecules and improves colloidal stability, required for vectorization applications. In very recent studies, our group has reported the use of TiONts as carrier for therapeutic molecules together with DTX (TiONts-DTX) into prostate tumor [43,44]. This nanocarrier was beforehand pre-functionalized with 3-aminopropyl triethoxysilane and with a hetero-bifunctional polymer (polyethylene glycol) to immobilize DTX by covalent linkages. In vivo tests with IT injections of TiONts-DTX showed that more than 70% of TiONt nanovectors were retained within the tumor for at least 7 days. In addition, the radiosensitizing effect of nanohybrids was evaluated on PC-3 tumors with and without RT. In both conditions, tumor growth was significantly slowed down in mice receiving TiONts-DTX compared to mice receiving free DTX. This work proved nanohybrids ability to remain inside the tumor, increasing therapeutic efficiency.

Encouraged by these results, it was necessary to further improve the radiosensitizing effect of these nanohybrids. Over the past decade an increasing interest to use gold nanoparticles (AuNPs) as radiosensitizers for radiation therapy [48,49] has arisen. AuNPs have the ability to combine imaging and therapy on the basis of the strong X-ray absorption cross section due to the high atomic number (Z) of gold [49,50]. They have been commonly used for imaging applications [51–54] and accumulate in tumors upon the delivery of diagnostic agents and therapeutic drugs, while being effectively excluded from healthy tissue [55–58]. AuNPs are biologically well-tolerated and present a low toxicity [49,58,59]. Among the numerous examples of gold nanoparticles, Au@DTDTPA NPs appear attractive for image-guided radiotherapy. The ultrasmall gold core confers to the nanoparticles an efficient radiosensitizing effect, which increased the efficiency of radiation therapy by twofold when tumor-bearing animals were treated by radiotherapy after IT injection of Au@DTDTPA NPs [60,61]. Moreover, the organic shell of these nanoparticles has been designed to immobilize gadolinium ions and radioisotopes (indium-111, ^{111}In). Consequently, the biodistribution of Au@DTDTPA NPs can be monitored by magnetic resonance imaging (MRI), and by nuclear imaging (positron emission tomography—PET, and single photon emission computed tomography—SPECT) [62–64]. Biodistribution studies, performed by a combination of MRI and SPECT, highlighted the safe behavior of Au@DTDTPA NPs after intravenous (IV) injection (accumulation in tumor, no undesirable accumulation in healthy tissue and renal clearance) and provided useful data to determine the ideal delay between the IV injection of Au@DTDTPA NPs and irradiation [60,64]. The radiosensitizing effect of Au@DTDTPA NPs can therefore be better exploited thanks to the possibility of following these nanoparticles by MRI. However, their potential is probably under-exploited due to their fast-renal clearance. The combination of Au@DTDTPA NPs with TiONts is expected to overcome this limitation by (i) the maintaining of nanotubes on site thanks to the design of nanohybrids compared to circulating nanovectors, (ii) improving the efficiency of nanohybrids in IT compared to IV even with the EPR effect, and (iii) the very possibility of combined injection of nanohybrids with radioactive iodine grains during brachytherapy [65]. Moreover, grafting gold nanoparticles onto TiONts, together with anticancer agents, paves the way to associate in the same entity, tumor retention, radiosensitization, and chemotherapy, and seems to be a new, attractive, and versatile platform.

This paper describes and analyzes each step required for the synthesis of a next generation nanohybrid. Analysis was performed using different characterization techniques (scanning transmission electron microscopy (STEM), thermogravimetric analysis (TGA), ζ-potential measurement, X-ray photoelectron spectroscopy (XPS), Fourier-transformed infrared (FTIR), UV-visible and inductively coupled plasma (ICP) spectroscopies) as well as biological tests to evaluate efficacy against prostate cancer. Herein, we also report in vitro bioassays carried out on a human PC-3 prostate adenocarcinoma cells using 3-(4,5-dimethylthiazol-2-yl)-5-(3-carboxymethoxyphenyl)-2-(4-ulfophenyl)-2H-tetrazolium (MTS) assay. In vivo biodistribution assays were performed in PC-3 xenografted prostate tumors, after IT injection, on Balb/c nude male mice. The radiosensitizing efficacy of TiONts-AuNPs-PEG$_{3000}$-DTX nanohybrids in association with RT, on a hormone-independent prostate cancer model, was also studied. Overall, these results describe the impact of a new generation TiONt-based treatment on a model of prostate cancer.

2. Results

The final nanohybrid (TiONts-AuNPs-PEG$_{3000}$-DTX) was synthesized step-by-step from titanate nanotubes (TiONts) according to Loiseau et al. [43]. The strategy used to engineer a very versatile platform, which could be used for both nuclear imaging and therapy, is presented in Figure 1, even if the final end product is intended only for therapy and imaging being used only for preclinical developments. In this report, each grafting step has been characterized by different techniques. After hydrothermal synthesis of TiONts, morphological conformity was highlighted by transmission electron microscopy (TEM). As expected, a coiled spiral-shaped structure and an internal cavity, as described in [41,43] and supporting information (Figure S1a) is shown. The observed dimensions are in agreement with literature on this compound, showing (10 ± 1) nm in outer diameter, (4 ± 1) nm in inner diameter, and (170 ± 50) nm in length [29–32,43]. TiONts present a large specific surface area due to their tubular shape ((174 ± 1) m^2.g^{-1}), which is necessary to graft an important number of organic compounds. These ligands improve colloidal stability, dispersion state, and circulation time within the organism.

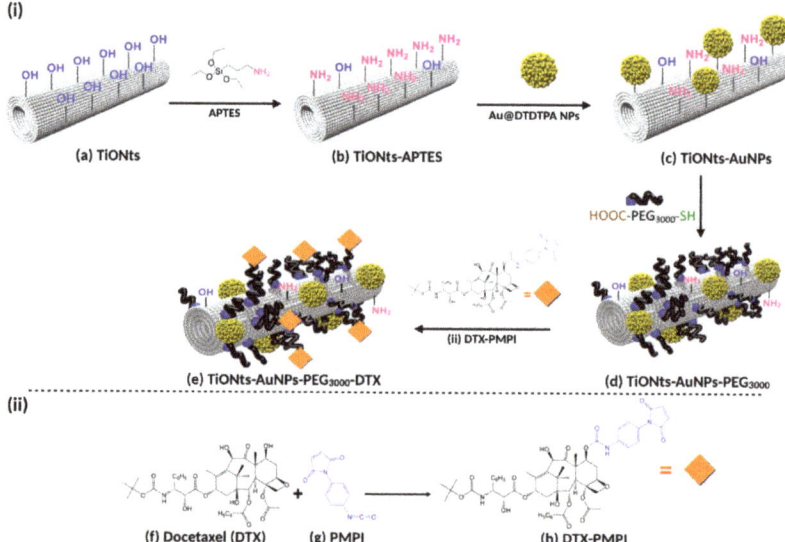

Figure 1. Illustration of (**i**) (**a**) titanate nanotubes (TiONts) and step-by-step pre-functionalization with (**b**) 3-aminopropyltriethoxysilane (APTES), (**c**) dithiolated diethylenetriaminepentaacetic acid-modified gold (Au@DTDTPA) nanoparticles (NPs), (**d**) α-acid,ω-thiol-polyethylene glycol (HS-PEG$_{3000}$-COOH), and (**e**) *p*-maleimidophenyl isocyanate (PMPI)-modified docetaxel (DTX-PMPI) to yield the final nanohybrid—TiONts-AuNPs-PEG$_{3000}$-DTX; (**ii**) this step corresponds to the modification of (**f**) DTX with (**g**) PMPI to form (**h**) DTX-PMPI (represented by an orange diamond).

In a previous work, TiONts, TiONts-APTES, and DTX-PMPI had already been characterized by several analysis techniques [30,39,43]. Briefly, grafting ratio on TiONts surface was determined by thermogravimetric analysis (TGA) (Figure 2). Results are reported in Table 1, and the details of the equations are given in Figures S2 and S3.

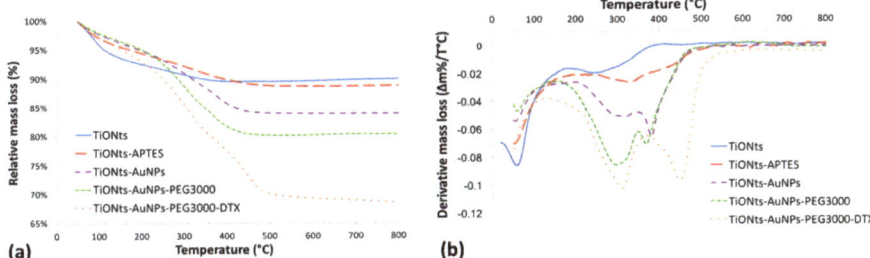

Figure 2. (a) Thermogravimetric analysis (TGA) and (b) derivative curves of bare TiONts and functionalized-TiONts under air atmosphere.

Table 1. Results of relative mass loss and graft ratio of bare TiONts and functionalized-TiONts.

Nanohybrid Name	Initial Temperature of Degradation (°C)	Relative Mass Loss (%)	Degraded Molecular Weight (g.mol^{-1})	Molecule.nm^{-2} (average)	Reproducibility (n)	Number of Grafted Molecules Per TiONt [1]
TiONts	190	2.6	18	10.2 (±1.5) OH	10	–
TiONts-APTES	175	6.3	58	2.6 (±0.2) NH$_2$	9	14,230
TiONts-AuNPs	150	12.4	511	0.40 (±0.05) DTDTPA	7	2,200
TiONts-AuNPs-PEG$_{3000}$	150	16.1	3,073	0.040 (±0.003) PEG$_{3000}$	4	220
TiONts-AuNPs-PEG$_{3000}$-DTX	150	27.4	1,049	0.30 (±0.01) DTX-PMPI	2	1,700

[1] The number of grafted molecules per TiONt was estimated by means of geometrical calculation considering only the external surface of TiONts.

Then, DTDTPA-modified gold nanoparticles were coupled with TiONts-APTES by peptide bond formation. Peptide coupling was performed between one of DTDTPA's carboxyl groups present in Au@DTDTPA NPs and an amine function on the TiONts-APTES surface. These Au@DTDTPA NPs are composed of a gold core with a diameter around 2.6 nm and a multilayered organic shell with approximately 120 DTDTPA per nanoparticle according to the literature [52,62,64]. Thanks to TGA, the graft ratio of DTDTPA on AuNPs was evaluated as 5.7 DTDTPA.nm^{-2} (Figure S4). The relative mass loss (Au@DTDTPA NPs) was 50%, which led to molar ratio of 1:2.5 between DTDTPA and AuNPs, respectively. HAADF-STEM (high angle annular dark field scanning transmission electron microscopy) images highlighted the presence of gold nanoparticles on the nanotube surface and nowhere else on the grid, suggesting a good purification of ungrafted Au@DTDTPA NPs (Figure 3a,b). The grafting rate of gold nanoparticles on the TiONt surface was calculated and estimated between 20 and 40 AuNPs/TiONt using several techniques: STEM (via a STEM counting of about several hundred of nanotubes), TGA (the relative mass loss is due to DTDTPA molecules and was 0.40 (±0.05) DTDTPA.nm^{-2} of TiONts; Table 1), and a dosage via ICP (inductively coupled plasma). Then, comparing HAADF-STEM images before (Figure 3c,d) and after (Figure 3e,f) reflected the grafting step of PEG$_{3000}$ on TiONts-AuNPs.

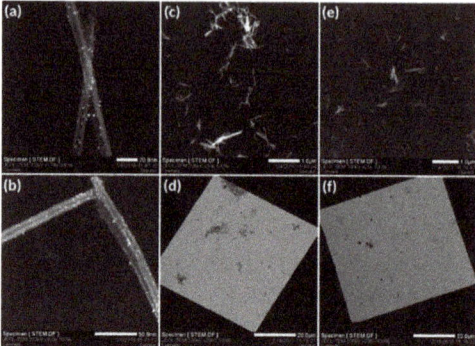

Figure 3. HAADF-STEM (high angle annular dark field scanning transmission electron microscopy) images showing (**a**,**b**) the grafting of Au@DTDTPA NPs on TiONts-APTES and the evolution of TiONts dispersion state (**c**,**d**) before (TiONts-AuNPs) and (**e**,**f**) after PEG$_{3000}$ grafting (TiONts-AuNPs-PEG$_{3000}$).

X-ray photoelectron spectroscopy (XPS) analyses were carried out to evaluate the chemical composition of the TiONts-AuNPs and TiONts-AuNPs-PEG$_{3000}$ surface (Figure 4 and Table 2).

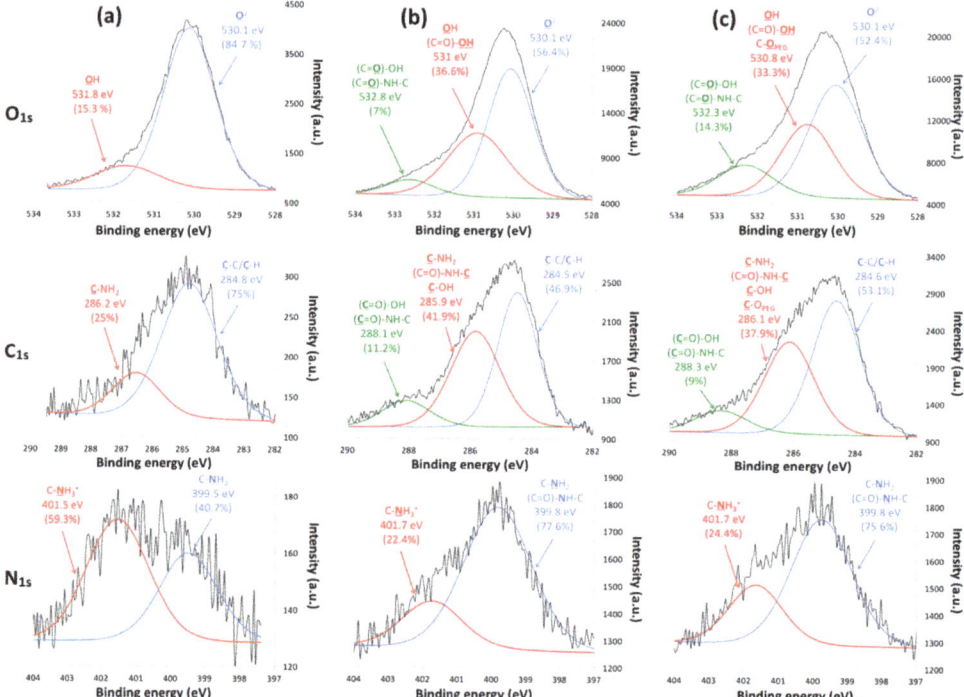

Figure 4. Fitted curves of O$_{1s}$, C$_{1s}$, and N$_{1s}$ peaks in XPS spectra for (**a**) TiONts-APTES, (**b**) TiONts-AuNPs, and (**c**) TiONts-AuNPs-PEG$_{3000}$.

Table 2. X-ray photoelectron spectroscopy (XPS) analyses: atomic concentration of bare TiONts, TiONts-APTES, TiONts-AuNPs, and TiONts-AuNPs-PEG$_{3000}$.

Atomic Concentration (%)	C_{1s}	O_{1s}	Na_{KLL}	Ti_{2p}	N_{1s}	Si_{2p}	Au_{4f}
TiONts	7.3	58.7	13.5	20.5	–	–	–
Elements (TiONts)/Ti (%)	0.3	2.9	0.7	1.0	–	–	–
TiONts-APTES	11.2	56.8	5.7	21.5	2.3	2.5	–
Elements (TiONts-APTES)/Ti (%)	0.5	2.6	0.3	1.0	0.1	0.1	–
TiONts-AuNPs	18.5	54.1	1.4	19.2	3.1	2.5	1.2
Elements (TiONts-AuNPs)/Ti (%)	1.0	2.8	0.1	1.0	0.2	0.1	0.1
TiONts-AuNPs-PEG$_{3000}$	23.8	52.1	0.5	17.5	2.9	2.0	1.2
Elements (TiONts-AuNPs-PEG$_{3000}$)/Ti (%)	1.4	3.0	≈ 0	1.0	0.2	0.1	0.1

FTIR spectroscopy was realized to confirm the effective coatings on TiONts (Figure 5a)—TiONts-APTES with the presence of amino-silane and the corresponding groups (Si-O-Si, C-C-NH$_2$, CH$_2$); TiONts-AuNPs following the grafting of gold nanoparticles onto TiONts by peptidic coupling ((C=O)-N-H formation as well as (C=O)-OH due to the DTDTPA coating of AuNPs); and finally PEG$_{3000}$ on TiONts-AuNPs-PEG$_{3000}$ with a new C-O$_{PEG}$ specific to the ethylene glycol repeat units. As far as surface modifications of TiONts are concerned, ζ-potential measurements were realized to evaluate changes in terms of isoelectric points (IEP) and potential values at the physiological pH (Figure 5b).

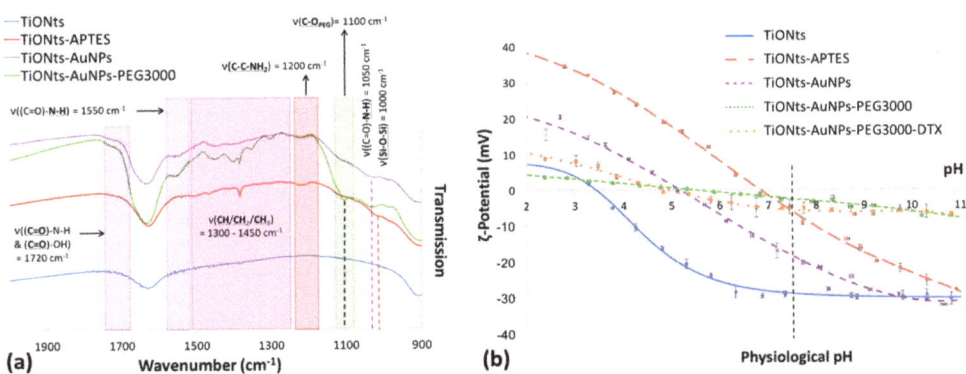

Figure 5. (a) FTIR spectra of TiONts, TiONts-APTES, TiONts-AuNPs, and TiONts-AuNPs-PEG$_{3000}$ between 2000–900 cm^{-1} and (b) ζ-potential curves of bare TiONts and different functionalized TiONts (the vertical dashed line corresponds to the physiological pH).

To study the colloidal stability of TiONts nanohybrids in physiological conditions (phosphate buffered saline (PBS) buffer, pH 7.4), tubidimetric studies were realized (Figure 6a) by comparing the decrease in absorbance over time at the wavelength of 600 nm. As expected, initial TiONts and simply modified TiONts-APTES exhibited the lowest stability compared to the further modifications of TiONts including AuNPs, PEG, and DTX, as can be seen also in the picture of the suspension of the final nanohybrids (Figure 6b).

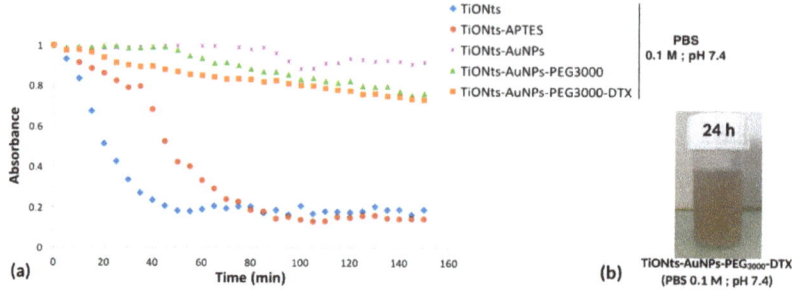

Figure 6. (a) Turbidimetric studies: colloidal stability of functionalized TiONt suspensions (phosphate buffered saline (PBS) 0.1 M; pH 7.4) over 150 min following their absorbance at 600 nm as a function of time. (b) Picture of a TiONts-AuNPs-PEG$_{3000}$-DTX suspension in PBS (0.1 M; pH 7.4) after 24 h.

MTS assays on a PC-3 human prostate cancer cell lines were performed to evaluate the cytotoxicity of DTX in the final nanohybrid (Figure 7a). Briefly, an increasing range of DTX (from 0.5 nM to 500 nM) was used to evaluate the cytotoxicity of free DTX and TiONts-AuNPs-PEG$_{3000}$-DTX. For a given DTX concentration, the committed quantity of TiONts-AuNPs-PEG$_{3000}$ (without DTX) (green curve) or Au@DTDTPA NPs (blue curve) corresponded to the quantity present on TiONts-AuNPs-PEG$_{3000}$-DTX (orange curve).

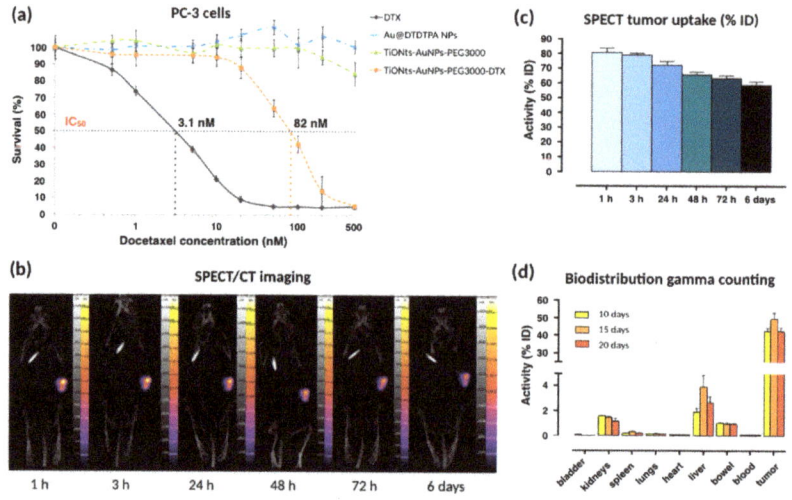

Figure 7. (a) Survival curves (3-(4,5-dimethylthiazol-2-yl)-5-(3-carboxymethoxyphenyl)-2-(4-ulfophenyl)-2H-tetrazolium (MTS) cytotoxicity assays) on PC-3 cell lines after incubation of DTX, Au@DTDTPA NPs, TiONts-AuNPs-PEG$_{3000}$, and TiONts-AuNPs-PEG$_{3000}$-DTX (mean ± SD). The studied range was from 0.5 to 500 nM in DTX concentration, which also corresponded to a concentration range of 4.1×10^{-3} to 4.1 µg.mL^{-1} for TiONts-AuNPs-PEG$_{3000}$ and 3×10^{-3} to 3 µg.mL^{-1} for Au@DTDTPA NPs, present on the TiONts-AuNPs-PEG$_{3000}$-DTX. The horizontal dotted line allows for an estimate of the different nanohybrids' IC$_{50}$. (b) Single photon emission computed tomography coupled with a conventional scanner (SPECT/CT) imaging of kinetics and (c) SPECT tumor uptake (mean value ± SD) achieved in Balb/c nude male mice after intratumoral (IT) injection of TiONts-AuNPs-PEG$_{3000}$-DTX-^{111}In at 1 h, 3 h, 24 h, 48 h, 72 h, and 6 days (as a function of ^{111}In injected activity (5.7–8.7 MBq) and corrected by ^{111}In radioactive decay). (d) TiONts-AuNPs-PEG$_{3000}$-DTX-^{111}In biodistribution in dissected organs (bladder, kidney, spleen, lung, heart, liver, bowel, blood, and tumor) by radioactivity detection using gamma counting 10, 15, and 20 days after IT injection (mean value ± SD).

The first in vivo biodistribution images, realized by SPECT coupled with a conventional scanner (SPECT/CT) after IT injection, showed that TiONts-AuNPs-PEG$_{3000}$-DTX rabiolabeled with ^{111}In were always retained within tumors six days after IT injection (Figure 7b). Moreover, from 24 h to 6 days, the remaining quantity of nanohybrids in tumors did not seem to decrease and proved the ability of the nanohybrid to maintain DTX and gold nanoparticles within tumors to increase their therapeutic efficacy, as more than 60% of the injected radiolabeled nanohybrids were still inside the tumor after 6 days (Figure 7c) and that there was therefore no release of the radiolabeled Au@DTDTPA (NPs)—they were still grafted to titanate nanotubes. Moreover, gamma counting confirmed these results because more than 42.5 ± 3.7% of nanohybrids were still kept inside tumors 20 days after IT injection (Figure 7d).

Finally, the therapeutic effects on TiONt nanohybrids were investigated by the study of tumor growth delay until a tumor volume of 1000 mm^3 was reached (Figure 8 and Figure S9) and in the presence or not of radiotherapy (RT). Differences were noted between treatments with or without RT and the final nanohybrids TiONts-AuNPs-PEG$_{3000}$-DTX associated with RT showed (i) the longest delay before tumor growth (over 55 days) and (ii) a significant difference in delay compared to similar nanohybrids without AuNPs (28% higher).

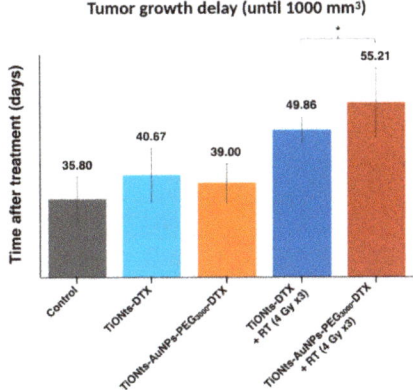

Figure 8. Therapeutic effect of control, TiONts-DTX, and TiONts-AuNPs-PEG$_{3000}$-DTX, associated or not with radiotherapy (RT) administered with three daily fractions of 4 Gy (3 groups, n = 6–7), after IT injection into PC-3 xenografted tumors. * p = 0.035 (TiONts-AuNPs-PEG$_{3000}$-DTX + RT vs. TiONts-DTX + RT); comparison performed using nonparametric Mann–Whitney test.

3. Discussion

The applied functionalization protocol with 3-aminopropyl triethoxysilane (APTES) tended to limit the multilayered formation of this molecule on the surface of TiONts [66,67]. Thus, the grafting ratio of APTES (2.6 NH$_2$.nm^{-2}) decreased significantly when compared to results available in the literature [39,43]. Moreover, TiONts-APTES enhanced tube individualization, as compared to bare nanotubes, for a suspension of equal concentration (Figure S1b,c). To some extent, a similar observation can be made on grafted AuNPs that did not seem to stick to each other and were relatively evenly distributed over the whole surface of TiONts.

From XPS analyses, gold was observed on TiONts-AuNPs and TiONts-AuNPs-PEG$_{3000}$, which was consistent with the presence of AuNPs (Table 2 and Figure S5). In addition, other atoms such as nitrogen and silicon corresponding to APTES or even chemical elements identical to those of bare TiONts (Ti, O, and Na) were found. Subsequently, the quantitative analysis revealed an increase in carbon and oxygen content for TiONts-AuNPs, in comparison to TiONts-APTES, consistent with the presence of DTDTPA on nanohybrid. Thereafter, increase of these same chemical elements also showed PEG$_{3000}$ grafting on TiONts-AuNPs-PEG$_{3000}$. A significant decrease for chemical elements such as Ti$_{2p}$, O$_{1s}$, and Na$_{KLL}$ was also observed, according to successive grafting. The decomposition of O$_{1s}$, C$_{1s}$, and N$_{1s}$ peaks in

XPS spectra highlighted the formation of secondary amide bonds, characteristic of AuNPs grafting on TiONts via peptide coupling (EDC/NHS) as well as carboxyl functions from DTDTPA (Figure 4a,b). These same peaks also suggested the evolution of components associated to PEG$_{3000}$ grafting via peptide coupling (PyBOP) on the remaining free amine functions, after covalent immobilization of Au@DTDTPA NPs (Figure 4c). Therefore, appearance of two new components was attributed to two types of bonds ((C=O)-NH-C and (C=O)-OH) concerning TiONts-AuNPs and TiONts-AuNPs-PEG$_{3000}$ samples compared to TiONts-APTES, one of which was located at 532.8 eV (7%) for the O$_{1s}$ peak and the other at 288.1 eV (11.2%) for the C$_{1s}$ peak [40,68]. Moreover, the O$_{1s}$ region of TiONts-AuNPs-PEG$_{3000}$ showed an increase for the component located at 532.3 eV, indicating a higher peptide coupling rate and more carboxyl functions (from 7% to 14.3% before and after PEG$_{3000}$ grafting, respectively). Moreover, other components may be also assigned to carboxyl groups ((O=C)-OH), such as those located at ≈531 eV (O$_{1s}$) and ≈286 eV (C$_{1s}$) [68]. These functions were responsible for the increase of these components in comparison to those observed at the same positions for TiONts-APTES—15.3% (O$_{1s}$) and 25% (C$_{1s}$), respectively. These analyses were consistent with what was observed for N$_{1s}$ peak for TiONts-AuNPs and TiONts-AuNPs-PEG$_{3000}$, due to the increase of the 399.8 eV component attributed to ((C=O)-NH-C) groups as well as C-NH$_2$ bonds at the expense of C-NH$_3^+$ (401.7 eV) with respect to the N$_{1S}$ region of TiONts-APTES [69]. With regards to TiONts-AuNPs-PEG$_{3000}$, the decomposition of C$_{1s}$ and the O$_{1s}$ threshold highlighted the grafting of the polymer. The component associated with C-C/C-H groups at 284.6 eV was more intense due to the PEGylated chains of PEG$_{3000}$ (from 46.9% to 53.1%). Regarding the contributions of the C-O$_{PEG}$ bond, they may be located at 530.8 eV (O$_{1s}$) and 286.1 eV (C$_{1s}$) [40,69].

FTIR spectroscopy confirmed the XPS results, thus showing the effective synthesis of TiONts-AuNPs and TiONts-AuNPs-PEG$_{3000}$ nanohybrids. Indeed, IR spectra show the appearance of new characteristic vibration bands in Figure 5a, corresponding to the formation of amide bonds located at 1050 and 1550 cm^{-1} ((C=O)-N-H) as well as 1720 cm^{-1} ((C=O)-N-H). Furthermore, IR analysis was consistent in that Au@DTDTPA NPs remained on the surface of TiONts even after last synthesis steps, with the persistence of functions attributed to (C=O)-N-H and (C=O)-OH of DTDTPA molecules (violet highlights on IR spectrum) [62]. This was corroborated by the HAADF-STEM images (Figure 3 and Figure S6). Moreover, the strong absorption band at 1100 cm^{-1} (C-O$_{PEG}$) was also observed (green highlights on IR spectrum) [47]. Finally, functions attributed to aliphatic carbon chains were increasingly intense due to the additional organic moieties after each grafting (APTES, Au@DTDTPA NPs, and PEG$_{3000}$) on TiONts, and were located between 1450 and 1300 cm^{-1}.

ζ-potential measurements indicated an isoelectric point (IEP) at pH 6.9 for TiONts-APTES. This value was higher than for bare TiONts (IEP 3.3) due to the coating of amine functions (Figure 5b). Therefore, the decrease in the number of amines partly engaged in Au@DTDTPA NPs coupling with TiONts-APTES and appearance of COO$^-$ groups from DTDTPA led to an IEP shifted downward to the lower pH value of 5.1 (violet curve). At pH 7.4, carboxylate functions significantly improved the ζ-potential, in absolute value, favoring the electrostatic repulsion—from −6 mV (TiONts-APTES) to −20 mV (TiONts-AuNPs). Nevertheless, a significant screening effect was observed concerning PEG$_{3000}$-functionalized TiONts (green curve) over the entire pH range studied (−2 mV at pH 7.4). These results were striking when compared to a previous study [43], thus suggesting that the steric effect mainly governs colloidal stability at physiological pH. The electrokinetic monitoring of TiONts-AuNPs-PEG$_{3000}$-DTX (orange curve) showed a less pronounced screening effect (−7 mV at pH 7.4), even if the evolution of ζ-potential measurements as a function of pH were very close to that of nanohybrid without DTX-PMPI. The strong screening effect was observed while the grafting of Au@DTDTPA NPs induced a less important grafting density of PEG$_{3000}$ on the surface of nanohybrid than without Au@DTDTPA NPs (0.04 PEG$_{3000}$.nm^{-2} for TiONts-AuNPs-PEG$_{3000}$ vs. 0.05 PEG$_{3000}$.nm^{-2} for TiONts-PEG$_{3000}$; Table 1) [43] due to the decrease in the number of free amines and steric hindrance. The lower coverage rate of polymer led to an area per chain of 25 nm^2 (the PEG$_{3000}$ radius of gyration is about 2.5 nm, which corresponded to a covering surface of 20 nm^2), indicating a mushroom conformation [70]. However, this calculation did not consider the TiONts surface already occupied by gold nanoparticles. Therefore, the polymer could also have been in brush conformation onto nanohybrid.

DTX was modified by *p*-maleimidophenyl isocyanate (PMPI) to obtain an adequate function for the combination with TiONts-AuNPs-PEG$_{3000}$. The reaction between PMPI and thiol groups was expected at pH 7.4 in PBS, as maleimide reacts specifically with thiol in a pH range from 6.5 to 7.5 (Figure S7), whereas the reaction was possible both with thiol and amine functions above a pH of 7.5. The functionalization of TiONts-AuNPs-PEG$_{3000}$ with DTX-PMPI was observed by TGA. The relative mass loss of final nanohybrids was greater than that of TiONts-AuNPs-PEG$_{3000}$, revealing the immobilization of therapeutic agent (DTX) on the surface of TiONts (Figure 2). The grafting ratio was estimated to 0.30 DTX-PMPI.nm^{-2} (Table 1) and higher than previously reported (0.20 DTX-PMPI.nm^{-2}) [43]. Indeed, thiol functions brought both by DTDTPA and PEG$_{3000}$ could react with the maleimide group of DTX-PMPI in PBS (0.1 M; pH 7.4). However, despite repeated purifications, it cannot be excluded that DTX-PMPI clung/adsorbed to amine groups of APTES not functionalized by Au@DTDTPA NPs in the cavity of nanotubes and/or was trapped within PEGylated chains (Figure S8). Consequently, this enhancement of DTX quantity could increase the therapeutic effect of nanohybrid on tumor cells in addition to AuNPs.

Functionalization with Au@DTDTPA NPs and PEG$_{3000}$ enhanced tube individualization as compared to bare nanotubes at similar concentration (Figure 3c–f). Even if the graft ratio of PEG$_{3000}$ was low, their presence seemed to limit nanohybrids agglomeration, comparing their dispersion with the STEM images of TiONts-AuNPs. The hypothesis, shown above, concerning the conformation of PEG$_{3000}$ on the surface of TiONts (polymer brush conformation), could then be confirmed.

Colloidal stability of different functionalized TiONt suspensions was also investigated under physiological conditions (PBS 0.1 M; pH 7.4) by turbidimetric analyses (Figure 6a) and correlated with STEM images. Results demonstrated a very good colloidal stability of TiONts-AuNPs and TiONts-AuNPs-PEG$_{3000}$ in comparison with TiONts and TiONts-APTES. Indeed, the measured absorbance did not significantly change after 150 min for AuNP-functionalized TiONts. The grafting of DTX-PMPI on the surface of TiONts-AuNPs-PEG$_{3000}$ also did not lead to any major change on the colloidal stability of the final nanohybrid in PBS. Thus, colloidal stability was dramatically improved at physiological pH and was largely sufficient over time to in vivo inject the nanohybrid after radiolabeling the DTDTPA by ^{111}In. Moreover, Figure 6b shows that brown TiONts-AuNPs-PEG$_{3000}$-DTX suspension was always stable after 24 h in PBS, proving the presence of gold nanoparticles (TiONts suspensions are white).

Initial results demonstrated that Au@DTDTPA NPs and TiONts-AuNPs-PEG$_{3000}$ did not exhibit any cytotoxicity in the studied range (either from 3×10^{-3} to 3 µg.mL^{-1} of Au@DTDTPA NPs and 4.1×10^{-3} to 4.1 µg.mL^{-1} of TiONts-AuNPs-PEG$_{3000}$), whereas unmodified DTX showed cytotoxicity (black curve), with a half-maximum inhibitory concentration (IC$_{50}$) of 3.1 nM, in agreement with results previously shown in literature [43,71]. TiONts-AuNPs-PEG$_{3000}$-DTX were still cytotoxic (IC$_{50}$: 82 nM) even though they were less toxic than free DTX. Nevertheless, the cytotoxic efficacy of the final nanohybrid was higher with gold nanoparticles than what was previously observed for TiONts-DTX (IC$_{50}$ = 360 nM), synthesized by Loiseau et al. [43]. Indeed, these nanohybrids being better dispersed and more stable in suspension have probably improved cell internalization by diffusion or endocytosis processes of current nanohybrids in sick cells [45] and led to a better access of DTX to microtubules. These achievements were very promising and allowed in vivo experiments on PC-3 xenografted tumors into Balb/c nude mice.

Twenty days after IT injection, a small amount of nanohybrids was found in other organs such as liver (2.4 ± 0.9%), kidney (1.2 ± 0.4%), lung (0.10 ± 0.01%), spleen (0.20 ± 0.05%), and bowel (0.90 ± 0.01%). Less than 0.1% of nanohybrids were detected in bladder, blood, and heart. The low quantities detected in different organs were correlated with the lack of toxicity shown during mice follow up, which lasted three months post-injection.

Using this in vivo approach, we observed that tumor volumes revealed a slight growth delay after IT injection in mice. Indeed, TiONts-DTX and TiONts-AuNPs-PEG$_{3000}$-DTX groups without radiotherapy (RT) reached a volume of 1000 mm^3 at a later time when compared with the control group (40.7 ± 5.4 days, 39 ± 4 days, and 35.8 ± 4.5 days, respectively) (Figure 8). This interesting effect may be explained by the retention of DTX within tumor cells by TiONt-based nanovectors improving therapeutic efficacy and preventing its diffusion throughout the body. Thus, these results are consistent with biodistribution analysis. Moreover, these observations have already been described in prior studies evaluating the efficacy of TiONts-DTX with and without RT, in comparison with groups receiving free DTX [43,44]. More importantly, we observed an improved therapeutic efficacy by combining TiONts-AuNPs-PEG$_{3000}$-DTX with RT. Indeed, tumor growth was significantly slowed by TiONts-AuNPs-PEG$_{3000}$-DTX associated with RT to reach a volume of 1000 mm^3 (55.2 ± 6.9 days), compared with TiONts-DTX with RT (49.9 ± 2.5 days) in the same conditions (p = 0.035). Thus, these results suggest that gold nanoparticles significantly improve the RT efficacy of nanohybrid even if the gold quantity injected (corresponding to 36.1 nmol of Au or 66.5 pmol of AuNPs and 15 µg of Au@DTDTPA/animal) was significantly less than the quantity used in previous publication on Au@DTDTPA NPs alone (160 µg of Au@DTDTPA/animal) [61], thus showing the synergistic effect of the association of TiONts and AuNPs nanohybrids fulfilling their role as carriers by concentrating the therapeutic and chelating agents within cancer cells.

4. Materials and Methods

4.1. Materials

Titanium dioxide (TiO$_2$) rutile precursor was purchased from Tioxide (Calais, France). Sodium hydroxide (NaOH), 3-aminopropyl triethoxysilane (APTES), ethanol, benzotriazole-1-yl-oxytripyrrolidinophosphonium hexafluorophosphate (PyBOP), N,N-diisopropylethylamine (DIEA), diethylenetriaminepentaacetic acid bis(anhydride) (DTPA-BA), tetrachloroauric acid trihydrate (HAuCl$_4$· 3H$_2$O), sodium borohydride (NaBH$_4$), acetic acid, methanol, dimethyl formamide (DMF), trimethylamine, and aminoethanethiol were acquired from Sigma-Aldrich (Saint-Quentin-Fallavier, France). A derivative of polyethylene glycol, named α-acid, ω-thiol-polyethylene glycol (HS-PEG$_{3000}$-COOH, MW = 3073 g.mol^{-1}), was purchased from Iris Biotech GmbH (Marktredwitz, Germany). N-hydroxysuccinimide (NHS), 1-ethyl-3-(dimethylaminopropyl) carbodiimide hydrochloride (EDC), p-maleimidophenyl isocyanate (PMPI), and tris(2-carboxyethyl)-phosphine hydrochloride (TCEP) were obtained from Thermo Scientific (Illkirch, France). Docetaxel (DTX) was purchased from BIOTREND Chemikalien GmbH (Cologne, Germany). Borate buffered saline was prepared from boric acid (99.8%). Phosphate buffered saline (PBS) 1× solution (Fisher Bioreagents, Illkirch, France), dimethyl sulfoxide (DMSO extra dry, anhydrous 99.99%) (Acroseal), and hydrochloric acid (HCl) were also obtained from Fisher Chemicals (Illkirch, France). Only Milli-Q water (ρ = 18 MΩ cm) was used in the preparation of aqueous solutions and to rinse gold nanoparticles. The ultrafiltration cell (Model 8400, 400 mL) and membranes (regenerated cellulose) were purchased from Merck Millipore (Molsheim, France). Gold nanoparticles were filtered using a 0.22 µm pore diameter polymer membrane purchased from Osmonics Inc (Penang, Malaysia). All chemicals were used without further purification.

4.2. Preparation of Bare TiONts and Amine-Functionalized TiONts (TiONts-APTES)

Bare TiONts were synthesized by a hydrothermal method. A total of 1 g of precursor (titanium dioxide rutile) was ultrasonicated (30 min, 375 W, Sonics Vibra-Cells (Newton, CT, USA) in a NaOH aqueous solution (10 M, 250 mL). Subsequently, the mixture was transferred into a Teflon reactor with mechanical stirring and heating at 155 °C for 36 h. TiONts were washed by centrifugation (24,000 × g for 10 min), dialysis (Cellu·Sep tubular membranes of 12–14 kDa), and ultrafiltration (regenerated cellulose membranes with a molecular weight cut-off (MWCO) of 100 kDa) [30,31,43]. Subsequently, TiONts were functionalized with silane-coupling agent, presenting high reactivity with hydroxyl groups on the surface of material. Consequently, TiONts were modified with APTES (the molar ratio between hydroxyl functions of TiONts and APTES was 1:3) via hydrolysis and condensation in a solution of water and ethanol (50:50 v:v) under magnetic stirring at 60 °C for 5 h (TiONts-APTES) [39,47,67]. After the reaction, suspension was ultrafiltered (100 kDa) to eliminate the excess of APTES. Finally, the TiONts-APTES were freeze-dried.

4.3. Synthesis of Dithiolated Diethylenetriaminepentaacetic Acid (DTDTPA) and Functionalized Gold Nanoparticles Synthesis (Au@DTDTPA NPs)

The synthesis of Au@DTDTPA NPs was described by Alric et al. [52,63]. Briefly, 5.6×10^{-3} mol of dithiolated diethylenetriaminepentaacetic acid bis(anhydride) (DTPA-BA) was dissolved in DMF and heated to 70 °C. Then, 1.23×10^{-2} mol of aminoethanethiol was dissolved in DMF and 1.74 mL of triethylamine. This solution was added and mixture was stirred magnetically at 70 °C overnight. Subsequently, the solution was cooled to 25 °C and placed in an ice bath. A white powder (NEt$_3$·HCl) was seen to precipitate out and was filtered. After filtration, chloroform washing, and drying under vacuum, DTDTPA was obtained as a white powder.

Gold nanoparticles were synthesized adapting Brust's protocol in the presence of DTDTPA to control size and colloidal stability [72]. In a typical preparation of gold nanoparticles, 5.1×10^{-5} mol of HAuCl$_4$·3H$_2$O was dissolved in methanol and mixed with 9.4×10^{-5} mol of DTDTPA in water, and acetic acid was added to the gold salt solution while continuously stirring the mixture. After 5 min, 5×10^{-5} mol of NaBH$_4$ dissolved in water was added to the orange mixture under vigorous stirring at 25 °C for 1 h, before adding HCl solution. After partial removal of the solvent under reduced pressure at a maximum temperature of 40 °C, the precipitate was filtered. The resulting black powder (Au@DTDTPA NPs) was dried and either stored as a solid or dispersed in 10 mL of 0.01 M NaOH solution.

4.4. AuNP-Coated TiONt (TiONts-AuNPs) Synthesis

TiONts-APTES were mixed with Au@DTDTPA NPs in 40 mL of phosphate buffered saline (0.1 M; pH 7.4). A large excess of EDC and NHS were added beforehand on water (pH 5), to activate the carboxylate functions of the DTDTPA on the surface of AuNPs, during 90 min under magnetic stirring. The molar ratio between amines on the surface of the TiONts-APTES and the carboxylate functions of the DTDTPA was 1:0.6. The reaction took place under magnetic stirring for 24 h. Then, TiONts-AuNPs were washed by ultrafiltration (500 kDa) and freeze-dried. Elimination of non-grafted AuNPs was optimized by UV-control of washing waters.

4.5. Grafting of Polyethylene Glycol (PEG$_{3000}$) on TiONts-AuNPs

Heterobifunctional polymers HS-PEG$_{3000}$-COOH were activated with PyBOP in a molar ratio of 1:1. The reaction took place in DMSO in the presence of the organic base DIEA (excess) under magnetic stirring and nitrogen flow for 30 min. TiONts-AuNPs were dispersed in DMSO and added to activation solution for 24 h under magnetic stirring and nitrogen flow at 25 °C. Polymers were grafted on the remaining amine functions of APTES. The molar ratio was 1:1 between amine functions (initially present on TiONts-APTES even if gold nanoparticles were present) and polymers. Finally, the product (TiONts-AuNPs-PEG$_{3000}$) was washed by centrifugation (20,000 × g for 20 min), then purified by ultrafiltration (500 kDa) and freeze-dried.

4.6. Activation and Grafting of the Therapeutic Agent: DTX

Activation and grafting of the therapeutic agent have been described by Loiseau et al. [43]. First, DTX and PMPI (DTX-PMP) were dissolved in DMSO and then added in borate buffered saline. The molar ratio was 1:4, respectively, under magnetic stirring at 25 °C for 24 h. The solution of DTX-PMPI was dialyzed (0.5–1 kDa) and freeze-dried to obtain a yellowish powder. TiONts-AuNPs-PEG$_{3000}$-DTX were synthesized from TiONts-AuNPs-PEG$_{3000}$ and DTX-PMPI (large excess) using TCEP in PBS

(0.1 M; pH 7.4). The mixture was homogenized beforehand in an ultrasonic bath and placed under magnetic stirring for 24 h at 25 °C. TiONts-AuNPs-PEG$_{3000}$-DTX were dialyzed, ultrafiltered (500 kDa), and freeze-dried.

4.7. Characterization Techniques of Nanohybrids

4.7.1. Thermogravimetric Analysis (TGA)

The amount of the molecules on the surface of the TiONts after each grafting step was determined by TGA (TA instrument, Discovery TGA (New Castle, DE, USA)). An air flow rate of 25 mL.min^{-1} and a temperature ramp of 10 °C.min^{-1} from 50 to 800 °C were used for measurements.

4.7.2. Surface Area Measurements

Specific surface area measurements were carried out using a Micromeritics Tristar II apparatus. Samples were outgassed in situ under 20 mTorr pressure for 16 h at 100 °C. Brunauer–Emmett–Teller (BET) method (S$_{BET}$) was used in the calculation of specific surface area value from N$_2$ gas adsorption.

4.7.3. Transmission Electron Microscopy (TEM)

Nanotube morphology and agglomeration state characterization were carried out with a JEOL JEM-2100F, operating at an accelerating voltage of 200 kV and fitted with an ultra-high pole-piece achieving a point-to-point resolution of 0.19 nm. HAADF-STEM micrographs of AuNP-loaded TiONts were taken on this instrument, equipped with a field emission gun (FEG) type cathode. Samples were prepared by dropping a dilute suspension of powders onto the carbon-coated copper grids.

4.7.4. Inductively Coupled Plasma (ICP) Spectroscopy

Determination of titanium and gold contents in final nanohybrids was performed by ICP coupled to mass spectrometry (ICP-MS) analysis (ThermoScientific iCAP 6000 series ICP Spectrometer (Waltham, MA, USA)). A total of 2 mg of final nanohybrids were dissolved in aqua regia at 40 °C. The resulting solutions were diluted in HNO$_3$ for analysis.

4.7.5. X-ray Photoelectron Spectroscopy (XPS)

XPS measurements were collected with a PHI 5000 Versaprobe apparatus from a monochromatic Al Kα_1 radiation (EKα_1 (Al) = 1486.7 eV with a 200 µm diameter spot size, accelerating voltage of 12 kV, and power of 200 W). Powders were deposited on an indium sheet and then pressed. A Shirley background was subtracted and Gauss (70%)–Lorentz (30%) profiles were applied. Data analysis and curve fittings were realized with CasaXPS processing, and MultiPak software was employed for quantitative analysis. Neutralization process was used to minimize charge effects. Titanium 2p peak (458.7 eV) was used as a reference and allowed the correction of charge effects. The resolution was 2.0 eV for global spectra and 1.3 eV for windows corresponding to selected lines.

4.7.6. Fourier Transformed Infrared (FTIR) Spectroscopy

FTIR spectra were recorded on a Bruker Vertex 70v using OPUS version 3.1. using the KBr method, in which the pellets were made by mixing 2 mg of sample within 198 mg of dried KBr.

4.7.7. ζ-Potential Measurements

A Malvern Nano ZS instrument supplied by DTS Nano V7.11 software was used to determine zeta potentials of nanoparticle suspensions. pH titrations were performed using aqueous solutions of HCl (0.1 M), NaOH (0.1 M), or NaOH (0.01 M) to adjust the pH from 3 to 11. Before each measurement, suspension was prepared in aqueous NaCl solution (10^{-2} M) and sonicated for 10 min.

4.7.8. UV-Visible

Shimadzu UV-2550 was used to measure UV-visible absorbance at 600 nm. Turbidimetric studies of nanoparticle suspensions were made in PBS (0.1 M; pH 7.4) at 25 °C (one measurement/5 min).

4.8. Radiolabeling with Indium-111

For in vivo biodistribution studies, DTDTPA molecules grafted on the nanohybrid were labeled using indium-111 radionuclide (^{111}In radioactivity half-life $t_{1/2}$ = 67.9 h) [73]. The preparation of ^{111}In-labelled nanohybrids was performed by adding ^{111}In chloride to TiONts-AuNPs-PEG$_{3000}$-DTX in ammonium acetate buffer. Briefly, 386 MBq of ^{111}InCl$_3$ in 0.05 M HCl (500 µL) were mixed with 50 µL of 1 M AcONH$_4$ pH 7.07 and 450 µL of 0.1 M AcONH$_4$ pH 5.8, and 2 mg of TiONts-AuNPs-PEG$_{3000}$-DTX was then added. The resulting mixture (pH 5) was stirred overnight (16 h) at 37 °C in a Thermomixer. Instant thin layer chromatography (ITLC) was performed to determine the radiolabeling yield and to assess the absence of free ^{111}In. A total of 1 µL of the nanohybrids mixture was spotted on the ITLC-silica gel (SG) strip, which was subsequently eluted with sodium citrate 0.1 M pH 5, and the strip was then analyzed using an AR-2000 radiochromatograph (Eckert and Ziegler, Berlin, Germany; Rf = 0 for radiolabeled nanoparticles whereas Rf = 1 for small ^{111}In-AcO). At the end of incubation, suspension was centrifuged (13,000 × g, 15 min) and supernatant was discarded. The radiolabeled nanohybrids were then suspended in saline prior to injection.

4.9. Cells and Animals

Human PC-3 prostate adenocarcinoma cells (ATCC, Manassas, VA, USA) were cultured in Dulbecco's modified Eagle medium (DMEM) with 10% fetal serum calf (Dutscher, France) at 37 °C, 5% CO$_2$, and 95% humidity.

Two days prior to mice injection with cancer cells, whole-body irradiation was performed with a γ-source (2 Gy, 60Co, BioMep, Bretenières, France). The injection unit included 10 × 106 PC-3 cells in 200 µL serum-free culture medium containing Matrigel (50:50, $V:V$, BD Biosciences). Injection was performed subcutaneously on the right flank of immunosuppressed athymic Balb/c nude male mice which were at least six weeks of age (Charles River, L'Arbresles, France). All mice were housed in our approved animal facility (Centre Georges–François Leclerc, Dijon, France) and all experiments followed the guidelines of the Federation of European Animal Science Associations. All animal studies were conducted in accordance with the European legislation on the use of laboratory animals (directive 2010/63/EU) and approved by accredited ethical committee of the Grand Campus (Dijon, France). The Ministry project agreement numbers are #13968 (for radiotherapy experiments) and #7830 (for imaging experiments), and the ethical committee agreement number is 105, with the official name "C2ea Grand Campus".

4.10. Treatments

Mice were randomized 20 days post cancer cells injection. To distribute mice among the different treatment groups, a randomization was performed. The aim was to obtain an equivalent average tumor volume (TV) in each treatment group (about 200 mm^3). Before and during irradiation, each mouse was anesthetized with 2.5% isoflurane mixed with oxygen (MINERVE system, Esternay, France).

One hour before the first RT fraction, NPs were delivered intratumorally (50 µL, 1.87 µg/µL for TiONts-DTX and 2 µg/µL for TiONts-AuNPs-PEG$_{3000}$-DTX, in order to have the same DTX concentration in both cases). Radiotherapy was delivered using three daily fractions of 4 Gy by a small animal irradiator (SARRP, Xstrahl, United Kingdom), with 225 kV energy X-ray photons and a dose rate of 3.1 Gy/min. For each RT session, an anterior field and a posterior field were used to irradiate the tumor in a targeted way with a homogeneous dose.

4.11. In Vitro Evaluation of Nanohybrid Cytotoxicity

To evaluate the cytotoxic activity of DTX on the surface of nanohybrids, androgen-independent PC-3 prostate cancer cells were seeded in 96-well plates at a concentration of 3000 cells/well and incubated at 37 °C in 190 µL of drug-free culture medium (DMEM) with 10% fetal bovine serum (FBS) for 24 h before treatment (when the cells were at around 20% confluence). Cytotoxicity assays were performed with four samples at each concentration of free DTX (positive control), Au@DTDTPA NPs, TiONts-AuNPs-PEG$_{3000}$, or TiONts-AuNPs-PEG$_{3000}$-DTX. Tumor cells were incubated (+10 µL of drug in 190 µL of culture medium) with a range of equivalent DTX concentrations from 0.5 to 500 nM (100 nM of DTX corresponds to 0.2 µg of nanohybrids per well from TGA, i.e., a nanohybrid concentration of 1.0 µg.mL^{-1}). After 96 h of incubation, cell viability was evaluated using MTS assay (Promega Corporation, Madison, WI, USA) according to Mirjolet et al. [44,45,74]. Results were expressed as relative absorption at 490 nm relative to the untreated control.

4.12. Analysis of TiONts-AuNPs-PEG$_{3000}$-DTX Biodistribution

Because the organic shell of Au@DTDTPA NPs ensures the immobilization of ^{111}In ions (due to the chelating properties of DTDTPA) [64], TiONts-AuNPS-PEG$_{3000}$-DTX can be radiolabeled. The location of these hybrid nanostructures can therefore be monitored by SPECT. After mice in vivo injection, TiONts were tracked using a NanoSPECT/CT small animal imaging tomographic gamma-camera (Bioscan Inc., Poway, CA, USA). TiONts-AuNPs-PEG$_{3000}$-DTX-^{111}In (50 µL, 40–60 µg; 5.7–8.7 MBq of activity) were injected into nine subcutaneous PC-3 human prostate tumor-bearing mice. In vivo biodistribution at 1 h, 3 h, 24 h, 48 h, 72 h, and 6 days after injection was analyzed using SPECT/CT imaging. Then, 10 days post-injection, the 3 imaged animals were sacrificed, and 15 days and 20 days after injection the other mice (three animals per group) were also sacrificed. Tumor, blood, lung, liver, kidney, spleen, bladder, bowel, and heart of each mouse were collected and radioactivity in these samples was measured using a gamma counter (Wizard 1480, Perkin Elmer, Waltham, MA, USA).

4.13. Evaluation of the Radiotherapeutic Efficacy of TiONts-DTX and TiONts-AuNPs-PEG$_{3000}$-DTX

To evaluate the benefit of nanohybrids, tumors were treated with an intratumoral injection of a 50 µL TiONts-DTX or TiONts-AuNPs-PEG$_{3000}$-DTX suspension (containing 10.5 nmol of DTX grafted onto 93.5 µg of TiONts-DTX and 100 µg of TiONts-AuNPs-PEG$_{3000}$-DTX). The gold quantity injected present on TiONts-AuNPs-PEG$_{3000}$-DTX was 15 µg Au@DTDTPA/animal (corresponding to 36.1 nmol of Au or 66.5 pmol of 2.6-nm AuNPs). After induction of PC-3 tumors in mice and as soon as the tumors had reached a mean volume of approximately 200 mm^3, mice were randomized according to their individual tumor volume into three groups of 67 mice (control IT injection, TiONts-DTX, and TiONts-AuNPs-PEG$_{3000}$-DTX).

To evaluate the effectiveness of treatment, tumor growth was evaluated by the growth retardation parameter (time to reach a volume of 1000 mm^3). The TV was recorded three times a week using calipers and calculated according to the following formula: TV = thickness × width × length × 0.5. Each group included six or seven mice; numbers were calculated considering inter-mouse variability. Tumor growth delay was compared between mice groups using the nonparametric Mann–Whitney test.

5. Conclusions

The elaborated nanohybrid (TiONts-AuNPs-PEG$_{3000}$-DTX) was prepared using a step-by-step synthesis allowing for the precise characterization of each grafting step. A thorough characterization of the latter led to substantial results, showing the originality and innovation of the associations, particularly the AuNPs/TiONts combination. Grafting of gold nanoparticles, functionalized with DTDTPA, on the surface of TiONts-APTES was successful thanks to peptidic coupling. This pathway of grafting limited AuNP and TiONt agglomeration and ensured an even distribution of Au@DTDTPA NPs over the surface of TiONts. Moreover, gold nanoparticles provided nanohybrids with a remarkable colloidal stability under physiological conditions, improving in vitro and in vivo behavior for targeted biomedical applications. The significant amount of therapeutic agent (DTX) modified by PMPI on the TiONts surface showed that DTX-PMPI were covalently bound with thiol functions (from PEG$_{3000}$ and DTDTPA) but also via free amine groups (APTES) depending on the pH. Thus, this study confirmed the potent therapeutic effect of our final nanohybrid after DTX grafting onto the surface of nanotubes. In vitro biological assays (MTS) highlighted the cytotoxic activity of DTX present on the surface of TiONts-AuNPs-PEG$_{3000}$-DTX on human PC-3 prostate adenocarcinoma cells. Although nanohybrids' cytotoxicity was lower than that of DTX alone (IC$_{50}$ = 82 nM versus 3.1 nM, respectively), cytotoxic activity remained very high. These results proved a better access of TiONts-AuNPs-PEG$_{3000}$-DTX to microtubules compared to first generation TiONts-DTX (without Au@DTDTPA NPs) (IC$_{50}$ = 390 nM) [43], possibly suggesting a better internalization. This observation was not surprising, as new functionalized nanomaterial was better dispersed at physiological pH, and was thus more stable in suspension even though it exhibited a lower ζ-potential indicating a screening effect (the steric hindrance should prevail in this case). In addition, we successfully developed a safe nanocarrier of DTX to directly deliver this drug into prostate tumors (by IT injection), able to maintain it inside tumor cells for longer (at least 20 days, as demonstrated by biodistribution results in Balb/c nude mice), and to prevent its diffusion throughout the body, avoiding side effects. Therefore, the effectiveness of the selected therapeutic agent was improved. After combined IT injection with radiotherapy, TiONts-AuNPs-PEG$_{3000}$-DTX nanohybrid improved treatment efficacy by delaying tumor growth compared to the homologous nanohybrids without gold nanoparticles. Gold can increase the effect already demonstrated for TiONts-DTX [49,52]. Finally, these functionalized TiONts appear as promising versatile tools in the biomedical field to fight cancer, prostate cancer in particular.

Supplementary Materials: The following materials are available online at http://www.mdpi.com/2072-6694/11/12/1962/s1. Figure S1: Transmission electron microscopy (TEM) images show (**a**) the spiral morphology with an internal cavity of titanate nanotubes and (**b**,**c**) the evolution of TiONt dispersion before and after APTES grafting, respectively, Figure S2: Theoretical calculation of the hydroxyl rates on bare TiONts, Figure S3: Theoretical calculation for functionalized TiONt rate of grafting, Figure S4: TGA and derivative curves of Au@DTDTPA NPs under air atmosphere, Figure S5: (**a**) Ti$_{2p}$ and (**b**) Au$_{4f}$ peaks in XPS spectra for TiONts-AuNPs, Figure S6: HAADF-STEM images of TiONts-AuNPs-PEG$_{3000}$, Figure S7: (**a**) Maleimide reacts specifically with a thiol function at pH <7.5 and (**b**) loses its specificity to react either with a thiol function or with amine function at pH >7.5, Figure S8: (**a**) Polymer (Boc-NH-PEG$_{3000}$-COOH; MW = 3,173 g.mol^{-1}) having an inactive function (Boc) and carboxyl function to react with an amine group via peptide coupling and (**b**) TGA curves showing the adsorption of DTX-PMPI upon contact between TiONts-PEG$_{3000}$-Boc and DTX-PMPI (TiONts-DTX were washed by dialysis and ultrafiltration (100 kDa)), Figure S9: Therapeutic effect as function of time of control, TiONts-PEG$_{3000}$-DTX, and TiONts-AuNPs-PEG$_{3000}$-DTX, associated or not with radiotherapy (RT) with three daily fractions of 4 Gy, 24 h after injection into PC-3 xenografted tumors (n = 6, 7).

Author Contributions: Conceptualization, N.M., J.B., S.R. and C.M. initiated, N.M. and C.M. directed the project and N.M. and C.M. contributed equally in this work; A.L., S.R. and J.B. designed the chemical experiments; A.L. performed the synthesis and characterization of nanohybrids; C.M. managed all biological experiments; A.O., M.M., and R.B. performed the ^{111}In-labelling of nanohybrids and biodistribution analysis; C.M. performed in vitro tests and evaluation of radiotherapeutic effect; R.C. investigated TEM and HAADF-STEM images; N.M.S. and S.R. provided samples of DTDTPA-modified gold nanoparticles. A.L. wrote the manuscript; J.B., C.M., and N.M. supervised and corrected the paper. All authors contributed to the final manuscript.

Funding: This work was supported by the Cancéropôle Est through the call "Emergence 2015" (Région Bourgogne Franche Comté). This work is also part of the project "Nano2Bio", funded by the "Université de Bourgogne" and the "Conseil Régional de Bourgogne" through the "Plan d'Actions Régional pour l'Innovation (PARI)", the European Union through the PO FEDER-FSE Bourgogne 2014/2020 programs and this work has been supported by the EIPHI Graduate School (contract "ANR-17-EURE-0002").

Acknowledgments: The authors would like to thank Olivier Heintz (ICB) for XPS measurements; Fadoua Sallem (ICB) for preparation; Myriam Heydel (Sayens) for ICP measurements; and Véronique Morgand (CGFL), Camille Drouet (CGFL), and Mélanie Guillemin (CGFL) for their help during in vitro and in vivo assays. This work was performed within a regional center of excellence in pharmaco-imaging (Pharmimage GIE, Pharmaco-imaging "groupement d'intérêt scientifique" (GIS). Finally, the authors also thank Isabel Gregoire (CGFL) for editorial assistance.

Conflicts of Interest: The authors declare no conflict of interest.

References

1. Shevchenko, E.V.; Talapin, D.V.; Murray, C.B.; O'Brien, S. Structural Characterization of Self-Assembled Multifunctional Binary Nanoparticle Superlattices. *J. Am. Chem. Soc.* **2006**, *128*, 3620–3637. [CrossRef]
2. Rawla, P. Epidemiology of Prostate Cancer. *World J. Oncol.* **2019**, *10*, 63–89. [CrossRef]
3. National Cancer Institute. Available online: http://seer.cancer.gov/statfacts/html/prost.html (accessed on 10 October 2019).
4. Ferlay, J.; Colombet, M.; Soerjomataram, I.; Dyba, T.; Randi, G.; Bettio, M.; Gavin, A.; Visser, O.; Bray, F. Cancer incidence and mortality patterns in Europe: Estimates for 40 countries and 25 major cancers in 2018. *Eur. J. Cancer* **2018**, *103*, 356–387. [CrossRef]
5. Kuroda, K.; Liu, H.; Kim, S.; Guo, M.; Navarro, V.; Bander, N.H. Docetaxel down-regulates the expression of androgen receptor and prostate-specific antigen but not prostate-specific membrane antigen in prostate cancer cell lines: Implications for PSA surrogacy. *Prostate* **2009**, *69*, 1579–1585. [CrossRef]
6. Armstrong, C.M.; Gao, A.C. Drug resistance in castration resistant prostate cancer: Resistance mechanisms and emerging treatment strategies. *Am. J. Clin. Exp. Urol.* **2015**, *3*, 64–76.
7. Galsky, M.D.; Vogelzang, N.J. Docetaxel-based combination therapy for castration-resistant prostate cancer. *Ann. Oncol.* **2010**, *21*, 2135–2144. [CrossRef]
8. Bolla, M.; Hannoun-Levi, J.M.; Ferrero, J.-M.; Maingon, P.; Buffet-Miny, J.; Bougnoux, A.; Bauer, J.; Descotes, J.-L.; Fourneret, P.; Jover, F.; et al. Concurrent and adjuvant docetaxel with three-dimensional conformal radiation therapy plus androgen deprivation for high-risk prostate cancer: Preliminary results of a multicentre phase II trial. *Radiother. Oncol.* **2010**, *97*, 312–317. [CrossRef]
9. Larsen, A.K.; Escargueil, A.E.; Skladanowski, A. Resistance mechanisms associated with altered intracellular distribution of anticancer agents. *Pharmacol. Ther.* **2000**, *85*, 217–229. [CrossRef]
10. Morgillo, F.; Lee, H.-Y. Resistance to epidermal growth factor receptor-targeted therapy. *Drug Resist. Update* **2005**, *8*, 298–310. [CrossRef]
11. Sahoo, S.K.; Parveen, S.; Panda, J.J. The present and future of nanotechnology in human health care. *Nanomedicine* **2007**, *3*, 20–31. [CrossRef]
12. Parveen, S.; Sahoo, S.K. Polymeric nanoparticles for cancer therapy. *J. Drug Target.* **2008**, *16*, 108–123. [CrossRef]
13. Parhi, P.; Mohanty, C.; Sahoo, S.K. Nanotechnology-based combinational drug delivery: An emerging approach for cancer therapy. *Drug Discov. Today* **2012**, *17*, 1044–1052. [CrossRef]
14. Lammers, T.; Kiessling, F.; Hennink, W.E.; Storm, G. Nanotheranostics and image-guided drug delivery: Current concepts and future directions. *Mol. Pharm.* **2010**, *7*, 1899–1912. [CrossRef]
15. Muthu, M.S.; Leong, D.T.; Mei, L.; Feng, S.-S. Nanotheranostics—Application and Further Development of Nanomedicine Strategies for Advanced Theranostics. *Theranostics* **2014**, *4*, 660–677. [CrossRef]
16. Maeda, H. The enhanced permeability and retention (EPR) effect in tumor vasculature: The key role of tumor-selective macromolecular drug targeting. *Adv. Enzyme Regul.* **2001**, *41*, 189–207. [CrossRef]
17. Allen, T.M. Ligand-targeted therapeutics in anticancer therapy. *Nat. Rev. Cancer* **2002**, *2*, 750–763. [CrossRef]
18. Cho, K.; Wang, X.; Nie, S.; Shin, D.M. Therapeutic nanoparticles for drug delivery in cancer. *Clin. Cancer Res.* **2008**, *14*, 1310–1316. [CrossRef]
19. Sun, T.; Zhang, Y.S.; Pang, B.; Hyun, D.C.; Yang, M.; Xia, Y. Engineered Nanoparticles for Drug Delivery in Cancer Therapy. *Angew. Chem. Int. Ed.* **2014**, *53*, 12320–12364. [CrossRef]
20. McDevitt, M.R.; Chattopadhyay, D.; Kappel, B.J.; Jaggi, J.S.; Schiffman, S.R.; Antczak, C.; Njardarson, J.T.; Brentjens, R.; Scheinberg, D.A. Tumor targeting with antibody-functionalized, radiolabeled carbon nanotubes. *J. Nucl. Med.* **2007**, *48*, 1180–1189. [CrossRef]
21. Lazzara, G.; Cavallaro, G.; Panchal, A.; Fakhrullin, R.; Stavitskaya, A.; Vinokurov, V.; Lvov, Y. An assembly of organic-inorganic composites using halloysite clay nanotubes. *Curr. Opin. Colloid Interface Sci.* **2018**, *35*, 42–50. [CrossRef]
22. Ji, S.-R.; Liu, C.; Zhang, B.; Yang, F.; Xu, J.; Long, J.; Jin, C.; Fu, D.-L.; Ni, Q.-X.; Yu, X.-J. Carbon nanotubes in cancer diagnosis and therapy. *Biochim. Biophys. Acta Rev. Cancer* **2010**, *1806*, 29–35. [CrossRef]
23. Liu, Z.; Sun, X.; Nakayama-Ratchford, N.; Dai, H. Supramolecular Chemistry on Water-Soluble Carbon Nanotubes for Drug Loading and Delivery. *ACS Nano* **2007**, *1*, 50–56. [CrossRef]

24. Chen, J.; Chen, S.; Zhao, X.; Kuznetsova, L.V.; Wong, S.S.; Ojima, I. Functionalized Single-Walled Carbon Nanotubes as Rationally Designed Vehicles for Tumor-Targeted Drug Delivery. *J. Am. Chem. Soc.* **2008**, *130*, 16778–16785. [CrossRef]
25. Vaisman, L.; Wagner, H.D.; Marom, G. The role of surfactants in dispersion of carbon nanotubes. *Adv. Colloid Interface Sci.* **2006**, *128–130*, 37–46. [CrossRef]
26. Lvov, Y.M.; Shchukin, D.G.; Möhwald, H.; Price, R.R. Halloysite Clay Nanotubes for Controlled Release of Protective Agents. *ACS Nano* **2008**, *2*, 814–820. [CrossRef]
27. Vergaro, V.; Abdullayev, E.; Lvov, Y.M.; Zeitoun, A.; Cingolani, R.; Rinaldi, R.; Leporatti, S. Cytocompatibility and Uptake of Halloysite Clay Nanotubes. *Biomacromolecules* **2010**, *11*, 820–826. [CrossRef]
28. Tarasova, E.; Naumenko, E.; Rozhina, E.; Akhatova, F.; Fakhrullin, R. Cytocompatibility and uptake of polycations-modified halloysite clay nanotubes. *Appl. Clay Sci.* **2019**, *169*, 21–30. [CrossRef]
29. Bavykin, D.V.; Walsh, F.C. *Titanate and Titania Nanotubes: Synthesis, Properties and Applications*; Royal Society of Chemistry: Cambridge, UK, 2010; p. 154.
30. Papa, A.-L.; Millot, N.; Saviot, L.; Chassagnon, R.; Heintz, O. Effect of Reaction Parameters on Composition and Morphology of Titanate Nanomaterials. *J. Phys. Chem. C* **2009**, *113*, 12682–12689. [CrossRef]
31. Sallem, F.; Chassagnon, R.; Megriche, A.; El Maaoui, M.; Millot, N. Effect of mechanical stirring and temperature on dynamic hydrothermal synthesis of titanate nanotubes. *J. Alloys Compd.* **2017**, *722*, 785–796. [CrossRef]
32. Kasuga, T.; Hiramatsu, M.; Hoson, A.; Sekino, T.; Niihara, K. Formation of titanium oxide nanotube. *Langmuir* **1998**, *14*, 3160–3163. [CrossRef]
33. Fenyvesi, F.; Kónya, Z.; Rázga, Z.; Vecsernyés, M.; Kása, P.; Pintye-Hódi, K.; Bácskay, I. Investigation of the Cytotoxic Effects of Titanate Nanotubes on Caco-2 Cells. *AAPS PharmSciTech* **2014**, *15*, 858–861. [CrossRef]
34. Oh, S.-H.; Finõnes, R.R.; Daraio, C.; Chen, L.-H.; Jin, S. Growth of nano-scale hydroxyapatite using chemically treated titanium oxide nanotubes. *Biomaterials* **2005**, *26*, 4938–4943. [CrossRef]
35. Niu, L.; Shao, M.; Wang, S.; Lu, L.; Gao, H.; Wang, J. Titanate nanotubes: Preparation, characterization, and application in the detection of dopamine. *J. Mater. Sci.* **2008**, *43*, 1510–1514. [CrossRef]
36. Papa, A.L.; Dumont, L.; Vandroux, D.; Millot, N. Titanate nanotubes: Towards a novel and safer nanovector for cardiomyocytes. *Nanotoxicology* **2013**, *7*, 1131–1142. [CrossRef]
37. Niu, H.; Cai, Y. Preparation of amino-modified titanate nanotubes and its striking adsorption ability to duplex DNA. *J. Nanoparticle Res.* **2011**, *13*, 39–43. [CrossRef]
38. Papa, A.-L.; Maurizi, L.; Vandroux, D.; Walker, P.; Millot, N. Synthesis of Titanate Nanotubes Directly Coated with USPIO in Hydrothermal Conditions: A New Detectable Nanocarrier. *J. Phys. Chem. C* **2011**, *115*, 19012–19017. [CrossRef]
39. Paris, J.; Bernhard, Y.; Boudon, J.; Heintz, O.; Millot, N.; Decreau, R.A. Phthalocyanine-titanate nanotubes: A promising nanocarrier detectable by optical imaging in the so-called imaging window. *RSC Adv.* **2015**, *5*, 6315–6322. [CrossRef]
40. Sallem, F.; Boudon, J.; Heintz, O.; Severin, I.; Megriche, A.; Millot, N. Synthesis and characterization of chitosan-coated titanate nanotubes: Towards a new safe nanocarrier. *Dalton Trans.* **2017**, *46*, 15386–15398. [CrossRef]
41. Sruthi, S.; Loiseau, A.; Boudon, J.; Sallem, F.; Maurizi, L.; Mohanan, P.V.; Lizard, G.; Millot, N. In vitro interaction and biocompatibility of titanate nanotubes with microglial cells. *Toxicol. Appl. Pharmacol.* **2018**, *353*, 74–86. [CrossRef]
42. Baati, T.; Kefi, B.B.; Aouane, A.; Njim, L.; Chaspoul, F.; Heresanu, V.; Kerkeni, A.; Neffati, F.; Hammami, M. Biocompatible titanate nanotubes with high loading capacity of genistein: Cytotoxicity study and anti-migratory effect on U87-MG cancer cell lines. *RSC Adv.* **2016**, *6*, 101688–101696. [CrossRef]
43. Loiseau, A.; Boudon, J.; Mirjolet, C.; Crehange, G.; Millot, N. Taxane-Grafted Metal-Oxide Nanoparticles as a New Theranostic Tool against Cancer: The Promising Example of Docetaxel-Functionalized Titanate Nanotubes on Prostate Tumors. *Adv. Healthc. Mater.* **2017**, *6*, 1700245. [CrossRef] [PubMed]
44. Mirjolet, C.; Boudon, J.; Loiseau, A.; Chevrier, S.; Boidot, R.; Oudot, A.; Collin, B.; Martin, E.; Joy, P.A.; Millot, N. Docetaxel-titanate nanotubes enhance radiosensitivity in an androgen-independent prostate cancer model. *Int. J. Nanomed.* **2017**, *12*, 6357–6364. [CrossRef]

45. Mirjolet, C.; Papa, A.-L.; Créhange, G.; Raguin, O.; Seignez, C.; Paul, C.; Truc, G.; Maingon, P.; Millot, N. The radiosensitization effect of titanate nanotubes as a new tool in radiation therapy for glioblastoma: A proof-of-concept. *Radiother. Oncol.* **2013**, *108*, 136–142. [CrossRef] [PubMed]
46. Decuzzi, P.; Godin, B.; Tanaka, T.; Lee, S.Y.; Chiappini, C.; Liu, X.; Ferrari, M. Size and shape effects in the biodistribution of intravascularly injected particles. *J. Control. Release* **2010**, *141*, 320–327. [CrossRef] [PubMed]
47. Papa, A.-L.; Boudon, J.; Bellat, V.; Loiseau, A.; Bisht, H.; Sallem, F.; Chassagnon, R.; Berard, V.; Millot, N. Dispersion of titanate nanotubes for nanomedicine: Comparison of PEI and PEG nanohybrids. *Dalton Trans.* **2015**, *44*, 739–746. [CrossRef]
48. James, F.H.; Daniel, N.S.; Henry, M.S. The use of gold nanoparticles to enhance radiotherapy in mice. *Phys. Med. Biol.* **2004**, *49*, N309.
49. Schuemann, J.; Berbeco, R.; Chithrani, D.B.; Cho, S.H.; Kumar, R.; McMahon, S.J.; Sridhar, S.; Krishnan, S. Roadmap to Clinical Use of Gold Nanoparticles for Radiation Sensitization. *Int. J. Radiat. Oncol. Biol. Phys.* **2016**, *94*, 189–205. [CrossRef]
50. Subiel, A.; Ashmore, R.; Schettino, G. Standards and Methodologies for Characterizing Radiobiological Impact of High-Z Nanoparticles. *Theranostics* **2016**, *6*, 1651–1671. [CrossRef]
51. Chen, J.; Saeki, F.; Wiley, B.J.; Cang, H.; Cobb, M.J.; Li, Z.-Y.; Au, L.; Zhang, H.; Kimmey, M.B.; Li, X.; et al. Gold Nanocages: Bioconjugation and Their Potential Use as Optical Imaging Contrast Agents. *Nano Lett.* **2005**, *5*, 473–477. [CrossRef]
52. Alric, C.; Serduc, R.; Mandon, C.; Taleb, J.; Le Duc, G.; Le Meur-Herland, A.; Billotey, C.; Perriat, P.; Roux, S.; Tillement, O. Gold nanoparticles designed for combining dual modality imaging and radiotherapy. *Gold Bull.* **2008**, *41*, 90–97. [CrossRef]
53. Park, J.-A.; Kim, H.-K.; Kim, J.-H.; Jeong, S.-W.; Jung, J.-C.; Lee, G.-H.; Lee, J.; Chang, Y.; Kim, T.-J. Gold nanoparticles functionalized by gadolinium–DTPA conjugate of cysteine as a multimodal bioimaging agent. *Bioorg. Med. Chem. Lett.* **2010**, *20*, 2287–2291. [CrossRef] [PubMed]
54. Mieszawska, A.J.; Mulder, W.J.M.; Fayad, Z.A.; Cormode, D.P. Multifunctional Gold Nanoparticles for Diagnosis and Therapy of Disease. *Mol. Pharm.* **2013**, *10*, 831–847. [CrossRef] [PubMed]
55. Yang, P.-H.; Sun, X.; Chiu, J.-F.; Sun, H.; He, Q.-Y. Transferrin-Mediated Gold Nanoparticle Cellular Uptake. *Bioconjugate Chem.* **2005**, *16*, 494–496. [CrossRef]
56. Ghosh, P.; Han, G.; De, M.; Kim, C.K.; Rotello, V.M. Gold nanoparticles in delivery applications. *Adv. Drug Deliv. Rev.* **2008**, *60*, 1307–1315. [CrossRef]
57. Dykman, L.; Khlebtsov, N. Gold nanoparticles in biomedical applications: Recent advances and perspectives. *Chem. Soc. Rev.* **2012**, *41*. [CrossRef]
58. Figueiredo, S.; Cabral, R.; Luís, D.; Fernandes, A.R.; Baptista, P.V. Conjugation of Gold nanoparticles and liposomes for combined vehicles of drug delivery in cancer. *Nanomedicine* **2014**, *48*, 48–69.
59. Brun, E.; Sanche, L.; Sicard-Roselli, C. Parameters governing gold nanoparticle X-ray radiosensitization of DNA in solution. *Colloids Surf. B Biointerfaces* **2009**, *72*, 128–134. [CrossRef]
60. Miladi, I.; Alric, C.; Dufort, S.; Mowat, P.; Dutour, A.; Mandon, C.; Laurent, G.; Bräuer-Krisch, E.; Herath, N.; Coll, J.L.; et al. The In Vivo Radiosensitizing Effect of Gold Nanoparticles Based MRI Contrast Agents. *Small* **2014**, *10*, 1116–1124. [CrossRef]
61. Butterworth, K.T.; Nicol, J.R.; Ghita, M.; Rosa, S.; Chaudhary, P.; McGarry, C.K.; McCarthy, H.O.; Jimenez-Sanchez, G.; Bazzi, R.; Roux, S. Preclinical evaluation of gold-DTDTPA nanoparticles as theranostic agents in prostate cancer radiotherapy. *Nanomedicine* **2016**, *11*, 2035–2047. [CrossRef]
62. Debouttière, P.J.; Roux, S.; Vocanson, F.; Billotey, C.; Beuf, O.; Favre-Réguillon, A.; Lin, Y.; Pellet-Rostaing, S.; Lamartine, R.; Perriat, P.; et al. Design of Gold Nanoparticles for Magnetic Resonance Imaging. *Adv. Funct. Mater.* **2006**, *16*, 2330–2339. [CrossRef]
63. Alric, C.; Taleb, J.; Le Duc, G.; Mandon, C.; Billotey, C.; Le Meur-Herland, A.; Brochard, T.; Vocanson, F.; Janier, M.; Perriat, P.; et al. Gadolinium chelate coated gold nanoparticles as contrast agents for both X-ray computed tomography and magnetic resonance imaging. *J. Am. Chem. Soc.* **2008**, *130*, 5908–5915. [CrossRef] [PubMed]
64. Alric, C.; Miladi, I.; Kryza, D.; Taleb, J.; Lux, F.; Bazzi, R.; Billotey, C.; Janier, M.; Perriat, P.; Roux, S.; et al. The biodistribution of gold nanoparticles designed for renal clearance. *Nanoscale* **2013**, *5*, 5930–5939. [CrossRef] [PubMed]

65. Laprise-Pelletier, M.; Lagueux, J.; Côté, M.F.; LaGrange, T.; Fortin, M.A. Low-Dose Prostate Cancer Brachytherapy with Radioactive Palladium–Gold Nanoparticles. *Adv. Healthc. Mater.* **2017**, *6*, 1601120. [CrossRef] [PubMed]
66. Zhu, M.; Lerum, M.Z.; Chen, W. How to Prepare Reproducible, Homogeneous, and Hydrolytically Stable Aminosilane-Derived Layers on Silica. *Langmuir* **2012**, *28*, 416–423. [CrossRef] [PubMed]
67. Pontón, P.I.; d'Almeida, J.R.M.; Marinkovic, B.A.; Savić, S.M.; Mancic, L.; Rey, N.A.; Morgado, E.; Rizzo, F.C. The effects of the chemical composition of titanate nanotubes and solvent type on 3-aminopropyltriethoxysilane grafting efficiency. *Appl. Surf. Sci.* **2014**, *301*, 315–322. [CrossRef]
68. Thomas, G.; Demoisson, F.; Boudon, J.; Millot, N. Efficient functionalization of magnetite nanoparticles with phosphonate using a one-step continuous hydrothermal process. *Dalton Trans.* **2016**, *45*, 10821–10829. [CrossRef]
69. Rouxhet, P.G.; Genet, M.J. XPS analysis of bio-organic systems. *Surf. Interface Anal.* **2011**, *43*, 1453–1470. [CrossRef]
70. Perry, J.L.; Reuter, K.G.; Kai, M.P.; Herlihy, K.P.; Jones, S.W.; Luft, J.C.; Napier, M.; Bear, J.E.; DeSimone, J.M. PEGylated PRINT nanoparticles: The impact of PEG density on protein binding, macrophage association, biodistribution, and pharmacokinetics. *Nano Lett.* **2012**, *12*, 5304–5310. [CrossRef]
71. Wang, X.; Ma, D.; Olson, W.C.; Heston, W.D. In vitro and in vivo responses of advanced prostate tumors to PSMA ADC, an auristatin-conjugated antibody to prostate-specific membrane antigen. *Mol. Cancer Ther.* **2011**, *10*, 1728–1739. [CrossRef]
72. Brust, M.; Fink, J.; Bethell, D.; Schiffrin, D.J.; Kiely, C. Synthesis and reactions of functionalised gold nanoparticles. *J. Chem. Soc. Chem. Commun.* **1995**, 1655–1656. [CrossRef]
73. Lee, D.S.; Im, H.J.; Lee, Y.S. Radionanomedicine: Widened perspectives of molecular theragnosis. *Nanomedicine* **2015**, *11*, 795–810. [CrossRef] [PubMed]
74. Mirjolet, J.; Barberi-Heyob, M.; Merlin, J.; Marchal, S.; Etienne, M.; Milano, G.; Bey, P. Thymidylate synthase expression and activity: Relation to S-phase parameters and 5-fluorouracil sensitivity. *Br. J. Cancer* **1998**, *78*, 62–68. [CrossRef] [PubMed]

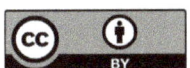

© 2019 by the authors. Licensee MDPI, Basel, Switzerland. This article is an open access article distributed under the terms and conditions of the Creative Commons Attribution (CC BY) license (http://creativecommons.org/licenses/by/4.0/).

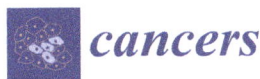

Article

Verteporfin-Loaded Lipid Nanoparticles Improve Ovarian Cancer Photodynamic Therapy In Vitro and In Vivo

Thierry Michy [1,2], Thibault Massias [1], Claire Bernard [1,2], Laetitia Vanwonterghem [1], Maxime Henry [1], Mélanie Guidetti [1], Guy Royal [3], Jean-Luc Coll [1], Isabelle Texier [4], Véronique Josserand [1,*,†] and Amandine Hurbin [1,*,†]

[1] Institute for Advanced Biosciences, Institut National de la Santé Et de la Recherche Médicale INSERM U1209, Centre National de la Recherche Scientifique CNRS UMR5309, Université Grenoble Alpes, F-38000 Grenoble, France; tmichy@chu-grenoble.fr (T.M.); thibault.massias@gmail.com (T.M.); claire.bernard95@laposte.net (C.B.); laetitia.vanwonterghem@univ-grenoble-alpes.fr (L.V.); maxime.henry@univ-grenoble-alpes.fr (M.H.); melanie.guidetti@univ-grenoble-alpes.fr (M.G.); jean-luc.coll@univ-grenoble-alpes.fr (J.-L.C.)
[2] Centre Hospitalier Universitaire CHU Grenoble Alpes, Université Grenoble Alpes, F-38000 Grenoble, France
[3] Centre National de la Recherche Scientifique CNRS UMR5250, Département de Chimie Moléculaire, Université Grenoble Alpes, F-38000 Grenoble, France; guy.royal@univ-grenoble-alpes.fr
[4] Commissariat à l'Energie Atomique et aux Energies Alternatives CEA, Laboratoire D'électronique et de Technologie de L'information, Département Technologies pour la Biologie et la Santé LETI-DTBS, Université Grenoble Alpes, F-38000 Grenoble, France; isabelle.texier-nogues@cea.fr
* Correspondence: veronique.josserand@univ-grenoble-alpes.fr (V.J.); amandine.hurbin@inserm.fr (A.H.); Tel.: +33-476-549-410 (V.J.); +33-476-549-553 (A.H.)
† These authors contributed equally.

Received: 17 September 2019; Accepted: 5 November 2019; Published: 8 November 2019

Abstract: Advanced ovarian cancer is the most lethal gynecological cancer, with a high rate of chemoresistance and relapse. Photodynamic therapy offers new prospects for ovarian cancer treatment, but current photosensitizers lack tumor specificity, resulting in low efficacy and significant side-effects. In the present work, the clinically approved photosensitizer verteporfin was encapsulated within nanostructured lipid carriers (NLC) for targeted photodynamic therapy of ovarian cancer. Cellular uptake and phototoxicity of free verteporfin and NLC-verteporfin were studied in vitro in human ovarian cancer cell lines cultured in 2D and 3D-spheroids, and biodistribution and photodynamic therapy were evaluated in vivo in mice. Both molecules were internalized in ovarian cancer cells and strongly inhibited tumor cells viability when exposed to laser light only. In vivo biodistribution and pharmacokinetic studies evidenced a long circulation time of NLC associated with efficient tumor uptake. Administration of 2 mg·kg^{-1} free verteporfin induced severe phototoxic adverse effects leading to the death of 5 out of 8 mice. In contrast, laser light exposure of tumors after intravenous administration of NLC-verteporfin (8 mg·kg^{-1}) significantly inhibited tumor growth without visible toxicity. NLC-verteporfin thus led to efficient verteporfin vectorization to the tumor site and protection from side-effects, providing promising therapeutic prospects for photodynamic therapy of cancer.

Keywords: photodynamic therapy; lipid nanoparticles; drug delivery system; tumor vectorization; verteporfin; ovarian carcinomatosis; spheroids

1. Introduction

Ovarian cancer accounts for about 4% of worldwide cancer incidence and is the most lethal gynecological cancer [1]. Seventy-five percent of ovarian cancer cases are detected in late stages, and the 5-year survival rate of patients in advanced-stages is barely 30% [2]. Due to its non-symptomatic advancement, high metastasis rate, and its resistance to chemotherapy, treatment of ovarian cancer constitutes a clinical challenge. Tumor growth and dissemination of ovarian cancer within the peritoneal cavity result in peritoneal carcinomatosis. Current treatments are based on tumor surgery combined with intravenous chemotherapy [2,3]. Unfortunately, most women with ovarian cancer relapse after the first-line therapy [2]. It is therefore critical to develop new approaches and treatment options to decrease the recurrence rate and to improve patient survival [2,3].

Photodynamic therapy (PDT) is an emerging and promising therapeutic modality for fighting cancer. PDT is based on the administration of a photosensitizer and its activation at the tumor site when exposed to light of a particular wavelength. The activated photosensitizer releases energy to generate highly toxic singlet oxygen ($^1O_2$) and reactive oxygen species (ROS). These products mediate microvascular damages, tumor cell toxicity, and anti-tumor immune responses [4–6]. PDT is used for the treatment of several cancers, in particular those that are accessible to laser light including skin, bladder, gastroesophageal, and lung cancers [4]. There are several photosensitizing agents currently approved by the US Food and Drug Administration. Among those, verteporfin (Visudyn®) is a second-generation photosensitizer approved for the PDT-based treatment of age related macular degeneration. It is now extensively studied as PDT agent for treatment of numerous cancer types [4,7–9]. Verteporfin is activated by near infrared (NIR) light (689 nm) that penetrates deeply into tissues and displays a very high yield of singlet oxygen production [7]. However, this photosensitizer lacks tumor specificity, resulting into adverse effects on healthy tissues and thus limiting its concentration of use [4,7,10]. Combining photosensitizing drugs with nanoparticles could overcome some of the limitations encountered with free photosensitizers [11–13], in particular because it is expected to increase their cellular uptake and passive accumulation into tumors due to the enhanced permeability and retention (EPR) effect [12,14]. Verteporfin loaded in mesoporous silica nanoparticles has been shown to inhibit the growth of melanoma cells in vitro [15], and in vivo in subcutaneous tumor bearing mice after topical administration and light exposure [16].

In the present study, verteporfin was encapsulated within nanostructured lipid carriers (NLC) for PDT of ovarian cancer after systemic administration. Lipid-based nanoparticles are used as drug nanocarriers because of their excellent biocompatibility, long circulation time, and high tumor accumulation due to the EPR effect [12,13,17–19]. The cell-uptake and phototoxicity of NLC-verteporfin were first assessed in vitro using 2D-monolayers and 3D-spheroids of human ovarian cancer cells. Biodistribution and pharmacokinetic studies of NLC-verteporfin were then evaluated in vivo after intravenous injection. Finally, the PDT efficacy of NLC-verteporfin was compared to free verteporfin in mice with ovarian cancer tumors. This study provides promising therapeutic prospects for PDT in ovarian cancer.

2. Results

2.1. Nanostructured Lipid Carriers Efficiently Encapsulate Verteporfin

NLC were used to encapsulate the photosensitizer verteporfin, or the NIR fluorophore Lipimage™815 as a drug delivery reporter. NLC formulation was performed as previously described [19], providing neutral nanoparticles with an hydrodynamic diameter of 47.9 ± 1.0 nm and a polydispersity index < 0.2 (Table 1). Verteporfin encapsulation yield in NLC was quantitative (>95%), with a final formulation payload of 943 µg of drug for 100 mg of lipids. This formulation was stable for at least 3 months (size variation < 10%, polydispersity index < 0.2), when stored at 4 °C in dark in water (concentration of ~100 mg·mL^{-1} of lipids) (Table 1).

Considering spectral properties, NLC-verteporfin displayed similar absorption profiles at 690 nm compared to free verteporfin in culture medium, in particular with an absorption peak at 690 nm (Figure S1a), and showed that verteporfin molecules were mainly in a monomeric form without aggregation inside the lipid core of the nanoparticles. The loading capability was also confirmed by comparable fluorescence emission signal intensity from verteporfin and NLC-verteporfin after excitation at 420 nm (Figure S1b).

Table 1. Physico-chemical and encapsulation properties of nanostructured lipid carriers (NLC).

Properties	NLC-Verteporfin		NLC-LipImage[TM]815
	T0	T0 + 3 Months	
Hydrodynamic diameter (nm) [a]	47.9 ± 1.0	54.4 ± 0.6	46.1 ± 0.7
Polydispersity index [a]	0.12 ± 0.02	0.18 ± 0.01	0.13 ± 0.01
Zeta potential (mV) [a]	−3.7 ± 0.9	−2.0 ± 1.3	−4.2 ± 4.3
Verteporfin (µg/mL) [b]	1026.2 ± 15.6	1037.5 ± 0.7	/
Verteporfin concentration (µM) [b]	1428	1443	/
LipImage[TM]815 concentration (µM)	/	/	302

[a] Dynamic Light Scattering DLC; [b] High Performance Liquid Chromatography HPLC.

2.2. Verteporfin and NLC-Verteporfin Bind and are Internalized in Ovarian Cancer Cells

The cellular uptake of verteporfin and NLC-verteporfin was evaluated in three different ovarian cancer cell lines, and was found to be slower for NLC-verteporfin than for free verteporfin. Indeed, flow cytometry analyses showed maximal binding of verteporfin in ovarian cancer cell lines SKOV3, IGROV1, and OVCAR3 after 2 h and 24 h incubation at 37 °C (Figure 1). In contrast, the binding of NLC-verteporfin was increased at 24 h compared to 2 h incubation in these cells. At 4 °C, the internalization process was inhibited for both verteporfin and NLC-verteporfin (Figure 1).

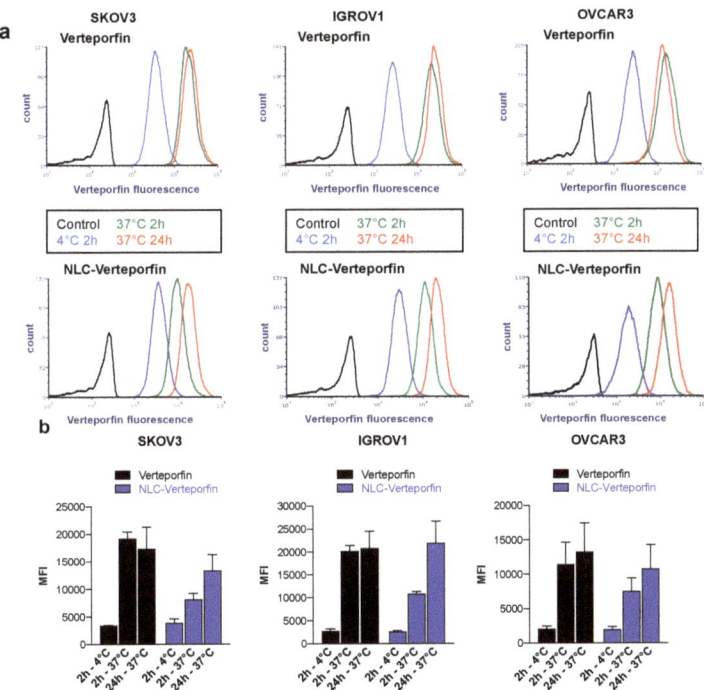

Figure 1. Verteporfin and NLC-verteporfin interact with ovarian cancer cells. Ovarian cancer SKOV3, IGROV1, and OVCAR3 cells were incubated with 1 µmol·L^{-1} verteporfin or NLC-verteporfin for 2 h or 24 h at 4 °C or 37 °C as indicated. (**a**) Histograms show cellular uptake assessed by flow cytometry. Black, control cells; blue, 4 °C for 2 h; green, 37 °C for 2 h; red, 37 °C for 24 h. (**b**) Median fluorescence intensity (MFI). Data are expressed as the mean ± standard deviation (SD) of three independent experiments.

Confocal microscopy showed that both verteporfin and NLC-verteporfin were mostly found in the cytoplasm of SKOV3 and OVCAR3 cells (Figure 2a and Figure S2), confirming their internalization in cells. In SKOV3 spheroids, which mimic solid tumors with appropriate cell–cell interactions as well as gradients of nutrients and oxygen [20], verteporfin, and NLC-verteporfin uptakes were observed in both at the periphery and at the center of the spheroids (Figure 2b).

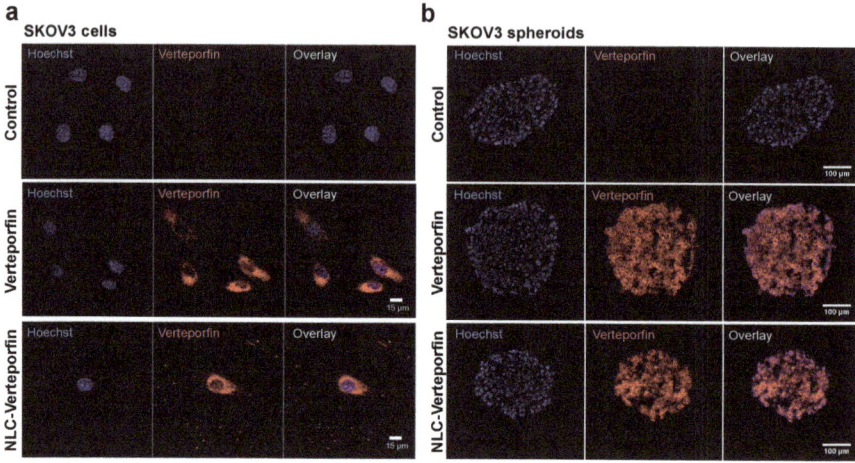

Figure 2. Verteporfin and NLC-verteporfin are internalized in SKOV3 cells and spheroids. Representative confocal microscopy images of SKOV3 cells (**a**) or sections of SKOV3 spheroids (**b**), incubated with 1 μmol·L^{-1} verteporfin or NLC-verteporfin for 24 h. Nuclei are stained with Hoechst 33342 (in blue). Verteporfin fluorescence is observed in red. Control: untreated cells or spheroids.

2.3. Verteporfin and NLC-Verteporfin Induce Phototoxicity in Ovarian Cancer Cells and Spheroids

Both free verteporfin and NLC-verteporfin induced high phototoxicity in ovarian cancer cells in vitro. Increasing concentrations of free verteporfin or NLC-verteporfin exposed to NIR light reduced the viability of SKOV3 and OVCAR3 cells cultured in monolayers and in spheroids, whereas they had no toxic effect on their proliferation in the dark (Figure 3). The OVCAR3 cells cultured in monolayer appeared to be less sensitive to verteporfin and NLC-verteporfin treatments as compared to SKOV3 cells (Figure 3a,b and Table 2), but interestingly OVCAR3 spheroids were highly sensitive to light exposure 2 h or 24 h after both treatments, with IC_{50} values similar to those of SKOV3 spheroids (Figure 3c,d, Table 2 and Figure S3).

The drug-light interval (light exposure 2 h or 24 h after treatment) had no influence on the phototoxicity of both treatments in 2D cell cultures (Figure 3a,b and Table 2). In contrast, both verteporfin and NLC-verteporfin had a stronger toxic effect on the viability of SKOV3 and OVCAR3 spheroids when exposed to the light 24 h after treatment as compared to 2 h (Figure 3c,d and Table 2).

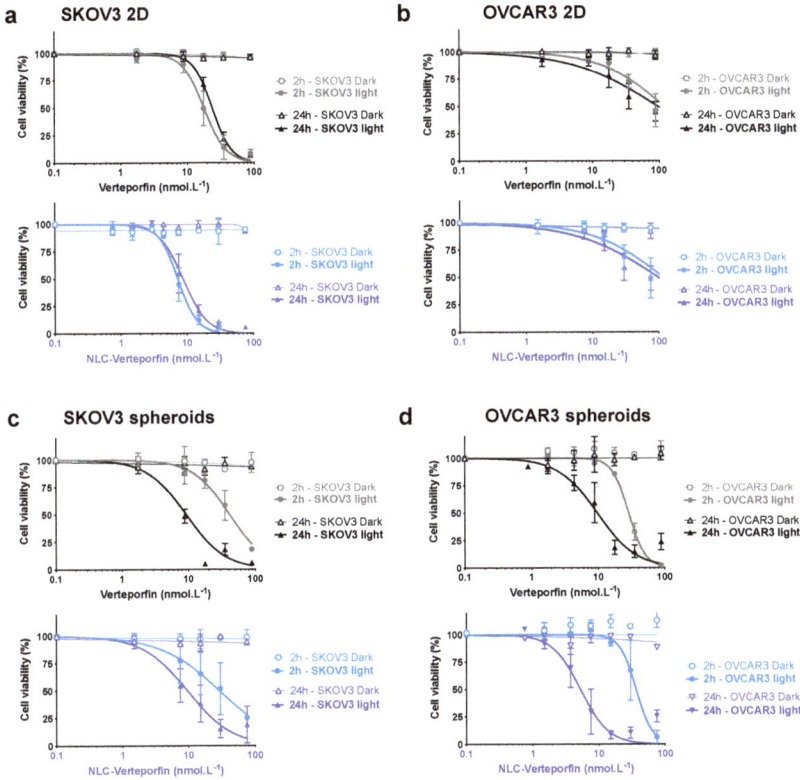

Figure 3. Verteporfin and NLC-verteporfin mediated phototoxicity in SKOV3 and OVCAR3 cells and spheroids. SKOV3 (left panels) and OVCAR3 (right panels) cells (**a**,**b**) or spheroids (**c**,**d**) were treated with increasing concentrations of free verteporfin (in grey/black) or NLC-verteporfin (in blue) for 2 h or 24 h before NIR light exposure at 690 nm (fluency 10 J·cm^{-2}). In parallel, cells or spheroids were maintained in the dark. (**a**,**b**) Cell viability was assessed 72 h following light exposure. Data are expressed as the mean ± SD of ≥ 3 independent experiments. (**c**,**d**) Cell viability in spheroids was assessed 72 h following light exposure. Data are expressed as the mean ± SD of ≥ 3 independent experiments in triplicate.

Table 2. Sensitivity of ovarian cancer cells to verteporfin and NLC-verteporfin.

Cell Lines	Culture Conditions		Verteporfin IC$_{50}$ (nmol·L^{-1})	NLC-Verteporfin IC$_{50}$ (nmol·L^{-1})
SKOV3	2D	2 h	17.8 ± 0.9	7.3 ± 0.4
		24 h	23.8 ± 0.9	8.8 ± 0.5
	3D	2 h	41.2 ± 4.2	29.3 ± 7.1
		24 h	9.3 ± 0.7	9.7 ± 1.1
OVCAR3	2D	2 h [#]	117.5 ± 14.4	116.4 ± 22.7
		24 h	94.9 ± 15.4	97.5 ± 17.4
	3D	2 h	28.9 ± 0.8	36.6 ± 3.2
		24 h	9.7 ± 1.0	5.3 ± 0.5

The drug concentrations required to inhibit cell growth by 50% (IC$_{50}$) at 2 h or 24 h in SKOV3 or OVCAR3 cells cultured in monolayer (2D) or spheroids (3D) and after light exposure (690 nm; 10 J·cm^{-2}). Data represent the mean ± SD (SKOV3, $n = 3$; OVCAR3, $n = 4$, except [#] $n = 2$). Each independent experiment was performed in triplicate.

2.4. NLC Accumulate in Ovarian Tumors In Vivo

The in vivo biodistribution and pharmacokinetics of NLC were assessed with particular interest on tumor uptake and specificity. While free verteporfin was rapidly eliminated from the bloodstream following intravenous administration (elimination half-life: 1.9 h) (Figure 4a), NLC circulated for several hours as shown by ex vivo fluorescence imaging of plasma samples from healthy mice after intravenous injection of fluorescent dye-loaded NLC (NLC-LipImage^{TM}815: elimination half-life: 6.5 h) or NLC-verteporfin (elimination half-life: 9.1 h) (Figure 4a).

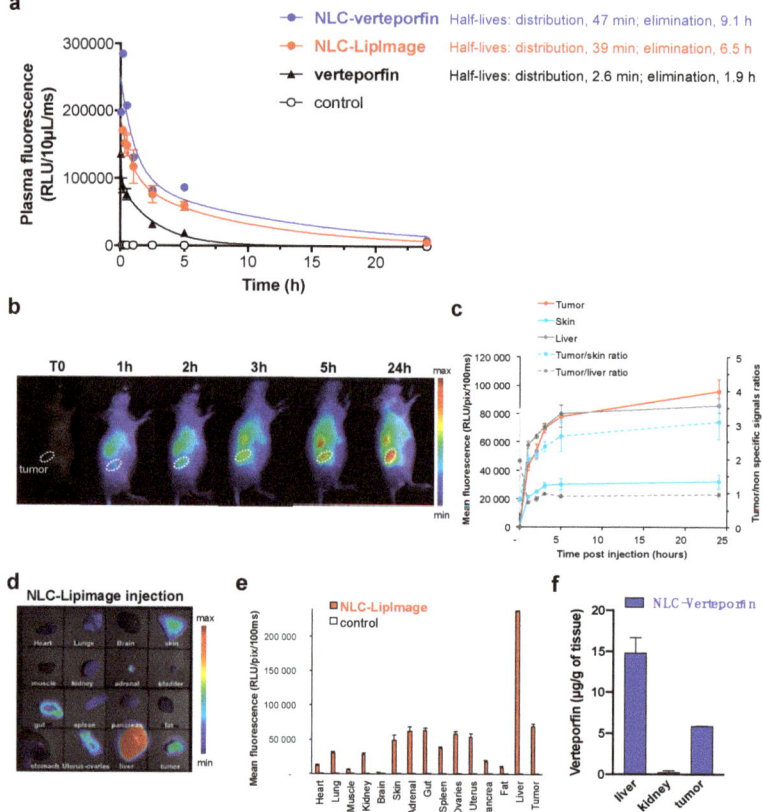

Figure 4. NLC circulated in the bloodstream and accumulated in subcutaneous SKOV3 tumors. (**a**) Healthy mice were injected intravenously with NLC-verteporfin (8 mg·kg^{-1} of verteporfin), dye-loaded NLC (LipImage^{TM}-815), or free verteporfin (2 mg·kg^{-1}). Fluorescence intensity measurements of verteporfin (for free verteporfin or NLC-verteporfin), or of LipImage^{TM}-815 (for NLC-LipImage) were performed on blood plasma samples taken at different time points. The results are expressed as the mean ± SD (n = 3). (**b–e**) Mice with SKOV3 subcutaneous tumors were injected intravenously with NLC-LipImage. (**b**) Representative fluorescence images (50 ms integration time) recorded using 2D-Fluorescence reflectance optical imaging (FRI) at different times after intravenous injection are shown (min-max: 4243-55869). Dotted lines show subcutaneous tumors. (**c**) Regions of interest (ROI) are defined on tumor, liver, and skin to semi-quantify the amount of photons detected per pixel. The results are expressed as the mean fluorescence ± SD in tumor, skin, and liver, and as the mean tumor/skin and tumor/liver fluorescence ratios ± SD (n = 3). (**d**) Fluorescence images were

performed on isolated organs 24 h after intravenous injection of NLC-LipImage. Representative fluorescence images of organs in injected and non-injected mice are shown (20 ms integration time; min-max: 1414-27109). (e) ROI are defined on the extracted organs to semi-quantify the amount of photons detected per pixel. The results are expressed as the mean ± SD in SKOV3 tumor-bearing mice (n = 3) and non-injected mice (control). (f) Mice with SKOV3 subcutaneous tumors were injected intravenously with NLC-verteporfin (8 mg·kg^{-1} of verteporfin). Verteporfin measurements were performed by HPLC at 24 h on tumors, livers, and kidneys. The results are expressed as the mean ± SD (n = 2).

In addition, in vivo biodistribution of NLC-LipImage in mice with subcutaneous SKOV3 tumors showed accumulation into the liver, as expected with lipid nanoparticles, reaching a plateau between 5 h and 24 h (Figure 4b,c). Nonetheless, NLC also progressively accumulated into the tumor, reaching a maximum 24 h after injection. Tumor specificity was illustrated by a tumor to skin ratio of 3.1 ± 0.5 at 24 h (Figure 4c). At this time, the mice were euthanized, and the collected organs were subjected to ex vivo fluorescence imaging (Figure 4d), confirming the strong fluorescence signal in the liver, but also the accumulation of NLC-LipImage into the tumor, with a high tumor to muscle ratio of 11.5 ± 0.8 (Figure 4e). High performance liquid chromatography (HPLC), as another quantification method, also confirmed these results in tissues and blood plasma (Figure 4f and Figure S4). Altogether, in vivo and ex vivo fluorescence imaging demonstrated long circulation time, liver uptake, and tumor accumulation of NLC-verteporfin after intravenous injection in mice.

2.5. NLC-Verteporfin Improves PDT, Free Verteporfin is Highly Toxic In Vivo

Mice with well-established subcutaneous SKOV3 ovarian tumors were treated by single intravenous injection of free verteporfin, NLC-verteporfin or vehicle (control group) (Figure 5a). Tumors were then exposed to NIR laser light and the tumor volume was monitored for 2 weeks.

We first assessed the PDT efficacy of free verteporfin. When tumors were exposed to laser light 15 min after free verteporfin injection (2 mg·kg^{-1}), their growth was rapidly and strongly reduced (Figure 5b). However, three mice died on the day of light exposure, and two others died one week after, showing the strong toxicity of circulating activated verteporfin (Figure 5b and Figure S5). Among the three remaining mice at the end of the experiment, two were totally cured, and one escaped the treatment. In contrast, in absence of light or when tumors were exposed to laser light 24 h after verteporfin injection, no effect was observed on either tumor growth or animal wellbeing, showing the high photospecificity and the short circulation half-life of verteporfin, respectively (Figure 5b and Figure S5). Similarly, intravenous administration of NLC-verteporfin (2 mg·kg^{-1} of verteporfin), in the dark or when tumors were exposed to laser light 24 h after NLC-verteporfin administration, was safe and did not induce any sign of toxicity. However, no effect on tumor growth was observed, suggesting inadequate PDT conditions (Figure 5c).

Since no undesirable toxicity had been observed using NLC-verteporfin (Figure S5), a new experiment was performed using higher NLC-verteporfin concentration and higher light fluency. We checked the innocuousness of light exposure at 200 J·cm^{-2} in a preliminary experiment, and observed no effect on mice tumor and skin (Figure S6a). Thereby, NLC-verteporfin (8 mg·kg^{-1} of verteporfin) was combined with 200 J·cm^{-2} light exposure 24 h after intravenous administration, and significantly inhibited tumor growth as compared to the control group or to NLC-verteporfin in the dark (Figure 5d). These treatments were well tolerated and no significant weight loss was observed (Figure S6b). In accordance with our preliminary experiment, the 200 J·cm^{-2} light exposure did not damage the skin (Figure S7). Moreover, in most tumors treated with NLC-verteporfin (7/8 tumors), a whitening of the tumor was observed during the days following light exposure that might indicate treatment activity (Figure S7). In addition, necrotic areas were observed in tumors treated with NLC-verteporfin combined with laser light only (Figure 5e). Macroscopic observation of the main organs did not show evidence of damage. In addition, liver sections did not show any evidence of necrosis or damage (Figure S8).

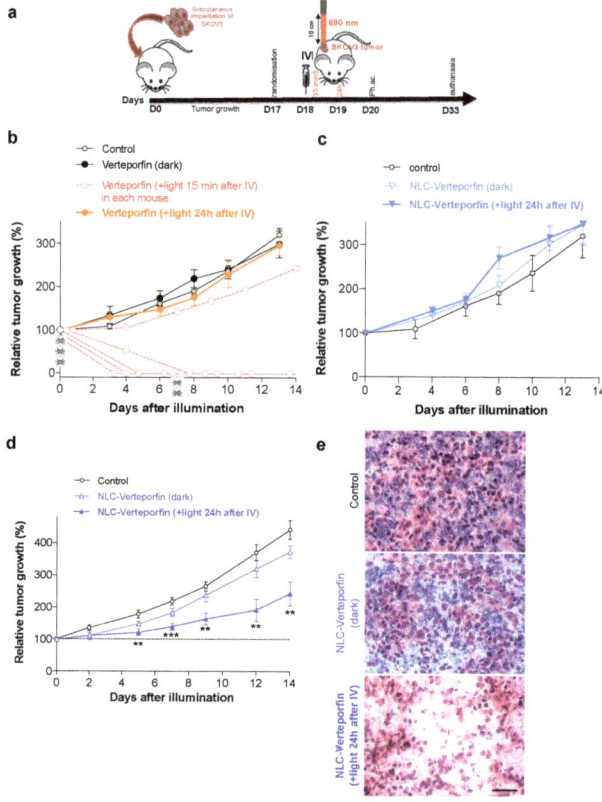

Figure 5. NLC-verteporfin improved PDT after intravenous administration in mice with ovarian cancer. (**a**) Mice with well-established SKOV3 subcutaneous tumors (125 ± 7 mm^3) were distributed into groups of 8 mice and treated by a single intravenous injection of free verteporfin, NLC-verteporfin or vehicle (control). Mice were maintained in the dark or submitted to a single NIR laser exposure 15 min or 24 h after injection. Non-invasive monitoring of tissue oxygenation (StO$_2$) was performed by in vivo photoacoustic imaging (Ph.ac.) on the tumors 24 h after light exposure. The tumor volume was evaluated by caliper measurements 3 times a week for 2 weeks. (**b**,**c**) Mice were injected with 1× PBS (control), free verteporfin (2 mg·kg^{-1}), or NLC-verteporfin (2 mg·kg^{-1} of verteporfin), and tumors were exposed to 50 J·cm^{-2} light 15 min or 24 h after the injection, as indicated. Data are expressed as the relative tumor growth (% of tumor volume on the day of light exposure) ± SEM in each group (n = 8, except in the group treated with free verteporfin and exposed to light 15 min after IV injection of verteporfin, in which 5 mice died during the experiment, as illustrated by skulls). Dotted red lines represent the tumor volume of each mouse from the group exposed to 50 J·cm^{-2} light, 15 min after free verteporfin injection. (**d**) Mice were intravenously injected with 1× PBS (control), or NLC-verteporfin (verteporfin 8 mg·kg^{-1}), and exposed to 200 J·cm^{-2} light, 24 h after the injection as indicated. Data are expressed as the relative tumor growth (% of tumor volume at the day of light exposure) ± SEM in each group (n = 8). p = 0.0003 ANOVA with Tukey post-hoc tests (**, ***, significantly different from the control group). (**e**) Hematoxylin and eosin staining on frozen tumor sections, Scale bar: 50 µm. Representative images in each group are shown.

Besides, tumor tissue oxygen saturation (StO$_2$) measured by non-invasive photoacoustic imaging 24 h after light exposure was decreased among mice treated with NLC-verteporfin as compared to the control group (Figure S9a), suggesting vascular impairment resulting in tissue hypoxia in the treated tumors. Interestingly, the two tumors from the treated group displaying the higher StO_2 values were the less-responsive tumors (Figure S9b).

Taken together, these results showed that NLC-verteporfin accumulation in tumor allowed a significant inhibition of tumor growth after light exposure with high fluency, and decreased side-effects.

2.6. NLC Accumulate in Disseminated Ovarian Tumor Nodules

Peritoneal carcinomatosis results from tumor growth and dissemination within the peritoneal cavity, and disseminated tumor nodules could be treated with PDT [3]. To evaluate tumor accumulation and drug delivery in disseminated small tumor nodules, NLC tumor uptake was assessed in an orthotopic mouse model of human peritoneal carcinomatosis from ovarian cancer. Luciferase-modified SKOV3 ovarian cancer cells were inoculated into one ovary, and tumor growth and peritoneal dissemination was monitored using non-invasive bioluminescence imaging in vivo (Figure 6a). When peritoneal carcinomatosis was established (4 to 5 weeks after tumor cells implantation), NLC-LipImage was administered intravenously. Despite the predictable high liver signal, NLC-LipImage provided clearly detectable signal spots in the peritoneal cavity (Figure 6b, Video S1 and Video S2). Furthermore, intraoperative fluorescence imaging was used simultaneously with bioluminescence imaging, and showed the colocalization of NLC with most tumor nodules (Figure 6c), demonstrating NLC tumor uptake in peritoneal carcinomatosis.

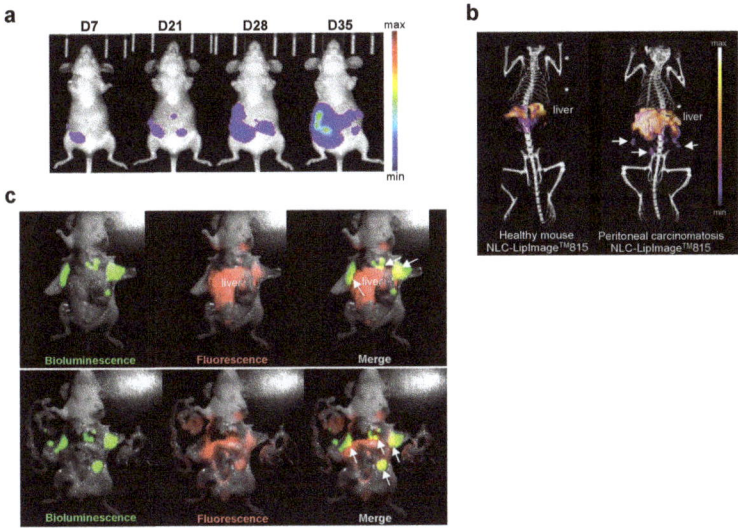

Figure 6. NLC-LipImage accumulated in ovarian tumor nodules after intravenous administration. (**a**) Orthotopic murine model of peritoneal carcinomatosis from ovarian cancer. Mice were inoculated with SKOV3-Luc cells into one ovary. Tumor growth and dissemination of tumor cells in the peritoneal cavity were followed by in vivo bioluminescence imaging over time. (**b**) Mice with peritoneal carcinomatosis or healthy mice were injected intravenously with NLC-LipImage^{TM}-815 for 24 h, and imaged with fluorescence tomography/micro-computed tomography (microCT). Arrows show NLC-LipImage fluorescence in tumor nodules. (**c**) Mice with established peritoneal carcinomatosis were injected intravenously with NLC-LipImage, and were submitted to intraoperative fluorescence in combination with bioluminescence after 24 h. Representative images of one operated mouse (upper panel), and with extended organs exposition after liver removal (lower panel) are shown. Bioluminescence showed SKOV3 cells in the peritoneal cavity (in green) and 2D-fluorescence imaging showed NLC-LipImage location (in red). Arrows show NLC-LipImage and SKOV3 tumor nodules signals colocation (in yellow).

3. Discussion

In this study, we showed that the encapsulation of the clinically approved photosensitizer verteporfin in NLC allowed cellular uptake and high phototoxicity in ovarian cancer cells cultured in monolayers and in 3D-spheroids. When injected intravenously in mice, these nanoparticles demonstrated tumor uptake, including in peritoneal small tumor nodules. Furthermore, NLC-verteporfin improved PDT efficacy in ovarian tumors in vivo with no phototoxic adverse effects compared to free verteporfin.

Lipid-based nanoparticles appear as nanocarriers of choice for lipophilic molecules such as the verteporfin photosensitizer [13,19]. We demonstrated here that verteporfin loading did not affect the colloidal properties of NLC. In addition, NLC showed high verteporfin encapsulation efficiency and stability for several months, as previously shown [21]. With solvent-free simple up-scalable fabrication process, NLC-verteporfin could easily be produced in large quantities for the clinic.

The cellular uptake of NLC-verteporfin involved endocytosis processes, taking more time than free verteporfin, part of which can rapidly diffuse across cell membranes. NLC-verteporfin uptake was also shown in tumor spheroids, which mimic in vivo tumors with tumor cell interactions and gradients of nutrients and oxygen [22–25]. The slower kinetic of NLC-verteporfin uptake compared to free verteporfin did not impair the efficiency of verteporfin phototoxicity. Indeed, verteporfin had the same phototoxicity when free or loaded in NLC in both SKOV3 and OVCAR3 ovarian cancer cells and spheroids. Accordingly, the phototoxic activity of verteporfin formulated in nanoparticles has recently been shown in ovarian carcinoma cells in vitro [26,27]. In addition, we observed that PDT was more efficient in spheroids than in monolayer-cultured cells, especially on OVCAR3 spheroids. The mechanism by which the OVCAR3 cells resisted to PDT in 2D culture but not in spheroids is still unknown. These results highlighted that the toxicity of drugs significantly varied depending on whether it is assessed in spheroids or in monolayer cell cultures, and this thus underlined the importance of using spheroids before moving forward in vivo experiments in mice [22,23,25]. Further experiments are needed to study NLC-verteporfin uptake and cytotoxicity in multicellular spheroids, which will reproduce both tumor cells and microenvironment [24]. Taking into account cellular and microenvironment heterogeneity within tumors is particularly important to enhance the accumulation of nanoparticles in the tumor.

Verteporfin therapy is the first-line therapy for serious ocular diseases, age-related macular degeneration and myopic choroidal neovascularization [28]. In these cases, the illumination of the retina is performed 15 min after intravenous injection of the photosensitizer, and the photodynamic reaction produces an anti-vascular effect that reduces disease progression. Because of its high NIR light-specific phototoxicity (in the nanomolar range), verteporfin is also extensively studied as PDT agent for the treatment of cancers, but mainly in vitro at the moment [4,7,9,27]. Yet, verteporfin has been evaluated in a phase I/II clinical study in patients with advanced pancreatic cancer, and has been shown to induce PDT-dependent tumor necrosis with high variability [8]. In our work, illumination of subcutaneous SKOV3 ovarian tumors 15 min after intravenous injection of a high dose of verteporfin led to strong tumor regression, illustrating the strong phototoxic effect of verteporfin on vasculature, but was associated with dramatic adverse effects and ultimately with death of most of the mice. The inhibitory effect of verteporfin on tumor vasculature and/or tumor cells, and its relationship to side-effects, remain to be formally investigated. Given the high photospecificity of verteporfin, no effect was observed in the absence of light. Furthermore, according to the short circulation half-life of free verteporfin, we did not observe any impact on tumors exposed to laser light 24 h after verteporfin injection. Altogether, this strongly suggested the need to formulate verteporfin to improve its tumor specificity and to decrease its side-effects.

A major issue for PDT is therefore to improve photosensitizer delivery efficiency and tumor specificity [7]. Many nanoparticle-based formulations have been proposed and developed, in order to exploit the EPR effect of tumors [7,13,14]. According to our data, and to the literature [12,13,17–19], NLC had a long circulation time and accumulate in subcutaneous tumors, as well as in peritoneal small tumor nodules 24 h after injection. This accumulation enabled tumor delivery of high concentrations of verteporfin, as demonstrated by tumor fluorescence imaging and HPLC dosing. These data and previous study [29] suggested that NLC were rapidly dissociated following their internalization in tumor cells, thus releasing verteporfin. Furthermore, photoactivation was performed 24 h after injection when circulating NLC-verteporfin concentration was low. This appeared to protect from post-illumination systemic adverse effects of verteporfin, since no toxicity was observed. In addition, no evidence of toxicity was observed in liver, despite the high hepatic accumulation of NLC, as it has been previously shown with dye-loaded NLC [30]. Nanoparticles-based encapsulation of verteporfin has been shown to promote anticancer activity in melanoma cells in vitro [15] and in vivo after topical administration and repeated light exposure [16]. In addition, co-encapsulation of verteporfin with chemotherapies, such as temozolomide in glioblastoma multiform cells in vitro [31], cisplatin in SKOV3 cells in vitro [32], or docetaxel in colon cancer cells in vitro and in vivo after six instances of light exposure [33], has also shown anticancer activity. Our study is the first, to our knowledge, to show PDT efficacy in subcutaneous ovarian tumors after single intravenous administration of NLC-verteporfin and laser light exposure. These results should be reinforced by using orthotopic model of peritoneal carcinomatosis from ovarian cancer.

The success of PDT mainly depends on total light dose, exposure time, and fluency rate [34]. Here, we demonstrated that tumor growth inhibition was related to the combination of NLC-verteporfin dose (8 mg·kg^{-1} of verteporfin) and laser light fluency (690 nm and 200 J·cm^{-2}), these factors yet needing further optimization. Optimal excitation wavelengths for PDT are described between 600 and 850 nm, and a fluency of 200 J·cm^{-2} is usually used to avoid thermal effect [34]. Our data showed that these PDT conditions induced tumor necrosis. A specific quantification of tumor necrosis should be performed to confirm these observations. However, in our experiment, although PDT significantly inhibited tumor growth, tumors still grew. A white coloring was observed on most of the tumors following light exposure, but it disappeared after 5 days, suggesting that some tumor cells escaped PDT or were incompletely treated, especially at the tumor periphery. With our illumination set-up, the area optimally covered by the laser light was 5 mm in diameter, and may not be large enough to treat the entire tumor (6.4 ± 1.0 mm mean diameter at the day of illumination). Tumor periphery thus received suboptimal illumination, which can explain the partial response and consequent relapse we observed. Delivering the activating light to allow PDT to uniformly treat all tumor cells is indeed challenging, but essential for optimal therapeutic efficacy [3,35,36]. In addition, NLC-verteporfin efficacy may be transient. Interestingly, repeating PDT, as experienced in colon cancer or melanoma [16,33], might reduce the risk of tumor recurrence with no accumulative toxicity, hypersensitivity or resistance [3,36]. This yet requires repeated access to the tumor, which may not be practical, depending on the tumor location and accessibility. Altogether, these data suggested that the dose regimen of NLC-verteporfin have to be optimized to achieve long-term antitumor efficacy. Furthermore, the effect of PDT on induction of inflammatory and immune response, as well as its combination with cancer immunotherapies might be investigated to enhance the PDT response [5,6,13,34].

We further used non-invasive photoacoustic imaging to measure tissue oxygenation in the tumor 24 h after PDT treatment. The reduced levels of StO$_2$ observed in tumors responding to the treatment suggested vascular impairment and tissue hypoxia, although this remains to be demonstrated by CD31 staining in tumors. In contrast, high levels of StO$_2$ were observed in tumors not responding to treatment. This suggested that tumor hypoxia monitoring by non-invasive photoacoustic imaging could be used to predict early tumor response to PDT, as soon as 24 h after light exposure. Similarly, photoacoustic imaging has been previously demonstrated to be predictive of tumor response to radiotherapy in head and neck cancer [37].

Our results offer new prospects for the management of ovarian cancer and in particular for the treatment of peritoneal carcinomatosis, in which conventional cytoreductive surgery often remains suboptimal for a number of patients [2,3]. Indeed, some tumor residues cannot be surgically removed because of their location or close contact with vital structures, and are responsible for relapse. Actually,

PDT has already been demonstrated to be combined with conventional surgical tumor resection to improve treatment outcome of peritoneal carcinomatosis despite a narrow therapeutic index [3]. Intraoperative PDT could be applied immediately following surgical tumor debulking and could treat residual peritoneal tumors in areas where surgical procedures pose a high risk of perioperative complications [38,39]. Significant toxicity induced by intraperitoneal PDT has been shown in Phase I and II clinical trials, owing to the heterogeneous population of patients, who had poor prognosis and failed to respond to first-line treatments, and to the non-specificity of photosensitizers for tumor cells [3]. We showed that NLC-verteporfin accumulated in small tumor nodules and provided tumor contrast that can be detected by intraoperative fluorescence imaging. Therefore, photoactivating laser light can be specifically delivered on identified tumor residue, thus further increasing treatment specificity and sparing healthy tissue, including the liver. Treating residual peritoneal metastases by PDT after cytoreductive surgery should thus be further investigated depending on metastatic tumor burden.

4. Materials and Methods

4.1. Materials

Suppocire™ NB was purchased from Gattefossé (Saint-Priest, France). Myrj™ S40 (poly(ethylene glycol) stearate surfactant with 40 ethylene glycol motifs, and Super-refined Soybean oil were supplied by CRODA (Chocques, France). Lipoid™ s75 was purchased from Lipoid GmbH (Ludwigshafen, Germany). HPLC grade solvents were obtained from VWR Scientific (Fontenay sous Bois, France) and other chemicals including verteporfin from Sigma-Aldrich (Saint-Quentin Fallavier, France).

HPLC-grade water (specific resistance = 18.2 MΩ cm) was obtained from a Classic DI MK2 water purification system (Elga, UK) and was used in all experiments. SpectraPor™ dialysis membrane 12–14,000 was purchased from Roth Sochiel EURL (Lauterbourg, France). Nanostructured lipid carriers (NLC) were formulated using a VCX750 Ultrasonic processor from Sonics (Newtown, CT, USA) equipped with a 3 mm diameter microtip.

4.2. Formulation of Nanostructured Lipid Carriers

The lipid phase was prepared by mixing solid (Suppocire™ NB, 255 mg) and liquid (Super-refined Soybean oil, 85 mg) lipids as well as the lipophilic surfactant Lipoid™ s75 (65 mg) and verteporfin (4 mg) while the aqueous phase was composed of the hydrophilic surfactant, Myrj™ S40 (345 mg) prepared in 1250 µL DI water. After homogenization at 50 °C, both lipid and aqueous phases were crudely mixed and sonication cycles were performed at 45 °C during 5 min. Non-encapsulated components were separated from NLC by dialysis (1× PBS, MWCO: 12–14 kDa, overnight). Dye-loaded NLC (LipImage™ 815) were synthetized by a similar process, as previously described [40]. Prior to characterization and injection, NLC dispersions were filtered through a 0.22 µm cellulose Millipore membrane for sterilization. Particle concentration was assessed by weighing freeze-dried samples of NLC obtained from a known volume. NLC formulation was stored in liquid suspension at 4 °C in dark.

4.3. Dynamic Light Scattering

The hydrodynamic diameter and zeta potential of the NLC were measured at 22 °C with a Malvern Zeta Sizer Nanoinstrument (NanoZS, Malvern, UK) in 0.1× PBS buffer. Physical stability was investigated by DLS measurements over 3 months with samples stored at 4 °C in dark. Mean average diameters and polydispersity indices reported were obtained from scattered light intensity results. Data were expressed in terms of mean and standard deviation of three independent measurements.

4.4. HPLC Analyses

Verteporfin was analyzed by HPLC using a Waters Alliance 2695 Separation module equipped with a Waters 2487 dual absorbance detector and a reverse-phase C18 column (Atlantis T3, 5 µm,

50 × 4.6 mm, 100 Å) (Waters, Milford, MA, USA). Data were processed using Empower™ 2 software. The elution used a gradient mobile phase consisting of (A) 0.05 mM monobasic sodium phosphate (pH 3.5) solution and (B) methanol, according to previously published method [41]. The gradient was applied as follows: 0–4 min from 50 to 65% eluent B; 4–8 min from 65 to 85% eluent B; 8–22 min from 85 to 99% eluent B; 22–27 min from 99 to 10% eluent B; 27–30 min from 10 to 50% eluent B; 30–40 min 50% eluent B. A flow rate of 1 mL/min was used with a 20 µL injection volume. Verteporfin was detected at 430 nm (Soret band) and linear calibration curve was established from 0 to 600 µg·mL^{-1} for quantification.

For analysis of the verteporfin payload in NLC, nanoparticles were disassembled. 100 µL of NLC was added to 100 µL of methanol. Samples were centrifuged to pellet lipids after precipitation, and the supernatant was taken for analysis. The lipid pellet was rinsed three times more with 100 µL methanol. The total supernatant, adjusted to 500 µL, was centrifuged once more to remove any remaining lipids and injected to HPLC analysis for verteporfin quantitation.

For plasma pharmacokinetics, plasma samples were diluted two-fold with (MeOH 90%/NaH$_2$PO$_4$ 0.05 mM 10%) and centrifuged for 1h at 13,000 rpm. The supernatant was injected on HPLC. For organ quantification, tumors, livers and kidneys were crudely crushed then incubated with 1 mL of (MeOH 90%/NaH$_2$PO$_4$ 0.05 mM 10%), for 4 days. After centrifugation for 1 h at 13,000 rpm, the supernatant was analyzed by HPLC.

4.5. Absorbance and Fluorescence Spectrum

Evolution 201 UV–visible spectrophotometer (Thermo Fisher Scientific, Waltham, MA, USA) and LS 55 Fluorescence Spectrometer (PerkinElmer, Waltham, MA, USA) were used to measure verteporfin and NLC-verteporfin absorbance in medium and fluorescence in 1× PBS, respectively.

4.6. Cell Lines and Culture

The human SKOV3 and OVCAR3 cell lines were obtained from LGC standard (Molsheim, France). The human IGROV1 cell line was obtained from Institut Gustave Roussy (Villejuif, France). All cells were routinely tested for the presence of mycoplasma (Mycoalert® Mycoplasma Detection Kit, Lonza, Rockland, ME, USA) and used within three months after thawing.

4.6.1. Two-Dimensions (2D) Cell Culture

Cells were maintained in culture at 37 °C in RPMI-1640 medium with 10% FBS (SKOV3 and IGROV1) or with 20% FBS and 0.01 mg·mL^{-1} insulin (OVCAR3) in a 5% CO$_2$ humidified atmosphere. The cell morphology was routinely checked.

4.6.2. Three-Dimensions (3D) Cell Culture

Spheroids were generated by plating 3000 cells/well, into 96-well round bottom ultra-low attachment (ULA) spheroid microplates (Corning, Tewksbury, MA, USA). The spheroid culture was performed in complete medium in a humidified atmosphere with 5% CO$_2$. Spheroid formation and growth were assessed by microscopic examination using an inverted microscope and by imaging the spheroids at each time point.

4.7. Flow Cytometry

Cells were plated on 6-well plates and treated with verteporfin or NLC-verteporfin for 2 h or 24 h at 37 °C or at 4 °C in the dark. After incubation cells were harvested and re-suspended in 1× PBS for flow cytometry analysis. Fluorescence emission of verteporfin was analyzed using flow cytometry LSRII and FCS Express software (BD Biosciences, San Jose, CA, USA).

4.8. Fluorescence Microscopy

Cells were plated on labtek® and treated with verteporfin or NLC-verteporfin for 2 h or 24 h in the dark at 37 °C before confocal imaging. Spheroids were treated with verteporfin or NLC-verteporfin incubation for 24 h at 37 °C, and harvested, washed, fixed in 4% paraformaldehyde, frozen in optimal cutting temperature (OCT) compound for embedding, and cut into 12-μm sections. Hoechst was used to counterstain the cell nuclei. Fluorescence microscopy was carried out using a confocal microscope (LSM 710; Carl Zeiss, Jena, Germany). An objective Plan Apochromat 20×/0.8 NA in air and an objective Plan Apochromat 63×/1.4 NA in oil were used. The excitation was at 405 nm and emission filter between 650 and 730 nm for verteporfin, and between 450 and 500 nm for Hoechst.

4.9. In Vitro Cytotoxicity Assays

Cell proliferation assays were conducted in 96-well culture plates. 2D-cultured cells and spheroids were cultured for 24 h and 72 h, respectively, prior to treatment with increasing concentration of verteporfin or NLC-verteporfin in complete medium. Illumination at 690 nm for 60 s with power output at 167 mW·cm^{-2} (fluency 10 J·cm^{-2}, High Power Devices Inc., North Brunswick, NJ, USA) was performed 2 h or 24 h after treatment. The cell viability was quantified 72 h after light exposure using Presto Blue™ (Invitrogen, Waltham, MA, USA) in 2D cell models, or using the CellTiter-Glo® 3D Cell Viability Assay (Promega, Charbonnière, France) in spheroids. Fluorescence was measured using a multilabel counter (Omega Fluostar, BMG Labtech, Champigny sur Marne, France) with the excitation and emission filter at 560 and 590 nm, and the bioluminescence was measured using counter (Victor^{3TM}, Perkin Elmer, Waltham, MA, USA). Cell viability was normalized to control cells (no drug and un-illuminated). The drug concentrations required to inhibit cell growth by 50% (IC$_{50}$) were interpolated from the dose-response curves.

4.10. In Vivo Experiments

All animal studies were performed in accordance with the European Economic Community guidelines and the "Principles of Laboratory Animal Care" (NIH publication N 86-23 revised 1985) and were approved by the institutional guidelines and the European Community (EU Directive 2010/63/EU) for the use of experimental animals (authorization for the experiment: apafis#15176-201808281433752 v1).

4.10.1. Subcutaneous Ovarian Tumor Model

Anesthetized (4% isoflurane/air for anesthesia induction and 1.5% thereafter) six-week-old female NMRI nude mice (Janvier Labs, Le Genest-Saint Isle, France) were injected subcutaneously in the flank with 10^7 luciferase-modified SKOV3 cells in 1× PBS. Tumor size was measured three times a week using a caliper, and the tumor volume was calculated as

$$\text{length} \times (\text{width})^2 \times 0.4$$

4.10.2. Pharmacokinetics Studies on Blood Plasma Samples

Healthy mice or mice with SKOV3 subcutaneous tumor were anesthetized using 4% isoflurane/air for anesthesia induction and 1.5% thereafter, and 200 μL NLC-LipImage™815 (50 μM of Lipimage™815) or NLC-verteporfin (8 mg·kg^{-1} of verteporfin) or free verteporfin (2 mg·kg^{-1}) were administered intravenously via the tail vein. Fifty microliters of blood were sampled from the tail vein before and at different times after injection, centrifuged 5 min at 8,000 g, and 10 μL of plasma were used for fluorescence imaging [23,42] or HPLC. Half-lives were measured from nonlinear regression fit analyses (two phase decay). Tumor, liver, and kidney samples were excised 24 h after treatments, and frozen for further HPLC analyses.

4.10.3. Biodistribution of Fluorescent NLC In Vivo

2D-fluorescence images were acquired at several time points after intravenous administration of NLC-LipImage^{TM}-815 (200 µL, 50 µmol·L^{-1}) using the Fluobeam800^{TM} (Fluoptics, Grenoble, France) that excites fluorescence at 780 nm and detects emitted light at wavelengths greater than 830 nm. At the end of the experiment, mice were sacrificed, and some organs were collected for ex vivo imaging using the Fluobeam800^{TM}. Semiquantitative data were obtained using the Wasabi® software (Hamamatsu, Massy, France) by drawing regions of interest (ROIs) on the different organs and were expressed as the number of relative light units per pixel per unit of exposure time and relative to the fluorescence signal in the skin or muscle [22,42].

4.10.4. Orthotopic Murine Model of Peritoneal Carcinomatosis from Ovarian Cancer

Six-week-old female NMRI nude mice (Janvier) were anesthetized (isoflurane/air 4% for induction and 2% then after) and placed on a heating mat at 37 °C. Buprenorphin 0.6 mg·kg^{-1} was injected subcutaneously for analgesia before and 16 h after surgery. An incision of 2 cm was performed in the peritoneum. Luciferase-modified SKOV3 cells were suspended in medium at 3×10^6 cells/50 µL and were slowly injected into the ovaries through lumen of the fallopian tube. The peritoneum and the skin were closed with synthetic absorbable suture (Optime® 4.0 for the peritoneum and Monocryl® 4.0 for the skin), and mice were placed on the right flank and were carefully observed until they woke up. Tumor growth and peritoneal invasion were weekly monitored by in vivo bioluminescence imaging (IVIS KINETIC, Perkin Elmer, Waltham, MA, USA) 5 min after the intraperitoneal injection of 150 mg·kg^{-1} of D-luciferin (Promega, Charbonnière, France).

Fluorescence diffuse optical tomography (fDOT) acquisitions were performed 24 h after intravenous administration of NLC-LipImage^{TM}-815 (200 µL, 50 µM) in mice with established peritoneal carcinomatosis or in healthy mice. This system consists of a 690 nm laser source, a CCD camera and a set of filters [42]. The light source is a 35-mW compact laser diode (Power Technology, Little Rock, AR, USA) equipped with a bandpass interference filter (685AF30OD6; Melles Griot, Albuquerque, NM, USA). Emitted fluorescence was filtered by 730/30 nm band-pass filter (RG9 OD5; Schott, Mainz, Germany) placed in front of a near infrared-sensitive CCD camera (Hamamatsu Photonics K.K., Shizuoka, Japan) mounted with a f/15-mm objective (Schneider Kreutznach, Bad Kreuznach, Germany). X-ray micro-computed tomography was performed using the vivaCT40 (Scanco Medical, Wangen-Brüttisellen, Switzerland) at 45 kV voltage and 177 µA intensity with an 80 µm isotropic voxel size and 200 ms integration time. 3D fluorescence and microCT reconstructed volumes were merged using external as well as anatomical landmarks from both imaging modalities. Immediately after 3D non-invasive fluorescence imaging, mice received an intraperitoneal injection of 150 mg·kg^{-1} of D-luciferin and were then quickly dissected so as to expose the main organs for sequential bioluminescence and fluorescence imaging (IVIS KINETIC (Perkin Elmer, Waltham, MA, USA) and Fluobeam®800 (Fluoptics, Grenoble, France)).

4.10.5. PDT In Vivo

When SKOV3 subcutaneous tumors of approximately 100 mm^3 were established (17 days after cells implantation), mice were distributed into groups of 8. Intravenous administration of 200 µL of free verteporfin (1.8 mg·kg^{-1}) or loaded in lipids nanoparticles (NLC-verteporfin, 2 or 8 mg·kg^{-1} of verteporfin) was performed in anesthetized mice (isoflurane/air 4% for induction and 1.5% thereafter). Control mice received the vehicle (1× PBS).

Either 15 m or 24 h after verteporfin or NLC-verteporfin injections, subcutaneous tumors were exposed to a near infrared laser emitting at 690 nm with a collimator (convex lens, 25 mm diameter) positioned at 10 cm distance from the tumor, for 5 min and 30 s (150 mW·cm^{-2}, fluency 50 J·cm^{-2}) or for 22 min and 15 s (150 mW·cm^{-2}, fluency 200 J·cm^{-2}). Injected groups and control group were then maintained in the dark for 6 days after injection. Mice were observed daily and weighed three times a week. Tumor size was measured three times a week using a caliper for 2 weeks after PDT. Mice bearing tumors ≥ 1.5 cm^3 were euthanized immediately. At the end of the experiment, tumors were excised and frozen for further analyses.

4.10.6. Photoacoustic Imaging

Photoacoustic imaging was performed 24 h after tumor exposure to light with the Vevo®LAZR system (Fujifilm, Visualsonics Inc., Toronto, ON, Canada) using the LZ201 transducer (256 elements linear array; 15 MHz center frequency, [9–18 MHz bandwith], 100 µm axial resolution; 220 µm lateral resolution; 30 × 30 mm^2 image size). All imaging experiments were conducted under gaseous anesthesia (isoflurane/air 4% for induction and 1.5% thereafter). 3D B-mode and oxyhemo (750 and 850 nm) scans were performed on the subcutaneous tumors. Total oxygen saturation rate (StO$_2$) was calculated from oxyhemo data as previously described [43].

4.10.7. Histology

Tumors and livers were frozen and sections of a 7-µm thickness were stained with hematoxylin and eosin (HE). Sections were observed under a Zeiss AxioImager M2 microscope by two researchers who were blinded to the treatment groups (four different samples per group).

4.11. Statistical Analyses

All analyses were performed using the GraphPad Prism software (GraphPad Software Inc., San Diego, CA, USA). Statistical comparisons between two groups or more were conducted with Mann–Whitney test, Kruskal–Wallis test, or Friedman test with Dunn's multiple comparisons post hoc test. Statistical comparisons between mice groups over time were determined by two-way ANOVA with Tukey's post hoc test. Statistical significance was defined for p values ≤ 0.05.

5. Conclusions

PDT is increasingly recognized as an emerging clinical tool in cancer therapy besides other therapies. There are several advantages for PDT, such as spatiotemporal control of treatment induction by light activation, reduced systemic cytotoxicity, conventional therapies synergy, chemoresistance reversing, and activation of the immune response. Our study established that the encapsulation of the photosensitizer verteporfin in NLC enhanced PDT in ovarian cancer cells cultured in monolayer, in spheroids, and in vivo in tumor bearing mice. Encapsulating verteporfin in NLC led to higher tumor specificity with both higher verteporfin concentration delivered to the tumor and lower circulating verteporfin at the time of illumination, thus protecting from photosensitizer systemic adverse effects. These results provided promising therapeutic perspectives for PDT in ovarian cancers and in peritoneal carcinomatosis from ovarian cancer in combination with conventional surgery.

Supplementary Materials: The following are available online at http://www.mdpi.com/2072-6694/11/11/1760/s1, Figure S1: Absorbtion and fluorescence spectra of verteporfin and NLC-verteporfin, Figure S2: Verteporfin and NLC-verteporfin are internalized in ovarian cancer cells and spheroids; Figure S3: Representative images of SKOV3 and OVCAR3 spheroids treated with verteporfin or NLC-verteporfin; Figure S4: Circulating verteporfin and NLC-verteporfin detected by HPLC after intravenous administration; Figure S5: Weight of mice from the implantation of the tumors to the end of the experiment; Figure S6: No side-effect of NIR light exposure at 200 J·cm^{-2} in mice with ovarian subcutaneous cancer; Figure S7: NLC-verteporfin enhances PDT after intravenous administration in mice with ovarian subcutaneous cancer; Figure S8: Hematoxylin and eosin staining on frozen liver sections; Figure S9: Tumor tissue oxygen saturation and tumor weight after NLC-verteporfin and PDT in mice with ovarian subcutaneous cancer; Video S1: Biodistribution of NLC-Lipimage after intravenous administration in healthy mouse; Video S2: Biodistribution of NLC-Lipimage after intravenous administration in mouse with SKOV3 peritoneal carcinomatosis.

Author Contributions: Conceptualization, A.H., V.J., I.T., and G.R.; Investigation, T.M. (Thibault Massias), C.B., L.V., M.H., and M.G.; Methodology, T.M. (Thierry Michy), L.V., M.G., and M.H.; Validation, T.M. (Thierry Michy), T.M. (Thibault Massias), L.V., and M.G.; Formal analysis, T.M. (Thibault Massias), L.V., M.G., and A.H.; Visualization, C.B., T.M. (Thibault Massias), L.V., M.G., M.H., and A.H.; Resources, J.-L.C., G.R., V.J., and I.T.; Writing—original draft preparation, A.H., I.T., and V.J.; Writing—review and editing, A.H., I.T., J.-L.C., and V.J.; Supervision, A.H., and V.J.; Project administration, A.H. and V.J.; Funding acquisition, J.-L.C., V.J., and G.R.

Funding: This research was funded by Cancéropôle Lyon Auvergne Rhône-Alpes, Oncostarter program and France Live Imaging (FLI-Grenoble; French program "Investissement d'Avenir"; grant "Infrastructure d'avenir en Biologie Santé," ANR-11-INBS-0006). LETI-DTBS is supported by the French National Research Agency in the framework of Arcane Labex program (CBH-EUR-GS, ANR-17-EURE-0003), and Glyco@Alps "Investissement d'avenir" program (ANR-15-IDEX-02).

Acknowledgments: We acknowledge the assistance of A. Grichine, J. Mazzega, and M. Pezet (Platform Optical microscopy—Cell Imaging, Centre de Recherche Institut National de la Santé et de la Recherche Médicale U1209). The in vivo evaluation was performed by the OPTIMAL facility, which is part of the France Live Imaging Program. We acknowledge the help of Marie Escudé for NLC synthesis and characterization. We acknowledge Xiaojie Jiang, Marianne Roche, and Guillaume Vayssière for their help in in vitro and in vivo experiments. We acknowledge Henri Josserand for English proofreading the manuscript.

Conflicts of Interest: The authors declare no conflict of interest. The funders had no role in the design of the study; in the collection, analyses, or interpretation of data; in the writing of the manuscript, or in the decision to publish the results.

References

1. Torre, L.A.; Islami, F.; Siegel, R.L.; Ward, E.M.; Jemal, A. Global Cancer in Women: Burden and Trends. *Cancer Epidemiol. Biomarkers Prev.* **2017**, *26*, 444–457. [CrossRef] [PubMed]
2. Narod, S. Can advanced-stage ovarian cancer be cured? *Nat. Rev. Clin. Oncol.* **2016**, *13*, 255–261. [CrossRef] [PubMed]
3. Almerie, M.Q.; Gossedge, G.; Wright, K.E.; Jayne, D.G. Treatment of peritoneal carcinomatosis with photodynamic therapy: Systematic review of current evidence. *Photodiagnosis Photodyn. Ther.* **2017**, *20*, 276–286. [CrossRef] [PubMed]
4. Yanovsky, R.L.; Bartenstein, D.W.; Rogers, G.S.; Isakoff, S.J.; Chen, S.T. Photodynamic therapy for solid tumors: A review of the literature. *Photodermatol. Photoimmunol. Photomed.* **2019**. [CrossRef] [PubMed]
5. Wachowska, M.; Muchowicz, A.; Demkow, U. Immunological aspects of antitumor photodynamic therapy outcome. *Cent. Eur. J. Immunol.* **2015**, *40*, 481–485. [CrossRef] [PubMed]
6. Shi, X.; Zhang, C.Y.; Gao, J.; Wang, Z. Recent advances in photodynamic therapy for cancer and infectious diseases. *Wiley Interdiscip. Rev. Nanomed. Nanobiotechnol.* **2019**, e1560. [CrossRef] [PubMed]
7. Baskaran, R.; Lee, J.; Yang, S.G. Clinical development of photodynamic agents and therapeutic applications. *Biomater. Res.* **2018**, *22*, 25. [CrossRef] [PubMed]
8. Huggett, M.T.; Jermyn, M.; Gillams, A.; Illing, R.; Mosse, S.; Novelli, M.; Kent, E.; Bown, S.G.; Hasan, T.; Pogue, B.W.; et al. Phase I/II study of verteporfin photodynamic therapy in locally advanced pancreatic cancer. *Br. J. Cancer* **2014**, *110*, 1698–1704. [CrossRef] [PubMed]
9. Liu, K.; Du, S.; Gao, P.; Zheng, J. Verteporfin suppresses the proliferation, epithelial-mesenchymal transition and stemness of head and neck squamous carcinoma cells via inhibiting YAP1. *J. Cancer* **2019**, *10*, 4196–4207. [CrossRef] [PubMed]
10. Akens, M.K.; Hardisty, M.R.; Wilson, B.C.; Schwock, J.; Whyne, C.M.; Burch, S.; Yee, A.J. Defining the therapeutic window of vertebral photodynamic therapy in a murine pre-clinical model of breast cancer metastasis using the photosensitizer BPD-MA (Verteporfin). *Breast Cancer Res. Treat.* **2010**, *119*, 325–333. [CrossRef] [PubMed]
11. Paszko, E.; Ehrhardt, C.; Senge, M.O.; Kelleher, D.P.; Reynolds, J.V. Nanodrug applications in photodynamic therapy. *Photodiagnosis Photodyn. Ther.* **2011**, *8*, 14–29. [CrossRef] [PubMed]
12. Naidoo, C.; Kruger, C.A.; Abrahamse, H. Photodynamic Therapy for Metastatic Melanoma Treatment: A Review. *Technol. Cancer Res. Treat.* **2018**, *17*, 1533033818791795. [CrossRef] [PubMed]
13. Debele, T.A.; Peng, S.; Tsai, H.C. Drug Carrier for Photodynamic Cancer Therapy. *Int. J. Mol. Sci.* **2015**, *16*, 22094–22136. [CrossRef] [PubMed]

14. Maeda, H.; Nakamura, H.; Fang, J. The EPR effect for macromolecular drug delivery to solid tumors: Improvement of tumor uptake, lowering of systemic toxicity, and distinct tumor imaging in vivo. *Adv. Drug Deliv. Rev.* **2013**, *65*, 71–79. [CrossRef] [PubMed]
15. Rizzi, M.; Tonello, S.; Estevao, B.M.; Gianotti, E.; Marchese, L.; Reno, F. Verteporfin based silica nanoparticle for in vitro selective inhibition of human highly invasive melanoma cell proliferation. *J. Photochem. Photobiol. B* **2017**, *167*, 1–6. [CrossRef] [PubMed]
16. Clemente, N.; Miletto, I.; Gianotti, E.; Invernizzi, M.; Marchese, L.; Dianzani, U.; Reno, F. Verteporfin-loaded mesoporous silica nanoparticles inhibit mouse melanoma proliferation in vitro and in vivo. *J. Photochem. Photobiol. B* **2019**, *197*, 111533. [CrossRef] [PubMed]
17. Laine, A.L.; Gravier, J.; Henry, M.; Sancey, L.; Bejaud, J.; Pancani, E.; Wiber, M.; Texier, I.; Coll, J.L.; Benoit, J.P.; et al. Conventional versus stealth lipid nanoparticles: Formulation and in vivo fate prediction through FRET monitoring. *J. Control. Release* **2014**, *188*, 1–8. [CrossRef] [PubMed]
18. Hirsjarvi, S.; Dufort, S.; Gravier, J.; Texier, I.; Yan, Q.; Bibette, J.; Sancey, L.; Josserand, V.; Passirani, C.; Benoit, J.P.; et al. Influence of size, surface coating and fine chemical composition on the in vitro reactivity and in vivo biodistribution of lipid nanocapsules versus lipid nanoemulsions in cancer models. *Nanomedicine* **2013**, *9*, 375–387. [CrossRef] [PubMed]
19. Navarro, F.P.; Creusat, G.; Frochot, C.; Moussaron, A.; Verhille, M.; Vanderesse, R.; Thomann, J.S.; Boisseau, P.; Texier, I.; Couffin, A.C.; et al. Preparation and characterization of mTHPC-loaded solid lipid nanoparticles for photodynamic therapy. *J. Photochem. Photobiol. B* **2014**, *130*, 161–169. [CrossRef] [PubMed]
20. Lovitt, C.J.; Shelper, T.B.; Avery, V.M. Advanced cell culture techniques for cancer drug discovery. *Biology* **2014**, *3*, 345–367. [CrossRef] [PubMed]
21. Gravier, J.; Navarro, F.P.; Delmas, T.; Mittler, F.; Couffin, A.C.; Vinet, F.; Texier, I. Lipidots: Competitive organic alternative to quantum dots for in vivo fluorescence imaging. *J. Biomed. Opt.* **2011**, *16*, 096013. [CrossRef] [PubMed]
22. Jeannot, V.; Gauche, C.; Mazzaferro, S.; Couvet, M.; Vanwonterghem, L.; Henry, M.; Didier, C.; Vollaire, J.; Josserand, V.; Coll, J.L.; et al. Anti-tumor efficacy of hyaluronan-based nanoparticles for the co-delivery of drugs in lung cancer. *J. Control. Release* **2018**, *275*, 117–128. [CrossRef] [PubMed]
23. Gilson, P.; Couvet, M.; Vanwonterghem, L.; Henry, M.; Vollaire, J.; Baulin, V.; Werner, M.; Orlowska, A.; Josserand, V.; Mahuteau-Betzer, F.; et al. The pyrrolopyrimidine colchicine-binding site agent PP-13 reduces the metastatic dissemination of invasive cancer cells in vitro and in vivo. *Biochem. Pharmacol.* **2019**, *160*, 1–13. [CrossRef] [PubMed]
24. Molla, A.; Couvet, M.; Coll, J.L. Unsuccessful mitosis in multicellular tumour spheroids. *Oncotarget* **2017**, *8*, 28769–28784. [CrossRef] [PubMed]
25. Nirmalanandhan, V.S.; Duren, A.; Hendricks, P.; Vielhauer, G.; Sittampalam, G.S. Activity of anticancer agents in a three-dimensional cell culture model. *Assay Drug Dev. Technol.* **2010**, *8*, 581–590. [CrossRef] [PubMed]
26. Rizvi, I.; Nath, S.; Obaid, G.; Ruhi, M.K.; Moore, K.; Bano, S.; Kessel, D.; Hasan, T. A Combination of Visudyne and a Lipid-anchored Liposomal Formulation of Benzoporphyrin Derivative Enhances Photodynamic Therapy Efficacy in a 3D Model for Ovarian Cancer. *Photochem. Photobiol.* **2019**, *95*, 419–429. [CrossRef] [PubMed]
27. Erdem, S.S.; Obeidin, V.A.; Yigitbasi, T.; Tumer, S.S.; Yigit, P. Verteporfin mediated sequence dependent combination therapy against ovarian cancer cell line. *J. Photochem. Photobiol. B* **2018**, *183*, 266–274. [CrossRef] [PubMed]
28. Battaglia Parodi, M.; La Spina, C.; Berchicci, L.; Petruzzi, G.; Bandello, F. Photosensitizers and photodynamic therapy: Verteporfin. *Dev. Ophthalmol.* **2016**, *55*, 330–336. [CrossRef]
29. Gravier, J.; Sancey, L.; Hirsjarvi, S.; Rustique, E.; Passirani, C.; Benoit, J.P.; Coll, J.L.; Texier, I. FRET imaging approaches for in vitro and in vivo characterization of synthetic lipid nanoparticles. *Mol. Pharm.* **2014**, *11*, 3133–3144. [CrossRef] [PubMed]
30. Sayag, D.; Cabon, Q.; Texier, I.; Navarro, F.P.; Boisgard, R.; Virieux-Watrelot, D.; Carozzo, C.; Ponce, F. Phase-0/phase-I study of dye-loaded lipid nanoparticles for near-infrared fluorescence imaging in healthy dogs. *Eur. J. Pharm. Biopharm.* **2016**, *100*, 85–93. [CrossRef] [PubMed]

31. Pellosi, D.S.; Paula, L.B.; de Melo, M.T.; Tedesco, A.C. Targeted and Synergic Glioblastoma Treatment: Multifunctional Nanoparticles Delivering Verteporfin as Adjuvant Therapy for Temozolomide Chemotherapy. *Mol. Pharm.* **2019**, *16*, 1009–1024. [CrossRef] [PubMed]
32. Bazylinska, U.; Kulbacka, J.; Chodaczek, G. Nanoemulsion Structural Design in Co-Encapsulation of Hybrid Multifunctional Agents: Influence of the Smart PLGA Polymers on the Nanosystem-Enhanced Delivery and Electro-Photodynamic Treatment. *Pharmaceutics* **2019**, *11*, 405. [CrossRef] [PubMed]
33. Jiang, D.; Xu, M.; Pei, Y.; Huang, Y.; Chen, Y.; Ma, F.; Lu, H.; Chen, J. Core-matched nanoassemblies for targeted co-delivery of chemotherapy and photosensitizer to treat drug-resistant cancer. *Acta Biomater.* **2019**, *88*, 406–421. [CrossRef] [PubMed]
34. Chilakamarthi, U.; Giribabu, L. Photodynamic Therapy: Past, Present and Future. *Chem. Rec.* **2017**, *17*, 775–802. [CrossRef] [PubMed]
35. Hahn, S.M.; Fraker, D.L.; Mick, R.; Metz, J.; Busch, T.M.; Smith, D.; Zhu, T.; Rodriguez, C.; Dimofte, A.; Spitz, F.; et al. A phase II trial of intraperitoneal photodynamic therapy for patients with peritoneal carcinomatosis and sarcomatosis. *Clin. Cancer Res.* **2006**, *12*, 2517–2525. [CrossRef] [PubMed]
36. Wilson, B.C.; Patterson, M.S. The physics, biophysics and technology of photodynamic therapy. *Phys. Med. Biol.* **2008**, *53*, R61–R109. [CrossRef] [PubMed]
37. Rich, L.J.; Miller, A.; Singh, A.K.; Seshadri, M. Photoacoustic Imaging as an Early Biomarker of Radio Therapeutic Efficacy in Head and Neck Cancer. *Theranostics* **2018**, *8*, 2064–2078. [CrossRef] [PubMed]
38. Fujwara, K.; Yoshino, K.; Enomoto, T.; Fujita, M.; Ueda, Y.; Miyatake, T.; Kimura, T.; Muraji, M.; Fujita, H.; Kimura, T.; et al. Usefulness of computed tomography in predicting cytoreductive surgical outcomes for ovarian cancer. *Arch. Gynecol. Obstet.* **2011**, *284*, 1501–1507. [CrossRef] [PubMed]
39. Glaser, G.; Torres, M.; Kim, B.; Aletti, G.; Weaver, A.; Mariani, A.; Hartmann, L.; Cliby, W. The use of CT findings to predict extent of tumor at primary surgery for ovarian cancer. *Gynecol. Oncol.* **2013**, *130*, 280–283. [CrossRef] [PubMed]
40. Jacquart, A.; Keramidas, M.; Vollaire, J.; Boisgard, R.; Pottier, G.; Rustique, E.; Mittler, F.; Navarro, F.P.; Boutet, J.; Coll, J.L.; et al. LipImage 815: Novel dye-loaded lipid nanoparticles for long-term and sensitive in vivo near-infrared fluorescence imaging. *J. Biomed. Opt.* **2013**, *18*, 101311. [CrossRef] [PubMed]
41. Zhang, H.; Ramakrishnan, S.K.; Triner, D.; Centofanti, B.; Maitra, D.; Gyorffy, B.; Sebolt-Leopold, J.S.; Dame, M.K.; Varani, J.; Brenner, D.E.; et al. Tumor-selective proteotoxicity of verteporfin inhibits colon cancer progression independently of YAP1. *Sci. Signal* **2015**, *8*, ra98. [CrossRef] [PubMed]
42. Jeannot, V.; Mazzaferro, S.; Lavaud, J.; Vanwonterghem, L.; Henry, M.; Arboleas, M.; Vollaire, J.; Josserand, V.; Coll, J.L.; Lecommandoux, S.; et al. Targeting CD44 receptor-positive lung tumors using polysaccharide-based nanocarriers: Influence of nanoparticle size and administration route. *Nanomedicine* **2016**, *12*, 921–932. [CrossRef] [PubMed]
43. Lavaud, J.; Henry, M.; Coll, J.L.; Josserand, V. Exploration of melanoma metastases in mice brains using endogenous contrast photoacoustic imaging. *Int. J. Pharm.* **2017**, *532*, 704–709. [CrossRef] [PubMed]

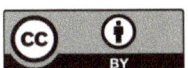

© 2019 by the authors. Licensee MDPI, Basel, Switzerland. This article is an open access article distributed under the terms and conditions of the Creative Commons Attribution (CC BY) license (http://creativecommons.org/licenses/by/4.0/).

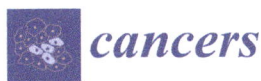

Article

Development and Mechanistic Insight into the Enhanced Cytotoxic Potential of Parvifloron D Albumin Nanoparticles in EGFR-Overexpressing Pancreatic Cancer Cells

Ana Santos-Rebelo [1,2], Pradeep Kumar [3], Viness Pillay [3], Yahya E. Choonara [3], Carla Eleutério [4], Mariana Figueira [4], Ana S. Viana [5], Lia Ascensão [6], Jesús Molpeceres [2], Patrícia Rijo [1,7], Isabel Correia [8], Joana Amaral [7], Susana Solá [7], Cecília M. P. Rodrigues [7], Maria Manuela Gaspar [7] and Catarina Pinto Reis [4,7,9,*]

1. CBIOS (Research Center for Biosciences and Health Technologies), Universidade Lusófona de Humanidades e Tecnologias, Campo Grande 376, 1749-024 Lisboa, Portugal; ana.rebelo1490@gmail.com (A.S.-R.); p1609@ulusofona.pt (P.R.)
2. Department of Biomedical Sciences, Faculty of Pharmacy, University of Alcalá, Ctra. A2 km 33,600 Campus Universitario, 28871 Alcalá de Henares, Spain; jesus.molpeceres@uah.es
3. Wits Advanced Drug Delivery Platform Research Unit, Department of Pharmacy and Pharmacology, Faculty of Health Sciences, School of Therapeutics Sciences, University of the Witwatersrand, Johannesburg, 7 York Road, Parktown 2193, South Africa; pradeep.kumar@wits.ac.za (P.K.); viness.pillay@wits.ac.za (V.P.); yahya.choonara@wits.ac.za (Y.E.C.)
4. Faculdade de Farmácia, Universidade de Lisboa, Av. Prof. Gama Pinto, 1649-003 Lisboa, Portugal; carlavania@ff.ul.pt (C.E.); mariana.selas.figueira@gmail.com (M.F.)
5. CQB, CQE, Faculdade de Ciências, Universidade de Lisboa, Campo Grande 1749-016 Lisboa, Portugal; apsemedo@fc.ul.pt
6. CESAM, Universidade de Lisboa, Faculdade de Ciências, Campo Grande 1749-016 Lisboa, Portugal; lmpsousa@fc.ul.pt
7. Research Institute for Medicines (iMed.ULisboa), Faculty of Pharmacy, Universidade de Lisboa, Av. Prof. Gama Pinto, 1649-003 Lisboa, Portugal; jamaral@ff.ulisboa.pt (J.A.); susana.sola@ff.ulisboa.pt (S.S.); cmprodrigues@ff.ulisboa.pt (C.M.P.R.); mgaspar@ff.ulisboa.pt (M.M.G.)
8. Centro de Química Estrutural, Instituto Superior Técnico, Departamento de Engenharia Química, Universidade de Lisboa,1049-001 Lisboa, Portugal; icorreia@tecnico.ulisboa.pt
9. IBEB, Faculdade de Ciências, Universidade de Lisboa, 1749-016 Lisboa, Portugal
* Correspondence: catarinareis@ff.ulisboa.pt; Tel.: +351-217-946-400; Fax: +351-217-946-470

Received: 5 October 2019; Accepted: 1 November 2019; Published: 5 November 2019

Abstract: Pancreatic cancer is one of the most lethal cancers, with an extremely poor prognosis. The development of more effective therapies is thus imperative. Natural origin compounds isolated from *Plectranthus* genus, such as parvifloron D (PvD), have cytotoxic and antiproliferative activity against human tumour cells. However, PvD is a very low water-soluble compound, being nanotechnology a promising alternative strategy to solve this problem. Therefore, the aim of this study was to optimize a nanosystem for preferential delivery of PvD to pancreatic tumour cells. Albumin nanoparticles (BSA NPs) were produced through a desolvation method. Glucose cross-linking and bioactive functionalization profiles of BSA platform were elucidated and analysed using static lattice atomistic simulations in vacuum. Using the optimized methodology, PvD was encapsulated (yield higher than 80%) while NPs were characterized in terms of size (100–400 nm) and morphology. Importantly, to achieve a preferential targeting to pancreatic cancer cells, erlotinib and cetuximab were attached to the PvD-loaded nanoparticle surface, and their antiproliferative effects were evaluated in BxPC3 and Panc-1 cell lines. Erlotinib conjugated NPs presented the highest antiproliferative effect toward pancreatic tumour cells. Accordingly, cell cycle analysis of the BxPC3 cell line showed marked accumulation of tumour cells in G1-phase and cell cycle arrest promoted by NPs. As a result, erlotinib conjugated PvD-loaded BSA NPs must be considered a suitable and promising carrier to deliver PvD at the tumour site, improving the treatment of pancreatic cancer.

Keywords: pancreatic cancer; parvifloron D; nanoparticles; albumin; erlotinib

1. Introduction

Pancreatic cancer remains one of the most lethal cancers worldwide [1]. Conventional therapy approaches such as surgery, radiation and chemotherapy have had discrete impact, as approximately 100% of patients develop metastases and end up dying [1]. Chemotherapy is still the most common option, although with minimal impact on survival [2–4]. The current first-line chemotherapy agent in pancreatic cancer is gemcitabine, which extends the overall survival by only 6 to 12 weeks [3,5,6]. Additionally, its benefits are generally compromised by a low half-life and relative low concentration around the tumour tissue [7]. Therefore, there is an urgent need for novel and more effective therapies [1].

Nowadays, approximately 60% of clinically used antitumor drugs are derivatives or come directly from natural products [8,9]. Terpenoids are the largest class of natural products with medicinal properties and they represent a rich source for drug discovery, especially anticancer drugs [10]. The majority induce tumour cell death by targeting apoptotic pathways [10]. Abietane diterpenoids are characteristic secondary metabolites from the Lamiaceae family reported to have cytotoxic and antiproliferative activity against tumour cell lines [11]. More specifically, *Plectranthus ecklonii* and its major compound, parvifloron D (PvD), caught our attention [12,13]. PvD has been shown to inhibit cancer proliferation by apoptosis in some cancer cell lines, such as human myeloid leukaemia, melanoma and breast cancer [12]. However, PvD presents very poor water solubility characteristics, as well as an apparent lack of selectivity toward cancer cells [12,14]. Since PvD also shows lack of specificity and cytotoxicity in noncancerous cell lines, the use of nanotechnology appears as a possible solution to deliver this drug to pancreatic cancer tissue without undesirable side effects.

Besides improving solubility and stability, nanoparticles (NPs) may extend formulation actions, combine activities with different degrees of hydrophilicity/lipophilicity, crucial for targeting and to deliver the drug at a specific tissue or organ [15–17]. In addition, NPs allow a better action of natural products, promoting a sustained release with reduced dose administration [15,18,19]. In this regard, albumin NPs (BSA NPs) are increasingly being used as drug delivery system for effective accumulation within tumour tissues through the enhanced permeability and retention (EPR) effect and albumin binding target proteins [6,20]. In fact, albumin is the most abundant protein in blood plasma, being biocompatible, biodegradable and nontoxic [6,20–22], and exhibiting active targeting and specific activity in the liver-pancreas system [7,23].

It has been shown that specific targeting of tumour cells can be guaranteed through different linkers or functional molecules [24,25]. Polyethylene glycol (PEG) is one of the most used polymers [26,27] since PEGylation has been shown to reduce NP immunogenicity and enhance accumulation in tumours by heightening the circulation time and promoting the EPR effect [24,27]. Further, the addition of antibodies, like cetuximab (CET) and erlotinib (ERL), was already shown to be necessary to promote targeted delivery. Indeed, the Epidermal Growth Factor Receptor (EGFR) is overexpressed in pancreatic cancer and both antibodies are EGFR inhibitors [28].

Therefore, due to the low water-solubility of PvD, we have encapsulated PvD into a biocompatible and hydrophilic nanomaterial as a possible drug delivery system. Bovine serum albumin (BSA) was chosen as encapsulating material. In order to produce our BSA NPs, a desolvation method was used. This method was chosen given its advantages, such as the fact that it does not require a temperature increase, being a suitable method for heat sensitive polymers, like BSA [29,30]. In the last step of desolvation method, glutaraldehyde is the most common added cross-linking agent [21,31,32].

However, due to glutaraldehyde's undesirable effects, we have tested more biocompatible alternative cross-linking methods including ultraviolet (UV) irradiation, addition of glucose, and combinations of both. Finally, to further optimize the NP preparation method, other different conditions were tested, including different stirring rates during the emulsion step (100 and 500 rpm), cross-linking times (30 min and 24 h) and type of organic solvent (hexane, acetone, DMSO and ethanol), and aqueous:organic solvent proportions (1:1, 2:1 and 3:1). The organic solvents tested were chosen for being the ones that best dissolve our compound with different ICH classification, i.e., grade of toxicity. All organic solvents were properly removed with centrifuge wash cycles after NP production.

To summarize, in the present work we produced PvD-loaded BSA NPs followed by their functionalization with ERL and/or CET for pancreatic cancer cell targeting.

2. Results

2.1. Optimization of BSA-Based NPs Preparation Method

To optimize the NP preparation method, different conditions were tested to select the best conditions to achieve BSA NPs with a mean size ranging between 100–400 nm, monodisperse size distribution, high cross-linking efficacy and the lowest negative zeta potential, to ensure high stability [33]. Table 1 shows the results obtained with all the conditions tested.

Table 1. BSA nanoparticle (NP) characterization in terms of size, zeta potential, polydispersity index (PdI) and cross-linking efficacy (CE (%))—influence of experimental conditions.

		Mean Size (nm) (± SD)	Zeta Potential	PdI	CE (%)
Cross-linking agent	Glutaraldehyde	178 (± 43)	−1	<0.220	54
	Glucose	**225 (± 60)**	−14	<0.250	97
	Glucose + UV	237 (± 70)	−4	<0.120	44
	UV	600 (± 116)	−1	<0.180	95
Stirring rate (rpm)	100	4396 (± 398)	0	<0.710	98
	500	**225 (± 25)**	−14	<0.250	97
Cross-linking time	24 h	129 (± 34)	11	<0.100	56
	30 min	**225 (± 25)**	−14	<0.250	97
Type of organic solvent	DMSO	153 (± 25)	0	<0.010	69
	Ethanol	145 (±42)	−2	<0.330	50
	Acetone	**244 (± 9)**	−8	**<0.260**	98
	Hexane	1346 (± 144)	−1	<0.180	88
Aqueous: Organic ratio	1:1	236 (± 62)	−1	<0.230	78
	2:1	898 (± 33)	0	<0.210	77
	3:1	**244 (± 9)**	−8	**<0.260**	98

After analysing the designed particles in terms of mean size, zeta potential and cross-linking efficacy [CE (%)], and testing different rpm (100 and 500 rpm), we conclude that the best outcomes were achieved with a stirring rate of 500 rpm with smaller particle size and lower PdI. Then, for the four cross-linking tested groups, the cross-linking with glucose showed the smallest size. However, when observing the cross-linking time (30 min and 24 h), we choose 30 min as the best cross-linking time, since the CE% drastically decreased over the time. Hereupon, comparing the results obtained for all organic solvents tested, we have elected acetone. Indeed, acetone is a ICH Class 3, i.e., regarded as less toxic and of lower risk to human health, and, of note, class 3 includes no solvent known as a human health hazard at levels normally accepted in pharmaceuticals. Finally, we tested different proportions of aqueous BSA: organic solvent ratios, and choose the 3:1. The resulting particle size was near 200 nm, presenting a negative zeta potential and high CE (up to 90%), close to the established goal. In bold (Table 1), is represented the best result in each condition tested.

2.2. Cytotoxicity Assay in a Saccharomyces Cerevisiae Model

The percentage of growth inhibition (GI) was calculated by the determination of the linear slope in the logarithmic phase for each sample (Figure 1).

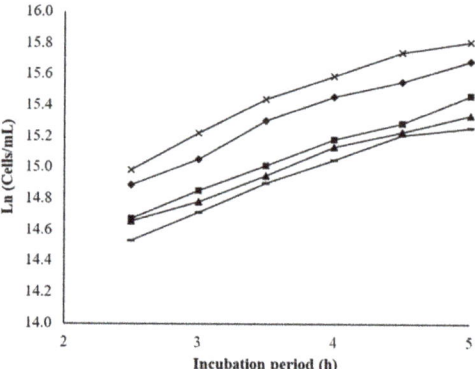

Figure 1. Growth curves of *Saccharomyces cerevisiae* cultures exposed to BSA NPs (x - negative control; ♦ - 3.0 µM; ■ - 3.9 µM; — - 4.6 µM; ▲ - 5.3 µM). Yeast growth is presented as the natural logarithm of cell concentration, which is expressed as number of yeast cells/mL. The interval 2–5 h was considered as the log growth phase (n = 4, mean ± SD).

Interestingly, the exposure to BSA NPs at the lowest concentration (3.0 µM) resulted in 3.2% of GI and at the highest concentration (5.3 µM) resulted in 15.6%. On the other hand, the negative control was assumed as producing zero percentage of GI (100% yeast growth), in each experiment.

2.3. Circular Dichroism Spectroscopy

Circular dichroism spectroscopy was used to analyse the secondary structure of the BSA protein in its native form (BSA), NPs (BSA NPs) and NPs with ERL (ERL conjugated BSA NPs). Samples of NPs that were randomly destroyed by ultra-sounds and heat (Destroyed NP) were also analysed to confirm if this method destroys the BSA secondary structure and consequently NPs.

All samples were quantified in water and the respective spectra were measured in the far UV with protein concentrations corresponding to 0.2 or 0.4 mg/mL. Figures 2 and 3 show the collected spectra. Typically, α-helix showed two maxima of negative signal at 208 and 222 nm. Antiparallel β-sheet shows one negative maximum at ca. 218 nm and a positive one at ca. 195 nm. Random coil is characterized by a negative maximum at ca. 208 nm.

Circular dichroism has been extensively applied to evaluate the secondary structure of proteins as different amounts of secondary structural elements, such as α-helix and β-sheets, correspond to different CD spectra. This is due to the protein CD spectrum being considered the sum of the spectra of the individual secondary structures present in the protein. In order to have the same intensity as the BSA spectrum, the spectra of all complexes in Figure 3 were multiplied by a constant.

BSA showed a typical CD spectrum with a high α-helical content - negative ellipticity at ~208 and ~220 nm in the far UV range. After aggregation and formation of the NPs the spectra lost intensity but kept their shape. This might indicate one of two possible effects, either the α-helical content decreased, or the protein concentration is lower. Without having a control experiment to accurately determine the protein concentration no conclusions can be made. However, the persistence of the band at 220 nm suggests that it is only a concentration decrease. Thus, the preparation process used to destroy the NP (ultra-sounds and increased heat) did not destroy the secondary structure of BSA, revealing that those methods are safe and do not affect BSA structure. Importantly, BSA secondary structure is maintained even when in particle form [34,35].

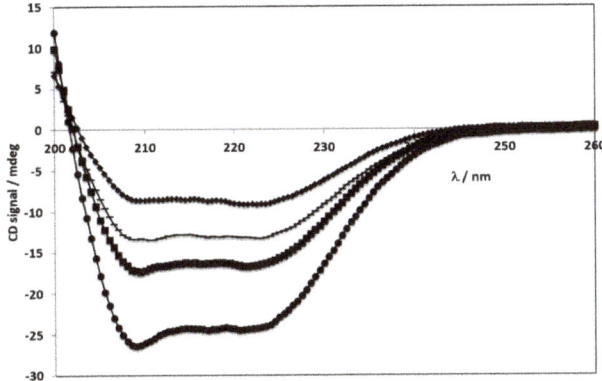

Figure 2. CD spectra measured in the far UV range for all samples: ● - BSA 0.2 mg/mL; ♦ - BSA NPs 0.4 mg/mL; ■ - ERL conjugated BSA NPs 0.4 mg/mL; — - Destroyed NPs 0.4 mg/mL.

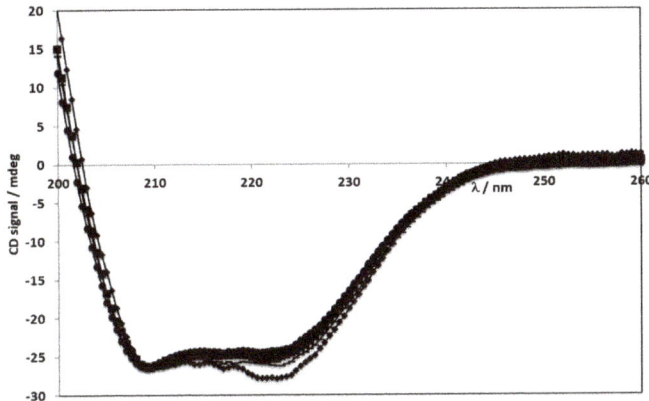

Figure 3. CD spectra measured in the far UV range after normalization – all spectra having the same intensity as BSA (● - BSA 0.2 mg/mL; ♦ - BSA NPs 0.4 mg/mL; ■ - ERL conjugated BSA NPs 0.4 mg/mL; — - Destroyed NPs 0.4 mg/mL).

2.4. Hemolytic Activity of Potential Injectable PvD-loaded BSA NPs Dosage Form

Understanding the interactions between NPs and blood components is critical for future clinical applications. One of the most fundamental studies on the interactions between NPs and blood components is to access their haemolytic properties. In fact, in vivo haemolysis can trigger several pathological conditions such as anaemia and jaundice. In vitro evaluation of NPs biocompatibility is a crucial step towards early preclinical development because the small size and unique physicochemical properties of NPs may cause damage in red blood cells (RBC). Thus, the US FDA recommends that an in vitro haemolysis study should be performed for compounds intended for injectable use, at the intended concentration for i.v. administration to test the possible haemolytic potential. This assay evaluates haemoglobin release in the plasma, as an indicator of RBC lysis, following the exposure to a test agent [36]. In this work, the haemolytic activity against RBCs was used as a marker of a general membrane toxicity effect of PvD. Since the concentration of haemoglobin depends both on the number of disintegrated RBCs in the sample and the volume of the fluid, the degree of haemolysis is often described as the percentage of free haemoglobin in relation to the total. The percentage of haemolysis of PvD in free form or incorporated in BSA NPs, as well as in empty NPs, was evaluated

2.5. PvD Encapsulation Efficiency

The encapsulation efficiency (EE, %) is one of the most important physicochemical characteristics of NPs-based formulations. Many methods have been used to evaluate the EE, including dialysis bag diffusion, gel filtration, ultrafiltration, and ultracentrifugation. Compared with the conventional drug delivery systems, the size of the reservoir of NPs in which the drug molecule is loaded is extremely small. Depending on this small capacity of NPs, the drug molecules interact with the polymeric structure to a certain degree. In this work, EE (%) was determined for all nanoformulations by measuring the non-encapsulated drug (lost PvD during the nanoencapsulation procedure) by centrifugation, i.e., through indirect quantification. Herein, we obtained 79.47%, 82.07%, 79.92%, 72.76%, for PvD-loaded BSA NPs, ERL conjugated PvD-loaded BSA NPs, CET conjugated PvD-loaded BSA NPs and ERL-CET conjugated PvD-loaded BSA NPs, respectively. For this assay, a calibration curve was firstly performed using previously isolated PvD as a standard. PvD solutions ranging from 4.4 to 44 µg/mL were evaluated and a calibration curve (y = 31316x − 66339) was obtained with $R^2 = 0.999$. Limit of Detection (LOD) and Limit of Quantification (LOQ) were calculated to be 2.2 µg/mL and 6.5 µg/mL, respectively.

2.6. ERL and CET Conjugated BSA NPs Conjugation Quantification

The ideal NP-based formulations should have a specific targeting to tumour cells, minimizing or even avoiding off-target effects of the drug on healthy tissues. In this field, much research has conjugated targeting ligands specific to cell surface components that are unique or upregulated in tumour tissues to NPs surfaces. In the current study, the presence of carboxylic and amino groups on the surface promotes the surface functionalization for BSA NPs. The ERL and CET conjugation quantification was determined by measuring the non-conjugated ligand, i.e., again through indirect quantification. The value was 40 µg/mL, for ERL conjugated PvD-loaded BSA NPs, ERL conjugated empty BSA NPs and ERL-CET conjugated empty BSA NPs, and 0.01 µg/mL for ERL-CET conjugated PvD-loaded BSA NPs. CET conjugated values were equivalent to those measured for ERL conjugation.

2.7. Static Lattice Atomistic Simulations (SLAS) in Vacuum

2.7.1. Molecular Mechanics Assisted Model Building and Energy Refinements

Molecular mechanics energy relationship (MMER), a method for analytical-mathematical representation of potential energy surfaces, was used to provide information about the contributions of valence terms, noncovalent Coulombic terms, and noncovalent van der Waals interactions for the BSA/cross-linker and BSA/bioactive interactions. The MMER model for potential energy factor in various molecular complexes can be written as follows in Equation (1):

$$E_{molecule/complex} = V_{\Sigma} = V_b + V_\theta + V_\varphi + V_{ij} + V_{hb} + V_{el} \quad (1)$$

where, V_{Σ} is related to total steric energy for an optimized structure, V_b corresponds to bond stretching contributions, V_θ denotes bond angle contributions, V_φ represents torsional contribution from dihedral angles, V_{ij} incorporates van der Waals interactions due to non-bonded interatomic distances, V_{hb} symbolizes hydrogen-bond energy function and V_{el} stands for electrostatic energy.

In addition, the total potential energy deviation, ΔE_{Total}, was calculated as the difference between the total potential energy of the complex system and the sum of the potential energies of isolated individual molecules, as in the following Equation (2):

$$\Delta E_{Total(A/B)} = E_{Total(A/B)} - (E_{Total(A)} + E_{Total(B)}) \quad (2)$$

The molecular stability can then be estimated by comparing the total potential energies of the isolated and complexed systems. If the total potential energy of complex is smaller than the sum of the potential energies of isolated individual molecules in the same conformation, the complexed form is more stable and its formation is favoured [37].

2.7.2. Fabrication of Glucose Cross-Linked BSA NPs

The energy relationships confirming the cross-linking of BSA with glucose are presented in Equations (3)–(5) and the corresponding energy minimized geometrical conformations are depicted in Figure 4:

$$E_{BSA} = -276.821 V_{\sum} = 4.001 V_b + 20.569 V_\theta + 29.478 V_\varphi - 23.961 V_{ij} - 6.478 V_{hb} - 300.432 V_{el} \quad (3)$$

$$E_{GLUCOSE} = 1.064 V_{\sum} = 0.556 V_b + 2.998 V_\theta + 1.696 V_\varphi + 6.820 V_{ij} - 0.000 V_{hb} + 11.008 V_{el} \quad (4)$$

$$E_{BSA\text{-}GLUCOSE} = -342.611 V_{\sum} = 5.383 V_b + 26.787 V_\theta + 38.058 V_\varphi - 21.609 V_{ij} - 4.323 V_{hb} - 386.908 V_{el} \quad (5)$$

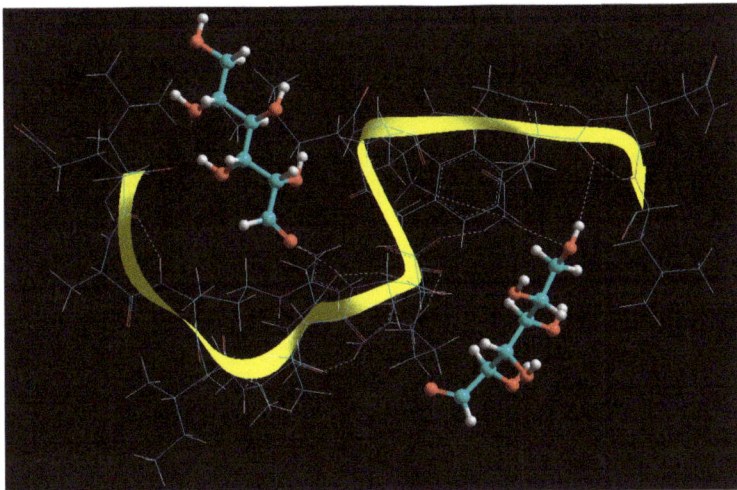

Figure 4. Visualization of geometrical preferences and functional interactions between BSA (stick rendering) in complexation with the glucose molecules (ball-and-tube rendering) after molecular mechanics simulations in vacuum. Colour codes: C (cyan), O (red), N (blue) and H (white).

It is evident from MMER that BSA-glucose formed a very stable complex, with $\Delta E_{BINDING}$ of −66.854 kcal/mol, wherein a major stabilizing role was played by electrostatic interactions ($\Delta E = -97.484$ kcal/mol) and partially by van der Waals forces ($\Delta E = -4.468$ kcal/mol). As expected from a cross-linked structure, the torsional strains caused by a small molecule cross-linking agent such as glucose may cause an internal stress arising from bond/angle stretching and bending, leading to a rigid structure and hence destabilization of the matrix as evident from the bonding energy terms viz V_b ($\Delta E = 0.826$ kcal/mol), V_θ ($\Delta E = 3.22$ kcal/mol) and V_φ ($\Delta E = 6.884$ kcal/mol). Interestingly, such constrained structure will bring the subpeptidic chains closer and hence enhancing the electrostatic interactions contributing to the final stabilized structure. It is worth noting that the H-bonding component of BSA was somewhat diminished ($\Delta E = 2.155$ kcal/mol) after cross-linking, which may be due to reduction in intramolecular H-bonding and introduction of intermolecular H-bonding. This observation is further confirmed by Figure 5 wherein: (1) the reducing sugar-derived carbonyl group of glucose formed an adduct with free amine group of BSA (–C=O . . . NH–) [38]; (2) –OH . . . O=C– hydrogen bonding; and (3) -OH . . .

NH– hydrogen bonding [39]. These findings further corroborate with the experimental data wherein it was proposed that longer cross-linking time may lead to reduced cross-linking efficiency which may further be attributed to the above inter- and intra-molecular H-bonding interplay.

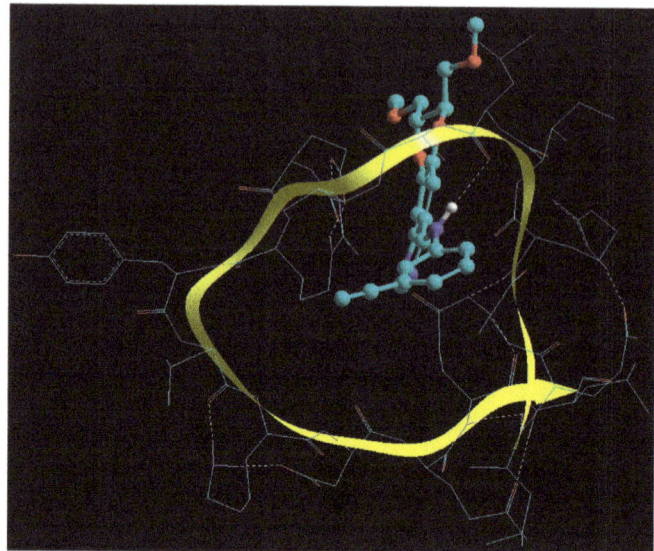

Figure 5. Visualization of geometrical preferences and functional interactions between BSA (stick rendering) in complexation with the ERL molecule (ball-and-tube rendering) after molecular mechanics simulations in vacuum. Colour codes: C (cyan), O (red), N (blue) and H (white).

2.7.3. Functionalization of BSA NPs with ERL

The geometrical visualization and MMER profiles for BSA-ERL complex are depicted in Equations (6)–(8) and Figure 5, respectively:

$$E_{BSA} = -276.821 V_{\sum} = 4.001 V_b + 20.569 V_\theta + 29.478 V_\varphi - 23.961 V_{ij} - 6.478 V_{hb} - 300.432 V_{el} \quad (6)$$

$$E_{ERL} = 17.719 V_{\sum} = 0.995 V_b + 1.991 V_\theta + 5.833 V_\varphi + 8.899 V_i \quad (7)$$

$$E_{BSA\text{-}ERL} = -284.457 V_{\sum} = 5.650 V_b + 45.119 V_\theta + 53.256 V_\varphi - 37.967 V_{ij} - 7.469 V_{hb} - 343.046 V_{el} \quad (8)$$

The aim of generating MMER in this case was to confirm the mode of interaction inherent to the peptide-bioactive complex. In case of bioactives' functionalization in a carrier, it is of utmost important that the functional groups responsible for their bioactivity are not involved in covalent bonding. In the current modelling exercise, it was established that the N atoms of ERL were H-bonded to the -C=O functionality of BSA. This is in line with previously developed ERL-functionalized carriers by Ali and co-workers, one of the first reports mentioning such functionalization [40]. The BSA-ERL complex was energetically stabilized with ΔE$_{binding}$ of −25.355 kcal/mol with both bonding and non-bonding interactions playing a significant part. The significant destabilization by the bonding interactions (V_b, V_θ and V_φ) led to significant geometrical changes in the BSA molecule further leading to apparent globalization which may further assist in *colloidation* of the nanosystem. The 41.158 kcal/mol destabilization by the bonding interactions was neutralized and exceeded by the non-bonding stabilization of 66.51 kcal/mol with electrostatic interactions playing the major role. Interestingly the close fit of the ERL molecule further stabilized the van der Waals contributions and hence the H-bonding.

2.7.4. Functionalization of BSA NPs with CET

In a study published in *PNAS*, Donaldson and co-workers provided an interesting proposition that can be quoted as follows "the identification and subsequent grafting of a unique peptide binding site within the Fab domain offers a unique means of adding functionality to monoclonal antibodies through a noncovalent interaction including improved pre-targeted imaging, alternative payload delivery, and cross-linking of mAbs on cell surfaces to enhance their therapeutic potential" [40]. Taking lead from the above proposition, the current study employed CET as the mAb and tested the potential of grafting BSA to the light (A, C) and heavy (B, D) chains of CET. As this study doesn't involve molecular docking, the light and heavy chains were individually interacted with the BSA molecule and thereby light chain A was selected for the final modelling paradigm based on preliminary geometrical and energetic interaction profiling (detailed docking studies are out-of-scope of this study). Similar to ERL, the BSA-CET molecular complex was destabilized by the bonding energy terms (bond, angle, and torsion) while significantly stabilized by the non-bonding energy components (van der Waals forces, H-bonding, and electrostatic interactions) as depicted in Equations (9)–(11):

$$E_{BSA} = -276.821 V_\Sigma = 4.001 V_b + 20.569 V_\theta + 29.478 V_\varphi - 23.961 V_{ij} - 6.478 V_{hb} - 300.432 V_{el} \quad (9)$$

$$E_{CET} = -959.541 V_\Sigma = 17.270 V_b + 124.263 V_\theta + 123.955 V_\varphi - 167.367 V_{ij} - 34.565_{hb} - 1023.1 V_{el} \quad (10)$$

$$E_{BSA\text{-}CET} = -1281.649 V_\Sigma = 23.443 V_b + 237.799 V_\theta + 203.402 V_\varphi - 238.943 V_{ij} - 44.723 V_{hb} - 1462.63 V_{el} \quad (11)$$

A close look at Figure 6 revealed an extensive molecular network with –C=O ... N-H amide linkages and –C=O ... O-H hydrogen bonds.

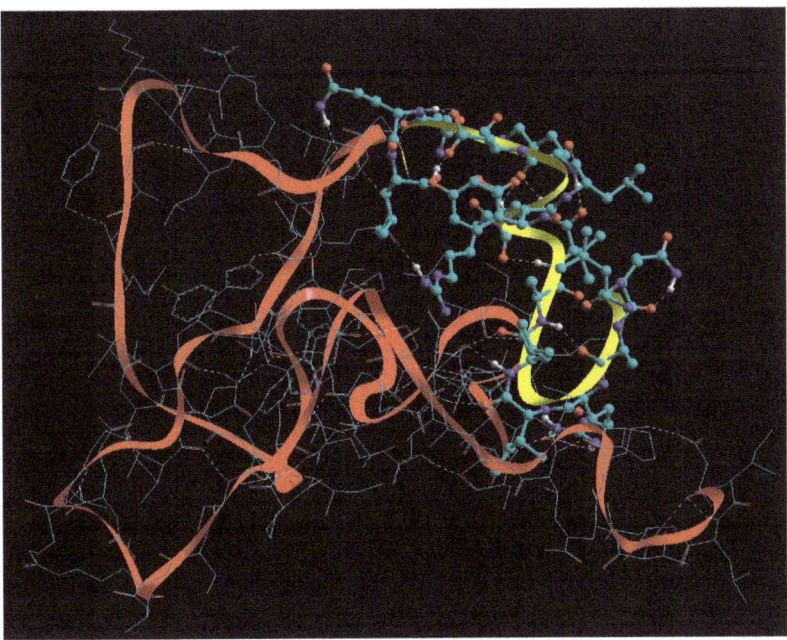

Figure 6. Visualization of geometrical preferences and functional interactions between BSA (yellow ribbon rendering) in complexation with the CET Chain A (red ribbon rendering) after molecular mechanics simulations in vacuum. Colour codes: C (cyan), O (red), N (blue) and H (white).

2.8. Physical and Morphological Characterization of the EGFR Inhibitors Conjugated BSA NPs

Table 2 shows DLS analysis of particle size and zeta potential of ERL conjugated empty BSA NPs, ERL conjugated PvD-loaded BSA NPs, CET conjugated empty BSA NPs, CET conjugated PvD-loaded BSA NPs, ERL-CET conjugated empty BSA NPs, ERL-CET conjugated PvD-loaded BSA NPs, PvD-loaded BSA NPs and Empty BSA NPs.

Table 2. Particle size, polydispersity index (PdI) and zeta potential of all EGFR inhibitors conjugated BSA nanoformulations by DLS analysis.

BSA Nanoformulations	Mean Diameter (nm) ± SD	Mean Zeta Potential (mV) ± SD	PdI
ERL-CET conjugated PvD-loaded BSA NPs	1466 (±155)	−48 (± 6)	<0.560
ERL-CET conjugated empty BSA NPs	502 (± 36)	−32 (± 6)	<1
ERL conjugated PvD-loaded BSA NPs	349 (± 59)	−39 (± 10)	<0.450
ERL conjugated empty BSA NPs	336 (± 91)	−36 (± 5)	<0.090
CET conjugated PvD-loaded BSA NPs	43 (± 4)	−43 (± 4)	<1
CET conjugated empty BSA NPs	42 (± 5)	−32 (± 6)	<1
PvD-loaded BSA NPs	280 (± 86)	−42 (± 4)	<0.370
Empty BSA NPs	393 (± 131)	−37 (± 6)	<0.120

AFM analysis confirmed that particles sizes were very close to those obtained by DLS analysis. Figures 7–10 show AFM images of all formulations prepared as well as their size and morphology.

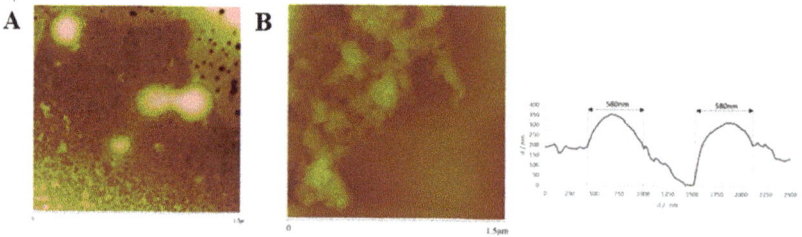

Figure 7. AFM images (2D and sectorial images) with size scale of (**A**) PvD-loaded, and (**B**) Empty ERL-CET conjugated NPs.

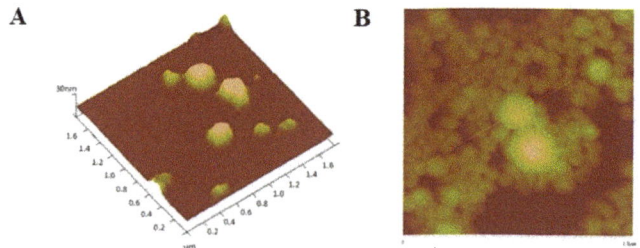

Figure 8. AFM images (3D and 2D images) with size scale of (**A**) PvD-loaded, and (**B**) empty ERL conjugated NPs.

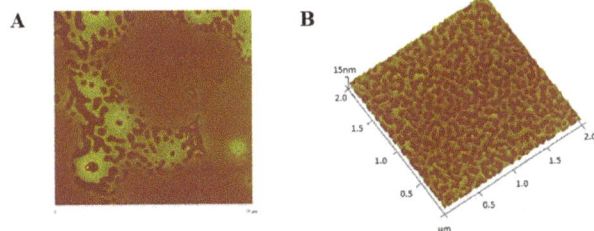

Figure 9. AFM images (2D and 3D images) with size scale of (**A**) PvD-loaded, and (**B**) empty CET conjugated NPs.

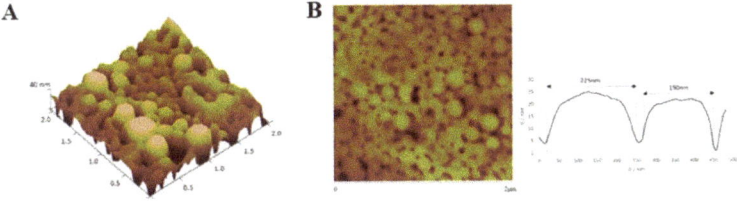

Figure 10. AFM images (3D and sectorial images) with size scale of (**A**) PvD-loaded, and (**B**) empty non-conjugated NPs.

AFM allows the optimization of biomaterials processes, performance, physical and chemical properties, offering a great contribution to the understanding of surface and interface properties, even at the nanoscale [41]. Considering DLS and AFM analysis, as well as the cell viability studies of PvD-loaded BSA NPs, we have decided to proceed only with the best particles in terms of mean size (between 100–400 nm, allowing a safe i.v. administration), zeta potential (higher than −30 mV, allowing a higher physical stability [33]), with monodisperse size distribution and lowest IC_{50} values as followed described. Thus, SEM and TEM focused on ERL conjugated NPs and non-conjugated NPs, confirming particle sizes and spherical morphology (Figures 11 and 12).

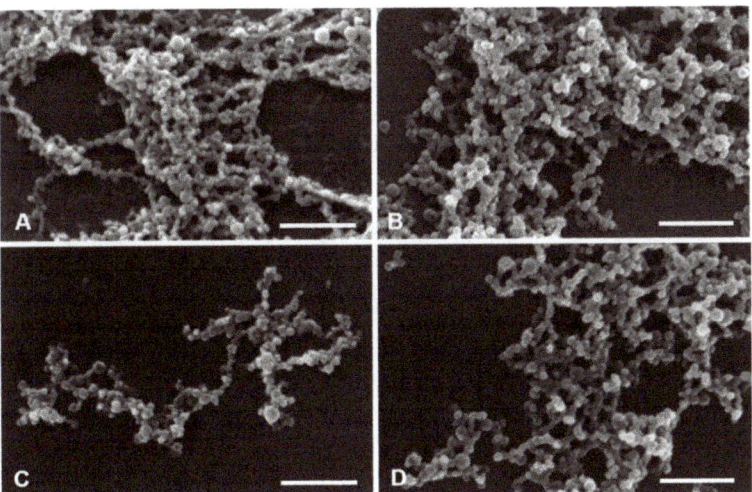

Figure 11. SEM images of BSA NPs. (**A**) empty ERL conjugated NPs; (**B**) PvD-loaded non-conjugated NPs; (**C**) ERL conjugated PvD-loaded NPs; (**D**) empty non-conjugated NPs. Scale bars = 1 µm.

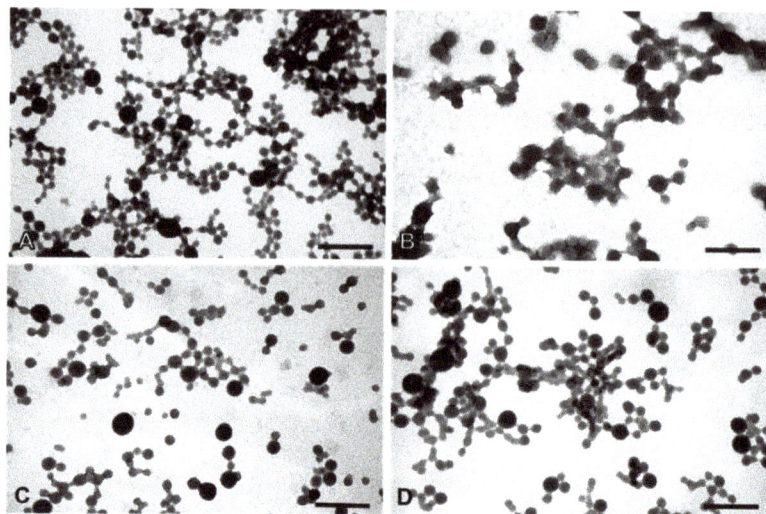

Figure 12. TEM images of BSA NPs. (**A**) empty ERL conjugated NPs; (**B**) PvD-loaded non-conjugated NPs; (**C**) ERL conjugated NPs PvD-loaded; (**D**) empty non-conjugated NPs. Scale bars = 0.5 μm.

2.9. Cell Viability Studies of PvD-loaded BSA NPs

Free PvD was shown highly cytotoxic for both cell lines, being particularly cytotoxic in BxPC3 cell line (Table 3).

Table 3. Antiproliferative effect (IC_{50}) of PvD in free form or nanoformulated in two human pancreatic adenocarcinoma cell lines (BXPC3 and PANC-1).

Formulation Tested	BxPC3	PANC-1
Free PvD	10.6 ± 3.6	21.7
Empty BSA NPs	>30	>40
PvD-loaded BSA NPs	>30	>40
ERL conjugated empty BSA NPs	<20	>40
ERL conjugated PvD-loaded BSA NPs	21.5 ± 2.2	16.8
CET conjugated empty BSA NPs	>30	>40
CET conjugated PvD-loaded BSA NPs	>30	>40
ERL-CET conjugated empty BSA NPs	<20	>40
ERL-CET conjugated PvD-loaded BSA NPs	6.9 ± 1.1	>40

Incubation period was 48 h. IC_{50} values are expressed in μM (n = 6).

However, the IC_{50} of PvD-loaded BSA NPs was higher than 30 μM, suggesting that at the end of the 48 h of incubation, PvD was not totally released from the particles. In fact, we know from previous in vitro studies (Santos-Rebelo et al. [13]) that total PvD particle release only occurs after 72 h of incubation. Indeed, NPs are possibly inducing its expected effect, since it would not be desirable that PvD cytotoxicity occurs during the administration, but only in the target tumor site. Nevertheless, IC_{50} of ERL conjugated PvD-loaded BSA NPs and ERL-CET conjugated PvD-loaded BSA NPs are lower than those of non-conjugated particles. However, when comparing ERL conjugated empty BSA NPs and ERL-CET conjugated empty BSA NPs, the IC_{50} values are also low, which leads us to hypothesize that the toxicity observed for ERL conjugated PvD-loaded BSA NPs and ERL-CET conjugated PvD-loaded BSA NPs may results from the ERL on the NP surface. In fact, this can increase particle internalization, allowing a higher drug release inside the target cells, particularly in the BxPC3 cell line. In vivo assays are needed to confirm targeting in a living organism.

2.10. Cell Cycle Assays

To go deeper into the mechanisms by which these different particles impact on tumour cell proliferation, we evaluated cell cycle progression in BxPC3 cells after incubation with free PvD, PvD-loaded BSA NPs and ERL conjugated PvD-loaded BSA NPs, and comparing with a blank control in which cells grew without any chemical influence. Figures 13 and 14 show the percentage of cells in different phases of the cell cycle after 24 h of particle incubation. As observed in Figure 14, exposure of cells to ERL conjugated PvD-loaded BSA NPs induced a marked accumulation of cells in the G1 phase, when compared with control ($p < 0.05$). Regarding PvD-loaded BSA NPs, the results show that these forms did not affect cell cycle progression. Importantly, this is in agreement with our previous hypothesis that total PvD is not totally released from the NPs at 24 h of incubation. Further, ERL in NPs surface probably increases particle internalization, allowing a higher drug release inside the target cells. In conclusion, these outcomes indicate that both PvD and ERL are responsible for driving tumour cells to arrest in the G1 phase of the cell cycle, preventing them from dividing and spreading.

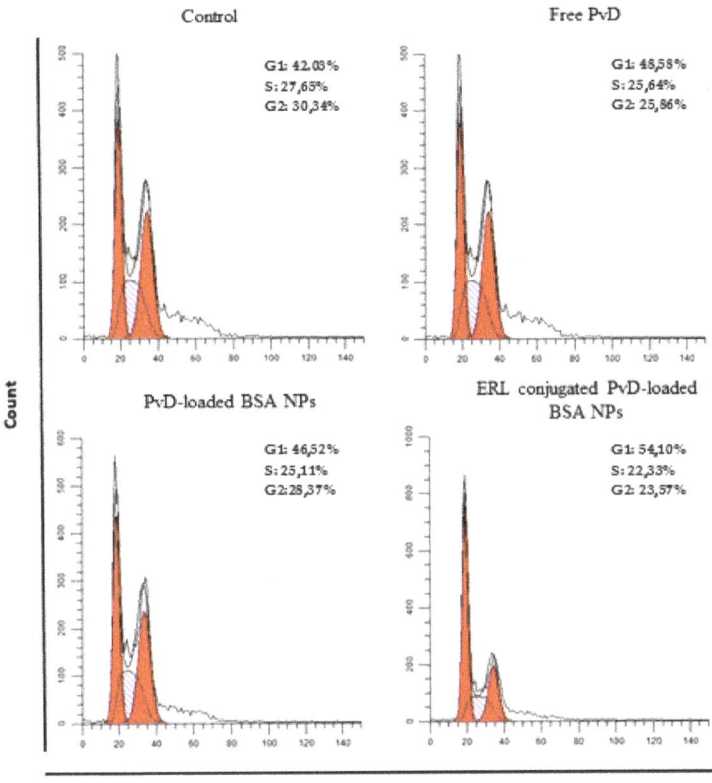

Figure 13. Effect of NPs on tumour cell cycle progression. Cellular DNA was stained with propidium iodide (PI) to determine cell cycle distribution. BxPC3 cells were treated with free PvD, PvD-loaded BSA NPs and ERL conjugated PvD-loaded BSA NPs, and compared with control, 24 h after incubation.

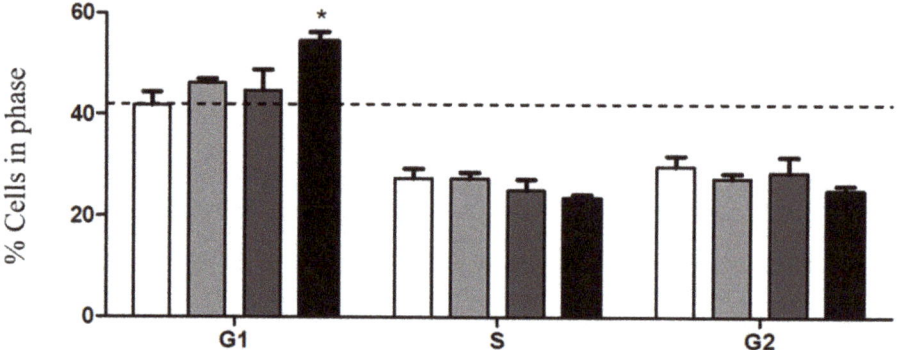

Figure 14. Effect of NPs on tumour cell cycle progression. Cellular DNA was stained with propidium iodide (PI) to determine cell cycle distribution. Percentage of cells in G1, S and G2 cell cycle phases in no addition (control; white), Free PvD (light grey), PvD-loaded BSA NPs (dark grey) and ERL conjugated PvD-loaded BSA NPs (black), after 24 h incubation. Results are expressed as mean ± SEM for three different experiments. * $p < 0.05$ from control by one-way ANOVA test.

2.11. Lactate Dehydrogenase Assay

To evaluate if PvD-dependent decrease of cell viability was due to either cell death or cell cycle arrest, we assessed lactate dehydrogenase release as a measure of cell membrane disruption, and therefore cell death (Figure 15).

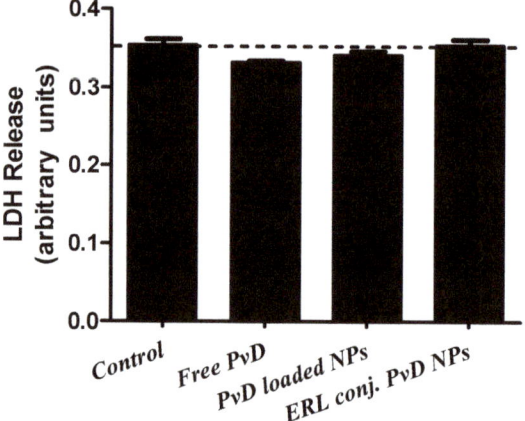

Figure 15. Lactate dehydrogenase (LDH) assay, using free PvD, ERL conjugated empty BSA NPs, ERL conjugated PvD-loaded BSA NPs. Results are expressed as mean ± SEM for three different experiments.

No significant differences were detected in membrane integrity between all samples tested, suggesting that the decrease of cell viability likely results from cell cycle arrest.

3. Discussion

Pancreatic cancer median survival after diagnosis ranges between 2–8 months, making this one of the most lethal types of cancer [2]. Moreover, the application of conventional drugs approved against pancreatic cancer is limited by drug resistance and a large number of adverse side effects [13]. Taking this into account, new therapies as nanoparticle applications could become a promising tool for sustained delivery of anticancer drugs.

We previously confirmed that PvD is a potential lead molecule mainly due to its specificity to pancreatic tumour cells [2]. However, PvD has very low water solubility and it strongly requires a suitable carrier like BSA NPs. In the present study, BSA NPs for PvD delivery were produced with an optimized method, where the conditions chosen include 500 rpm stirring rate, 30 min of cross-linking time and 3:1 aqueous/acetone ratio. These conditions resulted in particles with particle size ranging between 100–400 nm, monodisperse size distribution, high CE and negative zeta potential. BSA NPs were tested for toxicity in a *Saccharomyces cerevisiae* model, showing no relevant toxicity in the highest concentration tested, indicating promising carrier characteristics to deliver our drug. CD spectroscopy revealed the main structure of our NPs, where BSA secondary structure remained intact after nanoparticle arrangement. Previous studies by Differential Scanning Calorimetry [13] suggest that following NPs arrangement the structure modification of BSA chains may not involve changes in the protein secondary structure. Further, BSA secondary structure, even after NPs arrangement, seems to resist to heat and ultra-sounds. Finally, haemolytic activity was tested in BSA NPs as well as in free drug, to ensure that our formulation could be applied by i.v. administration. Since the haemolytic activity was below 1%, even for the highest concentrations tested, our formulation may be considered safe for i.v. administration, without any haemolytic risk.

The promising formulation, here developed, presented an EE greater than 80%, a value that is very high in comparison with other drug delivery systems. For example, in some micellar NPs the maximum capacity of the drug is only around 20–30% [42].

To target NPs to pancreatic cancer cells, we used EGFR inhibitors, ERL and CET, since EGFR overexpression has been found in 90% of pancreatic cancers [2]. NP conformation was further elucidated using SLAS in vacuum. Most studies with BSA NPs have used glutaraldehyde as cross-linking agent [43]. However, glutaraldehyde demonstrated toxicity to healthy cells [43]. We have proposed to use glucose as cross-linking agent and MMER confirmed that BSA-glucose formed a very stable complex. Moreover, MMER profiles for BSA-ERL complex showed that the functional groups responsible for bioactivity are not involved in covalent bonding, leaving them free to ensure their action in targeting tumour cells, and yet the BSA-ERL complex was considered energetically stabilized. When analysing BSA-CET molecular complex, it seems to be destabilized by the bonding energy terms, but significantly stabilized by the non-bonding energy components. Nevertheless, being CET a complex molecule with light and heavy chains, future molecular docking studies may better clarify those interactions.

When analysing ERL and CET conjugated empty and PvD-loaded BSA NPs by DLS, we concluded that ERL conjugated BSA NPs size, zeta potential and PdI values are better aligned with our goals. Accordingly, ERL-CET conjugated BSA NPs showed to have huge particle sizes as well PdI, which leads to a non-monodispersed suspension. On the other side, CET conjugated BSA NPs exhibit sizes that are too small. AFM analysis of those particles suggested a possible interaction between the compounds used that led to some kind of NP undoing process. In addition, CET conjugated BSA NPs showed low toxicity to pancreatic cancer cell lines, with IC_{50} values higher than 30 µM, compared to ERL conjugated BSA NPs, which showed IC_{50} values lower than 20 µM to BxPC3 cell line. Therefore, we choose to proceed our studies only with ERL conjugated BSA NPs. Thus, SEM, TEM, cell cycle and lactate dehydrogenase assays focused on ERL conjugated NPs and non-conjugated NPs. Cell cycle and lactate dehydrogenase assays suggested that the decrease of cell viability caused by NPs forms, as well as by free PvD, may occur by cell cycle arrest in the G1 phase and not by cell death, as membrane integrity remained intact.

Further in vivo testing is now required to characterize PvD pharmacokinetics and to evaluate its in vivo safety after the nanoencapsulation process. In a preliminary in vivo tolerability assay, a suspension of free PvD in 5% of DMSO (single dose 3 mg / kg) was intradermally injected in a small number of Wistar rats. Plasmatic concentration of PvD increased over the time (up to 6 h) and no animal death was verified till the end of the study (data not shown). In this preliminary study, the intradermal route was chosen mainly due to safety reasons. In vivo efficacy studies using the promising nanoformulation here developed are also warranted.

4. Materials and Methods

4.1. Optimization of BSA-Based NPs Development

Briefly, 50 mg of BSA was dissolved in 2.0 mL of purified water with the pH adjusted to 7–10 with NaOH solution. Subsequently, this solution was added dropwise into 8 mL of absolute ethanol solution under magnetic stirring (100 and 500 rpm). After the desolvation process, the cross-linking agent (glutaraldehyde, glucose, UV light and combination of both glucose and UV light methods) was added to induce particle cross-linking. The cross-linking process was performed under stirring of the suspension over a period of time (30 min and 24 h). First of all, the best stirring rate for NPs formation was defined. Then, after the desolvation process, four cross-linking groups were tested: the first in which 8% glutaraldehyde in water was added to induce particle cross-linking (1.175 µL/mg BSA); the second was placed in the UV chamber under UV light (wavelength 254 nm) for 30 min (the distance between the light source and the sample was 15 cm); on the third, 6 mM glucose was added (1.175 µL/mg BSA); for the forth, the addition of glucose was followed by immediate exposure to UV source in the same conditions mentioned in the second group [43]. After setting these first two steps, cross-linking process was tested under different time periods of stirring. Then, different organic solvents were added to BSA solution for further addition of the active compound in order to verify which one is the best solution for achieving the greatest nanoformulation in terms of size, zeta potential and cross-linking efficacy (CE, %).

4.2. NPs Cytotoxicity Assays on Saccharomyces Cerevisiae Model

The use of S. cerevisiae as an in vitro model organism has as main advantages the similarity with mammalian cells, the yeast fast growth, and the inexpensiveness and easy cultivation. Yeast is especially useful for toxicity studies involving oxidative stress-related mechanisms, since it can grow both in presence and absence of oxygen [44]. Through this assay, we aimed to study BSA NPs' potential cytotoxicity, testing the effects on the S. cerevisiae growth when contacting with different concentrations of BSA NPs samples. Saccharomyces cerevisiae (ATCC® 9763™) was cultivated in yeast extract peptone dextrose medium containing 1% yeast extract, 0.5% peptone and 2% glucose in disposable cuvettes, with a final volume of 2 mL. Non-treated cultures were used as negative control and BSA NPs samples were analysed at different concentrations (3.0 to 5.3 µM). Before adding the BSA NPs to the yeast cultures, an ultrasonic bath (Bandelin SONOREX Super RK510, Berlin, Germany) was used to homogenize the NP suspensions, for 3 min. Then, the assay was carried out as described by Roberto et al. [44]. Briefly, before each absorbance measurements in the spectrophotometer (Thermo Scientific model Evolution 300 BB, Waltham MA, USA) at 525 nm, the cultures were mixed in a vortex. The growth curve in the logarithmic phase for each sample, as well as for the control group was conducted by correlating the logarithm of the cell concentration (number of cells/mL) against the incubation time. Each group was tested in four replicates (n = 4). For each sample and corresponding concentration, the growth inhibition (GI, %) was calculated from the linear slope in the logarithmic phase of S. cerevisiae growth curve.

The cell concentrations (cells/mL) were calculated applying Equation (12):

$$n° \, cells/mL = \frac{(X * 1000mm^3)}{Y * w^2 * d} \quad (12)$$

where X = n.° cells counted; Y = n.° of smallest squares counted; d= depth of counting chamber and w= width of 1 square unit [44].

4.3. Evaluation of BSA NPs Secondary Structure by far UV Circular Dichroism

Circular dichroism (CD) spectra were recorded on a JASCO J-720 spectropolarimeter (JASCO, Hiroshima, Japan) equipped with a 180–700 nm photomultiplier (EXEL-308). CD spectra were recorded in the far UV range from 260 to 200 nm with quartz Suprasil® CD cuvettes (0.1 cm) at room temperature (ca. 25 °C). Each CD spectrum was the result of six scans recorded in degrees. The following acquisition parameters were used: data pitch, 0.5 nm; bandwidth, 2.0 nm; response, 2 s and scan speed, 50 nm/min.

4.4. Haemolytic Activity

The haemolytic activity of PvD in free and encapsulated forms as well as in empty NPs was determined using EDTA-preserved peripheral human blood [36]. Human peripheral blood was obtained from a voluntary donor, then it was EDTA-preserved and used in the same day of experiments. Plasma was removed by centrifugation at 1000× g for 10 min and the RBCs suspension was washed three-times in PBS at 1000× g for 10 min. The NPs formulations were suspended in PBS buffer (European Pharmacopeia 7.0) and free PvD was dissolved in DMSO and then diluted in PBS. Free PvD concentrations ranging from 0.03 to 51.27 µM and encapsulated PvD concentrations ranging from 0.04 to 80.11 µM were distributed in 96-well plates (100 µL/well). A DMSO control at the higher concentration used for free PvD was also tested. Then, 100 µL of RBCs suspension was added to all samples, microplates were incubated at 37 °C for 1 h and then centrifuged at 800× g for 10 min. Absorbance of supernatants was measured at 550 nm with a reference filter at 620 nm. The percentage of the haemolytic activity for each sample was calculated comparing each individual determination to a 100% haemolysis (erythrocytes in distilled water), positive control and negative control (erythrocytes in PBS) according to Equation (13):

$$(AbsS - AbsN)/(AbsP - AbsN) \times 100 \quad (13)$$

where AbsS is the average absorbance of the sample, AbsN is the average absorbance of the negative control and AbsP is the average absorbance of the positive control.

4.5. Synthesis of BSA NPs Conjugated with ERL or CET

In this step, we aimed to assess if the EGFR inhibitors and its conjugation with BSA NPs allow or not a targeting deliver of the system to pancreatic tumour cells. Thus, the synthesis of BSA NPs conjugated with ERL or CET was performed by incubating them with a NPs suspension [45,46]. Briefly, EGFR inhibitors (500 µL) were added dropwise into the NPs suspension, followed by a 2 h reaction under stirring (500 rpm). At the end of the reaction, the mixture was centrifuged (2800× g/10 min) and resuspended with purified water. The quantification of the EGFR inhibitors conjugation was then determined in the following section.

4.6. HPLC Method

A reverse-phase HPLC chromatographic method (stationary phase - LiChrospher RP 18 (5 µm), Lichrocart 250 – 4.6) at a detection wavelength of 254 nm, was used for PvD quantification. Briefly, we used a HPLC system (Hitachi LaCrom Elite, with column oven and a UV-Vis diode array detector, San Jose CA, USA) with a mobile phase containing methanol and trichloroacetic acid 0.1% (80:20, v/v) at a flow rate of 1.0 mL/min. The injection volume was 20 µL, the run-time was 15 min and the column conditions were maintained at 30 °C. Measurements were carried out in duplicate and PvD encapsulation efficiency was calculated according to Equation (14):

$$EE\ (\%) = (\text{Amount of encapsulated drug/Initial drug amount}) \times 100 \quad (14)$$

For ERL quantification, a reverse-phase HPLC chromatographic method on a NovaPak® C18 column (3.9 × 150 mm) from Waters (Milford, MA, USA) was used, at a detection wavelength of 346 nm, as previously described [47]. Briefly, the same HPLC system was used but with an isocratic mobile phase consisting of acetonitrile and acidified water pH 2.6 (40:60, v/v) and a flow rate of 1.0 mL/min.

Column conditions were maintained at 22 °C, with an injection volume of 20 μL and a retention time of 4.5 min. Measurements were carried out in duplicate.

4.7. LC-MS/MS Analysis for CET Quantification

LC-MS/MS analyses were performed as previously described by François et al. [48]. Briefly, a XEVO TQ-S triple quadrupole mass spectrometer (Waters) was used, controlled by Masslynx software (version 4.1) and an Acquity I-Class LC system (Waters) was linked to the instrument. Chromatography was performed using a gradient combining 0.1% formic acid in water with 0.1% formic acid in acetonitrile. Peptides separation was achieved on an Acquity UPLC BEH Shield C18 column, 2.1 mm × 50 mm, 1.7 μm, (Waters), using a gradient from 5 to 33% over 10 min, at a flow rate of 500 μL/min and the temperature was maintained at 50 °C.

4.8. Static Lattice Atomistic Simulations

Molecular simulations were performed using commercial software: HyperChemLite™ 8.0.8 Molecular Modeling System (Hypercube Inc., Gainesville, FL, USA) and ChemBio3D Ultra 11.0 (CambridgeSoft Corporation, Cambridge, UK). The structures of glucose and ERL were with natural angles as a 3D model while the structures of the peptide chains BSA (BSA; sequence: LQARILAVERYLKDQQL) and CET (CET; PDBID:4GW5; Chain A) were generated using the built-in sequence editor module of HyperChem. A progressive-convergence-strategy was applied for energy minimization with MM+ force field. The confirmers having lowest energy were employed for geometrical optimization and the molecular complexes were assembled by parallel disposition to generate the final models: BSA-glucose, BSA-ERL, and BSA-CET corresponding to BSA formulations with glucose cross-linking and ERL/CET functionalization, respectively. Full geometry optimization was carried out in vacuum employing the Polak–Ribiere conjugate gradient algorithm until an RMS gradient of 0.001kcal/mol was reached. For molecular mechanics calculations in vacuum, the force fields were utilized with a distance-dependent dielectric constant scaled by a factor of 1. The 1–4 scale factors were electrostatic = 0.5 and van der Waals = 0.5 [49].

4.9. Physical and Morphological Characterization of the EGFR Inhibitors Conjugated BSA NPs (Size, Surface and Morphology): Dynamic Light Scattering (DLS) and Atomic Force Microscopy (AFM), Scanning Electron Microscopy (SEM) and Transmission Electron Microscopy (TEM)

Freshly prepared nanoformulations were studied in terms of their structure, surface morphology, shape and size by DLS, AFM, SEM and TEM. The analysed samples were: empty BSA-NPs, PvD-loaded BSA NPs, ERL conjugated empty BSA NPs, ERL conjugated PvD-loaded BSA NPs, CET conjugated empty BSA NPs, CET conjugated PvD-loaded BSA NPs, ERL-CET conjugated empty BSA NPs ERL-CET conjugated PvD-loaded BSA NPs.

DLS (Coulter nano-sizer Delta Nano™, Brea, CA, USA) was used to perform a physical characterization of the NPs, evaluating mean particle size, polydispersity index (PdI) and zeta potential of the NPs' diluted suspension (n = 3). For DLS analysis, samples were diluted with purified water (1:10) and the measurements were carried out at room temperature (25 °C).

An atomic force microscope, Multimode 8 coupled to Nanoscope V Controller (Bruker, Coventry, UK) was used to acquire AFM images by using peak force tapping and ScanAssist mode. An aliquot of each sample (~30 μL) was mounted on a freshly cleaved mica sheet and left to dry before being analysed, in order to offer a clean and flat surface for AFM analysis. The images were obtained in ambient conditions, at a sweep rate close to 1 Hz, using Scanasyst-air 0.4 N/m tips, from Bruker.

For SEM, all samples were fixed with 2.5% glutaraldehyde in 0.1 M sodium phosphate buffer (European Pharmacopeia 7.0), at pH 7.2 during 1 h. After centrifugation, the pellets were washed three times in the fixative buffer and aliquots (10 μL) of the sample suspensions were scattered over a round glass coverslip previously coated with poly-L-lysine. The samples were then exposed to osmium tetroxide vapours in a fixative chamber during 30 min, dehydrated in a graded series of ethanol and dried with hexamethyldisilazane. After coated with a thin layer of gold, the samples were observed on a JEOL 5200LV scanning electron microscope (JEOL Ltd., Tokyo, Japan) at an accelerating voltage of 20 kV, and images were recorded digitally.

For TEM, the samples were fixed with glutaraldehyde as for SEM and aliquots (10 µL) of the samples' suspensions were dispersed on carbon-coated copper grids. Afterwards, the material was negative staining with 1% uranyl acetate and left to dry at room temperature. Observations were carried out on a JEOL 1200EX transmission electron microscope (JEOL Ltd.) at an accelerating voltage of 80 kV. Images were recorded digitally.

4.10. Cell Viability Studies of PvD-Loaded BSA NPs

In order to evaluate PvD selectivity and antiproliferative effects against human pancreatic tumour cells in its free form, as well as when encapsulated in BSA NPs, two different cell lines were tested, BxPC3 and PANC-1 (human pancreatic adenocarcinoma cell lines). Both BxPC3 and PANC-1 cell lines were obtained from the ATCC (Manassas, VA, USA).

The cell lines tested are typically adherent cell cultures. Evaluations were made in different experimental conditions regarding the different types of cells. Thus, BxPC3 cells were maintained in in RPMI 1640 medium with glutamax, supplemented with 10% (v/v) inactivated fetal bovine serum (iFBS), 50 U/mL penicillin and 50 µg/mL streptomycin. PANC-1 cells were maintained in Dulbecco's Modified Eagle's medium (DMEM) with high-glucose (4500 mg/L), supplemented with 10% iFBS, 50 U/mL penicillin and 50 µg/mL streptomycin. Both cell lines were maintained in an incubator at 37 °C in a humidified atmosphere of 5% CO_2.

The effect of PvD on cell proliferation was evaluated by MTT assay [50]. Briefly, cells were seeded in 96-well plates (1×10^4 cell per well for BxPC3 and for PANC-1) under normal conditions (5% CO_2 humidified atmosphere at 37 °C) and allowed to adhere overnight. The cells were then incubated for 48 h with free PvD, ERL conjugated empty BSA NPs, ERL conjugated PvD-loaded BSA NPs, CET conjugated empty BSA NPs, CET conjugated PvD-loaded BSA NPs, ERL-CET conjugated empty BSA NPs, ERL-CET conjugated PvD-loaded BSA NPs, PvD-loaded BSA NPs and Empty BSA NPs at different concentrations: between 5 and 30.0 µM for BxPC3 and to PANC-1 between 10.0 and 40.0 µM for all PvD-loaded nanoformulations and free PvD and between 20 and 30.0 µM for BxPC3 and to PANC-1 between 30.0 and 40.0 µM for all empty nanoformulations. The cells medium was removed after the incubation period and PBS was used to wash the wells. Then, MTT solution (50 µL of a 10%) was added to the cells and the plates were incubated for a 4 h period. After the incubation time, to solubilize the formazan crystals formed during the incubation period, DMSO was added to each well (100 µL).

Using a microplate reader, it was measured the absorbance of all samples at 570 nm and the IC_{50} was determined. The cytotoxic effect was evaluated by determining the percentage of viable/death cells for each formulation studied concentration. Cell proliferation analysis was carried out in GraphPad Prism®5 (GraphPad Software, San Diego, CA, USA). Values were plotted and fit to a standard inhibition log dose-response curve to generate the IC_{50} values. A total of three independent experiments, with six replicates per condition, were carried out.

4.11. Cell Cycle Assays

BxPC3 human pancreatic carcinoma cells were used as a tumour cell model to evaluate the effects of PvD-loaded NPs and PvD in its free form on cell cycle progression. Cell cycle progression was evaluated using a standard staining procedure with propidium iodide (PI) (Fluka, Sigma-Aldrich, Darmstadt, Germany) followed by flow cytometry. Briefly, BxPC3 cells were incubated with free PvD, PvD-loaded BSA NPs and ERL conjugated PvD-loaded BSA NPs at a PvD concentration of 10 µM for 24 h. Next, cells were detached with Tryple and collected by centrifugation at $800\times g$ for 5 min, at 4 °C. Cell pellets were resuspended in ice-cold PBS and fixed under gentle vortexing by dropwise addition of an equal volume of ice-cold 80% ethanol (−20 °C), followed by 30 min on ice. Subsequently, samples were stored at 4 °C for at least 18 h until data acquisition. For cell cycle analysis, cells were centrifuged at 850× g for 5 min, at 4 °C, and pellets resuspended in RNase A (50 μg/mL, in PBS) and PI (25 μg/mL) and further incubated for 30 min, at 37 °C. Sample acquisition and data analysis were performed using the Guava easyCyte™ Flow Cytometer (Merck Millipore, Darmstadt, Germany) and Guava analysis software, with the acquisition of at least 10,000 events per sample.

4.12. Lactate Dehydrogenase (LDH) Assay

The lactate dehydrogenase assay measures membrane integrity as a function of the amount of cytoplasmic LDH released into the medium. The assay is based on the reduction of NAD by LDH. Reduced NADH is then utilized in the conversion of a tetrazolium dye to a coloured product that is measured spectrophotometrically. The 24 h incubation medium collected in the cell cycle assay was used to perform this assay for the same samples used in the previous assay: free PvD, ERL PvD-loaded BSA NPs and ERL conjugated PvD-loaded BSA NPs at a PvD concentration of 10 μM. A 50 μL aliquot of each incubation medium was collected and transferred to a 96-well plate and 50 μL of Lactate Dehydrogenase Assay Mixture was added and gently mixed. The plate was covered with an opaque material to protect from light and incubated at room temperature for 10 min. Samples absorbance was measured at a wavelength of 490 nm in a MR 4000 plate reader (Model 680 Microplate reader, Bio-Rad Laboratories, Hercules, CA, USA).

4.13. Statistical Analysis

The significance of differences between samples was assessed using one-way analysis of variance (ANOVA) for mean comparisons (Tukey's test). A 0.05 significance level was adopted for every test.

5. Conclusions

BSA NPs were efficiently produced and PvD was successfully encapsulated. The BSA secondary structure was shown to be maintained after NP formation and after submitting BSA NPs to ultra-sounds and heat, which can be seen as verification of the formation of stable nanocarriers. Regarding haemolytic activity, PvD-loaded BSA NPs have shown to be safe to human RBCs, which allows this formulation to be administered in future injectable use. Static lattice atomistic simulations have proven that these nanocarriers are a stable formulation, suggesting that glucose was an excellent choice as a cross-linking agent, with lower toxicity than glutaraldehyde. Concerning physical and morphological characterization of the NPs there are considerable differences between all the formulations developed, being ERL conjugated BSA NPs and non-conjugated BSA NPs (empty and PvD-loaded) the formulations that have shown better results according to our goals: size ranging between 100–400 nm, with monodisperse size distribution, well-defined morphology, high cross-linking efficacy and negative zeta potential. Cell culture and cytotoxicity assays indicated that NPs can damage pancreatic tumour cells. However, the results of CET conjugated NPs, when comparing to ERL conjugated NPs, showed that ERL conjugated NPs were more efficient at reducing cell viability. Thus, ERL conjugated NPs were chosen to proceed to SEM and TEM analysis, as well as to cell cycle and lactate dehydrogenase assays. This formulation showed well-defined morphology by SEM and TEM analysis. Since there was no significant damage in cell membrane integrity, our results suggest that the decrease on cell viability by these particles may occur, at least in part, by a cell cycle arrest-dependent mechanism rather than by inducing cell death.

Further studies must be undertaken, including mechanistic studies of the optimized formulation, by performing in vivo assays to test ERLconjugated PvD-loaded BSA NPs targeting efficacy as well as safety.

Author Contributions: Conceptualization: A.S.-R. and C.P.R.; methodology and formal analysis: A.S.-R.; P.K.; V.P.; Y.E.C.; J.A.; M.F.; C.E.; A.S.V., L.A.; I.C.; J.A.; S.S.; M.M.G. and C.P.R.; investigation: A.S.-R.; writing—original draft preparation, A.S.-R.; P.K. and I.C.; writing, review and editing: C.P.R.; L.A.; S.S.; J.A.; C.M.P.R. and M.M.G.; supervision, C.P.R.; P.R. and J.M.; project administration: C.P.R.; funding acquisition: FCT, ULHT/CBIOS and UAH.

Funding: This research was funded by Fundação para a Ciência e Tecnologia (FCT) under the Reference UID/DTP/04138/2019, Portugal; SEM analysis was funded by Fundação para a Ciência e Tecnologia (FCT) with financial support to CESAM (UID/AMB/50017/2019), through FCT/MEC National funds, and the co-funding by the FEDER, within the PT2020 Partnership Agreement and Compete 2020; in this research, phytochemical section was funded by Fundação para a Ciência e Tecnologia (FCT) under the Reference UID/DTP/04567/2019; cell cycle assays received funding from European Structural & Investment Funds through the COMPETE Programme - Programa Operacional Regional de Lisboa under the Programme grant LISBOA-01-0145-FEDER-016405, and from National Funds through FCT – Fundação para a Ciência e a Tecnologia under the Programme grant SAICTPAC/0019/2015.

Acknowledgments: The authors would like to thank to Professor A. Roberto for his supervision in *Saccharomyces cerevisiae* assay and to Leonor Fonseca for her help in the optimization of BSA NPs preparation method.

Conflicts of Interest: The authors declare no conflict of interest.

References

1. Li, D.; Xie, K.; Wolff, R.; Abbruzzese, J.L. Pancreatic cancer. *Lancet* **2004**, *363*, 1049–1057. [CrossRef]
2. Rebelo, A.; Molpeceres, J.; Rijo, P.; Pinto Reis, C. Pancreatic Cancer Therapy Review: From Classic Therapeutic Agents to Modern Nanotechnologies. *Curr. Drug Metab.* **2017**, *18*, 346–359. [CrossRef] [PubMed]
3. Yu, X.; Zhang, Y.; Chen, C.; Yao, Q.; Li, M. Targeted drug delivery in pancreatic cancer. *Biochim. Biophys. Acta* **2010**, *1805*, 1–16. [CrossRef] [PubMed]
4. Rebelo, A.; Reis, C. Emerging therapeutic nanotechnologies in pancreatic cancer: Advances, risks and challenges. *Ther. Deliv.* **2018**, *9*, 691–694. [CrossRef] [PubMed]
5. McCarroll, J.; Teo, J.; Boyer, C.; Goldstein, D.; Kavallaris, M.; Phillips, P.A. Potential applications of nanotechnology for the diagnosis and treatment of pancreatic cancer. *Front. Physiol.* **2014**, *5*, 1–10. [CrossRef] [PubMed]
6. Yu, X.; Jin, C. Application of albumin-based nanoparticles in the management of cancer. *J. Mater. Sci. Mater. Med.* **2016**, *27*, 1–10. [CrossRef] [PubMed]
7. Yu, X.; Zhu, W.; Di, Y.; Gu, J.; Guo, Z.; Li, H.; Fu, D.; Jin, C. Triple-functional albumin-based nanoparticles for combined chemotherapy and photodynamic therapy of pancreatic cancer with lymphatic metastases. *Int. J. Nanomed.* **2017**, *12*, 6771–6785. [CrossRef] [PubMed]
8. Xu, H.; Liu, L.; Fan, X.; Zhang, G.; Li, Y.; Jiang, B. Bioorganic & Medicinal Chemistry Letters Identification of a diverse synthetic abietane diterpenoid library for anticancer activity. *Bioorg. Med. Chem. Lett.* **2016**, 1–6. [CrossRef]
9. Nicolai, M.; Pereira, P.; Vitor, R.F.; Pinto, C.; Roberto, A.; Rijo, P. Antioxidant activity and rosmarinic acid content of ultrasound-assisted ethanolic extracts of medicinal plants. *Measurement* **2016**, *89*, 328–332. [CrossRef]
10. Gali-muhtasib, H.; Hmadi, R.; Kareh, M.; Tohme, R. Cell death mechanisms of plant-derived anticancer drugs: Beyond apoptosis. *Apoptosis* **2015**. [CrossRef]
11. Fronza, M.; Lamy, E.; Gunther, S.; Heinzmann, B.; Laufer, S.; Merfort, I. Abietane diterpenes induce cytotoxic effects in human pancreatic cancer cell line MIA PaCa-2 through different modes of action. *Phytochemistry* **2012**, *78*, 107–119. [CrossRef] [PubMed]
12. Silva, C.O.; Molpeceres, J.; Batanero, B.; Fernandes, A.S.; Saraiva, N.; Costa, J.G.; Rijo, P.; Figueiredo, I.V.; Faísca, P.; Reis, C.P. Functionalized diterpene parvifloron D-loaded hybrid nanoparticles for targeted delivery in melanoma therapy. *Ther. Deliv.* **2016**, *7*, 521–544. [CrossRef] [PubMed]
13. Santos-rebelo, A.; Garcia, C.; Eleut, C.; Bastos, A.; Coelho, C.; Coelho, M.A.N.; Viana, A.S.; Ascensão, L.; Pinto, F.; Gaspar, M.M.; et al. Development of Parvifloron D-Loaded Smart Nanoparticles to Target Pancreatic Cancer. *Pharmaceutics* **2018**, *10*, 216. [CrossRef] [PubMed]
14. Burmistrova, O.; Perdomo, J.; Simões, M.F.; Rijo, P.; Quintana, J.; Estévez, F. The abietane diterpenoid parvifloron D from *Plectranthus ecklonii* is a potent apoptotic inducer in human leukemia cells. *Phytomedicine* **2015**, *22*, 1009–1016. [CrossRef] [PubMed]
15. Bonifácio, B.V.; Silva, P.B.; Aparecido dos Santos Ramos, M.; Maria Silveira Negri, K.; Maria Bauab, T.; Chorilli, M. Nanotechnology-based drug delivery systems and herbal medicines: A review. *Int. J. Nanomed.* **2014**, *9*, 1–15. [CrossRef] [PubMed]
16. Reis, C.P.; Damgé, C. Nanotechnology as a promising strategy for alternative routes of insulin delivery. *Methods Enzymol.* **2012**, *508*, 271–294. [CrossRef]

17. Reis, C.P.; Neufeld, R.J.; Ribeiro, A.J.; Veiga, F. Design of Insulin-Loaded Alginate Nanoparticles: Influence of Calcium Ion on Polymer Gel Matrix Properties. *Chem. Ind. Chem. Eng. Q.* **2006**, *12*, 47–52. [CrossRef]
18. Reis, C.P.; Figueiredo, I.V.; Carvalho, R.A.; Jones, J.; Nunes, P.; Soares, A.F.; Silva, C.F.; Ribeiro, A.J.; Veiga, F.J.; Damgé, C.; et al. Toxicological assessment of orally delivered nanoparticulate insulin. *Nanotoxicology* **2008**, *2*, 205–217. [CrossRef]
19. Pinto Reis, C.; Silva, C.; Martinho, N.; Rosado, C. Drug carriers for oral delivery of peptides and proteins: accomplishments and future perspectives. *Ther. Deliv.* **2013**, *4*, 251–265. [CrossRef]
20. Yu, X.; Di, Y.; Xie, C.; Song, Y.; He, H.; Li, H.; Pu, X.; Lu, W.; Fu, D.; Jin, C. An in vitro and in vivo study of gemcitabine-loaded albumin nanoparticles in a pancreatic cancer cell line. *Int. J. Nanomed.* **2015**, *10*, 6825–6834. [CrossRef]
21. Elzoghby, A.O.; Samy, W.M.; Elgindy, N.A. Albumin-based nanoparticles as potential controlled release drug delivery systems. *J. Control. Released* **2012**, *157*, 168–182. [CrossRef] [PubMed]
22. Abrantes, G.; Duarte, D.; Reis, C.P. An Overview of Pharmaceutical Excipients: Safe or Not Safe? *J. Pharm. Sci.* **2016**, *105*, 2019–2026. [CrossRef] [PubMed]
23. Tan, Y.L.; Ho, H.K. Navigating albumin-based nanoparticles through various drug delivery routes. *Drug Discov. Today* **2018**, *23*, 1108–1114. [CrossRef] [PubMed]
24. Karimi, M.; Bahrami, S.; Ravari, S.B.; Sahandi, P.; Mirshekari, H.; Bozorgomid, M.; Shahreza, S.; Sori, M.; Hamblin, M.R. Albumin nanostructures as advanced drug delivery systems. *Expert Opin. Drug Deliv.* **2016**, *13*, 1609–1623. [CrossRef]
25. Li, Q.; Liu, C.; Zhao, X.; Zu, Y.; Wang, Y.; Zhang, B.; Zhao, D.; Zhao, Q.; Su, L.; Gao, Y.; et al. Preparation, characterization and targeting of micronized 10-hydroxycamptothecin-loaded folate-conjugated human serum albumin nanoparticles to cancer cells. *Int. J. Nanomed.* **2011**, *6*, 397–405. [CrossRef]
26. Kouchakzadeh, H.; Shojaosadati, S.A.; Maghsoudi, A.; Farahani, E.V. Optimization of PEGylation Conditions for BSA Nanoparticles Using Response Surface Methodology. *AAPS PharmSciTech* **2010**, *11*, 1206–1211. [CrossRef]
27. Bobo, D.; Robinson, K.J.; Islam, J.; Thurecht, K.J.; Corrie, S.R.; Corrie, S.R. Nanoparticle-Based Medicines: A Review of FDA-Approved Materials and Clinical Trials to Date. *Pharm. Res.* **2016**, *33*, 2373–2387. [CrossRef]
28. Liu, Y.; Feng, N. Nanocarriers for the delivery of active ingredients and fractions extracted from natural products used in traditional Chinese medicine (TCM). *Adv. Colloid Interface Sci.* **2015**, *221*, 60–76. [CrossRef]
29. Pinto Reis, C.; Neufeld, R.J.; Ribeiro, A.J.; Veiga, F. Nanoencapsulation I. Methods for preparation of drug-loaded polymeric nanoparticles. *Nanomed. Nanotechnol. Biol. Med.* **2006**, *2*, 8–21. [CrossRef]
30. Weber, C.; Coester, C.; Kreuter, J.; Langer, K. Desolvation process and surface characterisation of protein nanoparticles. *Int. J. Pharm.* **2000**, *194*, 91–102. [CrossRef]
31. Kiani, K.; Shakeri, S.; Maryam, K. Preparation and in vitro investigation of antigastric cancer activities of carvacrol-loaded human serum albumin nanoparticles. *IET Nanobiotechnol.* **2015**, *9*, 1–6. [CrossRef]
32. Yan, S.; Zhang, H.; Piao, J.; Chen, Y.; Gao, S.; Lu, C.; Niu, L.; Xia, Y.; Hu, Y.; Ji, R.; et al. Studies on the preparation, characterization and intracellular kinetics of JD27-loaded human serum albumin nanoparticles. *Procedia Eng.* **2015**, *102*, 590–601. [CrossRef]
33. Bhattacharjee, S. DLS and zeta potential - What they are and what they are not? *J. Control. Released* **2016**, *235*, 337–351. [CrossRef] [PubMed]
34. Sun, S.F.; Maximos, A.S. Circular dichroism of bovine serum albumin in divalent salt solutions. *Int. J. Pept. Protein Res.* **1989**, *34*, 46–51. [CrossRef]
35. Micsonai, A.; Wien, F.; Kernya, L.; Lee, Y.; Goto, Y.; Réfrégiers, M.; Kardos, J. Accurate secondary structure prediction and fold recognition for circular dichroism spectroscopy. *Proc. Natl. Acad. Sci. USA* **2015**, *112*, 3095–3103. [CrossRef]
36. Nave, M.; Castro, R.E.; Rodrigues, C.M.; Casin, A.; Soveral, G.; Gaspar, M.M. Nanoformulations of a potent copper-based aquaporin inhibitor with cytotoxic effect against cancer cells. *Nanomedicine* **2016**, *11*, 1817–1830. [CrossRef]
37. Kumar, P.; Choonara, Y.E.; Pillay, V. In silico analytico-mathematical interpretation of biopolymeric assemblies: Quantification of energy surfaces and molecular attributes via atomistic simulations. *Bioeng. Transl. Med.* **2018**, 1–10. [CrossRef]

38. Vasan, S.; Zhang, X.; Zhang, X.; Kapurniotu, A.; Bernhagen, J.; Teichberg, S.; Basgen, J.; Wagle, D.; Shih, D.; Terlecky, I.; et al. An agent cleaving glucose-derived protein crosslinks in vitro and in vivo. *Nature* **1996**, *382*, 275–278. [CrossRef]
39. Govender, M.; Choonara, Y.E.; Van Vuuren, S.; Kumar, P. A Dual-Biotic System for the Concurrent Delivery of Antibiotics and Probiotics: In Vitro, Ex Vivo, In Vivo and In Silico Evaluation and Correlation. *Pharm. Res.* **2016**, *33*, 3057–3071. [CrossRef]
40. Atef, A.; Ali, A.; Hsu, F.; Hsieh, C.; Shiau, C.; Chiang, C.; Wei, Z.; Chen, C.; Huang, H. Erlotinib-Conjugated Iron Oxide Nanoparticles as a Smart Cancer - Targeted Theranostic Probe for MRI. *Nat. Publ. Gr.* **2016**, 1–16. [CrossRef]
41. Marrese, M.; Guarino, V.; Ambrosio, L. Atomic Force Microscopy: A Powerful Tool to Address Scaffold Design in Tissue Engineering. *J. Funct. Biomater.* **2017**, *8*, 7. [CrossRef] [PubMed]
42. Çalış, S.; Öztürk, A.K.; Arslan, F.B.; Eroğlu, H.; Çapan, Y. Nanopharmaceuticals as Drug-Delivery Systems: For, Against, and Current Applications Nanoscience and Nanotechnology. In *Drug Delivery Micro and Nano Technologies*; Elsevier: Amsterdam, The Netherlands, 2019; pp. 133–154.
43. Niknejada, H.; Mahmoudzadeh, R. Comparison of Different Crosslinking Methods for Preparation of Docetaxel-loaded Albumin Nanoparticles. *Iran. J. Pharm. Res.* **2015**, *14*, 385–394.
44. Roberto, A.; Caetano, P.P. A high-throughput screening method for general cytotoxicity part I: Chemical toxicity. *Rev. Lusófona Ciências Tecnol. Saúde* **2005**, *2*, 95–100.
45. Liu, Y.; Chen, M.; Luo, Z.; Lin, J.; Song, L. Investigation on the site-selective binding of bovine serum albumin by erlotinib hydrochloride. *J. Biomol. Struct. Dyn.* **2012**, 37–41. [CrossRef]
46. Domotor, O.; Pelivan, K.; Borics, A.; Keppler, B.K.; Kowol, C.R.; Enyedy, E.A. Comparative studies on the human serum albumin binding of the clinically approved EGFR inhibitors gefitinib, erlotinib, afatinib, osimertinib and the investigational inhibitor KP2187. *J. Pharm. Biomed. Anal.* **2018**, *154*, 321–331. [CrossRef]
47. Mandal, B. Design, Development and Evaluation of Erlotinib-Loaded Hybrid Nanoparticles for Targeted Drug Delivery to NonSmall Cell Lung Cancer Design, Development and Evaluation of Erlotinib-Loaded Hybrid. *Theses Diss.* **2015**. [CrossRef]
48. Becher, F.; Ciccolini, J.; Imbs, D.; Marin, C.; Dupuis, C.; Fakhry, N.; Pourroy, B.; Ghettas, A.; Junot, C.; Duffaud, F.; et al. A simple and rapid LC-MS/MS method for therapeutic drug monitoring of cetuximab: a GPCO- UNICANCER proof of concept study in head-and-neck cancer patients. *Sci. Rep.* **2017**, *7*, 1–11. [CrossRef]
49. Kumar, P.; Pillay, V.; Choonara, Y.E.; Modi, G.; Naidoo, D. In Silico Theoretical Molecular Modeling for Alzheimer's Disease: The Nicotine-Curcumin Paradigm in Neuroprotection and Neurotherapy. *Int. J. Mol. Sci.* **2011**, *12*, 694–724. [CrossRef]
50. Burmistrova, O.; Simões, M.F.; Rijo, P.; Quintana, J.; Bermejo, J.; Estévez, F. Antiproliferative activity of abietane diterpenoids against human tumor cells. *J. Nat. Prod.* **2013**, *76*, 1413–1423. [CrossRef]

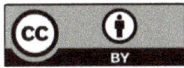

© 2019 by the authors. Licensee MDPI, Basel, Switzerland. This article is an open access article distributed under the terms and conditions of the Creative Commons Attribution (CC BY) license (http://creativecommons.org/licenses/by/4.0/).

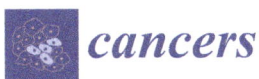

Article

Next-Generation Multimodality of Nanomedicine Therapy: Size and Structure Dependence of Folic Acid Conjugated Copolymers Actively Target Cancer Cells in Disabling Cell Division and Inducing Apoptosis

Manpreet Sambi [1], Alexandria DeCarlo [1], Cecile Malardier-Jugroot [2,*] and Myron R. Szewczuk [1,*]

[1] Department of Biomedical and Molecular Sciences, Queen's University, Kingston, ON K7L 3N6, Canada; 13ms84@queensu.ca (M.S.); 14ald4@queensu.ca (A.D.)
[2] Department of Chemistry and Chemical Engineering, Royal Military College of Canada, Kingston, ON K7K 7B4, Canada
* Correspondence: Cecile.Malardier-Jugroot@rmc.ca (C.M.-J.); szewczuk@queensu.ca (M.R.S.); Tel.: +16-13-541-6000 (ext. 6272) (C.M.-J.); Tel.: +16-13-533-2457 (M.R.S.); Fax: +16-13-542-9489 (C.M.-J.); Fax: +16-13-533-6796 (M.R.S.)

Received: 21 October 2019; Accepted: 30 October 2019; Published: 1 November 2019

Abstract: Nanomedicine as a multimodality treatment of cancer utilizes the advantages of nanodelivery systems of drugs. They are superior to the clinical administration of different therapeutic agents in several aspects, including simultaneous delivery of drugs to the active site, precise ratio control of the loading drugs and overcoming multidrug resistance. The role of nanopolymer size and structural shape on the internalization process and subsequent intracellular toxicity is limited. Here, the size and shape dependent mechanism of a functionalized copolymer was investigated using folic acid (FA) covalently bonded to the copolymer poly (styrene-*alt*-maleic anhydride) (SMA) on its hydrophilic exterior via a biological linker 2,4-diaminobutyric acid (DABA) to target folic acid receptors (FR) overly expressed on cancer cells actively. We recently reported that unloaded FA-DABA-SMA copolymers significantly reduced cancer cell viability, suggesting a secondary therapeutic mechanism of action of the copolymer carrier post-internalization. Here, we investigated the size and shape dependent secondary mechanism of unloaded 350 kDa and 20 kDa FA-DABA-SMA. The 350 kDa and 20 kDa copolymers actively target folic acid receptors (FR) to initialize internationalization, but only the large size and sheet shaped copolymer disables cell division by intracellular disruptions of essential oncogenic proteins including p53, STAT-3 and c-Myc. Furthermore, the 350 kDa FA-DABA-SMA activates early and late apoptotic events in both PANC-1 and MDA-MB-231 cancer cells. These findings indicate that the large size and structural sheet shape of the 350 kDa FA-DABA-SMA copolymer facilitate multimodal tumor targeting mechanisms together with the ability to internalize hydrophobic chemotherapeutics to disable critical oncogenic proteins controlling cell division and to induce apoptosis. The significance of these novel findings reveals copolymer secondary cellular targets and therapeutic actions that extend beyond the direct delivery of chemotherapeutics. This report offers novel therapeutic insight into the intracellular activity of copolymers critically dependent on the size and structural shape of the nanopolymers.

Keywords: nanomedicine; FA-DABA-SMA; self-assembly; oncogenic proteins; intracellular disruption; folic receptor alpha; active targeting; drug delivery

1. Introduction

Targeting strategies of nanopolymers are formulated to enhance the specific distribution of the therapeutic macromolecules in the treatment of cancer. Active targeting mechanisms utilize tumor-specific receptor ligands to achieve a degree of specificity and are therefore utilized as a promising complementary strategy to improve drug delivery. To this end, multifunctional "smart" nanopolymers combine several targeting strategies to increase treatment specificity and reduce systemic toxicities associated with conventional chemotherapeutics.

Recently, we reported on a biocompatible pH responsive, active targeting delivery system, fabricated using folic acid functionalized on an amphiphilic alternating copolymer poly (styrene-*alt*-maleic anhydride) via a biodegradable linker 2,4-diaminobutyric acid (FA-DABA-SMA) [1,2]. Active targeting strategies using folic acid (FA) have gained much attention in cancer because folic acid receptors (FR) are overexpressed on cancerous cells up to two orders in magnitude relative to non-malignant cells [2,3]. Additionally, the self-assembly of the FA-DABA-SMA copolymeric template was designed to be pH responsive, forming amphiphilic nanostructures at pH 7, allowing for the encapsulation of hydrophobic drugs in its interior core. This structure is stable at neutral pH, but collapses under acidic conditions consistent with the tumor microenvironment, thereby releasing the carrier drugs on-site from its core [4]. Nanopolymers can be selectively designed to alter the pharmacokinetic profile and tissue distribution characteristics of drug delivery vehicles. The size, shape and surface modifications, all of which alter the pharmacokinetics and intracellular mechanisms, can be chemically modified such that they can have a significant therapeutic impact in vivo [5].

Investigations into the toxic effects following nanopolymer internalization are minimal as many nanopolymers are designed to be inert delivery vehicles with little or no toxic effects when they release their contents. To this end, Albanese et al. provided a detailed review on the effect of the nanoparticle size, shape and surface chemistry on biological systems upon internalization [6]. Physical attributes of nanopolymers continued to be explored regarding their effects on therapeutic efficacy; however, the consensus remains that the effects and final properties of nanoparticles in the endo-lysosomal vesicles of cells remain unknown. For example, nanoparticles in the intracellular cytosol space can activate several biological functions, including disrupting mitochondrial function, eliciting the production of reactive oxygen species and activation of the oxidative stress mediated signaling cascade [7,8]. Other reports have demonstrated that nanoparticles such as hydrophilic titanium oxide TiO_2 nanoparticles are oncogenic [9]. It is known that large nanoparticles do not extravasate far beyond the blood vessel, whereas small nanoparticles travel deep into the tumor, but remain there only transiently. Therefore, it is essential to optimize the next generation of nanopolymers focusing on the intracellular therapeutic mechanisms after internalization to successfully translate these drug delivery systems to the clinic.

Recently, we demonstrated for the first time that FA-DABA-SMA can act as a "smart" cancer targeting drug delivery system able to penetrate the inner core of three-dimensional pancreatic and breast cancer tumor spheroids [4]. To elucidate the possibility of toxicity from the polymeric template design, we reported that the empty SMA and functionalized FA-DABA-SMA polymers reduced PANC-1 and MDA MB-231 cancer cell viability using the WST-1 cell proliferation reagent, the data of which indicated a concentration dependent cell death at 48 and 72 hours of incubation [1].

Unexpectedly, these results revealed a previously unknown mechanism(s) of action of the empty FA-DABA-SMA copolymer where it can reduce tumor spheroid volume. We propose that this is achieved through a possible intracellular mechanism of action that targets oncoproteins, thereby inducing apoptosis. The rationale for this is based on a seminal report by Boshnjaku et al. who reported on a novel role for FRα [10]. This report details that ability of FRα to translocate to the nucleus and to act as a transcription factor by binding to the cis-regulatory elements activating transcriptional developmental genes including *HES1* and *FGFR4* [10]. This finding suggests that FRα may influence the regulation of a variety of malignant processes such as cell migration, cell growth and epithelial to mesenchymal transition (EMT) [3]. Given this critical role of the FRα, we propose that FA-DABA-SMA remains bound to FRα and subsequently becomes internalized, leading to disruption of intracellular processes that regulate cell proliferation and survival, ultimately leading to apoptosis. This disruption of the intracellular processes by FA-DABA-SMA binding FRα may, therefore, translate into a potent multimodal therapeutic effect(s) by dysregulating the essential mechanisms of tumorigenesis.

In this report, the FA-DABA-SMA copolymer is found to bind FR, after which it is translocated intracellularly via receptor-mediated endocytosis. Due to the large size and nanostructure of the 350 kDa FA-DABA-SMA copolymer, it can disrupt critical oncogenic processes, including cell proliferation, and induce apoptosis. Here, the internalization of the 350 kDa FA-DABA-SMA was found to reduce cell viability, but also disabled the oncogenic p53, c-Myc and STAT-3 cell survival proteins, inducing apoptosis. The large sized 350 kDa FA-DABA-SMA has a single chain hydrodynamic radius (Rh) of 6 nm and self-assembles into sheets (Rh of the self-assembled SMA nanostructure of 850 nm in water), while the small sized 20 kDa polymer has a single chain Rh of 3 nm and self-assembles into cylinders (Rh of the self-assembled SMA structure of 120 nm in water). The large sized FA-DABA-SMA nanopolymers and not the 20 kDa copolymers were internalized by binding to FR and, subsequently, inhibited intracellular oncogenic proteins. These results support the next-generation multimodality and therapeutic potential of nanopolymers. It is known that nanomedicines conjugated with targeting macromolecules can recognize a specific target, bind and be internalized via a specific mechanism like receptor-mediated endocytosis [11,12]. The novelty of our findings suggests that the critical size and the unique nanostructure of the copolymer enable the active targeting of folic acid receptors to facilitate the internalization, transportation and cellular localization of the delivery vehicle, where it disables oncogenic survival proteins and induces apoptosis. The significance of these findings provides insight into the previously unknown secondary intracellular mechanisms of action of FA-DABA-SMA that may extend beyond simple delivery vehicles previously thought to be inert.

2. Results

2.1. Folic Acid Receptor Expression on DU-145 Prostate, PANC-1 Pancreatic and MDA-MB-231 Triple-Negative Breast Cancer Cells

The expression levels of FR were characterized in the prostate (DU-145), pancreatic (PANC-1) and breast (MDA-MB-231) cancer cells. It is well established in the literature that MDA-MB-231 and, to a lesser degree, PANC-1 cells overexpress FR, while DU-145 cells have minimal expression levels [13,14]. In Figure 1a, the immunocytochemistry staining of the FR using the anti-FR antibody showed varying expression levels of the FR on the different cancer cell lines (Figure 1b).

The MDA-MB-231 cells expressed high levels of FR in comparison to the PANC-1 pancreatic cancer cells. The DU-145 cells expressed minimal levels of FR. These different cell lines allowed for a better understanding of the behaviour of the nanopolymer interacting with the target FR receptor in a range from low to high FR expression levels to better evaluate the efficacy and targeting potential of FA-DABA-SMA. Flow cytometry analyses showed similar trends in FR expression for DU-145 and PANC-1 cells on the cell membrane; however, the expression levels of FR were much lower in the MDA-MB-231 breast cancer cells. The discrepancy between the results may be due to the staining of both external and internalized FR on permeabilized cells (Figure 1a, right) compared to only the surface staining of the receptor (Figure 1c, right). Typically, the majority of FR exists internally and is cycled to the surface dependent on growth related needs. It has been reported that the high expression of FR on MDA-MB-231 breast cancer cell lines may be due to the high metabolic activity of an aggressive invasive ductal adenocarcinoma and, therefore, may require more folate to sustain rapid cell growth [15]. Further research into FR expression has suggested that when cellular growth reaches a plateau and the growth rate slows, an increased expression of FR is observed [16]. Overall, the varying expression levels of the FR in these three cell lines provided valuable information on the efficacy and interactions of the FA conjugated nanopolymers targeting varying expression levels of FR and exerting their therapeutic effects, which will be discussed later.

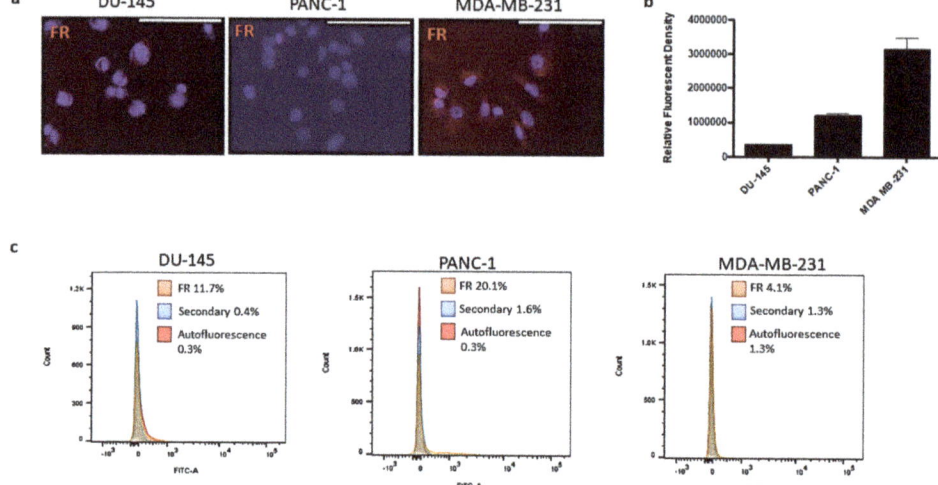

Figure 1. Folic acid receptor (FR) expression levels on DU-145 prostate, MDA-MB-231 breast and PANC1 pancreatic cancer cell lines. (**a**) Immunocytochemistry staining for FR in permeabilized DU-145, MDA-MB-231 and PANC-1 cells. The white scale bar represents 100 µm. Pictures were taken at 400× magnification. Blue DAPI stain represents the nuclei, and red staining is anti-FR antibody followed with AlexaFluor 594 secondary antibody for FR expression. (**b**) Quantification of expression levels by relative density corrected for average background staining of the AlexaFluor 594 secondary antibody. Error bar due to multiple images being quantified (n = 3–4). The data are a combination of two independent experiments with similar results. (**c**) Flow cytometry was used to confirm the expression level of the FR. Graphs represent an overlay of FR, secondary only control, and autofluorescence control.

2.2. Effect of Large and Small Sized FA-DABA-SMA Nanopolymers on the Cell Viability of DU-145, PANC-1 and MDA-MB-231 Cancer Cell Lines

Recently, we reported on the therapeutic efficacy of the 350 kDa FA-DABA-SMA and its ability to target FR actively and deliver hydrophobic anti-cancer agents [4,17]. Furthermore, the data in the report revealed that the empty nanopolymers reduced cell viability, penetrated tumor spheroids and decreased their volumes [4]. Here, we questioned whether the size of the nanopolymer could be a contributing factor to these therapeutically important effects of the nanopolymers [1,4,17]. We tested empty large (350 kDa) and small (20 kDa) sized FA-DABA-SMA nanopolymers on DU-145, PANC-1 and MDA-MB-231 cancer cell lines. As shown in Figure 2, both large and small FA-DABA-SMA at the effective dose of 3 µM as determined from our previous studies [1,17] did not affect DU-145 (Figure 2a) and PANC-1 (Figure 2b) cell viability. The MDA-MB-231 cell viability, however, was significantly reduced (p < 0.02) by the large nanopolymer when compared with the untreated control cells. These findings confirm the possibility of a novel dual therapeutic mechanism(s) of FA-DABA-SMA. It is proposed that the variation of the expression levels of the FR and the responsiveness of the MDA-MB-231 to the nanopolymer suggest that the binding avidity of the large sheet-like structure of FA-DABA-SMA interaction with FR might have a potent therapeutic effect, leading to FR stimulation and creating an enhanced sensitivity in cancer cells.

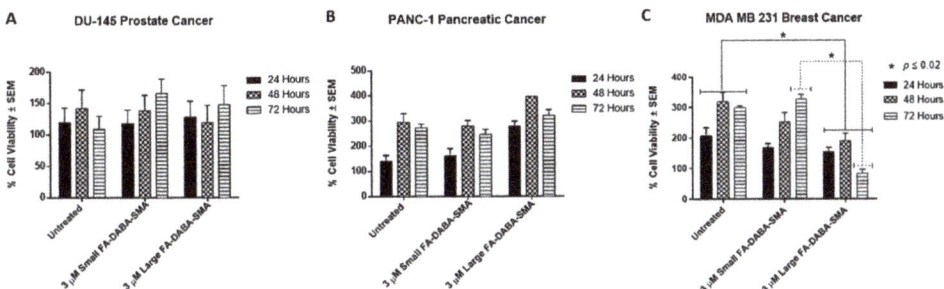

Figure 2. Differential effects of large and small FA-DABA-SMA nanopolymer on cell viability of DU-145 prostate, PANC-1 pancreatic and MDA-MB-231 breast cancer cells. Comparison of the cell viability of (**A**) DU-145, (**B**) PANC-1 and (**C**) MDA MB-231 cell lines at 24, 48 and 72 hours treated with a 20 kDa FA-DABA-SMA (small) and a 350 kDa FA-DABA-SMA (large) nanopolymer using the WST-1 assay. Results were compared by a one-way ANOVA at 95% confidence using Fisher's LSD test. The data (triplicates) are one of two separate experiments with similar results. The significance is reported in comparison to the untreated control at the respective time point (solid line) and as a comparison between 350 kDa and 20 kDa nanopolymers (dashed line).

2.3. Live Cell Fluorescence Microscopy of Curcumin Loaded 350 kDa FA-DABA-SMA Reveals FR Mediated Endocytosis and Translocation to the Nucleus

To track the nanopolymer's intracellular activity over 48 hours, the small and large sized FA-DABA-SMA nanopolymers were loaded with curcumin and applied on DU-145, PANC-1 and MDA-MD-231 cancer cells in culture. Within 24 hours, the large FA-DABA-SMA polymer was internalized and appeared to be translocated to the nucleus and released curcumin in the nucleus of MDA MB-231 cells after 48 hours (Figure 3). In contrast, the large nanopolymer was bound to FR on DU-145 prostate cancer cells with no evidence of internalization over 48 hours (Figure 3). As expected, there was no binding and internalization of the small (20 kDa) FA-DABA-SMA nanopolymer in the DU-145 cells. The PANC-1 cancer cells, on the other hand, appeared to interact with the small and large nanopolymer in a manner that was consistent with our previous studies [1,17]. These results suggest that the FR expression levels may not be a significant contributory factor, but more importantly, the size and nanostructure of the copolymer, which subsequently contribute to the therapeutic potential of FA-DABA-SMA, might be a more important factor to consider. To this end, the PANC-1 pancreatic and MDA-MB-231 breast cancer cells were used to investigate further the FR interactions and therapeutic potential of the FA-DABA-SMA copolymer size in delivering hydrophobic chemotherapeutic drugs.

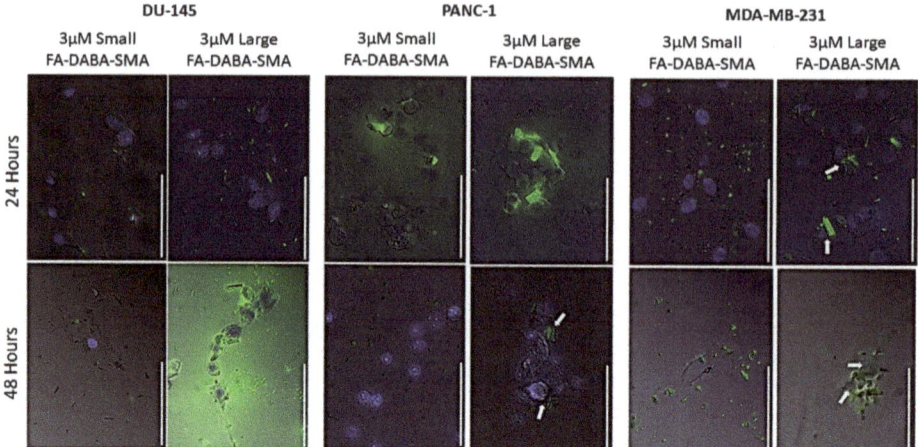

Figure 3. Live-cell fluorescence microscopy of curcumin-loaded FA-DABA-SMA binding FR mediating endocytosis and preferentially targeting the nucleus. Live cell tracking of the large (350 kDa) and small (20 kDa) curcumin loaded FA-DABA-SMA on DU-145, PANC1, and MDA MB-231 cells over 24 and 48 hours. Pictures were taken at 400× magnification. Blue DAPI stain represents the nuclei, and green fluorescence is the curcumin loaded nanopolymers. Results are a combination of two independent experiments with similar results. Arrows indicate nuclei.

2.4. The 350 kDa FA-DABA-SMA Delivers Hydrophobic Chemotherapeutic Drugs More Effectively Than the 20 kDa Copolymer to Reduce Cell Viability

In our initial studies, single chemotherapeutic agents demonstrated a decrease in cell viability; however, recent studies have suggested enhanced effectiveness of a combinatorial approach with nanopolymers [12,18]. Acetylsalicylic acid (ASA), a hydrophobic agent, is known to exert a synergistic effect when administered with conventional chemotherapeutics in several cancers [19,20]. To this end, ASA was chosen to be administered in combination with tamoxifen (Tmx) for MDA-MB-231 breast cancer cells and 5-fluorouracil (5-Fu) for PANC-1 cells.

PANC-1 pancreatic cancer cells were treated with small and large nanopolymers loaded with ASA and 5-Fu or with the respective drugs alone, and the cell viability was measured after 72 hours of treatment. In Figure 4, PANC-1 cells exhibited a significant ($p < 0.001$) decrease in cell viability when treated with the large nanopolymers loaded with 5-Fu compared with the 5-Fu drug alone. However, all other treatment conditions, including a combination treatment, did not show significant differences between free drugs or drug loaded nanopolymers. Drug loaded small nanopolymers also demonstrated no significant results when compared to cells treated with the drugs alone. Compared to the untreated control cells, all treatment groups except for 3 µM ASA loaded small FA-DABA-SMA and 2.5 mM ASA showed significant ($p < 0.01$ to $p \leq 0.0001$) decreases in cell viability.

In contrast, MDA-MB-231 cells treated with either ASA or tamoxifen (Tmx) loaded large nanopolymers showed a significant decrease ($p \leq 0.0001$) in cell viability when compared with the drugs alone. Consistent with previous results, MDA-MB-231 cells treated with Tmx loaded small nanopolymers exhibited a significant decrease in cell viability ($p \leq 0.0001$) when compared with Tmx alone. Compared to the untreated control cells, all treatment groups except for 3 µM ASA loaded small FA-DABA-SMA and 20 µM Tmx demonstrated significant ($p < 0.01$ to $p \leq 0.0001$) decreases in cell viability.

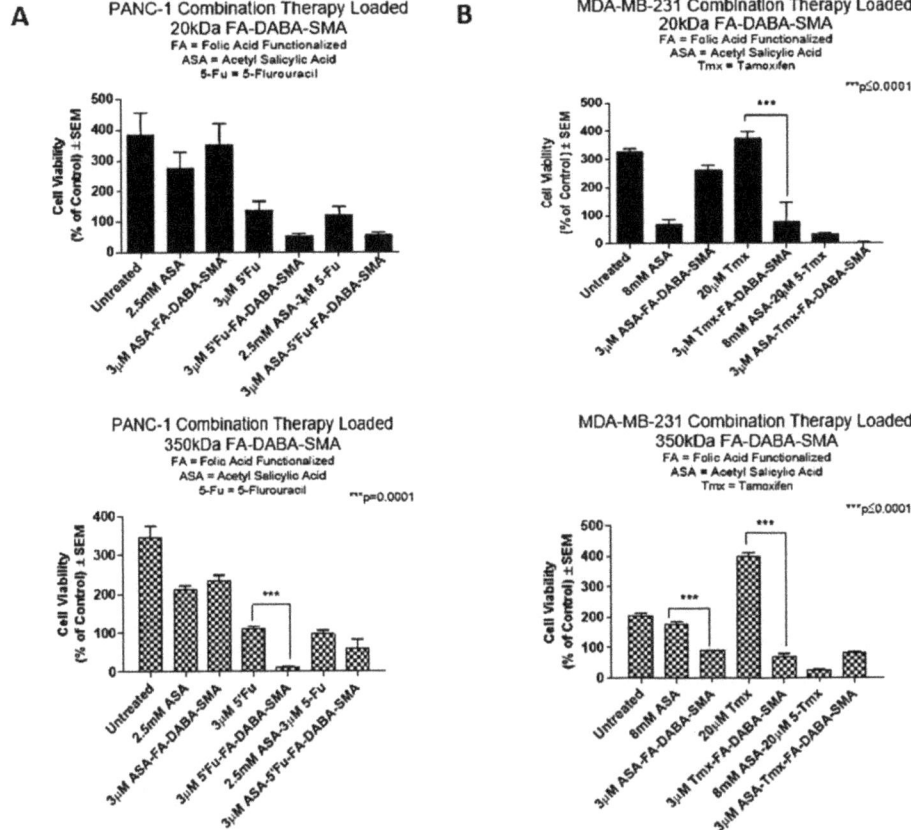

Figure 4. Large nanopolymers deliver hydrophobic therapeutic agents and reduces cell viability more efficiently than small nanopolymers. Comparison of the cell viability of (**A**) PANC-1 and (**B**) MDA-MB-231 cell lines at 72 hours treated with 20 kDa (small) and 350 kDa (large) FA-DABA-SMA nanopolymer loaded with hydrophobic agents, acetylsalicylic acid (ASA), 5-fluorouracil (5-Fu), and tamoxifen (Tmx) given individually or in combination using the WST-1 cell proliferation assay. Results were compared by a one-way ANOVA at 95% confidence using Fisher's LSD test ($n = 6$). The data are a combination of two independent experiments with similar results. The significance is in comparison to the nanopolymer delivered drug(s) and drug alone at the respective time point.

Collectively, these results indicate that the potency of both large and small nanopolymers, when loaded with hydrophobic drugs, may vary depending on the cancer type. For example, the MDA-MB-231 breast cancer cells demonstrated higher sensitivity to the treatment with both small and large nanopolymers when compared with PANC-1 pancreatic cancer cells. Interestingly, the potency of the combination drug therapy when delivered via the nanopolymers was comparable to the drugs alone across both cell lines. For example, tamoxifen is used to treat estrogen receptor positive breast cancer cases, as an important adjuvant hormonal therapy. However, tamoxifen induced side effects have been noted, in particular fatty liver, which is one of the most common side effects among them. Actively targeting cancer cells with drug loaded nanopolymers would upend any of these adverse side effects of the chemotherapeutics. Furthermore, the encapsulation of the hydrophobic drugs in an amphiphilic delivery system is expected to improve the solubility of the drug for enhanced access to cancerous cells. From these results, the size of the nanopolymer does not appear to affect the drug delivery ability of the nanopolymer as both the small and large therapy loaded nanopolymers were significantly able to reduce cell viability in both cell lines. Given these and earlier results, we further investigated the possibility of a novel dual therapeutic role of the large nanopolymers on both PANC-1 and MDA-MB-231 cancer cells.

2.5. Folic Acid-Functionalized Copolymer Disables Intracellular Expression of STAT3, p53 and c-Myc in MDA-MB-231 Breast Cancer Cells

To determine the possibility of a novel intrinsic therapeutic property of the large sized FA-DABA-SMA copolymer, it was important to consider its effects on critical oncogenic proliferation proteins that promote tumorigenesis.

Here, we treated PANC-1 and MDA-MB-231 cancer cells for 48 hours with large empty FA-DABA-SMA and investigated the effects of this nanopolymer on oncogenic proteins contributing to cell proliferation such as p53, activated phospho-p53, c-Myc and STAT3. In Figure 5a,b, the PANC-1 cells treated with the large empty nanopolymers exhibited a modest and insignificant decrease in expression levels of phospho-p53 along with p53, STAT-3 and c-Myc, when compared with untreated cells.

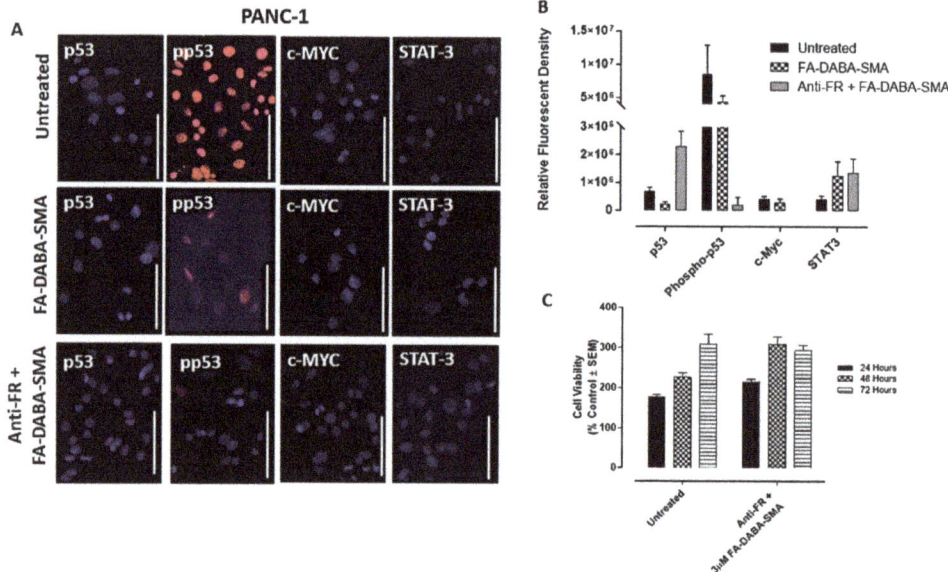

Figure 5. Dual role of FA-DABA-SMA copolymer targeting folic acid receptors (FR) and intracellular Inhibition of STAT3 and p53 and c-Myc in PANC-1 pancreatic cancer cells. (**A**) Immunocytochemistry staining of p53, phospho-p53, c-Myc and STAT3 on the PANC-1 cell line before (untreated), treated with large 350 kDa FA-DABA-SMA copolymer or pretreatment with the anti-FR antibody for two hours followed with large 350 kDa FA-DABA-SMA nanopolymer. The white scale bar represents 100 µm taken at 400× magnification. Blue DAPI stain represents the nuclei, and red staining is a primary antibody for the respective protein expression followed by AlexaFluor 594 secondary antibody. (**B**) Quantification of expression levels by relative density corrected for average background staining of the secondary antibody, mean ± S.E.M. of 3–4 different staining images. Results were compared by a one-way ANOVA at 95% confidence using Fisher's LSD test for a combination of two independent experiments. (**C**) Comparison of the cell viability of PANC-1 cells' pre-treatment with the anti-FR antibody for two hours followed by large 350 kDa FA-DABA-SMA nanopolymer at 24, 48 and 72 hours using the WST-1 assay. Results were compared by a one-way ANOVA at 95% confidence using Fisher's LSD test. The data presented are a combination of two independent experiments with triplicates ($n = 6$).

However, consistent with our previous results, the MDA-MB-231 breast cancer cells demonstrated increased responsiveness to treatment with the large empty nanopolymers. These results revealed that all oncogenic proliferation protein levels decreased after treatment of the large (350 kDa) FA-DABA-SMA with a significant decrease ($p < 0.05$) in p53, phospho-p53 and c-Myc expression levels (Figure 6a,b). These results suggest that upon internalization, the FA-DABA-SMA can disrupt the intracellular proliferation activities of critical oncogenic proliferation proteins in breast cancer cells.

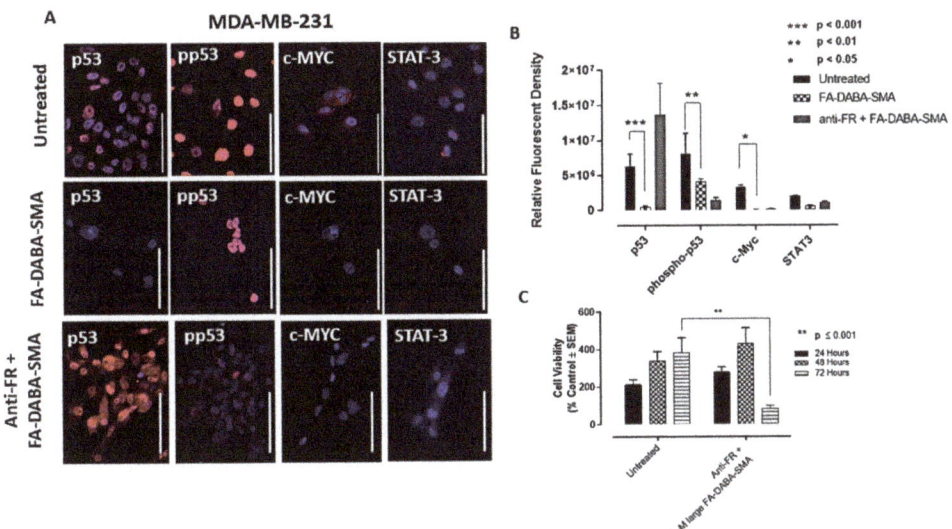

Figure 6. Dual role of FA-DABA-SMA copolymer targeting folic acid receptors (FR) and intracellular Inhibition of STAT3, p53 and c-Myc in MDA-MB-231 breast cancer cells. (**A**) Immunocytochemistry staining of p53, phosphor-53, c-Myc and STAT3 on the MDA-MB-231 cell line before (untreated), treated with large 350 kDa FA-DABA-SMA copolymer or pretreatment with an anti-FR antibody for two hours followed by large 350 kDa FA-DABA-SMA nanopolymer. The white scale bar represents 100 µm taken at 400× magnification. Blue DAPI stain represents the nuclei, and red staining is a primary antibody for the respective protein expression followed by AlexaFluor 594 secondary antibody. (**B**) Quantification of expression levels by relative density corrected for average background staining of the secondary antibody, mean ± S.E.M. of three to four different staining images. Results were compared by a one-way ANOVA at 95% confidence using Fisher's LSD test for a combination of two independent experiments. (**C**) Comparison of the cell viability of MDA-MB-231 cells' pretreatment with an anti-FR antibody for two hours followed by large 350 kDa FA-DABA-SMA nanopolymer at 24, 48 and 72 hours using the WST-1 assay. Results were compared by a one-way ANOVA at 95% confidence using Fisher's LSD test. The data presented are a combination of two independent experiments with triplicates ($n = 6$).

2.6. Anti-Folic Acid Receptor Blocking Antibody Reversed the Inhibitory Effects of the FA-DABA-SMA, Leading to an Increase in Expression Levels of p53 and STAT-3

To confirm that the resulting decrease in the expression levels of p53, phospho-p53 and c-Myc was facilitated by the nanopolymer's intracellular specific inhibitory actions FR, we treated PANC-1 and MDA-MB-231 cancer cells with anti-FR antibody and assessed the effects on cell viability and expression levels of p53, phospho-p53, STAT-3 and c-Myc. As shown in Figure 5c, the PANC-1 cells showed no significant decrease in cell viability with the large empty nanopolymers following anti-FR antibody blocking.

In contrast, the MDA-MB-231 cells, as depicted in Figure 6c, maintained cell growth up to 48 hours, followed by a significant ($p \leq 0.0001$) decrease in cell viability. This directly contrasts the results presented in Figure 2c, where significant decreases in cell viability following treatment with the large nanopolymers began immediately at the 24 hour time point. This finding may be attributed to the anti-FR blocking antibody being maintained in the presence of the large sized nanopolymer, resulting in a decrease in cell viability. To confirm these findings, immunocytochemistry analyses were performed following 48 hours of treatment with the FR antibody.

In Figures 5a and 6a (third row), the data revealed the increased expression of p53 in both PANC-1 and MDA-MB-231 cells, respectively, and STAT-3 expression in PANC-1 cells. This contrasts with the pre-treatment data presented in Figure 5a (first and second row), where p53 and STAT-3 expressions in PANC-1 cells were negligible. Similarly, in Figure 6a, the data showed low expression of p53 in MDA-MB-231 cells, whereas with the anti-FR blocking antibody, high expression levels of p53 were observed, as depicted in Figure 6a. Furthermore, the phospho-p53 expression was lower after anti-FR antibody blockage, which contrasts with the high expression levels observed in the data presented in Figures 5a and 6a for PANC-1 and MDA-MB-231 cells, respectively.

Collectively, these results indicate that the activity of the nanopolymer was due to specific inhibitory intracellular interactions, rather than the result of extracellular actions when the FR was inhibited. These findings support the concept of a new therapeutic action of the large FA-DABA-SMA bound to FR in addition to its cargo loaded with hydrophobic chemotherapeutic drugs.

2.7. FA-DABA-SMA Activates Early and Late Apoptosis in PANC-1 and MDA-MB-231 Cells

To assess the resultant effects of the intracellular inhibition of proliferative oncoproteins, we investigated apoptotic activity following treatment with 3 μM empty 350 kDa nanopolymers in PANC-1 and MDA-MB-231 cancer cells. As shown in Figure 7a, caspase 3/7 activity significantly increased after 48 hours of treatment when compared to the untreated control. Following 48 hours of treatment with nanopolymer, PANC-1 cells entered early apoptosis (13.9%) and late apoptosis/necrotic (5.9%) stages when compared to the untreated cells (early apoptosis 6.5% and late apoptosis/necrotic 4.9%)., as shown in Figure 7b. Furthermore, the number of viable cells in the untreated control was 88.3%, while the number of viable cells in the treatment group was 77.7%.

Caspase 3/7 activity did not significantly increase after 48 hours of treatment with 3 μM FA-DABA-SMA when compared to the untreated control in MDA-MB-231 breast cancer cells (Figure 8a). However, upon further investigation, a significant portion of MDA-MB-231 breast cancer cells entered early apoptosis (38.6%) and late apoptosis/necrotic (27.9%) stages when compared to the untreated cells (early apoptosis 4.2% and late apoptosis/necrotic 0.3%), as shown in Figure 8b.

Furthermore, the number of viable cells in the untreated control was 92.9%, while the number of viable cells in the treatment group was significantly reduced to 29.9%. These results indicate the intracellular interactions of FA-DABA-SMA with cell proliferative proteins, and possibly other critical molecules required to maintain cancer cell growth are irreversibly disrupted, leading to apoptosis. The consequences of intracellular protein disruptions were far more pronounced in the MDA-MB-231 breast cancer cells when compared to the PANC-1 cells, suggesting that this novel mechanism of action could represent a novel aspect of intrinsic therapeutic abilities that include cytotoxic activities of internalized nanopolymers that may be cell specific. However, the therapeutic delivery capabilities of the FA-DABA-SMA were relatively consistent between the PANC-1 and MDA-MB-231 cancer cell lines.

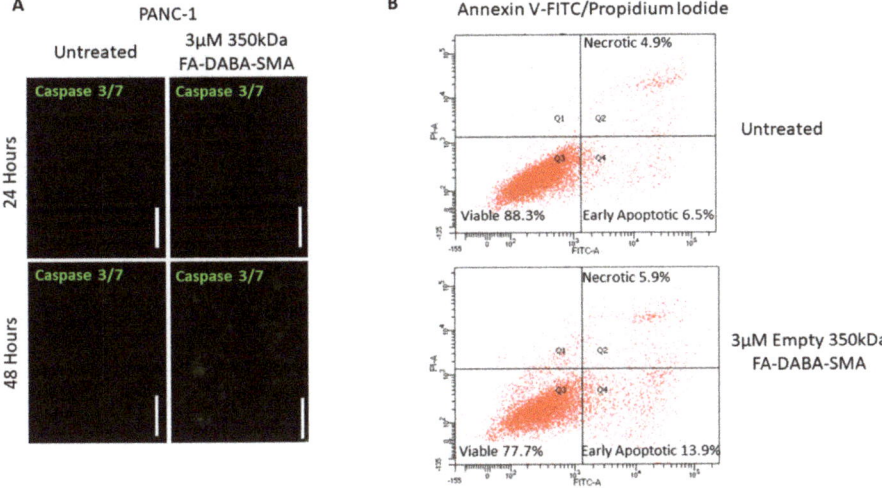

Figure 7. Caspase 3/7 and Annexin-V apoptotic activity post-treatment with 350 kDa FA-DABA-SMA on PANC-1 pancreatic cancer cells. (**A**) Immunocytochemistry staining for caspase on the PANC-1 cell line before after 24 and 48 hours of 3 μM FA-DABA-SMA (350 kDa) treatment. The white scale bar represents 100 μm, and pictures were taken at 400× magnification. Blue DAPI stain represents the nuclei, and green staining is caspase expression. (**B**) Flow cytometry of the Annexin-V apoptosis assay of untreated PANC-1 cells or 48 hours after treatment with 3 μM FA-DABA-SMA (350 kDa). An estimate of ~250,000 cells was collected and stained with Annexin V-FITC/propidium iodide to assess the stage of apoptosis.

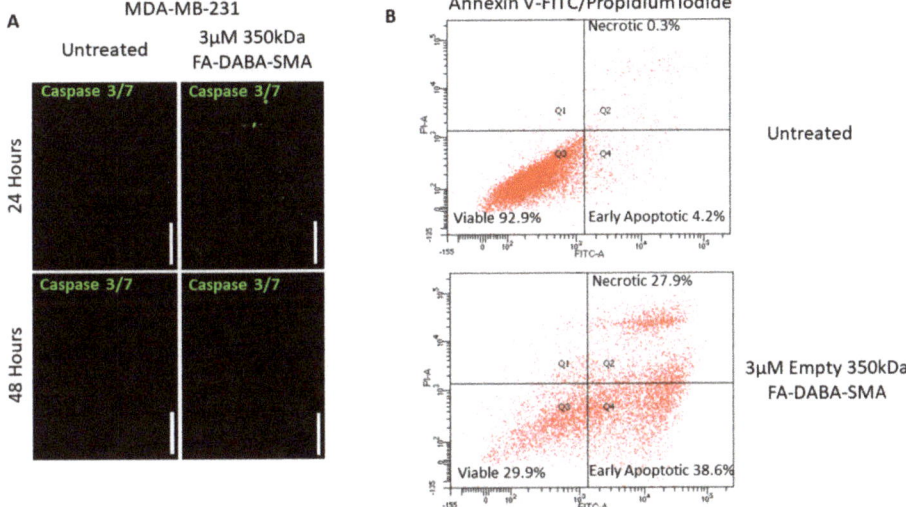

Figure 8. Caspase 3/7 and Annexin-V apoptotic activity post-treatment with 350 kDa FA-DABA-SMA on MDA-MB-231 breast cancer cells. (**A**) Immunocytochemistry staining for caspase on the MDA MB-231 cell line before and after 24 and 48 hours of FA-DABA-SMA (350 kDa) treatment. The white scale bar represents 100 μm, and pictures were taken at 400× magnification. Green staining is caspase expression. (**B**) Flow cytometry of Annexin-V apoptosis assay of untreated MDA-MB-231 cells or 48 hours after treatment with 3 μM FA-DABA-SMA (350 kDa). An estimate of ~250,000 cells was collected and stained with Annexin V-FITC/propidium iodide to assess the stage of apoptosis.

3. Discussion

Active targeting of overly expressed receptors and proteins on cancer cells is an important area of cancer research to increase the effectiveness of treatment regimens while at the same time reducing adverse side effects. This approach is equally valid of nanotechnology based drug carriers, which exploit overexpressed receptors to target cancer cells specifically and deliver the therapeutic drugs. Typically, these delivery nanoparticles are designed to be chemically inert and indirectly exert a therapeutic effect by delivering anti-cancer drugs. Advancements in research on the design and unique fabrication of nanopolymers with theranostic properties [21] focus on the physicochemical properties of the polymers, but cannot target cancer specific biological behavior in and around tumors and malignant cells [22]. Although there is robust research progress in the development of nanotechnology, knowledge of their intracellular tracking and endocytic pathway remains limited [5]. Therefore, the understanding of the intracellular mechanisms of nanopolymers is essential when developing the next generation of nano-delivery systems that can be successfully translated in the clinic. As such, this study was designed to further investigate the previously unknown intracellular mechanism of action of a pH responsive FA functionalized amphiphilic alternating copolymer (FA-DABA-SMA) on prostate DU-145, pancreatic PANC-1 and triple-negative breast MDA-MB-231 cancer cells [1]. FA-DABA-SMA has previously been shown to be a successful drug delivery system by actively targeting and penetrating tumor spheroids [4]. However, this study revealed a previously unknown therapeutic mechanism of action of empty FA-DABA-SMA in disabling cancer cell proliferation and survival.

The chemical design of the FA-DABA-SMA nanopolymer was initially fabricated to be pH-responsive, capable of self-assembly into ordered sheet like structures (large 350 kDa) or cylindrical structures (20 kDa) in a size dependent manner. Although this nanopolymer was designed to be inert when it was not loaded with chemotherapeutics, this study confirmed that the size and structure of FA-DABA-SMA contributed to its unusual intracellular therapeutic activity when unloaded. The influence of size and shape needs to be further investigated because the structure of the nanopolymer may be critical in facilitating the binding activity to the FR in order to promote the intrinsic therapeutic potential of FA-DABA-SMA.

Understanding the structure of FRα and its interactions with FA is important to consider in providing a potential explanation for the inherent therapeutic activity of FA conjugated nanopolymers. Under normal conditions, FA binds to FRα and is internalized through receptor mediated endocytosis [23]. Following internalization, the acidic environment of the endosome results in the release of folate from the receptor, followed by transportation to the cytoplasm by a proton coupled folate transporter [24]. Concerning the molecular interaction between FA and FRα, FA docks in a deep binding pocket of the receptor in a perpendicular orientation [24]. The critical finding by Chen et al. was that the pterin group located FRα binding pocket is critical in anchoring the folate to the receptor located in the binding pocket, while a glutamate group sticks out and can be readily conjugated with drugs. Given the critical role of FA orientation when binding to FRα, it is not surprising that the size and structure of FA conjugated nanopolymers is an important parameter to consider in order to facilitate adequate binding and subsequent internalization. However, the mechanistic features and properties for many nanopolymer delivery systems occurring after internalization remain unknown. These mechanistic profiles of nanopolymers may rely on the specific target that influences the pathophysiology of the tumour, including the accumulation, distribution, retention and efficacy of nanopolymers [22]. It is essential that key characteristics of nanopolymers, including size, shape and surface profiles be engineered to improve biodistribution and clearance of the nanopolymer for specific cancers and their characteristic tumor biology. For the first time, our findings support a next-generation multimodal potency of action of a nanopolymer, which depends on the cancer cell types. The MDA-MB-231 breast cancer cells were found to be most sensitive to the secondary multimodal effects, as depicted in Figure 9.

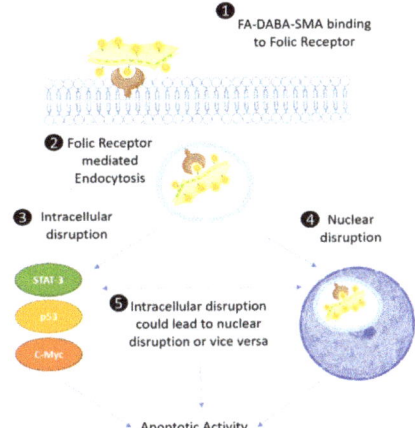

Figure 9. Proposed novel intrinsic therapeutic mechanism of FA-DABA-SMA. (1) FA-DABA-SMA binds to FRα. (2) Through receptor mediated endocytosis, the FRα-FA-SMA-DABA complex is internalized, where it could have two possible intrinsic therapeutic effects. It either (3) remains in the cytoplasm and disrupts the activity of key proliferation proteins such as STAT-3, p53 and c-Myc (and other proteins that maintain cancer growth and proliferation) or (4) the complex is translocated to the nucleus given the role of FRα as a transcription factor. Since FA-DABA-SMA is relatively large (350 kDa), the nanopolymer could theoretically block the binding of additional transcription factors, thus disrupting transcriptional processes of essential oncogenic proliferation proteins, resulting in the reduction of cell viability and activating apoptotic activity. Alternatively, (5) intracellular disruptions of critical cell proliferation proteins could lead to apoptotic events to be activated in the nucleus or, conversely, nuclear disruptions could lead to disruptions in the activity of critical oncogenic proteins. Overall, Steps 3, 4 and 5 could individually or collectively culminate and lead to the activation of apoptotic activity.

The proposed intracellular mechanism of FA-DABA-SMA bound to FR exhibited two possible therapeutic effects (Figure 9). It either remained in the cytoplasm and disrupted the activity of STAT-3, p53 and c-Myc and possibly other intracellular proteins, followed by translocating to the nucleus and inhibiting the FRα transcription factor from binding to the cis-regulatory elements and activating the transcription of developmental genes including *HES1* and *FGFR4*. This nanopolymer may affect multiple processes involved in tumorigenesis through varying, but similar mechanisms, such as disrupting epithelial to mesenchymal transition (EMT) via *HES1* inhibition [25]. HES1 is positively correlated with the levels of stem cell markers, suggesting that it may play a critical role in tumorigenesis through increasing the number of stem cell like cancer cells (CSCs) associated with mesenchymal phenotypes [3]. The large sized FA-DABA-SMA (350 kDa) may also block the binding of additional transcription factors in disrupting the transcriptional processes of essential oncogenic proteins. These resulting cytotoxic effects of the large sized and sheet like structured nanopolymer adds to the next-generation multimodality and therapeutic effects in reducing cancer cell viability and inducing apoptotic cell death.

FA-DABA-SMA is a smart drug delivery system specifically targeting the commonly overly expressed FR on cancer cells. In the present study, the characterization of the FR expression levels on all three cancer cell lines was essential to understand the underlying therapeutic mechanism(s) of the nanopolymer. As indicated in Figure 1a, MDA-MB-231 cells overly expressed FR when compared with DU-145 and PANC-1 cancer cells. The indicated quantification of the relative fluorescent density of the FR expression showed a consistent trend (Figure 1b). To further confirm the expression levels of FR on the cell membrane, flow cytometry analyses were conducted on all three cell lines. Surprisingly, these results were inconsistent with immunocytochemistry staining. The MDA-MB-231 cells are highly metabolically active and reflect an aggressive invasive ductal adenocarcinoma and, therefore, may require more folate to sustain rapid cell growth [15]. A possible explanation for the discrepancy can be attributed to the activity of FR in rapidly growing cells such as MDA-MB-231 [16]. Furthermore, the decreased need for folate when it is present in the environment also affects the FR expression levels. FR exists both on the cell surface and intracellularly dependent on cell specific growth needs, where 50 to 75% of FRα exists in endosomal compartments. However, the events leading to the trafficking of these receptors to the cell membrane remain unknown, and alterations in location could be attributed to growth specific needs or changes in the endocytic pathway events of GPI-anchored proteins [26]. The expression and binding activity of FR are regulated by the location of the receptor and the local environment, including pH, folate concentration and rate of receptor saturation and cycling [27]. The varying expression levels seen in the MDA-MB-231 cells may be a resulting differential receptor cycling, as the nanopolymer consistently targeted these cells. For the MDA-MB-231 breast cancer cells, the decreased membrane expression levels of FR observed in the present data may be due to more rapid cell growth and cell cycling when compared to the higher FR levels on DU-145 and PANC-1 cells. However, this merits further investigation and a deeper understanding of the stimulatory effects of folate and how this may influence the expression of the FR and in turn responsiveness to the action of FA-DABA-SMA.

Overall, the novel findings of this report highlight the importance of size and structure in possibly conferring intrinsic therapeutic abilities in FA-DABA-SMA that could potentially be extrapolated to other drug delivery vehicles and merit further investigation. Although both the 350 kDa and 20 kDa FA-DABA-SMA copolymers appeared to unload their hydrophobic payloads, only the 350 kDa nanopolymer can disrupt critical oncogenic proteins that are necessary for cancer growth. Furthermore, the activation of early apoptotic events, as well as caspase 3/7 enzymes, suggests that the dual therapeutic activity of the drug-loaded nanopolymers is irreversible and cytotoxic to rapidly proliferating cancer cells. Additional oncogenic proteins and critical survival activities that are necessary for cancer growth such as EMT and the selection of a CSC phenotype also merit further investigation.

4. Conclusions

This report presents next-generation multimodality and therapeutic effects of the size and structure dependence of functionalized folic acid conjugated amphiphilic alternating copolymer actively targeting cancer cells and disabling critical oncogenic proteins controlling cell division and apoptosis. Furthermore, this smart nanopolymer can effectively deliver hydrophobic chemotherapeutics to cancer cells preferentially to decrease the adverse side effects associated with cancer drug treatments. The large size and sheet like structure of FA-DABA-SMA allowed the nanopolymer to possess a previously unknown dual mechanism of disrupting the activity of intracellular oncogenic proteins and inducing apoptosis. The data suggest that FA-DABA-SMA is a potent delivery system capable of accurately targeting highly metabolic cancer cells and overcoming the barriers of conventional chemotherapy approaches. The size and structure of FA-DABA-SMA require further understanding of the full mechanistic potential of FA-DABA-SMA, specifically interacting with FR overly expressed in different cancer types.

5. Materials and Methods

5.1. Cell Lines and Culture Procedures

DU-145 (ATCC® HTB-81™) is a human prostate cancer cell line derived from a metastatic brain lesion from a 69-year older man with prostate cancer. PANC-1 (ATCC® CRL-1469™) is a human pancreatic cancer cell line whose site of origin was the duct in a 56-year old male with pancreatic ductal adenocarcinoma. PANC-1 has a genetic profile that has been characterized to express *KRAS*, *TP53*, and *CDKN2A* [28]. MDA-MB-231 (ATCC® HTB-26™) is a human triple-negative breast cancer cell line whose site of origin was a metastatic pleural effusion site of a 51-year-old woman with metastatic breast cancer. MDA-MB-231 is a highly aggressive invasive ductal adenocarcinoma and has a genetic profile that expresses *BRAF*, *CDKN2A*, *KRAS*, *NF2*, *TP53*, and *PDGFRA* mutations [29].

All three cell lines were grown in standard culture conditions containing 1× DMEM conditioned medium supplemented with 10% fetal bovine serum (FBS; HyClone, Logan, UT, USA) and 5 μg/mL plasmocin™ (InvivoGen, San Diego, CA, USA). All cells were incubated at 37 °C in a 5% CO_2 incubator. Cells were sub-cultured as needed (approximately every 4–5 days) using TrypLE Express (Gibco, Rockville, MD, USA).

5.2. Reagents

Acetylsalicylic acid (>99% pure, Sigma-Aldrich, Steinheim, Germany) was dissolved in dimethyl sulfoxide (DMSO) to prepare a 550 mM stock solution, which was stored in aliquots at −20°C. Tamoxifen citrate salt (≥99% pure, Sigma-Aldrich, Steinheim, Germany) was dissolved in methanol (99.8% pure, Sigma-Aldrich, Steinheim, Germany) to prepare a 1 mM stock solution, which was aliquoted, wrapped in aluminum foil (light-sensitive) and stored at 4°C. 5-Fluorouracil (>99% pure, Sigma-Aldrich, Steinheim, Germany) was dissolved in dimethyl sulfoxide (DMSO) to prepare a 28 mM stock solution and was stored at 4 °C.

Water-insoluble tamoxifen and 5-fluorouracil (5-Fu) were used for nanoparticle loading purposes. The powder forms of 5-Fu and tamoxifen were loaded in excess. Before the experiment, excess 5-Fu and tamoxifen were allowed to sediment, and the final concentrations of treatment loaded nanopolymers were 3 μM for both large FA-DABA-SMA (350,000 g/mol) and small FA-DABA-SMA (20,000 g/mol) made in the standard culture medium.

5.3. FA-DABA-SMA Alternating Copolymer

We previously reported on a novel polymer composed of a hydrophobic group (styrene) alternating with a hydrophilic group (maleic acid) along the polymeric chain (poly (styrene-*alt*-maleic anhydride) (SMA)). The polymer can self-assemble into nanostructures at physiological pH with a hydrophobic inner core that facilitates encapsulation of hydrophobic drugs [30,31]. The synthesis of this nanopolymer and characterization of this nanopolymer were reported by us [1,2,4]. For this study, two variations of this polymer were used to test the effects of size. The large polymer had a molecular weight of 350,000 g/mol (350 kDa) and a single chain hydrodynamic radius (Rh) of 6 nm and self-assembled into sheets (Rh of the self-assembled SMA structure of 850 nm in water). The small polymer had a molecular weight of 20,000 g/mol (20 kDa) with a single chain hydrodynamic radius (Rh) of 3 nm and self-assembled into cylinders (Rh of the self-assembled SMA structure of 120 nm in water).

5.4. WST-1 Assay

The water-soluble tetrazolium salt-1 (WST-1) assay is a direct measure of metabolically active cells, based on the reduction of a tetrazolium compound to its soluble formazan (orange) derivative by metabolically active cells [32]. The absorbance of the reaction at 420 nm directly correlates to the number of living cells in culture.

Cells were plated at a density of 10,000 cells/well in 96 well plates, incubated and allowed to adhere overnight. Adhered cells were treated with their respective concentrations of either curcumin loaded or empty FA-DABA-SMA or were left as the untreated controls. At the 24, 48 and 72 hour time-points following treatment (Days 1, 2 and 3, respectively), media was removed, and 100 μL of 10% WST-1 reagent (Roche Diagnostics, Laval-des-Rapides, QC, Canada) diluted in cell culture media were added to each well. The 96 well plate was then incubated at 37 °C for 2 hours before taking an absorbance reading using the SpectraMax250 machine and SoftMax software. Cell viability measured as a percentage of untreated control was illustrated as a bar graph using GraphPad Prism software (GraphPad Software, La Jolla, CA, USA).

The following formula was used to determine cell viability as a percentage of control (Day 0) after 24, 48 and 72 hours of drug treatment (Days 1, 2 and 3, respectively):

$$\frac{[(absorbance\ in\ given\ drug\ concentration\ on\ day\ 1,\ 2\ or\ 3) - (media\ absorbance)] \times 100}{(untreated\ absorbance\ on\ day\ 0) - (media\ absorbance)}$$

5.5. Immunocytochemistry

DU-145, PANC-1 and MDA-MB-231 cancer cells were plated at a density of 100,000 cells/mL on glass coverslips in 24 well plates. Cells were treated for 48 hours with empty FA-SMA-DABA or were blocked with FR antibody. At the end of the time point, cells were washed and fixed with 4% PFA for 30 minutes followed by blocking for 1 hour in 10% FBS + 0.1% Triton X-100 + 1× PBS (note: 0.1% Triton x-100 was omitted from blocking buffer for membrane only stains to prevent intracellular non-specific binding). Following blocking, cells were washed with 1× PBS 3× for 10 minutes, followed by the addition of the primary antibody, which was diluted to 1:250 using a 1% FBS + 1×PBS + 0.1% Triton X-100 (note: 0.1% Triton X-100 was omitted from antibody buffer for membrane only stains to prevent intracellular non-specific binding) overnight at 4 °C. Primary antibodies used for these studies were FR (sc-515521), STAT-3 (sc-8019), p53 (Bethyl Laboratories Inc., Montgomery, TX 77356 USA, A300-249A-T), phospho-p53 (R&D Systems, Minneapolis, MN 55413, USA) and c-Myc (sc-40). Cells were washed 5× for 10 minutes with 1× PBS and incubated for 1 hour with AlexaFluor 594 secondary antibodies. Cells were then washed 5× for 10 minutes with 1× PBS (note: one wash included 0.1% Triton X-100 to permeabilize cells for DAPI). DAPI containing mounting media (VECTH1200, MJS BioLynx Inc., P.O. Box 1150, 300 Laurier Blvd., Brockville, ON K6V 5W1, Canada) was added to slides, and coverslips were inverted on to the mounting media droplet and sealed.

5.6. Relative Fluorescence Density Quantification

Relative fluorescence density was quantified using images captured at 400× to ensure a wide field of view was obtained. Two representative images were taken at 400×. Background mean, mean and pixel measurements were obtained from Corel Photo-Paint X8. Red (AlexaFluor 594, Abcam Inc., c/o 913860, PO Box 4090 Stn A, Toronto, ON M5W 0E9, Canada) or green (AlexaFluor 488, Abcam Inc., c/o 913860, PO Box 4090 Stn A, Toronto, ON M5W 0E9, Canada) color channel images were quantified. The background means represent an unstained section of the image, and the mean represents the total fluorescence of the image. These measurements were then used to quantify the relative fluorescence density using the equation below:

$$density = (bkgd\ mean - mean) \times pixels$$

The relative fluorescence density was then corrected for unspecific staining by subtracting the relative fluorescence density of the secondary antibody control images. These corrected values are represented in Figures 1 and 5–8.

5.7. Immunofluorescence Live Cell Tracking

Cells were plated at a density of 150,000 cell/well on glass coverslips in 24 well plates. Cells were treated for 12, 24 and 48 hours with 300 µL of curcumin loaded FA-DABA-SMA. Curcumin represents a hydrophobic drug model in addition to acting as a fluorescent probe. At the end of each time point, glass coverslips were removed from the 24 well plates. Live cells were treated with the Hoechst 33342 nuclear counterstain to visualize nuclei and curcumin loaded FA-DABA-SMA at the respective time points. DAPI containing mounting media (ab104139, Abcam Inc., c/o 913860, PO Box 4090 Stn A, Toronto, ON M5W 0E9, Canada) diluted with 1× PBS + 0.1% Triton X-100 was added to slides, and coverslips were inverted on to the mounting media droplet. Pictures were taken at the respective time points using the green (AlexaFluor 488) color channel.

5.8. Caspase Assay

Cells were plated at a density of 100,000 cells/well on glass coverslips in 24 well plates. Cells were treated for 24 and 48 hours with 300 µL of empty FA-DABA-SMA. At the end of each time point, caspase staining (CellEvent™ Caspase 3/7 Green Detection Reagent, Thermo Fisher Scientific, 168 Third Avenue, Waltham, MA 02451, United States) was diluted to the manufacturer's recommended concentration of 5 µM in 5% FBS + 1× PBS from the stock solution of 2 mM. Stained cells were incubated for 30 minutes, then washed 2× in 1× PBS. The cells were then fixed with 4% paraformaldehyde solution diluted in 1× PBS for another 30 minutes. DAPI containing mounting media (Abcam ab104139) diluted with 1× PBS + 0.1% Triton X-100 was added to slides, and coverslips were inverted on to the mounting media droplet. Images were taken at the respective time points using the green (AlexaFluor 488) color channel.

5.9. Flow Cytometry

DU-145, PANC-1 and MDA-MB-231 cells were harvested and counted for a final concentration of 1.0×10^6 cells/mL. All subsequent steps were done on ice. Cells were washed 2× in 2% FBS + 1× PBS before primary antibody addition. The cells were treated with 100 µL of FR (sc-515521, Santa Cruz Biotechnology, Inc., 10410 Finnell Street, Dallas, Texas 75220, U.S.A.) primary monoclonal mouse antibody at a final concentration of 10 µg/mL and incubated for 60 minutes. Secondary control cells were treated with 100 µL of 2% FBS + 1× PBS and incubated for 60 minutes. The cells were then washed 2× with 2% FBS + 1× PBS followed by incubation for 60 minutes with 100 µL of secondary anti-mouse antibody AlexaFluor 488 at a final concentration of 10 µg/mL. The cells were then washed 2× with 2% FBS + 1× PBS and fixed in 1 mL of 4% paraformaldehyde solution before flow cytometry analysis.

5.10. Annexin V Assay

PANC-1 and MDA-MB-231 were plated at a density of 1×10^6 cells/mL in a T25 tissue culture flask. Cells were treated with empty FA-DABA-SMA for 48 hours or left untreated. The cells were then trypsinized, and ~250,000 cells/mL were analyzed for apoptotic, necrotic and viable cell populations using the Annexin V-FITC Apoptosis Kit (K101-25, BioVision, Inc., 155 S Milpitas Blvd. Milpitas, CA 95035, USA) following the manufacturer's manual. Briefly, the collected cells were resuspended in 500 µL of 1× binding buffer followed by 5 µL of each Annexin V-FITC and propidium iodide. The cells were incubated for 5 minutes at room temperature in the dark, followed by quantification by a flow cytometer.

5.11. Folic Receptor Blocking

PANC-1 and MDA-MB-231 cancer cells were plated at a density of 100,000 cells/mL on glass coverslips in 24 well plates for immunocytochemistry experiments or at a density of 10,000 cells/well for WST-1 experiments. For both experiments, cells were treated for 2 hours with the FR (sc-515521) antibody, followed by treatment with large empty nanopolymer. WST-1 experiments were performed according to the procedure outlined in Section 5.4, and immunocytochemistry experiments were performed after 48 hours of treatment following the procedure outlined in Section 5.5.

5.12. Statistical Analysis

Data are presented as the means ± the standard error of the mean (SEM) from two repeats of each experiment, each performed in triplicate. All statistical analyses were performed with GraphPad Prism software. All results were compared with one-way analysis of variance (ANOVA) and Fisher's LSD test, with the following asterisks denoting statistical significance: * $p \leq 0.05$, ** $p \leq 0.001$ and *** $p \leq 0.0001$.

Author Contributions: Conceptualization, M.S., A.D., C.M.-J. and M.R.S.; methodology, M.S., A.D., C.M.-J. and M.R.S.; software, M.S., A.D. and M.R.S.; validation, M.S., A.D., C.M.-J. and M.R.S.; formal analysis, M.S., A.D.,

C.M.-J. and M.R.S.; investigation, M.S., A.D., C.M.-J. and M.R.S.; resources, C.M.-J. and M.R.S.; data curation, M.S., A.D., C.M.-J. and M.R.S.; writing, original draft preparation, M.S., A.D., writing, review and editing, M.S., A.D., C.M.-J. and M.R.S.; visualization, M.S., A.D., C.M.-J. and M.R.S.; supervision, C.M.-J. and M.R.S.; project administration, C.M.-J. and M.R.S.; funding acquisition, C.M.-J. and M.R.S.

Funding: This work was supported in part by grants to C. Malardier-Jugroot and M.R. Szewczuk from the Natural Sciences and Engineering Research Council of Canada (NSERC). M. Sambi is the recipient of the Queen's University Graduate Award (QGA) and the R. Samuel McLaughlin Fellowship. A. DeCarlo is the recipient of the Queen's University Graduate Award (QGA).

Acknowledgments: We would like to thank Bessi Qorri and Xia Li for their diligent work in fabricating the nanopolymers that were used in this study. Their hard work and attention to detail in the fabrications of the small and large sized nanopolymers were essential to this study.

Conflicts of Interest: The authors report no conflicts of interest in this work.

References

1. Li, X.; Szewczuk, M.R.; Malardier-Jugroot, C. Folic acid-conjugated amphiphilic alternating copolymer as a new active tumor targeting drug delivery platform. *Drug Des. Devel. Ther.* **2016**, *10*, 4101–4110. [CrossRef] [PubMed]
2. Li, X.; McTaggart, M.; Malardier-Jugroot, C. Synthesis and characterization of a pH responsive folic acid functionalized polymeric drug delivery system. *Biophys. Chem.* **2016**, *214–215*, 17–26. [CrossRef] [PubMed]
3. Cheung, A.; Bax, H.J.; Josephs, D.H.; Ilieva, K.M.; Pellizzari, G.; Opzoomer, J.; Bloomfield, J.; Fittall, M.; Grigoriadis, A.; Figini, M.; et al. Targeting folate receptor alpha for cancer treatment. *Oncotarget* **2016**, *7*, 52553–52574. [CrossRef] [PubMed]
4. Li, X.; Sambi, M.; DeCarlo, A.; Burov, S.V.; Akasov, R.; Markvicheva, E.; Malardier-Jugroot, C.; Szewczuk, M.R. Functionalized Folic Acid-Conjugated Amphiphilic Alternating Copolymer Actively Targets 3D Multicellular Tumour Spheroids and Delivers the Hydrophobic Drug to the Inner Core. *Nanomaterials* **2018**, *8*, 588. [CrossRef]
5. Xu, C.; Haque, F.; Jasinski, D.L.; Binzel, D.W.; Shu, D.; Guo, P. Favorable biodistribution, specific targeting and conditional endosomal escape of RNA nanoparticles in cancer therapy. *Cancer Lett.* **2018**, *414*, 57–70. [CrossRef]
6. Albanese, A.; Tang, P.S.; Chan, W.C.W. The Effect of Nanoparticle Size, Shape, and Surface Chemistry on Biological Systems. *Annu. Rev. Biomed. Eng.* **2012**, *14*, 1–16. [CrossRef]
7. AshaRani, P.V.; Low Kah Mun, G.; Hande, M.P.; Valiyaveettil, S. Cytotoxicity and genotoxicity of silver nanoparticles in human cells. *ACS Nano.* **2009**, *3*, 279–290. [CrossRef]
8. Berneburg, M.; Kamenisch, Y.; Krutmann, J.; Rocken, M. 'To repair or not to repair—no longer a question': Repair of mitochondrial DNA shielding against age and cancer. *Exp. Dermatol.* **2006**, *15*, 1005–1015. [CrossRef]
9. Onuma, K.; Sato, Y.; Ogawara, S.; Shirasawa, N.; Kobayashi, M.; Yoshitake, J.; Yoshimura, T.; Iigo, M.; Fujii, J.; Okada, F. Nano-scaled particles of titanium dioxide convert benign mouse fibrosarcoma cells into aggressive tumor cells. *Am. J. Pathol.* **2009**, *175*, 2171–2183. [CrossRef]
10. Boshnjaku, V.; Shim, K.W.; Tsurubuchi, T.; Ichi, S.; Szany, E.V.; Xi, G.; Mania-Farnell, B.; McLone, D.G.; Tomita, T.; Mayanil, C.S. Nuclear localization of folate receptor alpha: A new role as a transcription factor. *Sci. Rep.* **2012**, *2*, 980. [CrossRef]
11. Xu, S.; Olenyuk, B.Z.; Okamoto, C.T.; Hamm-Alvarez, S.F. Targeting receptor-mediated endocytotic pathways with nanoparticles: Rationale and advances. *Adv. Drug Deliv. Rev.* **2013**, *65*, 121–138. [CrossRef] [PubMed]
12. Xu, X.; Ho, W.; Zhang, X.; Bertrand, N.; Farokhzad, O. Cancer nanomedicine: From targeted delivery to combination therapy. *Trends Mol. Med.* **2015**, *21*, 223–232. [CrossRef] [PubMed]
13. Ledermann, J.A.; Canevari, S.; Thigpen, T. Targeting the folate receptor: Diagnostic and therapeutic approaches to personalize cancer treatments. *Ann. Oncol.* **2015**, *26*, 2034–2043. [CrossRef] [PubMed]
14. Serpe, L.; Gallicchio, M.; Canaparo, R.; Dosio, F. Targeted treatment of folate receptor-positive platinum-resistant ovarian cancer and companion diagnostics, with specific focus on vintafolide and etarfolatide. *Pharmgenomics Pers. Med.* **2014**, *7*, 31–42. [CrossRef] [PubMed]

15. Necela, B.M.; Crozier, J.A.; Andorfer, C.A.; Lewis-Tuffin, L.; Kachergus, J.M.; Geiger, X.J.; Kalari, K.R.; Serie, D.J.; Sun, Z.; Moreno-Aspitia, A.; et al. Folate receptor-alpha (FOLR1) expression and function in triple negative tumors. *PLoS ONE* **2015**, *10*, e0122209. [CrossRef]
16. Doucette, M.M.; Stevens, V.L. Folate receptor function is regulated in response to different cellular growth rates in cultured mammalian cells. *J. Nutr.* **2001**, *131*, 2819–2825. [CrossRef] [PubMed]
17. Yang, M.; Yu, L.; Guo, R.; Dong, A.; Lin, C.; Zhang, J. A Modular Coassembly Approach to All-In-One Multifunctional Nanoplatform for Synergistic Codelivery of Doxorubicin and Curcumin. *Nanomaterials* **2018**, *8*, 167. [CrossRef]
18. Sambi, M.; Haq, S.; Samuel, V.; Qorri, B.; Haxho, F.; Hill, K.; Harless, W.; Szewczuk, M.R. Alternative therapies for metastatic breast cancer: Multimodal approach targeting tumor cell heterogeneity. *Breast Cancer* **2017**, *9*, 85–93. [CrossRef]
19. Zhang, X.; Feng, Y.; Liu, X.; Ma, J.; Li, Y.; Wang, T.; Li, X. Beyond a chemopreventive reagent, aspirin is a master regulator of the hallmarks of cancer. *J. Cancer Res. Clin. Oncol.* **2019**, *145*, 1387–1403. [CrossRef]
20. Hua, H.; Zhang, H.; Kong, Q.; Wang, J.; Jiang, Y. Complex roles of the old drug aspirin in cancer chemoprevention and therapy. *Med. Res. Rev.* **2019**, *39*, 114–145. [CrossRef]
21. Mukherjee, A.; Paul, M.; Mukherjee, S. Recent Progress in the Theranostics Application of Nanomedicine in Lung Cancer. *Cancers* **2019**, *11*, 597. [CrossRef]
22. Hare, J.I.; Lammers, T.; Ashford, M.B.; Puri, S.; Storm, G.; Barry, S.T. Challenges and strategies in anti-cancer nanomedicine development: An industry perspective. *Adv. Drug Deliv. Rev.* **2017**, *108*, 25–38. [CrossRef] [PubMed]
23. Chen, C.; Ke, J.; Zhou, X.E.; Yi, W.; Brunzelle, J.S.; Li, J.; Yong, E.L.; Xu, H.E.; Melcher, K. Structural basis for molecular recognition of folic acid by folate receptors. *Nature* **2013**, *500*, 486–489. [CrossRef] [PubMed]
24. Zhao, R.; Min, S.H.; Wang, Y.; Campanella, E.; Low, P.S.; Goldman, I.D. A role for the proton-coupled folate transporter (PCFT-SLC46A1) in folate receptor-mediated endocytosis. *J. Biol. Chem.* **2009**, *284*, 4267–4274. [CrossRef] [PubMed]
25. Gao, F.; Zhang, Y.; Wang, S.; Liu, Y.; Zheng, L.; Yang, J.; Huang, W.; Ye, Y.; Luo, W.; Xiao, D. Hes1 is involved in the self-renewal and tumourigenicity of stem-like cancer cells in colon cancer. *Sci. Rep.* **2014**, *4*, 3963. [CrossRef]
26. Sabharanjak, S.; Mayor, S. Folate receptor endocytosis and trafficking. *Adv. Drug Deliv. Rev.* **2004**, *56*, 1099–1109. [CrossRef]
27. Kamen, B.A.; Smith, A.K. A review of folate receptor alpha cycling and 5-methyltetrahydrofolate accumulation with an emphasis on cell models in vitro. *Adv. Drug Deliv. Rev.* **2004**, *56*, 1085–1097. [CrossRef]
28. Deer, E.L.; Gonzalez-Hernandez, J.; Coursen, J.D.; Shea, J.E.; Ngatia, J.; Scaife, C.L.; Firpo, M.A.; Mulvihill, S.J. Phenotype and genotype of pancreatic cancer cell lines. *Pancreas* **2010**, *39*, 425–435. [CrossRef]
29. Lehmann, B.D.; Bauer, J.A.; Chen, X.; Sanders, M.E.; Chakravarthy, A.B.; Shyr, Y.; Pietenpol, J.A. Identification of human triple-negative breast cancer subtypes and preclinical models for selection of targeted therapies. *J. Clin. Invest.* **2011**, *121*, 2750–2767. [CrossRef]
30. Malardier-Jugroot, C.; van de Ven, T.G.M.; Cosgrove, T.; Richardson, R.M.; Whitehead, M.A. Novel Self-Assembly of Amphiphilic Copolymers into Nanotubes: Characterization by Small-Angle Neutron Scattering. *Langmuir* **2005**, *21*, 10179–10187. [CrossRef]
31. McTaggart, M.; Malardier-Jugroot, C.; Jugroot, M. Self-assembled biomimetic nanoreactors I: Polymeric template. *Chem. Phys. Lett.* **2015**, *636*, 216–220. [CrossRef]
32. Ngamwongsatit, P.; Banada, P.P.; Panbangred, W.; Bhunia, A.K. WST-1-based cell cytotoxicity assay as a substitute for MTT-based assay for rapid detection of toxigenic Bacillus species using CHO cell line. *J. Microbiol Methods* **2008**, *73*, 211–215. [CrossRef] [PubMed]

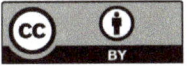

© 2019 by the authors. Licensee MDPI, Basel, Switzerland. This article is an open access article distributed under the terms and conditions of the Creative Commons Attribution (CC BY) license (http://creativecommons.org/licenses/by/4.0/).

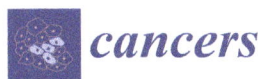

Article

Size Matters in the Cytotoxicity of Polydopamine Nanoparticles in Different Types of Tumors

Celia Nieto [1], Milena A. Vega [1], Jesús Enrique [1], Gema Marcelo [2,*] and Eva M. Martín del Valle [1,*]

[1] Departamento de Ingeniería Química y Textil, Facultad de Ciencias Químicas, Universidad de Salamanca, 37008 Salamanca, Spain; celianieto@usal.es (C.N.); mvega@usal.es (M.A.V.); j.enrique@usal.es (J.E.)
[2] Departamento de Química Analítica, Química Física e Ingeniería Química, Facultad de Farmacia, Universidad de Alcalá, 28801 Alcalá de Henares (Madrid), Spain
* Correspondence: gema.marcelo@uah.es (G.M.); emvalle@usal.es (E.M.M.d.V.); Tel.: +34-923-294-479 (E.M.M.d.V.)

Received: 8 October 2019; Accepted: 25 October 2019; Published: 29 October 2019

Abstract: Polydopamine has acquired great relevance in the field of nanomedicine due to its physicochemical properties. Previously, it has been reported that nanoparticles synthetized from this polymer are able to decrease the viability of breast and colon tumor cells. In addition, it is well known that the size of therapeutic particles plays an essential role in their effect. As a consequence, the influence of this parameter on the cytotoxicity of polydopamine nanoparticles was studied in this work. For this purpose, polydopamine nanoparticles with three different diameters (115, 200 and 420 nm) were synthetized and characterized. Their effect on the viability of distinct sorts of human carcinomas (breast, colon, liver and lung) and stromal cells was investigated, as well as the possible mechanisms that could be responsible for such cytotoxicity. Moreover, polydopamine nanoparticles were also loaded with doxorubicin and the therapeutic action of the resulting nanosystem was analyzed. As a result, it was demonstrated that a smaller nanoparticle size is related to a more enhanced antiproliferative activity, which may be a consequence of polydopamine's affinity for iron ions. Smaller nanoparticles would be able to adsorb more lysosomal Fe^{3+} and, when they are loaded with doxorubicin, a synergistic effect can be achieved.

Keywords: polydopamine nanoparticles; size; cytotoxicity; iron affinity; doxorubicin

1. Introduction

Nanomedicine has acquired an essential role in recent decades due to the urgent need for developing novel therapeutic strategies for cancer treatment. This multidisciplinary field, by taking advantage of nanotechnology, aims to overcome the pharmaceutical limitations of conventional chemotherapeutics. Thus, the improvement of their stability, aqueous solubility and dose limiting toxicity, as well as avoiding the apparition of multidrug resistances (MDR), are some of the objectives that are highly relevant for the scientific community today [1,2]. Moreover, with the employment of nanoparticles (NPs) for cancer treatment, increasing tumor retention of therapeutic molecules while reducing their non-specific distribution in normal tissues is being attempted [2].

In this manner, a considerable number of nanomaterials have been developed recently [3–5]. Among them, polydopamine (PD), a synthetic melanin, which is a black biopolymer produced by autoxidation of dopamine, has achieved great importance [6]. Thanks to their physical and chemical properties [5], their feasible surface functionalization, and their good degradation in vivo [7,8], PD NPs stand out for the development of new diagnosis and antiproliferative nanosystems [5,9–14].

Thus, there are only a few existing works that report nanoparticle systems devoid of drugs with an antineoplastic behavior in the literature [15,16]. However, in previous studies, it was demonstrated that PD NPs can also constitute themselves an antitumour strategy [17,18]. Thereby, unlike the majority of developed therapeutic nanocarriers, their use could help to reduce the administration of drugs. In one of these previous works, it was found that PD by itself had an antiproliferative capacity after developing a novel protocol to evaluate its cytotoxicity [18]. Furthermore, it was reported that such antiproliferative capacity could be related to a ferroptosis mechanism, since PD cytotoxicity was reduced in the presence of an iron chelator (deferoxamine, DFO) or a potent antioxidant compound involved in cellular ROS-protection (glutathione, GSH) [18–20]. As with other melanins [17,21], PD presents a great binding affinity for free metallic ions, especially for Cu^{2+} and Fe^{3+} [17,22,23]. These free ions, which are more abundant in cancer cells, are stored in lysosomes and, since PD NPs end up in these organelles when they are internalized [18], their metal affinity could be related to their cytotoxicity [24–28]. Precisely because of this fact, in another previous study, the antiproliferative ability of iron-loaded PD NPs was investigated, and it was observed that such systems had a strong cytotoxicity for breast carcinoma cells [17].

On the other hand, it is well accepted for the design of therapeutic nanosystems that size may determine their endocytosis rate and, therefore, their antiproliferative activity [29–31]. Cancer endothelium is known to present leaky fenestrations between vasculature cells, and these gaps have sizes ranging from 100 to 780 nm, depending on the tumor type. As a consequence, it is generally considered that the smaller the size of the administered NPs, the higher their rate of endocytosis and their accumulation in tumor sites [30–32].

For all these reasons, the size-dependent cytotoxicity effect of PD NPs was studied in the present work. PD NPs with three different sizes (115, 200 and 420 nm) were synthetized and characterized. Their antiproliferative activity was analyzed and compared in four distinct types of human carcinomas (breast, colon, liver and lung carcinomas) and in healthy stromal cells. Moreover, it was again proven that such antiproliferative effects may be related to their metal-loading ability. To do that, their cytotoxicity was studied in co-treatment experiments of PD with either DFO (iron chelator) and GSH (antioxidant compound), conducted with all of the previous mentioned cell lines [32–34]. Finally, doxorubicin (DOX), a conventional chemotherapy drug [35,36], was adsorbed on PD NPs in a very low concentration (10.6 ng DOX/mg PD NP) with the goal of enhancing their antitumor impact while reducing the necessary DOX therapeutic doses. The antitumor effect of the resulting nanosystem over the viability of breast carcinoma cells was also studied.

2. Results

2.1. Synthesis and Characterization of 115, 200 and 420 nm PD NPs

PD NPs of different sizes were synthetized through dopamine oxidative polymerization in a basic aqueous medium [17,18,37]. It contained fixed volumes of ethanol and water and different concentrations of ammonium hydroxide, on which the size of PD NPs depends (Figure 1a). To characterize them, transmission electron microscopy (TEM) images of all PD NPs were taken and size-range histograms were obtained (Figure 1b–d). As shown, their average sizes were 75 nm, 170 nm and 340 nm. Thus, the higher the ammonium hydroxide concentration employed, the smaller the synthetized PD NPs. In trizma base solution (50 mM, pH 10), such NPs remained stable with average hydrodynamic diameters of 115 ± 50 nm (PdI = 0.047), 199 ± 50 nm (PdI = 0.085) and 417 ± 50 nm (PdI = 0.012). Such values were analyzed by dynamic light scattering (DLS) and were higher than the ones obtained by TEM because of a possible PD NPs hydration.

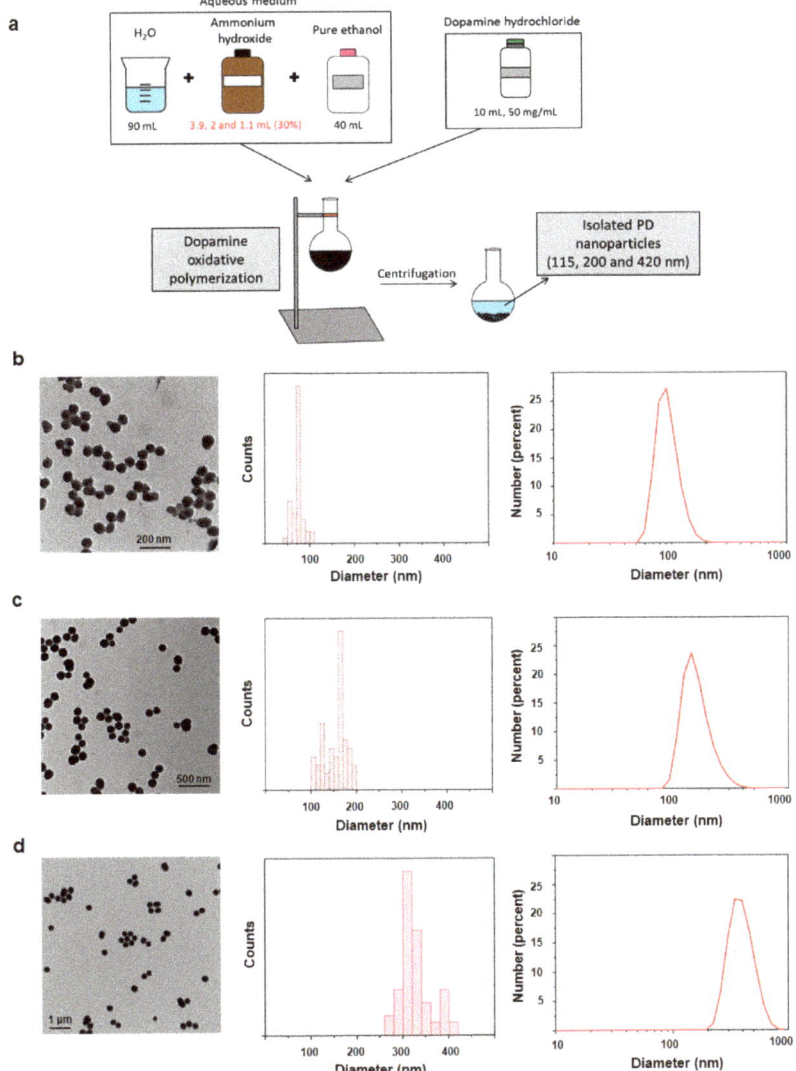

Figure 1. (**a**) Schematic representation of PD NPs synthesis by dopamine oxidative polymerization in a basic aqueous medium. (**b**–**d**) TEM images, size-range histograms and DLS number distributions of dispersions of PD NPs with three different diameters (pH = 7.0).

2.2. Cytotoxicity Effect of PD NPs Depends on Their Size

Since it was demonstrated that size of NPs plays an important role in their endocytosis rate and therapeutic effect [29–31], and that PD NPs are able to reduce the viability of cancer cells themselves [17,18], it was analyzed how the variation of PD NPs' diameter could affect to their cytotoxicity in different types of tumors. In this manner, BT474, HTC116, HEPG2 and H460 human cell lines were selected to carry out MTT assays with previously synthetized 115 and 200 nm PD NPs (Figure 2a–d and Figure S1a–d) [38]. Furthermore, such assays were also performed with a stromal human cell line, the HS5 one, in order to elucidate whether there were significant variations in the viability reduction of treated cancer and healthy cells (Figure 2e and Figure S1e). Four different concentrations of PD NPs were employed (from 0.0074 mg/mL to 0.042 mg/mL), and MTT assays were performed following a protocol which was previously developed in order to avoid the strong contribution of PD NPs absorbance to formazan salts absorbance values [18].

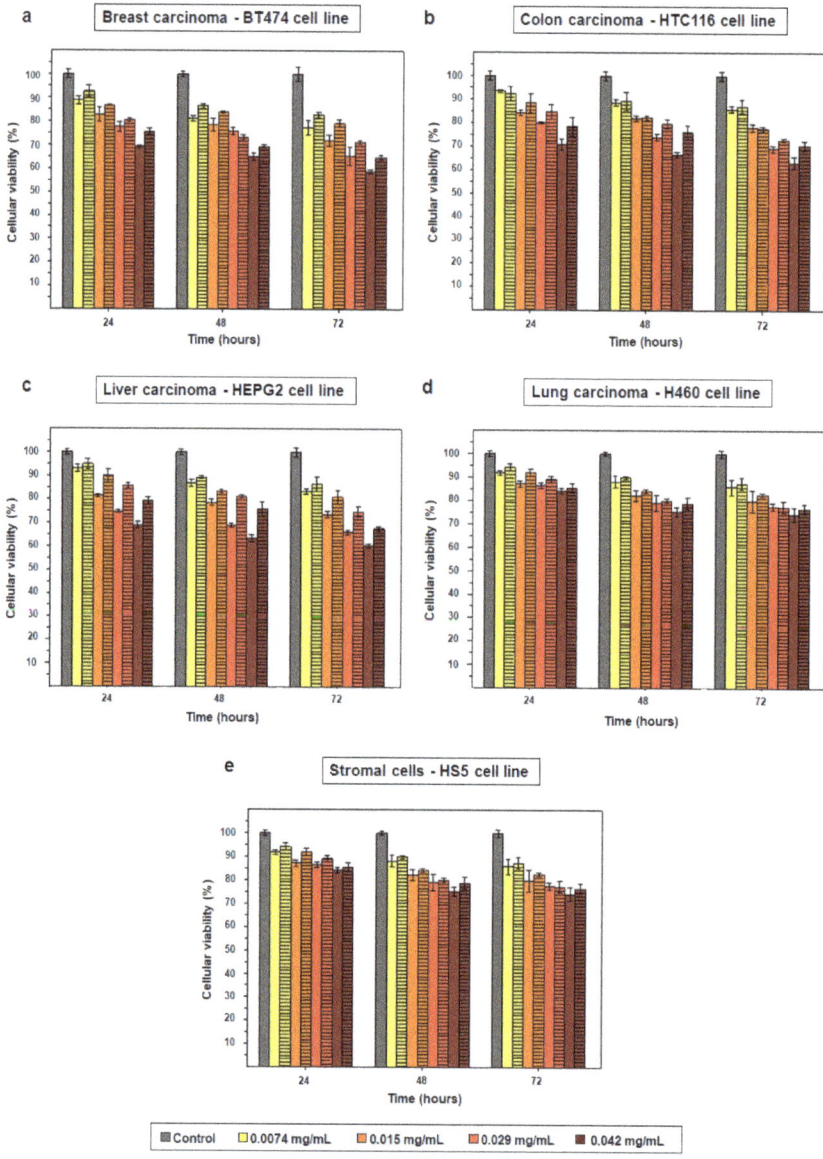

Figure 2. Obtained results in the MTT assays performed with the BT474 (**a**), HTC116 (**b**), HEPG2 (**c**), H460 (**d**) and HS5 (**e**) cell lines. Cells were treated with four different concentrations (0.0074, 0.015, 0.029 and 0.042 mg/mL) of PD NPs with a diameter of 115 nm (empty bars) and 200 nm (bars with the horizontal line pattern). The results shown are the mean ± SD of three replicates for each treatment.

As shown in Figure 2a and Figure S1a, when breast cancer cells (B7474 cell line) were treated with more elevated PD NPs concentrations, a more noticeable reduction in their viability was achieved. Thus, the best cytotoxic effect was obtained 72 h after treatment of the mentioned cells with 0.042 mg/mL of 100 nm PD NPs, which reduced their survival rate to 59%. The same concentration of 200 nm PD NPs decreased BT474 viability to 65% after 72 h.

In the case of the treatment of colon and liver carcinoma cells (HTC116 and HEPG2 cell lines) (Figure 2b,c and Figure S1b,c), it was analogously found that the best cytotoxic effect was accomplished when 0.042 mg/mL of 100 nm PD NPs were employed. With these experimental conditions, HTC116 survival rate was reduced to 63% after 72 h and HEPG2 viability, to 60%.

Likewise, a similar trend in the results obtained after the treatment of lung carcinoma cells (H460 cell line) can be observed in Figure 2d and Figure S1d. Nevertheless, the cytotoxicity of PD NPs was less remarkable than for the three previously mentioned tumor cell lines (BT474, HTC116 and HEPG2). Thereby, 72 h after the treatment with 0.042 mg/mL of 100 nm PD NPs, H460 survival rate decreased to 74%.

Positively, in the same manner, stromal cells' viability was not reduced as much as the carcinoma cell lines' viabilities when they were treated with PD NPs, neither those PD NPs with a size of 100 nm nor those with a size of 200 nm (Figure 2e and Figure S1e). Treatment with the highest concentration (0.042 mg/mL) of such NPs reduced, after 72 h, the viability of HS5 cells to 75–76%, but this value was higher than 80% 72 h after the treatment with the lowest concentrations of 100 and 200 nm PD NPs.

Therefore, in brief, it was found that the cytotoxicity of PD NPs was more noticeable, at all administered concentrations, for the HTC116, HEPG2 and, especially, for the BT474 cell line. The lowest concentration (0.0074 mg/mL) was barely toxic during the studied time for all treated cell lines. However, the two highest concentrations (0.029 and 0.042 mg/mL) achieved a notable decrease in cancer cell viability 72 h after a treatment of 35–40%, except for H460 viability, which was not so remarkably reduced. Furthermore, PD NPs did not decrease the viability of stromal cells in the same manner as the viability of cancer cells. In fact, the two lowest concentrations employed (0.0074 and 0.015 mg/mL) of PD NPs showed pretty specific results. Treatment with them almost had no affect on HS5 cellular viability, possibly because tumor cells present high intracellular iron levels [25,26]. Finally, it was generally observed that the smaller the diameter of the PD NPs, the more pronounced their cytotoxic effect. In comparison with the antiproliferative effect of the 200 nm PD NPs, those with a 115 nm diameter achieved a decrease in the viability of BT474 with a 3–8% improvement in efficacy, depending on the administered concentration. These differences in viability reduction, in the case of the HTC166, HEPG2, H460 and HS5 cells, were close to 2–9%, 3–12%, 2–5% and 1–11%, respectively, and could be explained by a larger endocytosis rate.

Next, since it was corroborated that size affected the therapeutic effect of PD NPs, MTT assays were again performed with synthetized 420 nm PD NPs [18]. For such assays, the BT474 cell line was chosen because the best previous MTT results were obtained with these breast carcinoma cells. As a result, and as shown in Figure 3, after the first 24 h of treatment, none of the concentrations employed were cytotoxic. The three lowest concentrations had virtually no effect on BT474 survival rate, and the highest one (0.042 mg/mL) only achieved a reduction in their viability to 92%. After 48 h of treatment, the cytotoxicity of the 420 nm PD NPs, in all concentrations, was neither pretty noticeable but, when 72 h had elapsed, it was more remarkable for the three highest chosen concentrations. In this manner, 0.015 mg/mL of PD NPs reduced breast cancer cells' survival to 84%, which was then decreased to 79% and 75% when 0.029 mg/mL and 0.042 mg/mL of PD NPs were employed for the treatment of BT474 cells. In any case, as expected, the cytotoxicity of 420 nm PD NPs was lower than that caused by the 115 and 200 nm PD NPs, with there being a difference of as high as 20–25% in cellular viability when the two most elevated NPs concentrations (0.029 and 0.042 mg/mL) were employed.

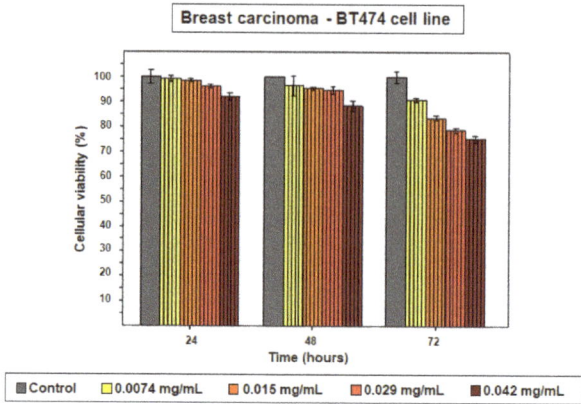

Figure 3. The results of the MTT assay carried out with PD NPs with a size of 420 nm (vertical lines—pattern bars) with BT474 cells. The same four concentrations (0.0074, 0.015, 0.029 and 0.042 mg/mL) of PD NPs as before were employed. The results shown are the mean ± SD of three replicates for each treatment.

Finally, in order to visually corroborate the cellular viability results obtained in the MTT assays, a live/dead assay with confocal laser scanning microscopy (CLSM) was performed. For this purpose, BT474 cells were again chosen and treated for 72 h with 0.042 mg/mL of 115 nm PD NPs, which were the NPs and the concentration that had previously reduced the survival of the breast carcinoma cell line the furthest. 24, 48 and 72 h after treatment, these cells were stained with calcein AM and propidium iodide (PI), and the resulting images are shown below in Figure 4 [39–41]. As can be observed, the survival rate of BT474 cells was reduced to 74% after the first 24 h of treatment and, after 48 and 72 h, 57% and 48% of the breast cancer cells remained alive, with these survival rates being similar to those that had been obtained when MTT assays were carried out previously (Figure 2a and Figure S1a). Thus, images of the live/dead assay corroborate the MTT results, wherein 115 nm PD nanoparticle cytotoxicity was more remarkable after 48 h of treatment.

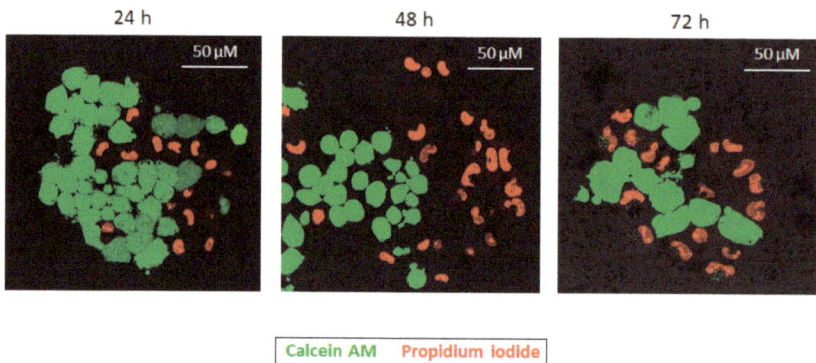

Figure 4. CMLS images taken 24, 48 and 72 h after the treatment of BT474 cells with 115 nm PD NPs (0.042 mg/mL). Calcein AM (in green, excited at 495 nm, indicator of cellular viability) and PI (in red, excited at 493 nm, indicator of cellular death) were selected to be performed in an alive/dead assay.

2.3. PD NPs Cytotoxicity in Tumor Cells Could be Related to Their Iron Affinity

PD NPs' ability to adsorb Fe^{3+} has been demonstrated in previous studies, as well as the fact that when these NPs are endocyted [17,42], they end up in cellular lysosomes. Such organelles are specifically responsible for the regulation of the concentration of free metallic cations and, as a consequence, when cells are treated with PD NPs, ROS production levels may be increased due to a possible imbalance in Fenton chemistry [18,24] (Figure 5).

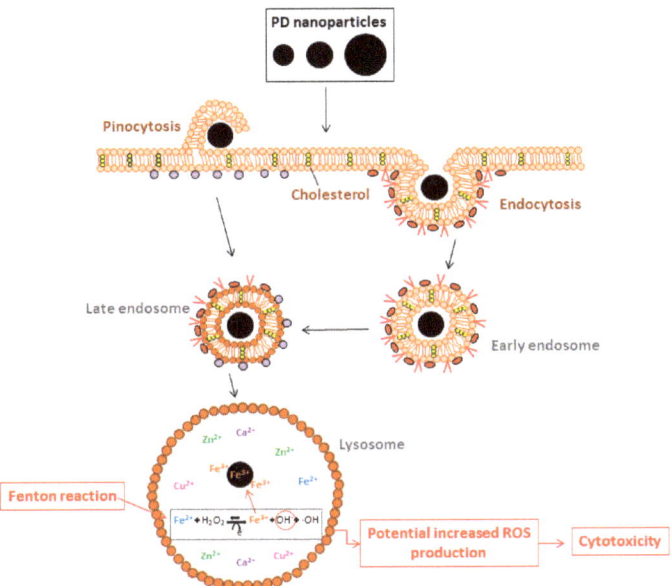

Figure 5. Schematic representation of the mechanism that could explain how PD NPs could be responsible for a reduction in cancer cells' viability after their cellular internalization in lysosomes.

For this reason, ferroptosis could be the process of cell death responsible for the cytotoxicity of PD NPs [32,34]. To demonstrate this fact, more MTT assays were performed with the same cell lines (BT474, HTC116, HEPG2, H460 and HS5) [17], treating cells with 115 and 200 nm PD NPs (0.029 mg/mL), but also with non-toxic concentrations of DFO (0.7 µM) and GSH (50 µM), an iron chelator and an antioxidant compound, respectively [19,20] (Figure 6a).

The results obtained with the BT474 and the HS5 cell lines when 115 nm PD NPs were employed are shown below (Figure 6b,c). It can be observed that, in both cell lines, the co-treatment with DFO and with GSH was able to decrease the antiproliferative effect of PD NPs at all measured times in all cell lines, with this fact becoming more noticeable after 24 h of treatment. For this reason, when BT474 cells were co-treated with DFO or GSH and with PD NPs, these last ones were around 12–18% less successful, depending on the time at which they were measured. In the case of the HS5 cell line, the cytotoxicity of PD NPs was reduced by 5–11%. This reduction could be lower because PD NPs were not as toxic for this cell line as for BT474 cells; however, despite this, with the administration of DFO and GSH, the toxicity of PD NPs was almost totally reduced for HS5 cells. Ultimately, with the other tumor cell lines (Figure S2) and with a co-treatment of DFO (0.7 µM) or GSH (50 µM) with 200 nm PD NPs (0.028 mg/mL), similar results as the ones obtained after the co-treatment of BT474 cells were also observed.

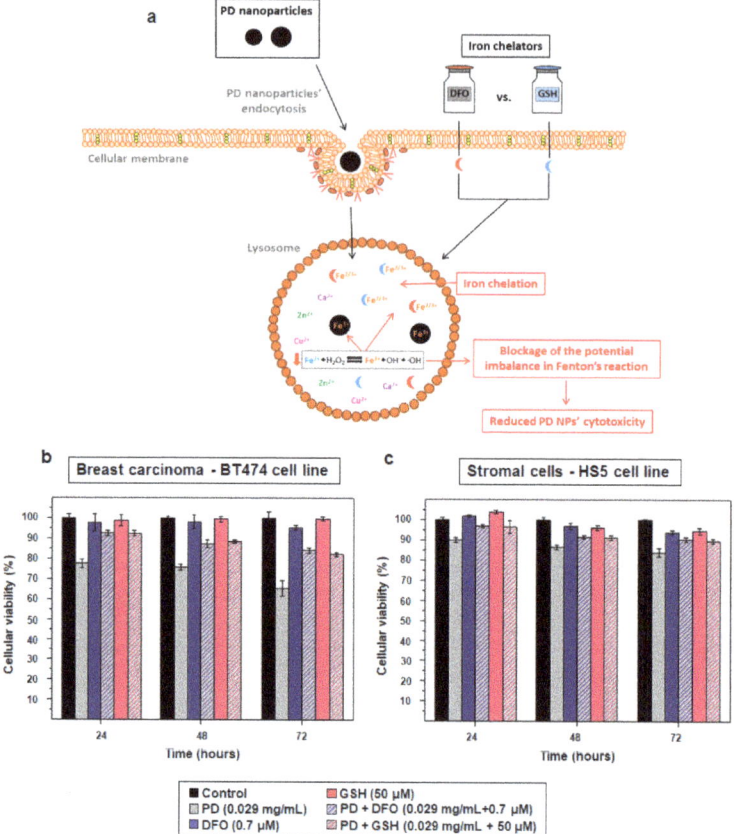

Figure 6. (**a**) Scheme that represents how DFO and GSH could be able to reduce the cellular death caused by the treatment with PD NPs. (**b**,**c**) Results of the MTT assays carried out with BT474 and HS5 cells after a co-treatment of 115 nm PD NPs (0.029 mg/mL, gray) with DFO (0.7 µM, blue) and GSH (50 µM, pink). The results shown are again the mean ± SD of three replicates of each treatment.

2.4. DOX-Adsorbed PD NPs (DOX@PD NPs) Presented a Notable Antiproliferation Activity

DOX is one of the most widely employed antineoplastic agents for the treatment of different types of cancers today, but its administration is currently limited due to the severe adverse effects that it has for patients. In this manner, many strategies are being developed to encapsulate this drug in order to improve its side toxicity [43,44]. Among these, PD-modified DOX-nanocarriers can already be found in the literature [45,46]. This issue, together with the fact that DOX is related to the formation of iron-related free radicals in cells [35,36], propitiated its selection for loading on the PD NPs synthetized here. For this purpose, 115 nm PD NPs were chosen because, as has been shown (Figure 2 and Figure S1), they present a more remarkable antiproliferative activity. In this manner, these NPs were mixed with a diluted DOX solution (10 nM), and the concentration of DOX adsorbed on PD NPs was determined by difference, by measuring the absorbance (λ = 494 nm) of the filtered supernatant once the DOX@PD NPs were isolated. As a result, it was found that the PD NPs were able to be loaded with 10.6 ng DOX/mg PD NPs.

Based on this data, three distinct concentrations of DOX@PD NPs (0.029, 0.035 and 0.045 mg/mL) were tested in BT474 cells, which were again chosen because the best MTT assay results had been achieved with this breast carcinoma cell line. Likewise, treatment with equivalent DOX concentrations

(0.5, 0.7 and 0.8 nM), which were pretty low in comparison to those employed in other works [11,44], was performed.

The results of these experiments indicated that, as shown in Figure 7, after only 24 h of treatment, DOX@PD NPs presented noticeable cytotoxicity, especially at the two highest concentrations (0.035 mg/mL + 0.7 nM and 0.042 mg/mL + 0.8 nM). While PD NPs achieved reductions in BT474 survival rate to 76%, 74% and 68%, the same concentrations of DOX@PD NPs achieved reductions of 73%, 62% and 50%, respectively. Moreover, the increase in the cytotoxicity of the two highest concentrations was more potent after 48 and 72 h of treatment. On the one hand, after 48 h had elapsed, 0.035 and 0.042 mg/mL of DOX@PD NPs decreased breast carcinoma cell viability to around 52% and 44%, while viability was approximately 72% and 64% when the same concentrations of non-loaded PD NPs were employed. On the other hand, after 72 h of treatment with the mentioned concentrations of DOX@PD NPs, BT474 viability was around 42% and 37%, while the corresponding values for similar treatment with PD NPs were 65% and 58%. In this way, at all measured times, cellular viability reduction caused by DOX@PD NPs was more remarkable than that caused by the non-loaded PD NPs, chiefly when cells were treated with 0.035 and 0.042 mg/mL of NPs. Furthermore, DOX@PD NPs were even more effective than the equivalent treatment with DOX concentrations, especially during the first 24 h. After this time, the highest concentration of free DOX only achieved a reduction in BT474 survival to 91%, and the other two presented almost no cytotoxicity. Then, 48 and 72 h after treatment, the reduction in cellular viability caused by free DOX was more noticeable but, in any case, it did not exceed that resulting from equivalent treatment with DOX@PD NPs. Such results could be explained by a likely more remarkable ferroptosis-dependent ROS production that could take place together with DOX-dependent DNA damage [35,36]. In this manner, the use of DOX@PD NPs could enhance the therapeutic activity of both PD and DOX, resulting in lower DOX doses being required for potential treatment, partially avoiding the severe adverse effects that this drug has for patients, as mentioned above [43,44].

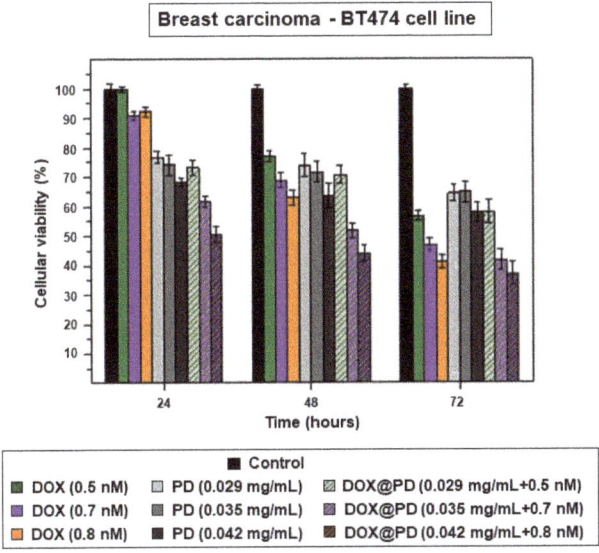

Figure 7. Results of the MTT assay carried out with the BT474 cell line, previously treated with free DOX (0.5 (green), 0.7 (purple) and 0.8 (orange) nM), 115 nm PD NPs (0.029, 0.035 and 0.042 mg/mL (grayscale)) and DOX@PD NPs (grayscale with colored patterns) in equivalent concentrations. The results shown are the mean ± SD of three replicates for each treatment.

3. Discussion

Since nanomedicine's occupation of a fundamental role in the development of novel therapeutic systems, the scientific community has been aware of the importance possessed by size in determining their effect [29–31,47]. For this reason, in the present work, the influence of size on the cytotoxicity of PD NPs, previously reported for breast and colon carcinoma cells [17,18], was studied in different tumor and stromal cell lines.

Thus, PD NPs with three different diameters (115, 200 and 420 nm) were synthetized. Once they had been characterized by TEM and DLS, the cytotoxicity of four different concentrations of the two smallest types of PD NPs (115 and 200 nm) was studied in different types (breast, colon, liver and lung) of human carcinomas and in stromal cells. Furthermore, the largest PD NPs' (420 nm) effect on cellular viability was also tested with the breast carcinoma cell line, BT474. The results obtained showed that, in all cases, the smaller the size of the NPs, the more noticeable their antiproliferative activity, with this being even more noticeable in BT474 cells. In addition, with such experiments, it could be noticed that the lowest tested concentrations of PD NPs had a tumor-selective effect. In this manner, employing low doses of these NPs could be a possible strategy for achieving greater treatment specificity and overcoming the any undesirable side effects. So far, most developed therapeutic nanosystems are vehicles for the delivery of cytotoxic drugs and, in this way, the employment of PD NPs could represent an awesome strategy for reducing the administration of chemotherapeutics [15]. Likewise, the size of PD NPs could be selected according to the antiproliferative effect that would be desired.

On the other hand, it was demonstrated that the adsorption of iron could be responsible for the cytotoxic effect of such PD NPs. Their affinity for different metallic cations has been described in numerous studies, and the ability of PD NPs to load lysosomal Fe^{3+} cations once they have been endocyted could explain the death of cells treated with them by means of Fenton chemistry [17,18,24,34]. To corroborate that this ferroptosis process could take place in the present study, more viability assays were carried out, treating cells of the different carcinomas simultaneously with PD NPs and with two iron chelators, DFO and GSH. In this manner, it was demonstrated that this co-treatment affected the cytotoxicity of PD NPs, decreasing it at all measured times and in all types of treated cells.

Finally, 115 nm PD NPs were loaded with DOX. This drug was chosen because it is one of the most commonly used chemotherapeutic drugs, and because it has also been associated with ferroptosis processes in recent toxicity-related studies [35,36]. The cytotoxicity of the resulting NPs (DOX@PD NPs') was analyzed with BT474 cells and compared with the viability values obtained with equivalent concentrations of free-DOX and non-loaded PD NPs. On the basis of this comparison, it could be seen that the antiproliferative effect of DOX@PD NPs was considerably greater. Actually, these NPs were even more effective than free DOX, possibly because of the occurrence of a synergist effect. Additionally, the DOX doses employed were much lower than those used so far in literature, and this fact could be important in avoiding the side effects, too [12,20].

4. Materials and Methods

4.1. Chemicals

Dopamine Hydrochoride, Ammonium Hydroxide (NH_4OH), Phosphate Buffered Saline (PBS, 0.01 M, pH 7.4), Dulbecco's Modified Eagle's Medium (DMEM), Fetal Bovine Serum (FBS, USA origin), Thiazolyl Blue Tetrazolium Bromide (MTT reagent), L-glutathione Reduced (GSH) and Deferoxamine Mesilate CRS (DFO) were all supplied by Sigma-Aldrich (Darmstadt, Germany). Ethanol absolute was purchased from VWR International Eurolab S.L. (Llinars del Vallés, Barcelona, Spain). Penicillin-Streptomycin (5000 U/mL), Calcein AM, Propidium Iodide (PI) ReadyProbes™ reagent and Doxorubicin Hydrochloride Solid (DOX) were obtained from Thermo Fisher Scientific (Eugene, OR, USA).

4.2. Synthesis and Characterization of PD NPs of Different Sizes

PD NPs with average diameters of 115, 200 and 420 nm were synthetized by mixing distinct volumes of NH_4OH aqueous solution (3.9, 2 and 1.1 mL, respectively, 28–30%) with ethanol (40 mL) and deionized water (90 mL). In all cases, the obtained mixture was left under magnetic stirring at room temperature for 30 min, and a dopamine hydrochloride aqueous solution (10 mL, 50 mg/mL) was later added. The reaction was allowed to react for 24 h. PD NPs were isolated and purified by several centrifugation-redispersion cycles in deionized water (35 mL). Finally, NPs were re-suspended in PBS at final concentrations of 2, 3.2 and 1 mg/mL, respectively [17,18,35].

To characterize them, TEM images (Tecnai Spirit Twin, Fei Company, Hillsboro, OR, USA) were taken, employing a voltage acceleration of 120 kV. The synthetized PD NPs were dispersed in deionized water (pH = 6.0) in a concentration of less than 0.01% (WT), and a drop of this dispersion was deposited on a copper grid with a collodium membrane and dried for 24 h. Images were recorded after this time, and histograms exhibiting the size ranges were obtained. To this end, the size of a minimum of 300 PD NPs in different images was determined (using ImageJ software, NIH, Bethesda, MD, USA) in order to build each histogram. Moreover, the hydrodynamic diameter of the PD NPs was analyzed using DLS (on the basis of their intensity–average size distribution) (Zetasizer Nano ZS90, Malvern Instruments Inc., Royston, Hertfordshire, UK) when they were re-suspended in a trizma base solution (pH = 10.0) in a concentration that was also less than 0.01% (WT).

4.3. Cell Culture

BT474, HTC116, HEPG2, H460 and HS5 cell lines were cultured with medium supplemented with FBS (10%) and antibiotics (penicillin-streptomycin) (1%) as instructed (ATCC, Wesel, Germany). All cells were cultured at 37 °C in a humidified atmosphere in the presence of CO_2 (5%).

4.4. Size-Dependent Cytotoxicity Effect of PD NPs

The antitumor activity of 115 and 200 nm PD NPs was firstly studied based on MTT assays [37]. BT474, HTC116, HEPG2, H460 and HS5 cells were seeded in 24-well plates and cultured with supplemented medium overnight. The next day, the culture medium was replaced by supplemented medium containing PBS (control) and four different concentrations (from 0.0074 mg/mL to 0.042 mg/mL) of 115 and 200 PD NPs. In addition, BT474 cells were also treated with the same concentrations of 420 nm PD NPs. In all cases, cellular survival was analyzed for 4 days (EZ Reader 2000, Biochrom, Cambridge, UK), every 24 h, following the protocol described by Nieto et al. [18]. The results shown are the mean ± SD of three replicates for each different treatment.

Secondly, the reduction of viability caused by 115 nm PD NPs was corroborated in BT474 cells by CLSM (Leica TCS SP5, Leica Microsystems, L'Hospitalet de Llobregat, Spain) with an alive/dead cellular assay [36]. The cells were seeded in crystal-bottom plates (8000 cells/mL) and cultured with supplemented medium overnight. Over the following days, the culture medium was replaced by supplemented medium containing PBS (control) and 115 nm PD NPs (0.042 mg/mL). After 24, 48 and 72 h, calcein AM (1.25 mM) and PI (1 drop/1 mL culture media) were added and, after 30 min, CLSM images were taken [37,38].

4.5. PD Iron-Affinity could Explain the Cytotoxicity of PD NPs in Tumor Cells

To demonstrate that the iron affinity of PD could be implicated in the cytotoxicity of cells treated with PD NPs, HTC116, HEPG2, H460, BT474 and HS5 cells were seeded in 24-well plates and cultured with supplemented medium overnight. After 24 h, the culture medium was replaced by supplemented medium containing PBS (control), DFO (0.7 µM), GSH (50 µM), 115 and 200 nm PD NPs (0.029 mg/mL) and PD NPs plus DFO and GSH at the same concentrations. Again, cell viability was analyzed every 24 h for 4 days, following the same protocol as before [18]. The results shown are also the mean ± SD of three replicates for each different treatment.

4.6. DOX Adsorption onto PD NPs

With the aim of adsorbing DOX onto PD NPs, an aqueous solution (1% DMSO) of the drug was prepared at a final concentration of 10 nM. PD NPs (0.75 mL, 0.035 mg/mL) with a diameter of 115 nm were mixed with DOX solution, and the mixture was kept under stirring overnight [17]. Next, DOX@PD NPs were isolated through centrifugation and re-suspended in PBS at a final concentration of 2 mg/mL. The resulting supernatant was preserved, and its DOX concentration was determined in order to quantify PD NPs DOX adsorption. To this end, the supernatant was filtered several times with 0.1 µM syringe filters (GE Healthcare Life Sciences, Buckinghamshire, UK) and its absorbance was measured at 494 nm (UV-1800 Spectrophotometer, Shimadzu Corporation, Soraku-gun, Kyoto, Japan). Finally, taking into account the absorbance value of the initial DOX solution at such wavelength, the DOX adsorption onto PD NPs was quantified.

4.7. Antiproliferative Activity of DOX@PD NPs

To study the reduction in tumor cells' viability caused by DOX@PD NPs, the BT474 cell line was chosen to carry out further MTT assays. Following the steps described above, the cells were again seeded in 24-well plates and, 24 h later, they were treated with medium supplemented with PBS (control), different concentrations of 115 nm DOX@PD NPs (0.029, 0.035 and 0.042 mg/mL) and equivalent adsorbed DOX concentrations (0.5, 0.7 and 0.8 nM). Cellular viability was measured every day for 72 h, always following the same protocol as before [18]. The results shown are again the mean ± SD of three replicates for each different treatment.

4.8. Statistical Analysis

Data related to the size of the PD NPs is the mean ± SD of three different measurements. Otherwise, results of the different MTT assays are represented as the mean ± SD of three replicates for each treatment of three different experiments, and the results were considered statistically significant where $p < 0.05$.

5. Conclusions

In this work, it has been demonstrated that size plays an important role in the cytotoxic effect of PD NPs. This was demonstrated on the basis of viability assays carried out with different human carcinoma cell lines and with stroma cells, in which the therapeutic action of two or three PD NPs of different sizes was analyzed (115, 200 and 420 nm). In all cell lines, and with all of the tested PD NP concentrations, it was shown that the smaller the diameter of the NPs, the more enhanced their antiproliferative activity. Therefore, the size of PD NPs could be tailored depending on the desired application.

With respect to the cytotoxic effect of PD NPs, it was observed that this may be related to a process of ferroptosis. PD NPs are able to load Fe^{3+} in lysosomes, and this fact could originate an abnormal cellular ROS production. However, when either an iron chelator (DFO) or a potent antioxidant (GSH) were employed, their antiproliferative ability was notably decreased. For this reason, when PD NPs were loaded with DOX, their antiproliferative effect was enhanced. Apart from triggering DNA damage, DOX cytotoxicity is also a consequence of a process of ferroptosis which, in addition to the one potentially produced by PD NPs, may result in the achievement of a synergist effect.

Supplementary Materials: The following are available online at http://www.mdpi.com/2072-6694/11/11/1679/s1. Figure S1: Data corresponding to MTT results shown in Figure 2 with the BT474 (a), HTC116 (b), HEPG2 (c), H460 (d) and HS5 (e) cell lines. Shown results are the average cellular viability percentage ± SD of three replicas for each treatment; Figure S2: Results of the MTT assays carried out with HTC116 (a), HEPG2 (b) and H460 (c) cells after a co-treatment of 115 nm PD NPs (0.029 mg/mL, blue) with DFO (0.7 µM, green) and GSH (50 µM, pink). Shown results are again the mean ± SD of three replicas for each treatment.

Author Contributions: Conceptualization, G.M. and M.A.V.; Methodology, C.N., J.E., G.M. and M.A.V; Investigation, C.N., J.E., G.M. and M.A.V.; Resources, E.M.M.d.V.; Writing—original draft preparation, C.N.; Writing—review and editing, C.N., G.M., M.A.V. and E.M.M.d.V.; Supervision, G.M., M.A.V. and E.M.M.d.V; Funding acquisition, E.M.M.d.V.

Funding: This research has been funded by the Spanish Ministry of Economy and Competitiveness (CTQ2016-78988-R) and by the Ramón Areces Foundation ("Development and validation of an aerosol with vectorized nanoparticles to human lung cancer treatment"). In addition, C.N. is recipient of a predoctoral contract from the Junta de Castilla y León, co-funded by the European Social Foundation (EDU/602/2016).

Acknowledgments: The authors would like to thank all the funding sources that have made possible this work.

Conflicts of Interest: The authors declare no conflict of interest.

References

1. Awasthi, R.; Roseblade, A.; Hansbro, P.M.; Rathbone, M.J.; Dua, K.; Bebawy, M. Nanoparticles in Cancer Treatment: Opportunities and Obstacles. *Curr. Drug Targets* **2018**, *19*, 1696–1709. [CrossRef] [PubMed]
2. Liu, J.; Cheng, Q.; Feng, L.; Liu, Z. Nanomedicine for tumor microenvironment modulation and cancer treatment enhacement. *Nano Today* **2018**, *21*, 55–73. [CrossRef]
3. Quader, S.; Kataoka, K. Nanomaterial-enabled cancer therapy. *Mol. Ther.* **2017**, *25*, 1501–1513. [CrossRef] [PubMed]
4. Liu, J.; Dong, J.; Zhang, T.; Peng, Q. Graphene-based nanomaterials and their potentials in advanced drug delivery and cancer therapy. *J. Control. Release* **2018**, *286*, 64–73. [CrossRef]
5. Wu, H.; Hu, H.; Wan, J.; Li, Y.; Wu, Y.; Tang, Y.; Xiao, C.; Xu, H.; Yang, X.; Li, Z. Hydroxyethyl starch stabilized polydopamine nanoparticles for cancer chemotherapy. *Chem. Eng. J.* **2018**, *349*, 129–145. [CrossRef]
6. Liu, H.; Qu, X.; Tan, H.; Song, J.; Lei, M.; Kim, E.; Payne, G.F.; Liu, C. Role of polydopamine's redox-activity on its pro-oxidant, radical-scavenging and antimicrobial activities. *Acta Biomater.* **2019**, *88*, 181–196. [CrossRef]
7. Liu, X.; Cao, J.; Li, H.; Li, J.; Jin, Q.; Ren, K.; Ji, J. Mussel-inspired polydopamine: A biocompatible and ultrastable coating for nanoparticles in vivo. *ACS Nano* **2013**, *7*, 9384–9395. [CrossRef]
8. Bettinger, C.J.; Bruggeman, J.P.; Misra, A.; Borestein, J.T.; Langer, R. Biocompatibility of biodegradable semiconducting melanin films for nerve tissue engineering. *Biomaterials* **2009**, *30*, 3050–3057. [CrossRef]
9. Dong, Z.; Gong, H.; Gao, M.; Zhu, W.; Sun, X.; Feng, L.; Fu, T.; Li, Y.; Liu, Z. Polydopamine nanoparticles as a versatile molecular loading platform to enable imaging-guided cancer combination therapy. *Theranostics* **2016**, *6*, 1031–1042. [CrossRef]
10. Mrowczynski, R. Polydopamine-based multifunctional (nano)materials for cancer therapy. *ACS Appl. Mater. Interfaces* **2018**, *10*, 7541–7561. [CrossRef]
11. Wang, L.; Dai, W.; Yang, M.; Wei, X.; Ma, K.; Song, B.; Jia, P.; Gong, Y.; Yang, J.; Zhao, J. Cell membrane mimetic copolymer coated polydopamine nanoparticles for combined pH-sensitive drug release and near-infrared photothermal therapeutic. *Colloids Surf. B Biointerfaces* **2019**, *176*, 1–8. [CrossRef] [PubMed]
12. Lei, Z.; Mengying, Z.; Dongdong, B.; Xiaoyu, Q.; Yifei, G.; Xiangtao, W.; Meihua, H. Alendronate-modified polydopamine-coated paclitaxel nanoparticles for osteosarcoma-targeted therapy. *J. Drug Deliv. Sci. Technol.* **2019**, in press. [CrossRef]
13. Zhang, H.; Sun, Y.; Huang, R.; Cang, H.; Cai, Z.; Sun, B. pH-sensitive prodrug conjugated polydopamine for NIR-triggered synergistic chemo-photothermal therapy. *Eur. J. Pharm. Biopharm.* **2018**, *128*, 260–271. [CrossRef] [PubMed]
14. Zhou, J.; Jiang, Y.; Hou, S.; Upputuri, P.K.; Wu, D.; Li, J.; Wang, P.; Zhen, X.; Pramanik, M.; Pu, K.; et al. Compact plasmonic blackbody for cancer theranosis in the near-infrared II window. *ACS Nano* **2018**, *12*, 2643–2651. [CrossRef]
15. Kim, S.E.; Zhang, L.; Ma, K.; Riegman, M.; Chen, F.; Ingold, I.; Conrad, M.; Turker, M.Z.; Gao, M.; Jiang, X.; et al. Ultrasmall nanoparticles induce ferroptosis in nutrient-deprived cancer cells and suppress tumour growth. *Nat. Nanotechnol.* **2016**, *11*, 977–985. [CrossRef]
16. Sarna, M.; Krzykawska-Serda, M.; Jakubowska, M.; Zadlo, A.; Urbanska, K. Melanin presence inhibits melanoma cell spread. *Sci. Rep.* **2019**, *9*, 9280–9289. [CrossRef]
17. Vega, M.A.; Nieto, C.; Marcelo, G.; Martín del Valle, E.M. Cytotoxicity of paramagnetic cations-loaded polydopamine nanoparticles. *Colloids Surf. B Biointerfaces* **2018**, *167*, 284–290. [CrossRef]

18. Nieto, C.; Vega, M.A.; Marcelo, G.; Martín del Valle, E.M. Polydopamine nanoparticles kill cancer cells. *RSC Adv.* **2018**, *8*, 36201–36208. [CrossRef]
19. Liu, P.; He, K.; Song, H.; Ma, Z.; Yin, W.; Xu, L.X. Deferoxamine-induced increase in the cellular iron levels in highly aggressive breast cancer cells leads to increased cell migration by enhancing TFN-α dependent NF-κB signaling and TGF-β signaling. *J. Inorg. Biochem.* **2016**, *160*, 40–48. [CrossRef]
20. Couto, N.; Wood, J.; Barber, J. The role of glutathione reductase and related enzymes on cellular redox homeostasis network. *Free Radic. Biol. Med.* **2016**, *95*, 27–42. [CrossRef]
21. Ball, V.; Bour, J.; Michel, M. Step-by-step deposition of synthetic dopamine-eumelanin and metal cations. *J. Colloid Interface Sci.* **2013**, *405*, 331–335. [CrossRef] [PubMed]
22. Cho, S.; Park, W.; Kim, D.H. Silica-coated metal chelting-melanin nanoparticles as a dual-modal contrast enhacement imaging and therapeutic agent. *ACS Appl. Mater. Interfaces* **2017**, *9*, 101–111. [CrossRef] [PubMed]
23. Ge, R.; Lin, M.; Li, X.; Liu, S.; Wang, W.; Li, S.; Zhang, Z.; Liu, Y.; Liu, L.; Shi, F.; et al. Cu^{2+}-loaded polydopamine nanoparticles for magnetic resonance imaging-guided pH- and near-infrared-light-stimulated thermochemotherapy. *ACS Appl. Mater. Interfaces* **2017**, *9*, 19706–19716. [CrossRef] [PubMed]
24. Kurz, T.; Eaton, J.W.; Brunk, U.T. The role of lysosomes in iron metabolism and recycling. *Int. J. Biochem. Cell. Biol.* **2011**, *43*, 1686–1697. [CrossRef] [PubMed]
25. Zhong, X.Z.; Yang, Y.; Sun, X.; Dong, X.-P. Methods for monitoring Ca^{2+} and ion channels in the lysosome. *Cell Calcium* **2017**, *64*, 20–28. [CrossRef] [PubMed]
26. Jung., M.; Mertens, C.; Tomat, E.; Brüne, B. Iron as a central player and promising target in cancer progression. *Int. J. Mol. Sci.* **2019**, *20*, 273. [CrossRef] [PubMed]
27. Manz, D.H.; Blanchette, N.L.; Paul, B.T.; Torti, F.M.; Torti, S.V. Iron and cancer: Recent insights. *Ann. N. Y. Acad. Sci.* **2016**, *1368*, 149–161. [CrossRef]
28. Liou, G.Y.; Storz, P. Reactive oxygen species in cancer. *Free Radic. Res.* **2010**, *44*, 479–496. [CrossRef]
29. Dreaden, E.C.; Austin, L.A.; Mackey, M.A.; El-Sayed, M.A. Size matters: Gold nanoparticles in targeted cancer drug delivery. *Ther. Deliv.* **2012**, *3*, 457–478. [CrossRef]
30. Gaument, M.; Vargas, A.; Gurny, R.; Delie, F. Nanoparticles for drug delivery: The need for precision in reporting particle size parameters. *Eur. J. Pharm. Biopharm.* **2008**, *69*, 1–9. [CrossRef]
31. Jo, D.H.; Kim, J.H.; Lee, T.G.; Kim, J.H. Size, surface charge and shape determine therapeutic effects of nanoparticles in brain and retinal diseases. *Nanomedicine* **2015**, *11*, 1603–1611. [CrossRef] [PubMed]
32. Mai, T.T.; Hamai, A.; Hienzsch, A.; Cañeque, T.; Müller, S.; Wicinski, J.; Cabaud, O.; Leroy, C.; David, A.; Acevedo, V.; et al. Salinomycin kills cancer stem cells by sequestering iron in lysososmes. *Nat. Chem.* **2017**, *9*, 1025–1033. [CrossRef] [PubMed]
33. Corcé, V.; Gouin, S.G.; Renaud, S.; Gaboriau, F.; Deniaud, D. Recent advances in cancer treatment by iron chelators. *Bioorg. Med. Chem. Lett.* **2016**, *26*, 251–256. [CrossRef] [PubMed]
34. Dixon, S.J.; Lemberg, K.M.; Lamprecht, M.R.; Skouta, R.; Zaitsev, E.M.; Gleason, C.E.; Patel, D.N.; Bauer, A.J.; Cantley, A.M.; Yang, W.S.; et al. Ferroptosis: An iron-dependent form of nonapoptotic cell death. *Cell* **2012**, *149*, 1060–1072. [CrossRef]
35. Zeng, X.; Cai, H.; Yang, J.; Qiu, H.; Cheng, Y.; Liu, M. Pharmacokinetics and cardiotoxicity of doxorubicin and its secondary alcohol metabolites in rats. *Biomed. Pharmacother.* **2019**, *116*, 108964. [CrossRef]
36. Koleini, N.; Nickel, B.E.; Edel, A.L.; Fandrich, R.R.; Ravandi, A.; Kardami, E. Oxidized phospholipids in doxorubicin-induced cardiotoxicity. *Chem. Biol. Interact.* **2019**, *303*, 35–39. [CrossRef]
37. Liu, Y.; Ai, K.; Liu, J.; Deng, M.; He, Y.; Lu, L. Dopamine-melanin colloidal nanospheres: An efficient near-infrared phototermal therapeutic agent for in vivo cancer therapy. *Adv. Mater.* **2013**, *25*, 1353–1359. [CrossRef]
38. Mosmann, T. Rapid colorimetric assay for cellular growth and survival: Application to proliferation and cytotoxicity assays. *J. Immunol. Methods* **1983**, *65*, 55–63. [CrossRef]
39. Boulos, L.; Prévost, M.; Barbeau, B.; Coallier, J.; Desjardins, R. LIVE/DEAD® Baclight™: Application of a new rapid staining method for direct enumeration of viable and total bacteria in drinking water. *J. Microbiol. Methods* **1999**, *34*, 77–86. [CrossRef]
40. Li, Y.; Khuu, N.; Gevorkian, A.; Sarfinsky, S.; Therien-Aubin, H.; Wang, Y.; Cho, S.; Kumacheva, E. Supramolecular nanofibrillar thermoreversible hydrogel for growth and release of cancer spheroids. *Angew. Chem. Int.* **2016**, *55*, 1–6.

41. Chung, S.; Nguyen, V.; Lin, Y.L.; Kamen, L.; Song, A. Thaw-and-use target cells pre-labeled with calcein AM for antibody-dependent cell-mediated cytotoxicity assays. *J. Immunol. Methods* **2017**, *447*, 37–46. [CrossRef] [PubMed]
42. Ding, L.; Zhu, X.; Wang, Y.; Bingyang, S.; Ling, X.; Chen, H.; Nan, W.; Barrett, A.; Guo, Z.; Tao, W.; et al. Intracellular fate of nanoparticles with polydopamine surface engineering and a novel strategy for exocytosis-inhibiting, lysosome impairment-based cancer therapy. *Nano Lett.* **2017**, *17*, 8790–8801. [CrossRef] [PubMed]
43. Ibsen, S.; Zahavy, E.; Wrasdilo, W.; Berns, M.; Chan, M.; Esener, S. A novel doxorubicin prodrug with controllable photolysis activation for cancer therapy. *Pharm. Res.* **2010**, *27*, 1848–1860. [CrossRef] [PubMed]
44. Chen, Y.; Wan, Y.; Wang, Y.; Zhang, H.; Jiao, Z. Anticancer efficacy enhancement and attenuation of side effects of doxorubicin with titanium dioxide nanoparticles. *Int. J. Nanomed.* **2011**, *6*, 2321–2326.
45. Bi, D.; Zhao, L.; Li, H.; Guo, Y.; Wang, X.; Han, M. A comparative study of polydopamine modified and conventional chemical synthesis method in DOX liposomes form the aspect of tumor targeted therapy. *Int. J. Pharm.* **2019**, *559*, 76–85. [CrossRef]
46. Ji, F.; Sun, H.; Qin, Z.; Zhang, E.; Cui, J.; Wang, J.; Li, S.; Yao, F. Engineering polyzwitterion and polydopamine decorated doxorubicin-loaded mesoporous silica nanoparticles as a pH-sensitive drug delivery. *Polymers* **2018**, *10*, 326. [CrossRef]
47. Win, K.-Y.; Feng, S.-S. Effects of particle size and surface coating on cellular uptake of polymeric nanoparticles for oral delivery of anticancer drugs. *Biomaterials* **2005**, *26*, 2713–2722. [CrossRef]

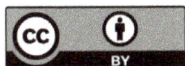

© 2019 by the authors. Licensee MDPI, Basel, Switzerland. This article is an open access article distributed under the terms and conditions of the Creative Commons Attribution (CC BY) license (http://creativecommons.org/licenses/by/4.0/).

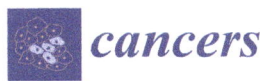

Article

Folate Receptor-Targeted Albumin Nanoparticles Based on Microfluidic Technology to Deliver Cabazitaxel

Fanchao Meng [1,†], Yating Sun [1,†], Robert J. Lee [1,2], Guiyuan Wang [1], Xiaolong Zheng [1], Huan Zhang [1], Yige Fu [3], Guojun Yan [4], Yifan Wang [5], Weiye Deng [5], Emily Parks [5], Betty Y.S. Kim [6], Zhaogang Yang [5,*], Wen Jiang [5,*] and Lesheng Teng [1,*]

1. School of Life Sciences, Jilin University, Changchun, Jilin 130012, China
2. Department of Pharmaceutics, College of Pharmacy, The Ohio State University, Columbus, OH 43210, USA
3. Department of Pharmaceutical Sciences, St. John's University, Queens, NY 11439, USA
4. School of Pharmacy, Nanjing University of Chinese Medicine, Nanjing, Jiangsu 210023, China
5. Department of Radiation Oncology, The University of Texas Southwestern Medical Center, Dallas, TX 75390, USA
6. Department of Neurosurgery, The University of Texas MD Anderson Cancer Center, Houston, TX 77030, USA
* Correspondence: zhaogang.yang@utsouthwestern.edu (Z.Y.); wen.jiang@utsouthwestern.edu (W.J.); tenglesheng@jlu.edu.cn (L.T.); Tel.: +86-431-85155320 (L.T.)
† These authors contributed equally to this work.

Received: 23 July 2019; Accepted: 6 October 2019; Published: 16 October 2019

Abstract: Microfluidic technology (MF) has improved the formulation of nanoparticles (NPs) by achieving uniform particle size distribution, controllable particle size, and consistency. Moreover, because liquid mixing can be precisely controlled in the pores of the microfluidic chip, maintaining high mixing efficiency, MF exerts higher of NP encapsulation efficiency (EE) than conventional methods. MF-NPs-cabazitaxel (CTX) particles (MF-NPs-CTX) were first prepared by encapsulating CTX according to MF. Folate (FA)- Polyethylene glycol (PEG)-NPs-CTX particles (FA-PEG-NPs-CTX) were formulated by connecting FA to MF-NPs-CTX to endow NPs with targeted delivery capability. Accordingly, the mean particle size of FA-PEG-NPs-CTX increased by approximately 25 nm, as compared with MF-NPs-CTX. Upon morphological observation of FA-PEG-NPs-CTX and MF-NPs-CTX by transmission electron microscopy (TEM), all NPs were spherical and particle size distribution was uniform. Moreover, the increased delivery efficiency of CTX in vitro and its strong tumor inhibition in vivo indicated that FA-PEG-NPs-CTX had a powerful tumor-suppressive effect both in vitro and in vivo. In vivo imaging and pharmacokinetic data confirmed that FA-PEG-NPs-CTX had good drug delivery efficiency. Taken together, FA-PEG-NPs-CTX particles prepared using MF showed high efficient and targeted drug delivery and may have a considerable driving effect on the clinical application of targeting albumin NPs.

Keywords: folate receptor; albumin nanoparticle; microfluidic; cabazitaxel

1. Introduction

After the Food and Drug Administration (FDA) approved Abraxane (Abraxis BioScience, Los Angeles, CA, USA) in 2010, albumin NPs have increasingly been attracting researchers' attention [1]. Nano-formulation delivery systems have been widely used because of their unique biocompatibility and stability [2]. Moreover, sufficient drug binding sites are contained in human serum albumin (HSA) molecules, endowing albumin NPs with a high drug-loading capacity [3–5].

Albumin NPs have been exploited to deliver various drugs, such as antineoplastic agents, gene drugs, peptide drugs, and hormone drugs [6,7]. NPs have been prepared by emulsification, desolvation, or nab-technology, but disadvantages included toxic reagent residues, complicated preparation processes, and poor repeatability between batches. Recently, excellent progress has been made in preparing NPs based on MF technology [8,9]. MF enables precise manipulation of liquid flow in the micron size range, allowing the organic and aqueous phases to be rapidly mixed to produce NPs with uniform particle size distribution, high drug encapsulation efficiency (EE), and small batch-to-batch variation.

Normally, conventional albumin NPs can only passively deliver drugs to tumor sites through the enhanced permeability and retention (EPR) effect, which severely limits their delivery efficiency. Because many malignant tumor cells express highly specific receptors such as human epidermal growth factor receptor 2 (HER2) [10], transferrin receptor (TfR) [8], and FA receptor (FR) [11], albumin NPs can be chemically modified with the corresponding ligands to provide targeted tumor delivery(Figure 1). FR is highly expressed on the surface of various tumor cells. Additionally, its ligand FA is not immunogenic and has high structural stability and a strong affinity with FR. NPs linked with FA can specifically bind to FR and enter the cytoplasm by endocytosis.

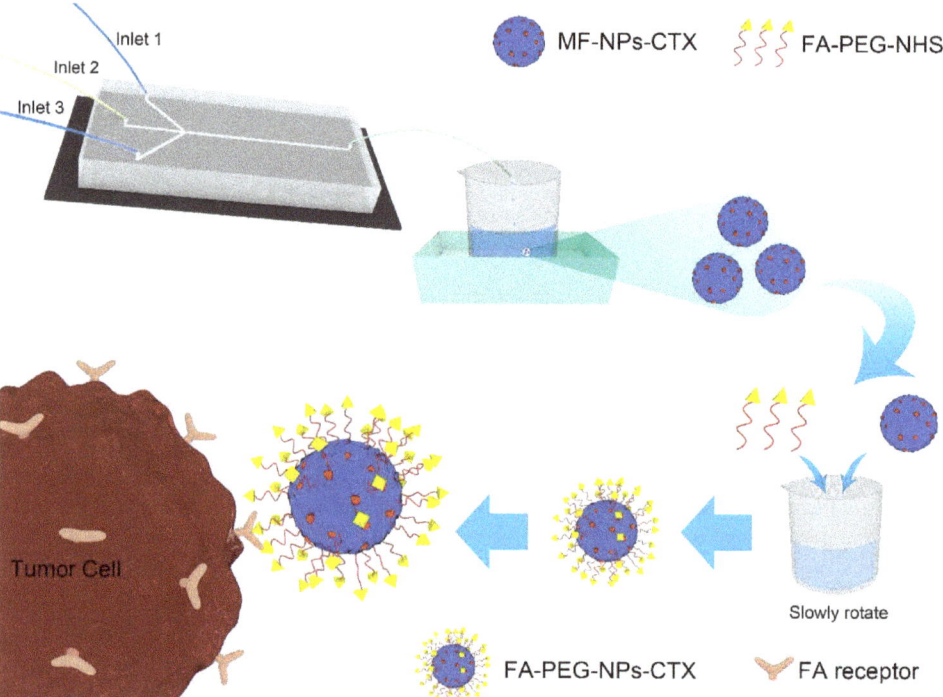

Figure 1. Preparation and function of FA-PEG-NPs-CTX. The aqueous phase was injected through the microfluidic chips at inlet 1 and inlet 3, and the organic phase was injected from inlet 2. MF-NPs-CTX were formed by high shear force mixing in the chip. Folate- Polyethylene glycol -NHS (FA-PEG-NHS) was allowed to react with -NH$_2$ of MF-NPs-CTX to form FA-PEG-NPs-CTX. FA-PEG-NPs-CTX were then taken up by tumor cells through FR-mediated endocytosis.

2. Results

2.1. Characterization

The in vitro characterization of MF-NPs-CTX, FA-PEG-NPs-CTX, and traditionally-prepared NPs (Tr-FA-PEG-NPs-CTX) is shown in Table 1: after FA-PEG attachment, the average of the NP particle size increased by about 25 nm. Because of FA-PEG's negative charge, FA-PEG-NPs-CTX's ζ-potential increased from -20.3 ± 0.5 mV to -27.8 ± 0.6 mV. During the FA-PEG-NHS - MF-NPs-CTX reaction, some CTX leaked, and the EE and drug-loading capacity (EC) of FA-PEG-NPs-CTX were both decreased. While polymer dispersity index (PDI) showed no obvious change, FA-PEG-NPs-CTX particles were still uniformly distributed.

Table 1. Characterization of FA-PEG-NPs-CTX vitro properties ($n = 3$).

Sample Name	Size (nm)	ζ-potential (mV)	PDI	EE (%)	EC (%)
MF-NPs-CTX	139.8 ± 2.6	-20.3 ± 0.5	0.093 ± 0.061	84.5 ± 1.8	15.7 ± 0.4
FA-PEG-NPs-CTX	162.4 ± 3.1	-27.8 ± 0.6	0.102 ± 0.032	81.3 ± 1.6	15.3 ± 0.3
Tr-FA-PEG-NPs-CTX	168.8 ± 8.3	-28.6 ± 0.9	0.248 ± 0.31	49.8 ± 0.6	5.2 ± 0.8

The morphology of FA-PEG-NPs-CTX (Figure 2A) was observed by transmission electron microscopy (TEM); particles were spherical and uniformly distributed. FA-PEG-NPs-CTX and FA-PEG-NHS had a unique absorption peak at 366 nm (Figure 2B). The FA content of FA-PEG-NPs-CTX was measured after trypsin treatment and found to be 9.28 µg/mg, while the connection efficiency of FA-PEG-NHS was 22.8%. The stability of MF-NPs-CTX and FA-PEG-NPs-CTX in a simulated plasma environment (37 °C, 10% of fetal bovine serum, FBS) is shown in Figure 2C. The particle size of the two NPs increased by about 20 nm within 8 h, and then stabilized. Within 48 h, the average particle size was increased by about 30 nm. These results indicate that MF-NPs-CTX and FA-PEG-NPs-CTX had good stability in serum.

To analyze the cumulative drug release, the preparations were incubated with PBS containing 0.1% Tween-80. Released CTX was measured by HPLC at fixed time points. The in vitro release results of Tween-CTX (CTX was formulated in Tween 80 and ethanol mixed solution according to JEVTANA®, 13% ethanol: Tween 80 = 4:1), MF-NPs-CTX, and FA-PEG-NPs-CTX are shown in Figure 2D. CTX was slowly released from MF-NPs-CTX and FA-PEG-NPs-CTX but not from Tween-CTX. Through the release profiles of CTX in MF-NPs-CTX and FA-PEG-NPs-CTX, FA-PEG linkage did not affect the release of FA-PEG-NPs-CTX. Both MF-NPs-CTX and FA-PEG-NPs-CTX had slow drug release behavior. After reaching the tumor site, CTX was gradually released from NPs and killed the tumor cells.

2.2. Cell Viability Assay

The cytotoxicity of FA-PEG-NPs-CTX was evaluated in both HeLa and A549 cells (Figure 3). Free CTX, MF-NPs-CTX, and FA-PEG-NPs-CTX killed cells in both dose- and time-dependent manners. Moreover, the vectors without CTX (MF-NPs and FA-PEG-NPs) were almost non-toxic to HeLa and A549 cells (Figure S1), thus, we inferred that FR could mediate its uptake by HeLa cells, FA-PEG-NPs-CTX was more cytotoxic to these cells than MF-NPs-CTX. Because of the targeted delivery of CTX by FA-PEG-NPs-CTX and higher EE, FA-PEG-NPs-CTX was more toxic for both cell types than Free CTX.

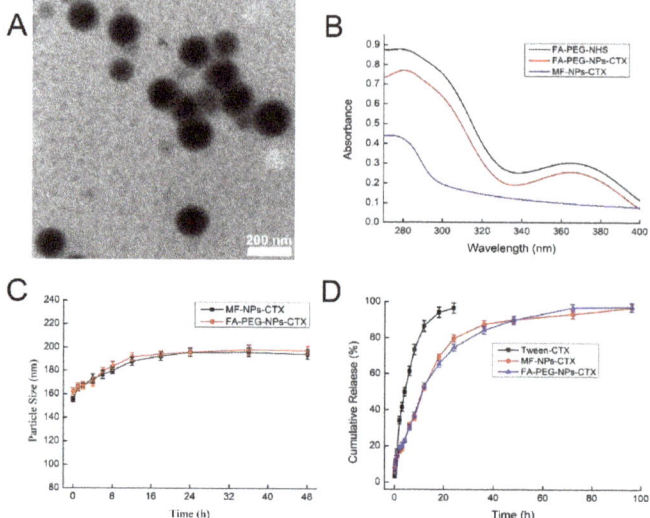

Figure 2. In vitro properties of MF-NPs-CTX and FA-PEG-NPs-CTX. (**A**) FA-PEG-NPs-CTX were observed by TEM. (**B**) The absorption curve of FA-PEG-NHS, FA-PEG-NPs-CTX, and MF-NPs-CTX determined by Ultraviolet–visible spectroscopy (UV-vis). (**C**) Stability of MF-NPs-CTX and FA-PEG-NPs-CTX in vitro. MF-NPs-CTX and FA-PEG-NPs-CTX were dissolved in 10% fetal bovine serum (FBS) ($n = 3$) and placed in a constant temperature shaker at 37 °C, 150 rpm; the particle sizes were measured by Zetasizer Nano particle size analyzer. (**D**) In vitro release of Tween-CTX, MF-NPs-CTX, and FA-PEG-NPs-CTX ($n = 3$). Release solution is 0.1% v/v Tween 80/PBS (pH 7.4).

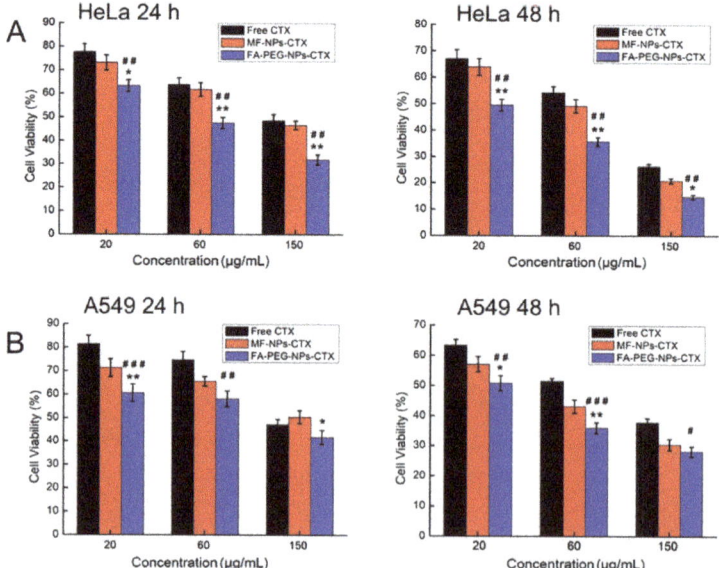

Figure 3. Evaluation FA-PEG-NPs-CTX cytotoxicity by HeLa and A549 cells ($n = 5$). (* $p < 0.05$, ** $p < 0.01$, Student's t-test, FA-PEG-NPs-CTX versus MF-NPs-CTX. ## $p < 0.01$, ### $p < 0.001$, Student's t-test, FA-PEG-NPs-CTX versus Free CTX).

2.3. Cellular Uptake Assay

Flow cytometry was used to analyze the cellular uptake of FA-PEG-NPs-CTX labeled by fluorescein isothiocyanate (FITC) (FA-PEG-FITC-NPs-CTX) (Figure 4). The uptake of FA-PEG-FITC-NPs-CTX by HeLa (Figure S2A) and A549 (Figure S2B) cells increased over 1–4 h, and the uptake of FA-PEG-FITC-NPs-CTX by HeLa was 2.73 times that of MF-FITC-NPs-CTX within 4 h (Figure 4A,B). After FA was blocked, the uptake of FA-PEG-FITC-NPs-CTX by HeLa cells was not significantly different from that of MF-FITC-NPs-CTX. To some extent, the uptake of FA-PEG-NPs-CTX by HeLa cells was enhanced by FR mediation. For A549 cells with low FR expression, the uptake of FA-PEG-FITC-NPs-CTX and MF-FITC-NPs-CTX only increased over time. At the same time point, no significant difference was observed in the uptake of A549 cells.

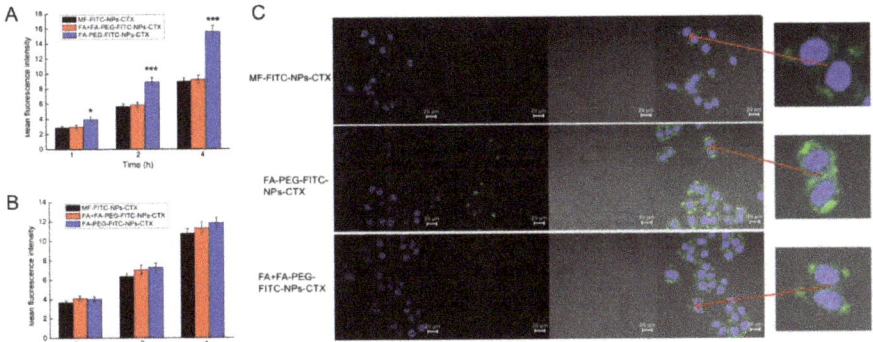

Figure 4. Detection of FA-PEG-FITC-NPs-CTX cellular uptake in vitro. Flow cytometry was used to quantitatively detect the uptake of FITC-labeled FA-PEG-NPs-CTX by HeLa (**A**) and A549 (**B**) ($n = 3$) cells, (* $p < 0.05$, *** $p < 0.001$, Student's t-test, FA-PEG-FITC-NPs-CTX versus MF-FITC-NPs-CTX). (**C**) LCSM was used to qualitatively observe the effect of FA block on the uptake of the CTX-loaded formulation by HeLa cells (×400); the rightmost side was an enlarged view of the area indicated by the arrow. The nucleus was dyed by 4′,6-diamidino-2-phenylindole (DAPI) (blue). FA-PEG-FITC-NPs-CTX and MF-FITC-NPs-CTX were labelled green.

Laser scanning confocal microscope (LCSM) was used to qualitatively observe the effect of FA block on the uptake of NPs by HeLa cells (Figure 4C). The fluorescence intensity of cells treated with FA-PEG-FITC-NPs-CTX after 4 h was significantly stronger than that those treated with MF-FITC-NPs-CTX, and no significant differences in fluorescence intensity were observed between the FA-PEG-FITC-NPs-CTX treatment group and the MF-FITC-NPs-CTX treatment group after FA block. The uptake of FA-PEG-FITC-NPs-CTX by HeLa cells was enhanced by FR mediation.

2.4. Biosafety Evaluation

The biosafety of FA-PEG-NPs-CTX was evaluated by hemolytic assay. The erythrocyte hemolysis rate results are shown in Table 2. Because of the strong hemolytic activity of the cosolvent Tween 80 in Tween-CTX, when the CTX concentration was 5.0 µg/mL in the Tween-CTX treatment group, 59.37 ± 0.88% hemolytic cells were counted, and the amount of hemolysis increased as the CTX concentration also increased. For MF-NPs-CTX and FA-PEG-NPs-CTX treatment groups, cell hemolysis rates were all less than 5.0%, in the range of 5.0–200.0 µg/mL. MF-NPs-CTX and FA-PEG-NPs-CTX showed good biosafety results and could be safely administered intravenously.

Table 2. Cell hemolysis rate results ($n = 3$).

Sample Name	5.0 µg/mL	10.0 µg/mL	25.0 µg/mL	50.0 µg/mL	100.0 µg/mL	200.0 µg/mL
MF-NPs-CTX	0.33 ± 0.07	0.46 ± 0.12	0.68 ± 0.12	2.15 ± 0.17	3.67 ± 0.28	4.37 ± 0.36
FA-PEG-NPs-CTX	0.36 ± 0.09	0.65 ± 0.13	0.73 ± 0.14	2.54 ± 0.16	3.35 ± 0.23	4.14 ± 0.45
Tween-CTX	59.37 ± 0.88	70.17 ± 0.67	78.23 ± 1.37	83.47 ± 1.42	89.95 ± 1.46	94.9 ± 1.27

2.5. In Vivo Distribution Experiment

The results of 1,1-dioctadecyl-3,3,3,3-tetramethylindotricarbocyanine iodide (DiR) content for MF-NPs-CTX-DiR, PEG-NPs-CTX-DiR, and FA-PEG-NPs-CTX-DiR after tail vein injection are shown in Figure 5. The fluorescence intensity of MF-NPs-CTX-DiR, PEG-NPs-CTX-DiR, and FA-PEG-NPs-CTX-DiR increased over time at the tumor site (Figure 5A), indicating that both particle types gradually accumulated near the tumor tissue because of the EPR effect. Moreover, FA-PEG-NPs-CTX-DiR had stronger fluorescence intensity in tumor tissues than MF-NPs-CTX-DiR and PEG-NPs-CTX-DiR. The distribution of fluorescence intensity in organ tissues and tumor tissues after euthanasia are shown in Figure 5B. The fluorescence intensity of tumor tissues in the FA-PEG-NPs-CTX-DiR treatment group was much stronger than that in the MF-NPs-CTX-DiR or PEG-NPs-CTX-DiR treatment group (Figure 5C). Furthermore, FA-PEG-NPs-CTX could be directly localized to the tumor site after targeted chemical modification.

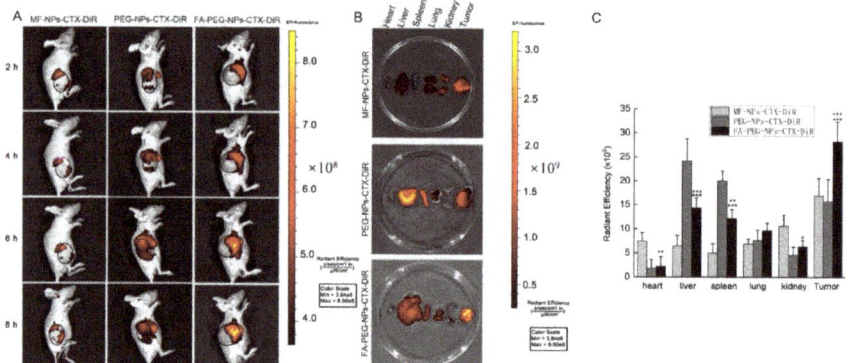

Figure 5. Biodistribution of MF-NPs-CTX-DiR, PEG-NPs-CTX-DiR, and FA-PEG-NPs-CTX-DiR. (**A**) In vivo distribution of HeLa tumor-bearing nude mice at 2, 4, 6, and 8 h after injection via the tail vein with three nanoparticle types with the same DiR content ($n = 3$). (**B**) Distribution of MF-NPs-CTX-DiR, PEG-NPs-CTX-DiR, and FA-PEG-NPs-CTX-DiR in organs and tumors of tumor-bearing nude mice after 8 h. (**C**) Ex vivo radiant fluorescence efficiency at organs and tumor tissues (* $p < 0.05$, ** $p < 0.01$, *** $p < 0.001$, Student's *t*-test, FA-PEG-NPs-CTX-DiR versus MF-NPs-CTX-DiR, ## $p < 0.01$, ### $p < 0.001$, Student's *t*-test, FA-PEG-NPs-CTX-DiR versus PEG-NPs-CTX-DiR).

2.6. In Vivo Therapeutic Efficacy of FA-PEG-NPs-CTX

Once the average tumor volume of HeLa tumor-bearing mice reached 180 mm³, the drug was injected via the tail vein. Tween-CTX, MF-NPs-CTX, and FA-PEG-NPs-CTX significantly inhibited tumor growth (*** $p < 0.001$) compared with the saline group (Figure 6). The inhibition rate of FA-PEG-NPs-CTX on tumor growth was 74.1%, which was significantly higher than that of MF-NPs-CTX (44.2%) and Tween-CTX (59.3%) (Figure 6A). Moreover, tumor weight in the FA-PEG-NPs-CTX treatment group was significantly lower than that of the MF-NPs-CTX treatment group (Figure 6C). Additionally, the average tumor volume in the FA-PEG-NPs-CTX treatment group was the smallest of all groups (Figure 6D). During the administration period, the bodyweight of the nude mice in the

FA-PEG-NPs-CTX treatment group did not change significantly, but the weight of the Tween-CTX treatment group decreased significantly (Figure 6B). Therefore, Tween-CTX was highly toxic to tumor-bearing nude mice. In general, FA-PEG-NPs-CTX had higher biosafety and also achieved better tumor inhibition. Thus, FA-PEG-NPs-CTX may be used successfully to treat tumors.

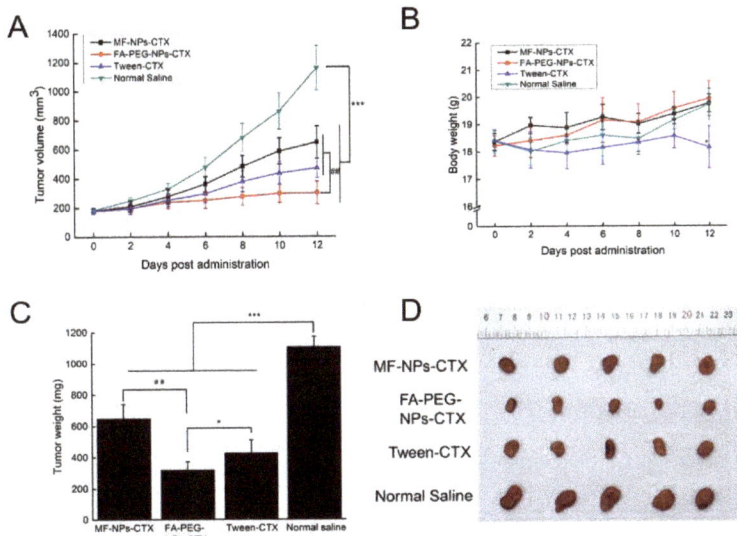

Figure 6. In vivo antitumor effect of MF-NPs-CTX, FA-PEG-NPs-CTX, and Tween-CTX. (**A**) Tumor volume change after 4 days of injection in different administration groups (*** $p < 0.001$, Student's t-test, Tween-CTX, MF-NPs-CTX and FA-PEG-NPs-CTX versus Normal saline. ## $p < 0.01$, Student's t-test, FA-PEG-NPs-CTX versus MF-NPs-CTX and Tween-CTX). (**B**) Bodyweight curves of different treatment groups ($n = 5$) (* $p < 0.05$, Student's t-test, FA-PEG-NPs-CTX versus Tween-CTX). (**C**) Tumor weight of different groups after treatment (*** $p < 0.001$, Student's t-test, Tween-CTX, MF-NPs-CTX and FA-PEG-NPs-CTX versus Normal saline. * $p < 0.05$, Student's t-test, FA-PEG-NPs-CTX versus Tween-CTX. ## $p < 0.01$, Student's t-test, FA-PEG-NPs-CTX versus Tween-CTX). (**D**) Tumor from different groups.

2.7. Pathological Analysis

After multiple administrations, the internal organs of the tumor-bearing nude mice in the Tween-CTX group were shown to be severely damaged (Figure 7): the myocardial fibers were loosely arranged, individual nuclei appeared concentrated, and large areas of hepatocyte necrosis were observed. Additionally, renal tubular epithelial cells showed a high number of eosinophils, and glomerular capillary dilatation was evident. In contrast, only partial lesions appeared in the kidneys of animals from the MF-NPs-CTX and FA-PEG-NPs-CTX treatment groups. Lesions were related to the strong renal toxicity of CTX itself. Thus, FA-PEG-NPs-CTX were shown to have good biosafety.

2.8. Plasma Pharmacokinetic Analysis

Pharmacokinetic parameters were calculated using the Winnonlin 5.3 software in a non-modal model. After intravenous injection, Tween-CTX was rapidly cleared in plasma (Table 3). Distribution (V) and clearance (CL) volumes were 4.46 times (*** $p < 0.001$) and 4.27 times (*** $p < 0.001$) greater than those of FA-PEG-NPs-CTX, respectively. At the same time, the area under the curve (AUC) of FA-PEG-NPs-CTX was 4.46 times greater than that of Tween-CTX (*** $p < 0.001$). Thus, FA-PEG-NPs-CTX significantly increased the blood concentration of CTX after administration. From the curve of CTX blood concentration over time (Figure 8), FA-PEG-NPs-CTX exhibited the best pharmacokinetic properties after administration of the three-drug preparations via the tail vein.

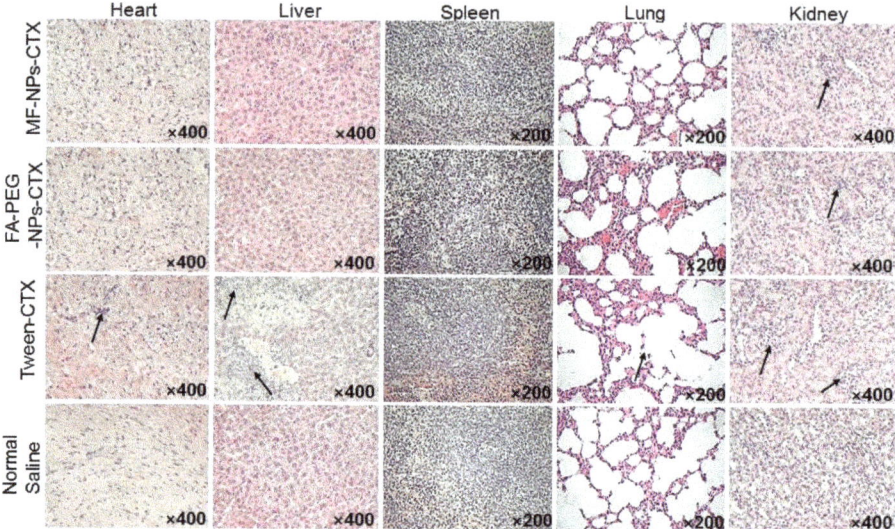

Figure 7. Pathological section analysis of heart, liver, spleen, lung, and kidney by H & E staining after MF-NPs-CTX, FA-PEG-NPs-CTX and Tween-CTX treatment. The arrows indicated the site of the damaged organ.

Table 3. Pharmacokinetic parameters of CTX after intravenous injection of different drugs ($n = 5$).

Parameters	Tween-CTX	MF-NPs-CTX	FA-PEG-NPs-CTX
C_{max} (ng/mL)	3426.00 ± 476.52	4573.33 ± 537.41	6618.38 ± 783.66
AUC (ng/mL/h)	1419.07 ± 120.61	4688.60 ± 489.83 ###	6329.06 ± 776.64 ***
V (mL)	1990.87 ± 179.36	635.39 ± 137.45 ###	446.03 ± 80.51 ***
CL (mL/h)	832.72 ± 131.41	254.13 ± 35.83 ###	194.96 ± 38.47 ***

(*** $p < 0.001$, Student's t-test, FA-PEG-NPs-CTX versus Tween-CTX. ### $p < 0.001$, Student's t-test, MF-NPs-CTX versus Tween-CTX).

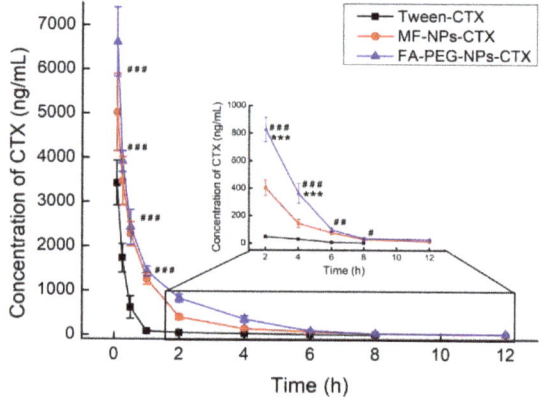

Figure 8. Pharmacokinetic curves of blood concentration of CTX for different drug administration groups ($n = 5$), *** $p < 0.001$, Student's t-test, FA-PEG-NPs-CTX versus MF-NPs-CTX. # $p < 0.05$, ## $p < 0.01$, ### $p < 0.001$, Student's t-test, FA-PEG-NPs-CTX versus Tween-CTX).

2.9. Pharmacokinetic Analysis of Drug Distribution in Various Tissues and Organs

After Tween-CTX, MF-NPs-CTX, and FA-PEG-NPs-CTX were injected into HeLa tumor-bearing nude mice via the tail vein, CTX distribution was determined in various organs and tumors (Figure 9). After intravenous injection, Tween-CTX was mainly found in the liver, lung, and kidney, while MF-NPs-CTX and FA-PEG-NPs-CTX accumulated in relatively smaller amounts in the liver and lung. In the tumor tissue, as shown in Figure S3, the CTX content of FA-PEG-NPs-CTX in the tumor site gradually increased within 0.5–6 h and reached a higher concentration at 8 h. The tumor site AUC of FA-PEG-NPs-CTX was 3.43 times greater than that of Tween-CTX and 1.75 times greater than that of MF-NPs-CTX. FA-PEG-NPs-CTX exhibited significant tumor-targeted aggregation ability.

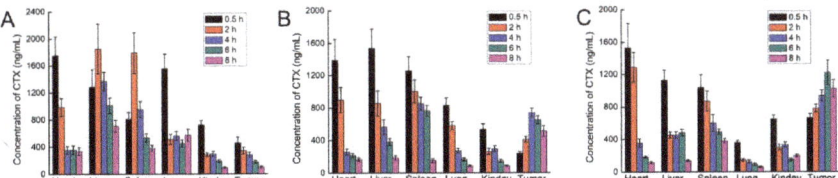

Figure 9. Pharmacokinetic analysis of tissue distribution of CTX at 0.5, 2, 4, 6, 8 h after Tween-CTX (**A**), MF-NPs-CTX (**B**), and FA-PEG-NPs-CTX (**C**) were injected into HeLa tumor-bearing nude mice via the tail vein ($n = 3$).

3. Discussion

Chemotherapy is one of the major strategies used to clinically manage malignant tumors [12–14]. As a second-generation taxane, CTX can prevent cell proliferation by binding to tubulin, and because of its low affinity with P-glycoprotein, it can overcome malignant tumor resistance [15,16]. Although CTX has good application prospects for treating malignant tumors, its inability to selectively kill cells leads to severe side effects in patients. Low solubility and side effects of cosolvents also limit the application of CTX. Albumin NPs have certain tumor-targeting properties that can improve in vivo drug distribution and reduce drug toxicity. Although NPs have good biosafety and biocompatibility levels [17–19], those prepared by conventional methods present disadvantages such as large batch-to-batch variation, wide particle size distribution, and lack of tumor targeting, which limit their clinical application [20,21]. To solve these problems, we applied microfluidic technology (MF) to encapsulate CTX into NPs [22]. Then, we attached FA-PEG to the NPs as a targeting ligand. FA-PEG had a characteristic absorption at 366 nm, while MF-NPs-CTX did not absorb at this wavelength. Results of the UV-vis absorption comparison and folate content analysis of FA-PEG-NPs-CTX (FA content was 9.28 µg/mg) both indicated that FA-PEG was attached to MF-NPs-CTX. Moreover, because of increased mixing efficiency and shearing force of the organic phase and the aqueous phase in the microfluidic chip, the EE of the prepared nanoparticles was 80% higher than that of the control, and the drug loading was 15% higher. Therefore, the same amount of nanoparticles was swallowed by the cells, and the dose of drugs that enter the cells will be higher, indicating the potential to increase the efficiency of drug entry into cells. The particle size distribution of the NPs was uniform and the PDI < 0.1. Currently, the yield of nanoparticles produced by our MF chip in one batch was around 40%, which is lower than the traditional emulsion method. However, according to our previous studies, MF can significantly improve the uniformity of the nanoparticles. The improved size distribution may further increase drug efficiency. Moreover, to increase the yield by MF, the multi-channel microfluidic chip is being investigated in our lab.

Results of in vitro stability experiments showed that the particle size of MF-NPs-CTX and FA-PEG-NPs-CTX increased by about 30 nm in plasma within 16 h, mainly because of adsorption in plasma of proteins such as opsonin and low-density lipoprotein [23]. However, after 16 h, the particle size tended to stabilize: first, because albumin is part of plasma and is stable in plasma; second, after the drug adsorbed on the nanoparticle's surface was released, the nanoparticles became more stable [24]. This result could be confirmed by conducting stability experiments. Therefore, we speculate that the NPs were still stable after injection into the bloodstream and could be safely administered through the tail vein.

Results of erythrocyte hemolysis tests showed that when CTX concentration was 5–200 µg/mL, the erythrocyte hemolysis rate of MF-NPs-CTX and FA-PEG-NPs-CTX treatments was still less than 5%, which is in line with the standards. Encapsulation of CTX in the nanoparticles removes the strong hemolysis properties of Tween 80 and improves drug safety[25]. This result confirmed that MF-NPs-CTX and FA-PEG-NPs-CTX had good biosafety levels. The results of in vitro cytotoxicity experiments showed that FA-PEG-NPs-CTX was significantly more cytotoxic to HeLa cells than MF-NPs-CTX at the same CTX concentration. Moreover, cellular uptake experiments by flow cytometry and LCSM showed that the cellular uptake of FA-PEG-NPs-CTX by HeLa and A549 cells were time-dependent. FA blocking profiles indicated that the uptake of FA-PEG-NPs-CTX by HeLa cells was significantly reduced by FA blockage, with no significant difference with the uptake of MF-NPs-CTX. FA blocking had no significant effect on the uptake of A549 cells with low FR expression. Cellular uptake experiments showed that cell-mediated uptake of FA-PEG-NPs-CTX could be enhanced by FR. Combined with cytotoxicity experiments, we concluded that FR mediates endocytosis of more nanoparticles to enhance drug toxicity to cells, possibly leading to more effective treatment in vivo.

Evaluation of the antitumor profile showed that FA-PEG-NPs-CTX have strong tumor-suppressive effects on HeLa-tumor mice with high FR expression. FA-PEG-NPs-CTX's inhibition rate on tumor growth was 74.1%, which was significantly higher than that of both MF-NPs-CTX (44.2%) and Tween-CTX (59.3%) groups. This was consistent with HeLa cells' enhanced cellular uptake results. After completing the entire administration course, the weight of mice in the FA-PEG-NPs-CTX and MF-NPs-CTX groups showed little change, while in the Tween-CTX group, the body weight decreased significantly after treatment, showing strong biotoxicity. This was also reflected in the histopathological analysis. FA-PEG-NPs-CTX and MF-NPs-CTX showed targeting effects. Additionally, their aggregation amount in normal tissues and organs was less than that of Tween-CTX, thus, toxicity to normal cells was low. Pharmacokinetic experiments further explored in vivo distribution. Tumor inhibition results showed that nanoparticles were more suitable for treating tumors than Tween-CTX. Additionally, FA-PEG-NPs-CTX had better therapeutic effects than MF-NPs-CTX.

After intravenous injection, the distribution of CTX in vivo was qualitatively and quantitatively examined by imaging and pharmacokinetic experiments, respectively. For in vivo imaging, because the situation of nanoparticles in the body is more complicated, in order to clarify the targeting effect of FA-NPs-CTX-DiR via FR in vivo, the PEG-NPs-CTX-DiR group was added. In vivo imaging showed that MF-NPs-CTX-DiR, PEG-NPs-CTX-DiR, and FA-PEG-NPs-CTX-DiR gradually accumulated at the tumor site after tail vein injection, but FA-PEG-NPs-CTX-DiR showed better accumulation than MF-NPs-CTX-DiR and PEG-NPs-CTX-DiR; thus, we believe this was likely due to the active targeting of FA to the FA-receptor [26]. After 4 h, mice were euthanized to collect the heart, liver, spleen, lung, kidney, and tumors. The fluorescence of FA-PEG-NPs-CTX-DiR at the tumor site was stronger than that of NPs-CTX-DiR, which also indicated that the active targeting of FA to the FA-receptor. Fluorescence also occurred in normal organs because of inevitable reticuloendothelial system (RES) action and renal excretion. Pharmacokinetic experiments were used to quantitatively investigate the distribution of different formulations of CTX in plasma and tissues to explore the reasons why the two nano-formulations were more effective than Tween-CTX. From the CTX plasma pharmacokinetic profile, we could see that its concentration in the FA-PEG-NPs-CTX and MF-NPs-CTX groups decreased less than that of Tween-CTX. The nano-formulations exhibited a slow release of CTX as well as a protective effect on the encapsulated drug. Combined with the distribution of CTX in tissues, we hypothesized two possible reasons for this difference. First, Tween-CTX was rapidly cleared by RES after intravenous injection. In contrast, albumin nano-formulations could only be partially removed by RES because of good biocompatibility and low immunogenicity. Second, during drug absorption, the apparent distribution volume of Tween-CTX was large and was absorbed by whole-body organ tissues; thus, the CTX concentration decreased rapidly at the same time. When CTX was loaded into NPs, the apparent distribution volume was small and the tissue clearance rate was reduced. As such, more NPs were accumulated into the tumor site by the EPR effect. Compared with MF-NPs-CTX, FA-PEG-NPs-CTX had FR targeting, and the modification of PEG prolonged its blood circulation time. This further increased the aggregation of CTX at the tumor site, and thus allowed FA-PEG-NPs-CTX to achieve a better tumor-suppressive effect. We also evaluated the PEGylation effect on the cellular uptake of this ligand-target nanoparticle in vitro. Interestingly, no statistical differences were observed by MTT in either Hela cells (48.7 ± 5.3% versus 46.8 ± 8.3%, MF-NPs-CTX versus MF-PEG-NPs-CTX, 48 h) or A549 cells (44.6 ± 4.6% versus 46.1 ± 7.0%, MF-NPs-CTX versus MF-PEG-NPs-CTX, 48 h) treated with MF-NPs-CTX or MF-PEG-NPs-CTX. The MF-PEG-NPs-CTX was prepared according to the method described in the FA-PEG-NPs-CTX part, with the FA-PEG-NHS replaced with PEG-NHS. This was consistent with our previous finding that FA can significantly improve the targeting effect of the nanoparticles [27]. It is generally believed that PEGylation can significantly increase the nanoparticle systemic circulation time by avoiding rapid clearance by reticuloendothelial system. However, recent studies also indicated that PEGylation may have no direct effect or even inhibit the cellular uptake of ligand-target nanoparticles [28]. Further investigation may shed light on the precise molecular mechanisms involved in the PEGylation effect on cellular uptake of ligand-target nanoparticles.

4. Materials and Methods

4.1. Materials and Animals

FA-PEG-NHS and MeO-PEG-NHS were purchased from Shanghai Ziqi Biotechnology Co. Ltd (Shanghai, China). CTX was purchased from Jiangsu Taxus Biotechnology Co. Ltd (Jiangsu, China). Carbamazepine was provided by Yuanye Biotechnology Shanghai Co. Ltd (Shanghai, China). Human serum albumin (HSA) was obtained from Octapharma (Vienna, Austria). The microfluidic chip was designed independently and customized at the Dalian Institute of Chemical Physics, Chinese Academy of Sciences (Dalian, China). Dulbecco's Modified Eagle's Medium (DMEM), fetal bovine serum (FBS), and penicillin-streptomycin were obtained from Gibco (Gaisburg, MD, USA). Fluorescein isothiocyanate (FITC), 4′,6-diamidino-2-phenylindole (DAPI) and acetonitrile were purchased from Sigma. 1,1-dioctadecyl-3,3,3,3-tetramethylindotricarbocyanine iodide (DiR iodide) was purchased from Thermo Fisher Scientific (Eugene, OR, USA). Tween-CTX was formulated in Tween 80 and ethanol mixed solution according to JEVTANA® (Eugene, OR, USA). The rest of the chemical reagents were of analytical or chromatographic purity.

Cervical cancer (HeLa) and lung cancer (A549) cells were obtained from ATCC and cultured in DMEM medium containing 10% FBS, 100 μg/mL streptomycin, and 100 mg IU/mL penicillin. The cells were cultured at 37 °C in a humidified incubator in 5% CO_2.

Six to eight weeks old female BALB/c nude mice were purchased from Beijing Vital River Laboratory Animal Technology Co, Ltd. (Beijing, China). Female SD rats (200 g) were purchased from Liaoning Changsheng Biotechnology Co. Ltd. (Benxi, China). All animal procedures were performed in accordance with the Guidelines on Humane Treatment of Laboratory Animals and procedures for the care and use of laboratory animals. All animal experiments were approved by the Institutional Animal Ethics Committee (Jilin University) (number 201810023).

4.2. Preparation of FA-PEG-NPs-CTX

According to previous research, the inverted W-type microfluidic chip was designed independently[9], MF-NPs-CTX were prepared by the microfluidic chip. Specifically, a 20.0 mg/mL CTX ethanol solution and a 12.5% sodium chloride solution were prepared and incubated in a 40 °C water bath with HSA (200 mg/mL). Deionized water was placed in a 60 °C water bath and heated to a constant temperature.

1.0 mL and 10.0 mL syringes were each attached to a microinjection pump: the 1.0 mL syringe was connected to inlet 2 of the microfluidic chip and the 10.0 mL syringes was connected to inlets 1 and 3. The entire microfluidics chip line was cleaned with deionized water before preparing the NPs. Then, 20.0 mg/mL CTX solution, 12.5% NaCl solution, and HSA were mixed at a volume ratio of 2:1:1 and placed in the 1.0 mL syringe, at a flow rate of 40.0 μL/min. Moreover, deionized water was placed in the 10.0 mL syringe at 60 °C with a flow rate of 600.0 μL/min. After mixing in the channel of the inverted W-type passive microfluidics chip, MF-NPs-CTX were obtained from the chip by connecting the tube and rapidly cooling in an ice water bath. MF-NPs-CTX were concentrated through a hollow fiber ultrafiltration column with a molecular weight cut off of 50 kD.

Concentrated MF-NPs-CTX was chemically modified with FA-PEG-NHS, and FA-PEG was attached to the MF-NPs-CTX via an amide bond. The bond was formed by dissolving 50.0 mg of FA-PEG-NHS in 2.0 mL of 2.0 M pH 10.0 Na_2CO_3/$NaHCO_3$ buffer solution, and slowly adding it dropwise to MF-NPs-CTX, which was also dissolved in 2.0 M pH 10.0 Na_2CO_3/$NaHCO_3$ buffer solution. The reaction was stirred at room temperature for 2 h. Then, the reacted NP solution was placed in an ultrafiltration centrifuge tube with a molecular weight cut off of 50 kDa and centrifuged at 3214× g for 10 min. The solution was repeatedly washed with deionized water to remove unreacted FA-PEG-NHS, concentrated by centrifugation to obtain FA-PEG-NPs-CTX, lyophilized, and set aside.

4.3. Characterization

Lyophilized MF-NPs-CTX and FA-PEG-NPs-CTX were re-dissolved with deionized water, and the particle size and ζ-potential were measured by a laser particle size analyzer. EE and EC of MF-NPs-CTX and FA-PEG-NPs-CTX were determined by high-performance liquid chromatography (HPLC) and calculated by the equation below. The morphology of MF-NPs-CTX and FA-PEG-NPs-CTX were observed by TEM (JEOL JEM 2100, Tokyo, Japan). To achieve this, MF-NPs-CTX and FA-PEG-NPs-CTX were dissolved and diluted with deionized water, then added dropwise to a copper mesh, dried, and observed by TEM. To assess the stability of FA-PEG-NPs-CTX in plasma after intravenous injection, the stability of FA-PEG-NPs-CTX was evaluated in a simulated plasma environment. FA-PEG-NPs-CTX were dissolved in 10% FBS and then placed in a constant temperature shaker at 37 °C, 150 rpm. A certain amount of sample was taken out at regular intervals to measure particle size by Zetasizer Nano particle size analyzer (Zetasazer Nano ZS90, Malvern, UK) [29].

$$EE = \frac{\text{weight of CTX in NPs}}{\text{weight of CTX in NPs} + \text{weight of CTX in the filtrate}} \times 100\%, \quad (1)$$

$$EC = \frac{\text{weight of CTX in NPs}}{\text{weight of NPs}} \times 100\%. \quad (2)$$

To evaluate the in vitro release of the formulation, MF-NPs-CTX and FA-PEG-NPs-CTX with a CTX content of 5.0 mg were accurately weighed (m) and dissolved in 2.0 mL of saline. The NPs were then transferred to dialysis bags with a molecular weight cut off of 8000–10,000 Da. In the meantime, 5.0 mg CTX was accurately weighed, dissolved in 2.0 mL of mixed solvent (13% ethanol: Tween 80 = 4:1), transferred to a dialysis bag, and placed in 80 mL of PBS release solution (V_0) that contained 0.1% Tween 80 [30]. The solution and the dialysis bag were set to rotate at 200 rpm, 37 °C. At a specific time point, 1.0 mL of each solution (V) was taken to determine CTX concentration (C_i) by HPLC, and 1.0 mL of fresh release solution was added. The cumulative release rate ($Q\%$) was calculated by the equation below:

$$Q(\%) = \frac{V_0 \times C_i + V \times \sum_{i=1}^{i-1} C_{i-1}}{m \times EE} \times 100\%. \quad (3)$$

4.4. Cellular Uptake Assay

The cellular uptake of FA-PEG-NPs-CTX by HeLa and A549 cells was analyzed by laser confocal microscopy. HSA was first labeled with FITC and then dissolved in 25.0 mM $Na_2CO_3/NaHCO_3$ buffer solution at pH = 9.8 with a concentration of 5.0 mg/mL. FITC was added to the HSA solution with a concentration of 0.1 mg/mL. The solution was incubated overnight at room temperature with constant stirring, and the mixed solution was passed through an ultrafiltration centrifuge tube with a molecular weight cut off of 50 kDa. The solution was centrifuged at $12857\times g$ for 10 min, and the concentrate was washed several times with $Na_2CO_3/NaHCO_3$ buffer solution to obtain FITC-labeled HSA. FA-PEG-FITC-NPs-CTX was prepared by labeled HSA with the same procedure used for FA-PEG-NPs-CTX.

In the FA blockage experiment, cells from the FA-blocked group were cultured in complete medium with an FA content of 5.0 mg/mL one week earlier. HeLa, FA-blocked HeLa, and A549 cells in the logarithmic growth phase were planted at a density of 1.0×10^5 cells/dish and cultured for 24 h. Then, the same FA-PEG-FITC-NPs-CTX protein content was added to each well. After incubating for 1, 2, and 4 h, the medium was removed and washed with cold PBS. Cells were fixed with 4% paraformaldehyde for 15 min. Nuclei were stained with 400.0 µL 1.0 µg/mL DAPI for 10 min, washed, and covered with cold PBS. The difference in fluorescence intensity after uptake of nanoparticles by cells was determined by LCSM.

Flow cytometry was used to analyze the uptake of FA-PEG-NPs-CTX by HeLa and A549 cells. First, both cell types were added at a cell density of 1.0×10^5 cells/well in a 12-well plate. Cells in the FA-blocked group were cultured in complete medium with an FA content of 5.0 mg/mL one week in advance. After the two cell lines were cultured in a 12-well plate for 24 h, the same protein contents of FA-PEG-FITC-NPs-CTX and MF-FITC-NPs-CTX were added to each well. At 1, 2, and 4 h, the cell culture medium was aspirated and cells were washed with PBS. Two hundred microliters of trypsin were then added to each well to digest the cells, and the medium was neutralized and centrifuged at $82\times g$ for 5 min. Cells were fixed with 500.0 µL of 4% paraformaldehyde, untreated cells were used as a control, and fluorescence intensity was measured by flow cytometry [31].

4.5. Analysis of Surface Folate Content

FA-PEG-NHS was dissolved in a 2.0 M pH = 10.0 $Na_2CO_3/NaHCO_3$ buffer solution, then diluted to 200.0, 100.0, 50.0, 20.0, 10.0, 5.0, and 2.0 µg/mL. UV-vis (scanning wavelength: 366 nm) was used to determine the absorbance of different FA-PEG-NHS concentrations. The standard curve was drawn by taking concentration X (µg/mL) of FA-PEG-NHS as the abscissa and absorbance Y as the ordinate. Lyophilized FA-PEG-NPs-CTX (10.0 mg) was dissolved in phosphate buffer solution at pH = 7.4. Then, a certain amount of trypsin was added and digested for 4 h, and the absorbance was measured by UV-vis at 366 nm. MF-NPs-CTX with the same protein content was dissolved in phosphate buffer, and the same procedure was conducted and used as a matrix to perform zero calibration of the absorbance.

4.6. Cell Viability Assay

Cells in the logarithmic growth phase were added at a density of 5000–8000 cells/well to 96-well plates. After 24 h, FA-PEG-NPs-CTX, MF-NPs-CTX, and free CTX with CTX concentrations of 20.0, 60.0, and 150.0 µg/mL were added. After 24 h and 48 h, respectively, 10.0 µL of 5.0 mg/mL MTT [3-(4,5-dimethylthiazol-2-yl)-2,5-diphenyltetrazolium bromide] reagent were added to each well and incubated for 4 h. Then, the medium was removed and 100 µL of DMSO was added to dissolve the formazan crystals. Absorbance at 490 nm was read on a microplate reader, and the half-maximal inhibitory concentration (IC50) was calculated by SPASS 17.0 software analysis (SPASS, Chicago, IL, USA) [32].

4.7. Hemolytic Evaluation

The biosafety of FA-PEG-NPs-CTX was evaluated via the hemolysis test. Tween-CTX, FA-PEG-NPs-CTX, and MF-NPs-CTX with CTX concentrations of 5.0, 10.0, 20.0, 50.0, 100.0, and 200.0 µg/mL were added to 1.0 mL of 2% mouse erythrocytes in 1.5 mL EP tubes and incubated for 2 h. The saline-treated group and the 1.0% Triton X-100-treated group served as negative and positive controls, respectively. After incubation, the EP tubes were centrifuged at 43× g for 5 min, and 100.0 µL of the supernatant were taken to a 96-well plate. The absorbance was measured at 540 nm using a microplate reader. The hemolysis rate was calculated according to the following equation:

$$\text{Hemolysis Rate} = \frac{\text{Absorbance} - \text{Negative Group}}{\text{Positive Group} - \text{Negative Group}} \times 100\%. \tag{4}$$

4.8. In Vivo Distribution Experiment

The in vivo distribution of the nano-formulations was examined by in vivo imaging experiments. MF-NPs-CTX-DiR and FA-PEG-NPs-CTX-DiR were prepared by encapsulating DiR and CTX following the same protocol as that used for MF-NPs-CTX and FA-PEG-NPs-CTX. The preparation method of PEG-NPs-CTX-DiR was the same as that of FA-PEG-NPs-CTX-DiR, except that FA-PEG-NHS was replaced by MeO-PEG-NHS, MF-NPs-CTX-DiR, PEG-NPs-CTX-DiR, and FA-PEG-NPs-CTX-DiR with the same DiR content were injected into nude mice through the tail vein. The nude mice were anesthetized with pentobarbital sodium at 1, 2, 4, and 8 h, and fluorescence distribution was observed using an IVIS in vivo imaging system. The excitation wavelength was 745 nm and the emission wavelength was 820 nm. After 8 h, the nude mice were euthanized to evaluate fluorescence intensity in the heart, liver, spleen, lung, kidney, and tumor tissues.

4.9. In Vivo Therapeutic Efficacy of FA-PEG-NPs-CTX

The anti-tumor effect of FA-PEG-NPs-CTX was evaluated using a HeLa tumor-bearing nude mouse model. About 5.0×10^6 HeLa cells were injected subcutaneously into the lower right side of each nude mouse. When the average tumor volume reached 100–200 mm^3, the nude mice were randomly divided into 4 groups ($n = 5$) for Tween-CTX, MF-NPs-CTX, FA-PEG-NPs-CTX, and saline treatment. On days 0, 4, and 8, the nude mice were injected with a CTX dose of 2.0 mg/kg via the tail vein. The body weight of the mice in each group and the length and width of the tumors were measured every 2 days. On day 12, five mice from each group were euthanized to harvest heart, liver, spleen, lung, kidney, and tumor tissues.

4.10. Pathological Section Analysis

Heart, liver, spleen, lung, and kidney obtained in "4.9" were fixed with 4% paraformaldehyde and analyzed by H & E staining to determine whether the drug preparation had damaged the internal organs of the nude mice[33].

4.11. Plasma Pharmacokinetic Analysis

Pharmacokinetic studies were performed by using SD rats of about 300 g that were randomly divided into 3 groups ($n = 5$). Tween-CTX, MF-NPs-CTX, and FA-PEG-NPs-CTX were injected into the tail veins at a dose of 5.0 mg/kg. At 0.083, 0.25, 0.5, 1, 2, 4, 6, 8, and 12 h after administration, about 500 µL of blood were taken from the orbital venous plexus, placed in a previously prepared EP tube treated with heparin sodium, and centrifuged at around 13,000× g for 5 min. The supernatant was taken to obtain plasma. The plasma sample was measured by UPLC-MS/MS, and the peak area was input into the standard curve of the CTX plasma sample to calculate the CTX concentration in the plasma sample. The curve was obtained by taking time X (h) after administration as the abscissa and plasma concentration Y (ng/mL) of CTX as the ordinate. Pharmacokinetic parameters were calculated by using the Winnonlin 5.3 software (CERTARA, Princeton, NJ, USA) in a non-modal model.

4.12. Pharmacokinetic Analysis of Drug Distribution in Various Tissues and Organs

Pharmacokinetics were analyzed to investigate drug accumulation in various tissues and organs of HeLa tumor-bearing nude mice after tail vein injection. Forty-five HeLa tumor-bearing nude mice were randomly divided into three groups of 15 rats each. Tween-CTX, MF-NPs-CTX, and FA-PEG-NPs-CTX were injected through the tail vein at a dose of 2.0 mg/kg. Three nude mice were euthanized from each group at 0.5, 2, 4, 6, and 8 h to harvest heart, liver, spleen, lung, kidney, and tumor tissues. Organs and tumor tissues were weighed and homogenized by adding two times the weight of saline. Tissue homogenates were sampled by UPLC-MS/MS by the established CTX tissue content analysis method.

4.13. Statistic and Analysis

Data analysis was performed using the SPSS 17.0 software (SPASS, Chicago, IL, USA), and all chart data were expressed as mean ± standard error (Mean ± SD). Significance was calculated by Student's *t*-test. When * $p < 0.05$ or # $p < 0.05$, a statistical difference between the two groups of data was noted. When ** $p < 0.01$ or ## $p < 0.01$, a significant difference between the two groups of data was noted. When *** $p < 0.001$ or ### $p < 0.01$, a highly significant difference between the two sets of data was noted.

5. Conclusions

Albumin NPs were prepared in a self-assembled manner based on MF technology (MF-NPs-CTX), and, accordingly, the inverted W-type microfluidic chip was designed independently. Our results indicated that FA-PEG-NPs-CTX had a significantly stronger tumor-suppressive effect with high FR expression both in vitro and in vivo. The modification of FA-PEG not only enhances NP tumor-targeting but also prolongs blood circulation time to some extent. We believe that targeted NPs prepared by MF technology have broad application prospects in clinically treating patients with cancer.

Supplementary Materials: The following are available online at http://www.mdpi.com/2072-6694/11/10/1571/s1, Figure S1: Cytotoxicity study with vector (MF-NPs and FA-PEG-NPs), Figure S2: LCSM was used to qualitatively detect the uptake of FA-PEG-FITC-NPs-CTX by HeLa (A) and A549 (B) cells at 1, 2, and 4 h, Figure S3: Distribution of CTX in tumor tissues after tail vein injection of Tween-CTX, MF-NPs-CTX, and FA-PEG-NPs-CTX ($n = 3$).

Author Contributions: Conceptualization, B.Y.S.K.; Z.Y., W.J., and L.T.; methodology, F.M., Y.S., G.W., G.Y., and X.Z.; formal analysis, W.D.; investigation, F.M., H.Z., and X.Z.; writing—original draft preparation, F.M., E.P., and Y.F.; writing—review and editing, R.J.L., Y.W., Z.Y., W.J., and L.T.

Funding: This work was partially supported by the National Natural Science Foundation of China for L.T. (No. 81502999).

Acknowledgments: The authors thank Damiana Chiavolini for editing the manuscript.

Conflicts of Interest: The authors declare no conflict of interest.

References

1. Miele, E.; Spinelli, G.P.; Miele, E.; Tomao, F.; Tomao, S. Albumin-bound formulation of paclitaxel (Abraxane ABI-007) in the treatment of breast cancer. *Int. J. Nanomed.* **2009**, *4*, 99–105.
2. Yang, Z.; Ma, Y.; Zhao, H.; Yuan, Y.; Kim, B. Nanotechnology platforms for cancer immunotherapy. *Wiley Interdiscip. Rev. Nanomed. Nanobiotechnol.* **2019**, *11*, e1530. [CrossRef]
3. Gradishar, W.J. Albumin-bound paclitaxel: A next-generation taxane. *Expert Opin. Pharmacother.* **2006**, *7*, 1041–1053. [CrossRef] [PubMed]
4. Von Storp, B.; Engel, A.; Boeker, A.; Ploeger, M.; Langer, K. Albumin nanoparticles with predictable size by desolvation procedure. *J. Microencapsul.* **2012**, *29*, 138–146. [CrossRef]
5. Satya Prakash, S. Human serum albumin nanoparticles as an efficient noscapine drug delivery system for potential use in breast cancer: Preparation and in vitro analysis. *Int. J. Nanomed.* **2010**, *5*, 525–532. [CrossRef]

6. Elzoghby, A.O.; Samy, W.M.; Elgindy, N.A. Albumin-based nanoparticles as potential controlled release drug delivery systems. *J. Control. Release* **2012**, *157*, 168–182. [CrossRef]
7. Lomis, N.; Westfall, S.; Farahdel, L.; Malhotra, M.; Shum-Tim, D.; Prakash, S. Human Serum Albumin Nanoparticles for Use in Cancer Drug Delivery: Process Optimization and In Vitro Characterization. *Nanomaterials* **2016**, *6*, 116. [CrossRef]
8. Yang, Z.; Yu, B.; Zhu, J.; Huang, X.; Xie, J.; Xu, S.; Yang, X.; Wang, X.; Yung, B.C.; Lee, L.J.; et al. A microfluidic method to synthesize transferrin-lipid nanoparticles loaded with siRNA LOR-1284 for therapy of acute myeloid leukemia. *Nanoscale* **2014**, *6*, 9742. [CrossRef]
9. Li, Y.; Lee, R.J.; Huang, X.; Li, Y.; Lv, B.; Wang, T.; Qi, Y.; Hao, F.; Lu, J.; Meng, Q.; et al. Single-step microfluidic synthesis of transferrin-conjugated lipid nanoparticles for siRNA delivery. *Nanomedicine* **2017**, *13*, 371–381. [CrossRef]
10. Iqbal, N.; Iqbal, N. Human Epidermal Growth Factor Receptor 2 (HER2) in Cancers: Overexpression and Therapeutic Implications. *Biochem. Mol. Biol. Int.* **2014**, *2014*, 1–9. [CrossRef]
11. Zwicke, G.L.; Ali Mansoori, G.; Jeffery, C.J. Utilizing the folate receptor for active targeting of cancer nanotherapeutics. *Nano Rev.* **2012**, *3*, 18496. [CrossRef] [PubMed]
12. Zhou, C.; Yang, Z.; Teng, L. Nanomedicine based on nucleic acids: Pharmacokinetic and pharmacodynamic perspectives. *Curr. Pharm. Biotechnol.* **2014**, *15*, 829–838. [CrossRef] [PubMed]
13. Kang, C.; Sun, Y.; Zhu, J.; Li, W.; Zhang, A.; Kuang, T.; Xie, J.; Yang, Z. Delivery of Nanoparticles for Treatment of Brain Tumor. *Curr. Drug Metab.* **2016**, *17*, 745–754. [CrossRef] [PubMed]
14. Chen, Y.; Liu, X.; Yuan, H.; Yang, Z.; von Roemeling, C.A.; Qie, Y.; Zhao, H.; Wang, Y.; Jiang, W.; Kim, B.Y.S. Therapeutic Remodeling of the Tumor Microenvironment Enhances Nanoparticle Delivery. *Adv. Sci.* **2019**, *6*, 1802070. [CrossRef]
15. Azarenko, O.; Smiyun, G.; Mah, J.; Wilson, L.; Jordan, M.A. Antiproliferative mechanism of action of the novel taxane cabazitaxel as compared with the parent compound docetaxel in MCF7 breast cancer cells. *Mol. Cancer Ther.* **2014**, *13*, 2092–2103. [CrossRef]
16. Paller, C.J.; Antonarakis, E.S. Cabazitaxel: A novel second-line treatment for metastatic castration-resistant prostate cancer. *Drug Des. Devel. Ther.* **2011**, *5*, 117–124. [CrossRef]
17. Xie, J.; Yang, Z.; Zhou, C.; Zhu, J.; Lee, R.J.; Teng, L. Nanotechnology for the delivery of phytochemicals in cancer therapy. *Biotechnol. Adv.* **2016**, *34*, 343–353. [CrossRef]
18. Sun, J.; Kormakov, S.; Liu, Y.; Huang, Y.; Wu, D.; Yang, Z. Recent Progress in Metal-Based Nanoparticles Mediated Photodynamic Therapy. *Molecules* **2018**, *23*, 1704. [CrossRef]
19. Hao, F.; Li, Y.; Zhu, J.; Sun, J.; Marshall, B.; Lee, R.J.; Teng, L.; Yang, Z.; Xie, J. Polyethylenimine-based Formulations for Delivery of Oligonucleotides. *Curr. Med. Chem.* **2019**, *26*, 2264–2284. [CrossRef]
20. Chen, Z.; Zhang, A.; Yang, Z.; Wang, X.; Chang, L.; Chen, Z.; James Lee, L. Application of DODMA and Derivatives in Cationic Nanocarriers for Gene Delivery. *Curr. Org. Chem.* **2016**, *20*, 1813–1819. [CrossRef]
21. Chen, Z.; Chen, Z.; Zhang, A.; Hu, J.; Wang, X.; Yang, Z. Electrospun nanofibers for cancer diagnosis and therapy. *Biomater. Sci.* **2016**, *4*, 922–932. [CrossRef] [PubMed]
22. Jahn, A.; Vreeland, W.N.; DeVoe, D.L.; Locascio, L.E.; Gaitan, M. Microfluidic directed formation of liposomes of controlled size. *Langmuir* **2007**, *23*, 6289–6293. [CrossRef] [PubMed]
23. Ho, Y.T.; Azman, N.A.; Loh, F.W.Y.; Ong, G.K.T.; Engudar, G.; Kriz, S.A.; Kah, J.C.Y. Protein Corona Formed from Different Blood Plasma Proteins Affects the Colloidal Stability of Nanoparticles Differently. *Bioconjugate Chem.* **2018**, *29*, 3923–3934. [CrossRef] [PubMed]
24. Sun, Q.H.; Zhou, Z.X.; Qiu, N.S.; Shen, Y.Q. Rational Design of Cancer Nanomedicine: Nanoproperty Integration and Synchronization. *Adv. Mater.* **2017**, *29*, 18. [CrossRef]
25. Qu, N.; Lee, R.J.; Sun, Y.T.; Cai, G.S.; Wang, J.Y.; Wang, M.Q.; Lu, J.H.; Meng, Q.F.; Teng, L.R.; Wang, D.; et al. Cabazitaxel-loaded human serum albumin nanoparticles as a therapeutic agent against prostate cancer. *Int. J. Nanomed.* **2016**, *11*, 3451–3459. [CrossRef]
26. Tong, L.X.; Chen, W.; Wu, J.; Li, H.X. Folic acid-coupled nano-paclitaxel liposome reverses drug resistance in SKOV3/TAX ovarian cancer cells. *AntiCancer Drugs* **2014**, *25*, 244–254. [CrossRef]
27. Zhao, J.; Zhao, M.; Yu, C.; Zhang, X.; Liu, J.; Cheng, X.; Lee, R.J.; Sun, F.; Teng, L.; Li, Y. Multifunctional folate receptor-targeting and pH-responsive nanocarriers loaded with methotrexate for treatment of rheumatoid arthritis. *Int. J. Nanomed.* **2017**, *12*, 6735–6746. [CrossRef]

28. Estelrich, J.; Busquets, M.A.; del Carmen Morán, M. Effect of PEGylation on Ligand-Targeted Magnetoliposomes: A Missed Goal. *ACS Omega* **2017**, *2*, 6544–6555. [CrossRef]
29. Favela-Camacho, S.E.; Perez-Robles, J.F.; Garcia-Casillas, P.E.; Godinez-Garcia, A. Stability of magnetite nanoparticles with different coatings in a simulated blood plasma. *J. Nanopart. Res.* **2016**, *18*, 9. [CrossRef]
30. Zhu, Z.S.; Li, Y.; Li, X.L.; Li, R.T.; Jia, Z.J.; Liu, B.R.; Guo, W.H.; Wu, W.; Jiang, X.Q. Paclitaxel-loaded poly(N-vinylpyrrolidone)-b-poly(epsilon-caprolactone) nanoparticles: Preparation and antitumor activity in vivo. *J. Control. Release* **2010**, *142*, 438–446. [CrossRef]
31. Yang, Z.; Xie, J.; Zhu, J.; Kang, C.; Chiang, C.; Wang, X.; Wang, X.; Kuang, T.; Chen, F.; Chen, Z.; et al. Functional exosome-mimic for delivery of siRNA to cancer: In vitro and in vivo evaluation. *J. Control. Release* **2016**, *243*, 160–171. [CrossRef] [PubMed]
32. Xie, J.; Teng, L.; Yang, Z.; Zhou, C.; Liu, Y.; Yung, B.C.; Lee, R.J. A polyethylenimine-linoleic acid conjugate for antisense oligonucleotide delivery. *Biomed Res. Int.* **2013**, *2013*, 710502. [CrossRef] [PubMed]
33. Yang, Z.; Wang, L.; Yu, H.; Wang, R.; Gou, Y.; Zhang, M.; Kang, C.; Liu, T.; Lan, Y.; Wang, X.; et al. Membrane TLR9 Positive Neutrophil Mediated MPLA Protects Against Fatal Bacterial Sepsis. *Theranostics* **2019**, *9*, 6269–6283. [CrossRef] [PubMed]

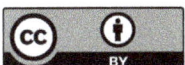

© 2019 by the authors. Licensee MDPI, Basel, Switzerland. This article is an open access article distributed under the terms and conditions of the Creative Commons Attribution (CC BY) license (http://creativecommons.org/licenses/by/4.0/).

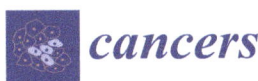

Article

Cocktail Strategy Based on NK Cell-Derived Exosomes and Their Biomimetic Nanoparticles for Dual Tumor Therapy

Guosheng Wang [†], Weilei Hu [†], Haiqiong Chen, Xin Shou, Tingting Ye and Yibing Xu *

Institute of Translational Medicine, Zhejiang University School of Medicine, Hangzhou 310029, China; 21518460@zju.edu.cn (G.W.); weileihu@zju.edu.cn (W.H.); 182594@zju.edu.cn (H.C.); shouxin@zju.edu.cn (X.S.); tingtingye@zju.edu.cn (T.Y.)
* Correspondence: yibingxu@zju.edu.cn
† These authors contributed equally to this work.

Received: 19 September 2019; Accepted: 9 October 2019; Published: 14 October 2019

Abstract: Successful cancer therapy requires drugs being precisely delivered to tumors. Nanosized drugs have attracted considerable recent attention, but their toxicity and high immunogenicity are important obstacles hampering their clinical translation. Here we report a novel "cocktail therapy" strategy based on excess natural killer cell-derived exosomes (NKEXOs) in combination with their biomimetic core–shell nanoparticles (NNs) for tumor-targeted therapy. The NNs were self- assembled with a dendrimer core loading therapeutic miRNA and a hydrophilic NKEXOs shell. Their successful fabrication was confirmed by transmission electron microscopy (TEM) and confocal laser scanning microscopy (CLSM). The resulting NN/NKEXO cocktail showed highly efficient targeting and therapeutic miRNA delivery to neuroblastoma cells in vivo, as demonstrated by two-photon excited scanning fluorescence imaging (TPEFI) and with an IVIS Spectrum in vivo imaging system (IVIS), leading to dual inhibition of tumor growth. With unique biocompatibility, we propose this NN/NKEXO cocktail as a new avenue for tumor therapy, with potential prospects for clinical applications.

Keywords: antitumor strategy; biomimetic core–shell nanoparticles; NK cell-derived exosomes; drug delivery system

1. Introduction

Targeted drug delivery systems for cancer therapy have attracted considerable recent attention owing to their high delivery efficiency along with minimal side effects [1–3]. Polymers are of great significance in targeted drug delivery as nanocarriers for biomacromolecular agents. Among them, polyamidoamine (PAMAM), the first reported and commercialized dendrimers, are hyperbranched polymers with a globular structure, which efficiently transfer nucleic acids (DNA, siRNA, miRNA, etc.) to various cell types and are safer than other cationic polymers [4–6]. PAMAM dendrimers have a distinctive structural feature with positively charged amino groups present at internal cavities, which can interact with negatively charged nucleic acids to form dendriplexes [7,8]. In order to improve their biocompatibility and targeting ability, many strategies have been taken to modify the PAMAM surface, including peptide conjugation, carbohydrate conjugation, acetylation and PEGylation [9].

More recently, biomembrane camouflage strategies have been investigated in cancer therapy. This strategy refers to nanocarriers coated with natural biomembrane components, making them highly versatile in cargo encapsulation and surface functionalization. Many types of membranes have been used to fabricate membrane-camouflaged nanoparticles, including membranes from red blood cells, platelets, white blood cells, cancer cells and bacteria [10–15]. Meanwhile, incorporation of membrane proteins within the bilayer of biomimetic nanovesicles using a microfluidic-based platform offers a one-step solution to endow nanoparticles with multiple biological feature such as evading the mononuclear phagocytic system, crossing the biological barriers or targeting inflamed tissues [16–18]. However, without exception, fabrication of core–shell nanoparticles has required extraction of plasma membrane materials by cell lysis and membrane purification, a process that greatly increases the risk of contamination and destruction of functional surface proteins. Therefore, it is of paramount importance for their clinical application to obtain functional off-the-shelf and highly biocompatible materials and establish an efficient and handy synthetic process [19].

Natural killer (NK) cells, known to play a critical role in tumor immunology [20,21] secret exosomes expressing killer proteins, including FASL and perforin, cytotoxic to multiple tumors [22–25]. Previous studies have also demonstrated that natural killer cell-derived exosomes (NKEXOs) have tumor-specific accumulation with no cytotoxic activity against normal tissues [22,23]. Meanwhile, acidic tumor microenvironment facilitates the accumulation of this nanoparticles [26]. Hence, NKEXOs can perform a dual function: They can facilitate tumor targeting and act as direct antitumor agent. More importantly, NK cell-based therapies can act as a renewable product in an allogeneic setting and be given to patients without causing graft-versus-host disease [27]. For these advantages, we ask whether intact NKEXOs could be used directly as camouflage material to greatly simplify synthetic steps and avoid contamination of immunogenic substances due to the destruction progress of membrane extraction.

2. Results

2.1. Characterization and Function of Isolated NKEXOs

To prepare the nanoparticle (NN)/NKEXO cocktail, we expanded the NK cells to a 94% purity level by co-culturing peripheral blood mononuclear cells with artificial antigen-presenting cells (aAPC) as previously reported (Figure 1a) [25,28]. Then, NKEXOs were isolated and purified from the culture supernatants of NK cells by differential centrifugation [29]. Their size was further measured by dynamic light scattering, showing a mean particle diameter of 100 nm (Figure 1b). In the purified extracts, typical exosome structures were observed by transmission electron microscopy TEM (Figure 1c). Western blot (WB) analysis indicated that NKEXOs contain typical exosomal proteins (Alix, TSG101 and CD63), together with the absence of cytochrome C (Figure 1d). These data are consistent with those previously reported for typical exosomes [30]. To verify their cytotoxicity towards tumor cells, MDA-MB-231-luc and CHLA-255-luc cells were incubated with NKEXOs for 24 h. As reported previously [22–25], cell viability decreased in both tumor cell lines in a dose-dependent manner (Figure 1e). Internalization of PKH26-labeled NKEXOs into tumor cells was also observed with confocal laser scanning microscopy (CLSM) with a rotating 3D rendering of z-stack images (Figure S1; Video S1).

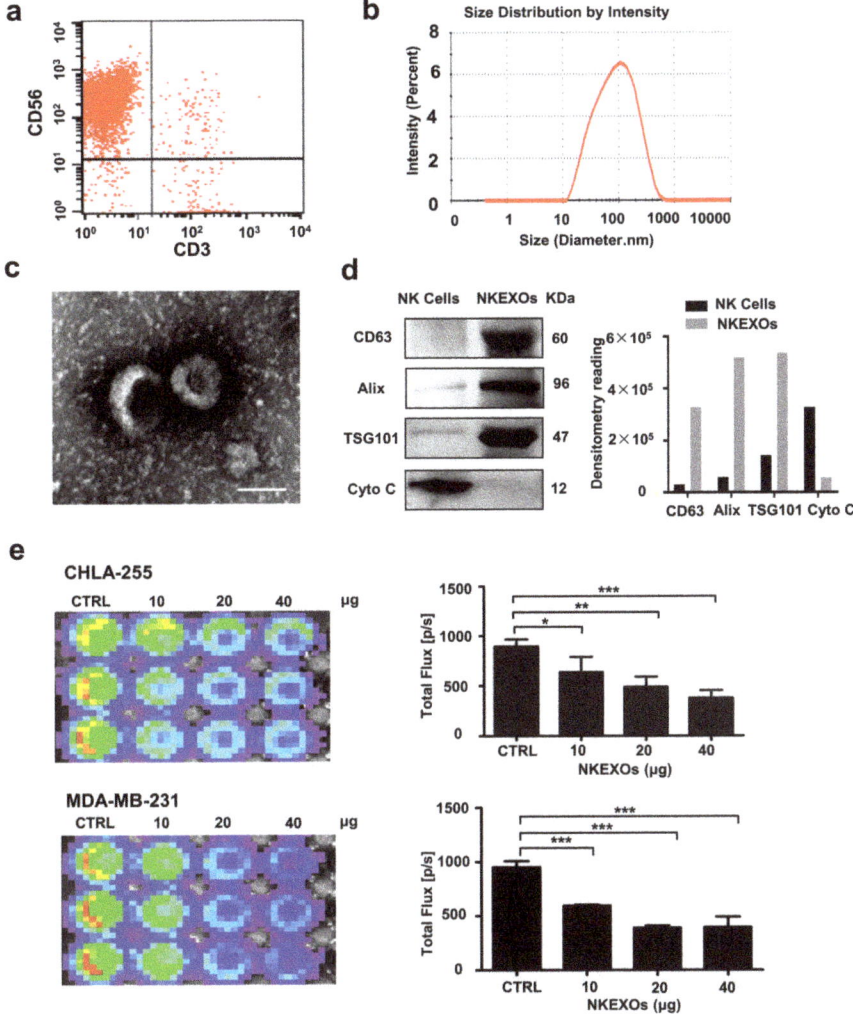

Figure 1. Characterization and function of isolated NKEXOs. (**a**) Flow cytometric analysis of NK cells (CD3− and CD56+) grown for a total of 21 days. (**b**) Size distributions of NKEXO measured by dynamic light scattering show peak diameters at 100 nm. (**c**) The morphology of exosomes was analyzed by transmission electron microscopy. (**d**) Western blot analysis of CD63, ALIX, TSG101 and cytochrome c (Cyto C) expression level in NK cells and NKEXOs. (**e**) MDA-MB-231luc and CHLA-255luc cell lines (10^4 cells per well) were incubated with control medium and different amounts of NKEXOs (10, 20 and 40 μg) for 24 h. Cell viability was assessed by bioluminescence imaging. Each bar represents the mean ± SD of three replicates. * $p < 0.05$; ** $p < 0.01$ and *** $p < 0.001$.

2.2. Fabrication and Characterization of the NN/NKEXO Cocktail

PAMAM dendrimer have been used previously for nucleic acid delivery [4–6]. Using the intrinsic hydrophobicity of the lipid bilayers in the exosome, tyrosine was linked to the dendrimers to promote the binding process [31]. Meanwhile, the phenyl groups of the tyrosine are able to disrupt the endosomal membrane, facilitating release of the therapeutic miRNA [32,33]. The NN/NKEXO cocktail was then prepared by simple incubation of the purified NKEXOs with tyrosine-coupled dendrimers preloaded with let-7a mimics (Figure 2a). The resulting NNs were further characterized by TEM, displaying a core–shell structure indicating the presence of the dendrimers in the core and NKEXOs in the shell (Figure 2b). More importantly, the precipitated NNs contained typical intracellular proteins including TSG101 and Alix, indicating the shell was made of intact exosomes (Figure 2c). Furthermore, the successful coating of the NKEXOs was confirmed by colocalization of the PKH26 (red)-labeled NKEXOs and Fluorescein phosphoramidites FAM (green)-labeled dendrimers (Figure 2d).

In order for the dendrimer core to be fully encapsulated, it is necessary to ensure that the exosomes are always in an excessive state. As an easy and reliable quality control, we used a high-content screening (HCS) system (Operetta, PerkinElmer, Massachusetts, USA) combined with fluorescent staining to determine the parameters for the cocktail synthesis. The module and parameter settings of the instrument were set as shown in Table S1. In each quality control process, we first fixed the amount of exosomes and used different amounts of let-7a mimics. Thus, the amount of let-7a mimics corresponding to the highest NNs synthesis rate was the maximum amount that could be loaded, and this amount or below was optional.

As shown in Figure 2e, for instance, we used fixed amounts of NKEXOs 10 µg and varied the amount of let-7a mimics and the synthesis time. Using HCS screening, we observed that the coupling efficiency of NNs increased over time and reached a peak of nearly 59.67% (±6.69%) at 24 h. In contrast, the highest NNs synthetic rate was observed when the amount of the let-7a mimics was 0.13 µg (10 µL at 1 µM concentration; Figure 2f). This was considered the maximum rate to prepare a single batch of the NN/NKEXO cocktail over a 24 h period. All the cocktails used in this study were subject to the same progress to ensure that NKEXOs are excess at any time.

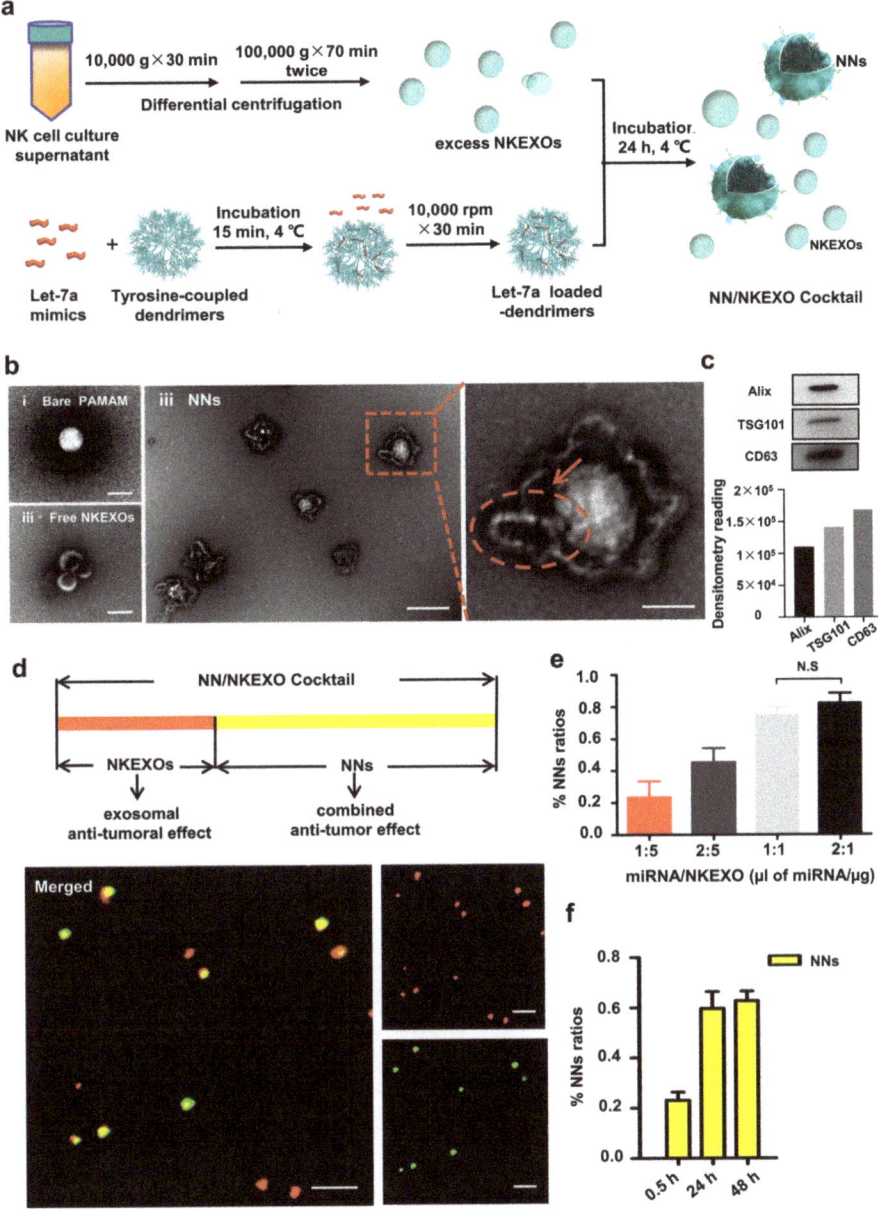

Figure 2. Fabrication and characterization of the NN/NKEXO cocktail. (**a**) Schematic design of the NN/NKEXO cocktail. (**b**) TEM images of bare PAMAM dendrimers (i), NNs (ii) and free NKEXO in supernatant (iii). The arrow indicates an integrated NKEXO. (**c**) NNs contain typical intracellular proteins markers (ALIX, TSG101), confirmed by Western blot (WB). (**d**) CLSM images of the fabricated NN/NKEXO cocktail illustrating the colocalization of let-7a loaded dendrimers (green) and NKEXO (red). (**e**) Percentages of NNs in the NN/NKEXO cocktail at different miRNA to NKEXO ratios. (**f**) Percentages of NNs in NNs-NKEXO cocktail at different synthesis times at a 1:1 miRNA to NKEXO ratio.

2.3. Binding and Cytotoxicity of the NN/NKEXO Cocktail to a Human Neuroblastoma Cell Line In Vitro

Next, we evaluated the nanoparticle cocktail kinetics in human neuroblastoma CHLA-255 cells at different incubation times with the dual labeled cocktail (miRNA loaded dendrimers: FAM, green and NKEXOs: PKH-26, red), followed by observation via CLSM. As shown in Figure 3a, the internalization of both NKEXOs and let-7a inside tumor cells increased from 12 to 24 h. Additional quantitative measurements were performed using flow cytometry. Equivalent exosomes derived from human embryonic kidney cell line 293T were obtained and 293N/293EXO cocktail was synthesized as control. The fluorescence intensity of let-7a mimics in CHLA-255 cells increased along with the NKEXO fluorescence in a time-dependent manner. Neither fluorescence intensities weakened until cells were incubated for at least 48 h. Importantly, CHLA-255 cells treated with the NN/NKEXO cocktail showed a prominent right shift in the cytometric analysis, suggesting a higher cellular uptake of exosomes than 293N/293EXO cocktail (Figure 3b). Furthermore, more CHLA-255 cells internalized miRNA, with the mean fluorescence intensity value higher than in the control cocktail at any time point (Figure 3c,d). This indicates that the NKEXO based outer shell plays a critical role in improving the cancer target drug delivery efficiency. We also used the bioluminescence assay to substantiate the synergistic apoptosis-inducing capability of the cocktail in vitro. Since let-7a, a therapeutic microRNAs, is closely involved in the proliferation of neuroblastomas [34,35]. As shown in Figure 3e, after 24 h of incubation, NN/NKEXO cocktail-let-7a exhibited significantly higher cytotoxicity compared with NKEXO alone in neuroblastoma cells. In contrast, no significant inhibition of cell growth was observed in let-7a or dendrimers treated groups, indicating that the NNs mediated delivery of therapeutic let-7a enhances the anti-tumor effect of the cocktail by triggering a synergistic induction of apoptosis.

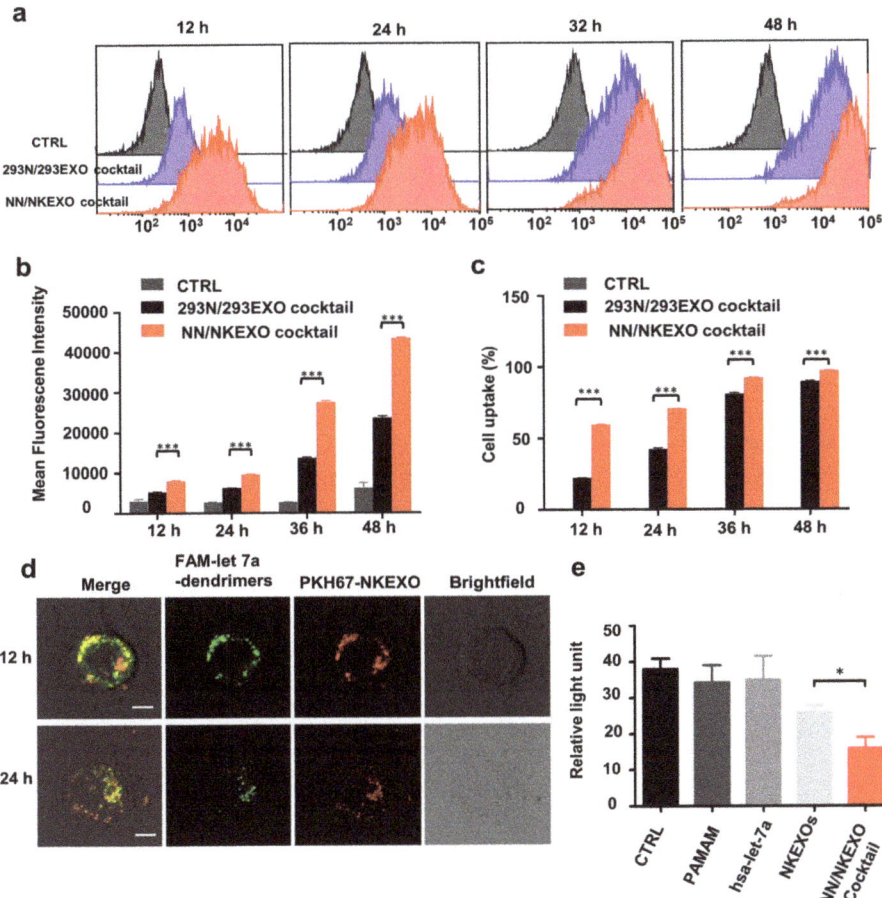

Figure 3. Binding and cytotoxicity of the NN/NKEXO cocktail to a human neuroblastoma cell line in vitro. (**a**) Representative confocal fluorescence images of CHLA-255 cells after treatment with NN/NKEXO cocktail for 12 and 24 h (let-7a-dendrimer: Green; NKEXO: Red). (**b**) Quantitative flow cytometric analysis of CHLA-255 cells incubated with control medium, 293N-293Exo cocktail and NN/NKEXO cocktail both made of let-7a (0.5 μg) and their exosomes (50 μg) for 12, 24, 36 and 48 h; $n = 3$. (**c**) Mean fluorescence intensity of CHLA-255 cells after 12, 24, 36 or 48 h incubation with control medium and different cocktails; $n = 3$. (**d**) Percentages of cells with increased miRNA fluorescence; $n = 3$. (**e**) Cell viability of CHLA-255 cells (10^4 cells per well) after treatment with PBS (CTRL), PAMAM, let-7a, NKEXOs and NN/NKEXO cocktail (40 μg NKEXOs and 0.05 μg let-7a) for 24 h. Data are presented as mean ± SD; $n = 3$.

2.4. In Vivo Biodistribution and Anti-Tumor Effect of the NN/NKEXO Cocktail

To evaluate the tumor targeting capability of the cocktail, let-7a was labeled with Cy5 and the cocktail was administrated intravenously into the CHLA-255-luc tumor-bearing nonobese diabetic/severe combined immunodeficient (NOD/SCID) mice. After removal of the tumors and organs of interest 6 h after injection, ex vivo fluorescence imaging showed strong fluorescence signals of let-7a loaded dendrimers in the tumor tissues and relatively strong signals in the kidneys. In contrast, no specific fluorescence was detected in tumor tissues of mice treated with miRNA alone or miRNA loaded dendrimers (Figure 4a). These results indicate that the NN/NKEXO cocktail have highly efficient targeting and miRNA delivery to tumor cells. NKEXOs showed tumor-specific accumulation as early as 24 h post-injection in vivo [6]. Here, we labeled NKEXOs with DiR (red) to prepare the cocktail administrated intravenously. Interestingly, using ex vivo fluorescence imaging (Figure 4b), NKEXOs showed tumor-specific accumulation as early as 6 h post-injection. In the second method, a subcutaneous tumor mice model was used. The dual fluorescently labeled cocktail (let-7a loaded dendrimers: FAM, green and NKEXOs: PKH-26, red) was intravenously injected. As demonstrated by two-photon excited scanning fluorescence imaging (TPEFI), miRNA loaded dendrimers were found in the tumor tissues as early as 20 min after administration (Figure 4c; Video S2). These results indicate that our cocktails are suitable for highly efficient tumor-targeted delivery. In this regard, CXCR4 presence in NKEXOs has been shown which intimately linked to the accumulation at specific organs, and CD47 presence is a "don't eat me" signal for phagocytic cells to achieve longer circulation times (Figure 4d) [36–38]. Both molecules potentially promoted NNs to target primary tumors and organ specific metastasis more accurately and actively.

Finally, we evaluated the in vivo antitumor effect of the cocktails. Mice bearing tumors induced by CHLA-255-luc cells were randomly sorted into five groups ($n = 3$ per group). As indicated in Figure 4e, a pronounced suppression of tumor growth was observed in the animals treated with cocktail-let-7a. Notably, the signal intensity of the cocktail treatment group was significantly lower than that of the NKEXO group ($p < 0.05$), further indicating that the let-7a was efficiently and successfully carried to tumor cells by NNs and exerted a synergistic antitumor effect with NKEXOs (Figure 4f,g).

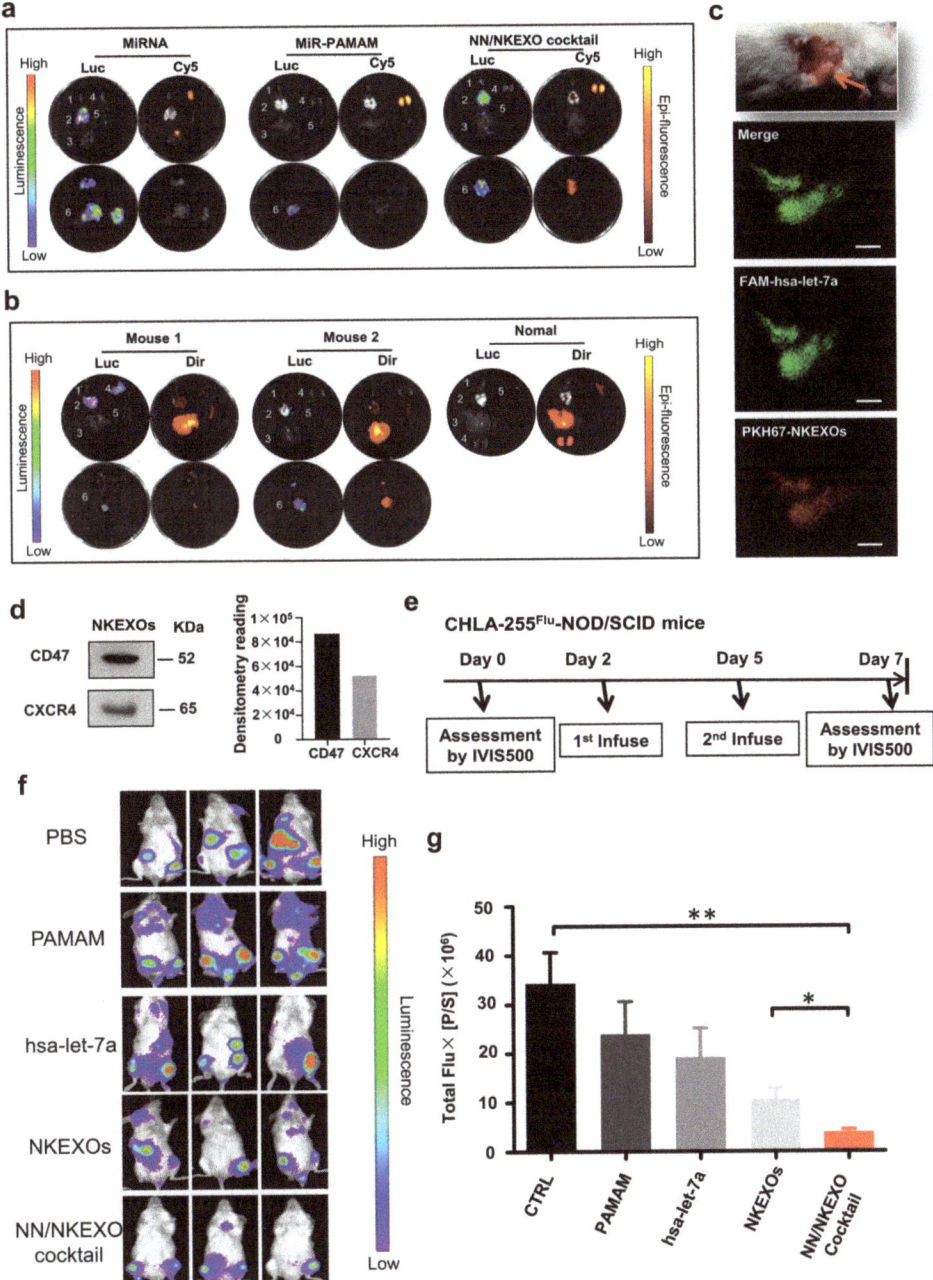

Figure 4. In vivo biodistribution and anti-tumor effect of the NN/NKEXO cocktail. (**a**) Bioluminescence (Luc) and miRNA fluorescence (Cy5) images of major organs of the NOD/SCID mice bearing systemic CHLA-255-luc tumors 6 h after intravenous (i.v.) injection of Cy5-let-7a, Cy5-let-7a-dendrimers and Cy5-labeled NN/NKEXO cocktail: 1) Heart; 2) lung; 3) liver; 4) kidney; 5) spleen and 6) tumor.

(**b**) Bioluminescence (Luc) and fluorescence images of major organs 6 h after i.v. injection of DiR-labeled NN/NKEXO cocktail made of 5.28 µg of let-7a and 100 µg of NKEXOs. (**c**) In vivo two-photon excitation fluorescence images of the CHLA-255^{luc} subcutaneous tumor model 20 min after i.v. injection of 400 µL dual fluorescently labeled NN/NKEXO cocktail made of 5.28 µg of let-7a and 100 µg of NKEXOs. (**d**) Expression of functional proteins (CD47 and CXCR4) was confirmed by WB. (**e**) Experimental protocol for CHLA-255^{luc}-NOD/SCID mice shown in (**f**). (**f**) Bioluminescence imaging (BLI) performed in CHLA-255^{luc}-NOD/SCID mice treated with different cocktail formulations at let-7a dose of 5.28 µg and NKEXO dose of 100 µg (n = 3). (**g**) Quantification of BLI results. Each bar represents mean ± SD of three replicates. * $p < 0.05$ and ** $p < 0.001$.

3. Discussion

An ideal nanomedicine for cancer therapy should elicit minimal immunogenicity. In the traditional membrane preparation processes, the use of integrated NKEXOs as shells of nanoparticles avoids potential contamination with immunogenic substances. The advantage of NK cells, a source of NKEXOs, is that it can act as an off-the-shelf product for allogeneic settings [27]. NKEXOs also exhibit the benefits of being stable vesicles that maintain their biological activities for at least two years at −80 °C [39]. These properties make them more suitable for clinical applications.

Although the exact mechanisms by which NKEXOs specifically target tumors are not clear, the following clues may explain this targeting and guide further research in this area. CXCR4 is one of the best-characterized chemokine receptors mediating leukocyte trafficking [40]. Moreover, its ligand, SDF-1a, is released in large amounts by some tumor or organs, such as the lung and liver [36,37]. The interaction between SDF-1 and CXCR4 also plays an important role in cancer metastasis [41,42]. NKEXOs, expressing CXCR4 as determined in our study, likely induced NNs to leave systemic circulation and traffic into tumors or organs. In this context, NNs had the potential to become "prophylactic" anti-metastatic agents.

However, we note that in our experiments the number of experimental animals was relatively small with a short observation period. Besides, more details of the coating progress from a chemical standpoint were not provided.

Given the distinct advantage of being easy to generate and having good clinical application prospects, we believe further research in this field will resolve the aforementioned limitations. To this end, this cocktail strategy is expected to offer new opportunities for the advancement of cancer nanomedicine.

4. Materials and Methods

4.1. Cell Culture

The human breast cancer cell lines MDA-MB-231 and human embryonic kidney cell lines 293T were propagated in DMEM (Gibco, Grand Island, NY, USA) supplemented with 10% FBS (Gibco) and 1% penicillin-streptomycin (Hyclone, Logan, UT, USA). Human neuroblastoma cells CHLA-255 were incubated in IMDM (Gibco) with 20% FBS and 1% penicillin-streptomycin. All cell lines were purchased from the American Type Culture Collection (ATCC). Both MDA-MB-231 and CHLA-255 cells were transfected by Nucleofection™ (Lonza, Cologne, Germany) with a firefly luciferase expression plasmid. All cells were maintained in a humidified 5% CO_2 atmosphere at 37 °C.

4.2. Preparation and Function of NK Cell Derived Exosomes

4.2.1. Isolation of Exosomes

We isolated NK cell-derived exosomes using differential ultracentrifugation according to the literature. On day 21, NK cell culture supernatants were harvested after a preliminary centrifugation at 400× g for 10 min to eliminate cells. The supernatants were centrifuged first at 2000× g for 10 min and then at 10,000× g for 70 min to remove dead cells and cell debris, followed by an additional centrifugation step at 100,000× g for 70 min in a 70Ti ultracentrifuge rotor (Optima™XPN-100, Beckman, Brea, CA, USA) to obtain pellets containing raw exosomes. The pellets were then purified by washing them with PBS and centrifuged at 100,000× g for another 70 min. The isolated exosomes were resuspended in PBS (100:1 enrichment) and stored at −80 °C before use. All procedures were carried out at 4 °C. We isolated exosomes from the 293T culture medium in the same way.

4.2.2. Measurement of Particle Size

A dynamic light scattering (DLS) system equipped with a 532-nm laser (Malvern Instruments, Malvern, UK) was used for exosome particle size analysis. Samples were diluted before analysis (10 µL, 1:100 diluted in PBS) and each sample was measured three times. Data was collected and analyzed by Dispersion Technology Software (Malvern Instruments). The size distribution was measured by signal intensity and the Z-average diameter obtained from the autocorrelation function using the general-purpose mode.

4.2.3. Determination of Protein Concentration

Protein concentration in isolated exosomes was calculated by the bicinchoninic acid protein assay. Briefly, 25 µL of an aqueous suspension of isolated exosomes after lysis were added to 200 µL of standard working reagent in wells of a 96-well plate. Absorbance of the mixture was determined at 562 nm with a microplate reader and the protein concentration estimated. A calibration curve was constructed using bovine serum albumin as protein standard.

4.2.4. Western Blotting (WB) Analysis

Presence of marker proteins in exosomes was analyzed and confirmed by WB. Proteins from lysed cells or isolated exosomes were denatured and loaded onto sodium dodecyl sulfate polyacrylamide gels, transferred to polyvinylidene difluoride membranes (Millipore, Billerica, MA, USA), and subsequently stained with the corresponding primary and secondary antibodies. The following antibodies were used for WB analysis according to manufacturer's instructions: Anti-ALIX polyclonal antibody (12422-1-AP, Proteintech, Rosemont, IL, USA), anti-CD47 polyclonal antibody (ab108415, Abcam, Cambridge, MA, USA), anti-CXCR4 polyclonal antibody (35-8800, Invitrogen, Waltham, MA, USA), anti-TSG101 monoclonal antibody (4A10, Abcam), anti-human CD63 polyclonal antibody (556019, BD Biosciences) and anti-cytochrome C antibody (10993-1-AP, Proteintech). The BioRad ChemiDoc Touch imaging system (BioRad, Hercules, CA, USA) was used to analyze the bands after incubation with the corresponding goat anti-mouse- or goat anti-rabbit-HRP secondary antibody conjugates (1:5000 dilutions). The densitometry readings of each band were calculated by ImagJ (NIH, Bethesda, MD, USA).

4.2.5. Transmission Electron Microscopy (TEM)

Morphology of the isolated NKEXOs was studied by TEM. A small drop (about 10 µL) of exosomes was dropped onto the Formvar/carbon-coated TEM grid. After settling for approximately 1 min, excess water was removed by touching the grid with a piece of filter paper. Next, the grid was covered with a small drop of 2% uranyl acetate. After drying for ten seconds, the copper nets were examined with a Tecnai T10 TEM (FEI, Oregon, OH, USA) operated at 120 kV. The morphology of the PAMAM dendrimers and NNs was also imaged by TEM following similar steps.

4.2.6. Samples Labeling

To label isolated exosomes and let-7a loaded PAMAM, different labeling assays were performed. We added 2 µL of red lipophilic fluorescent dye PKH26 (Sigma-Aldrich, St. Louis, MO, USA) to 500 µL of Diluent C (Sigma-Aldrich). The mixture was then added to the isolated NK derived exosomes and mixed gently for 5 min at room temperature followed by addition of 1% BSA

(1 mL) to facilitate the binding of the excess dye. Next, samples were washed with PBS and ultracentrifuged at 100,000 g for 70 min and the pellets resuspended in PBS. The fluorescent dye 1,10-dioctadecyl-3,3,30,30-tetramethylindotricarbocyanine iodide (DiR; Invitrogen) was also used to label exosomes. Purified exosomes were incubated in 1 µM DiR at a concentration of approximately 350 µg of exosomes per mL for 15 min at 37 °C, and washed as described above. FAM-labeled miRNA and cy5-labeled miRNA were both synthesized by Genepharma (Shanghai, China).

4.3. Cellular Uptake Assay

PKH26-labeled NKEXOs were incubated with MDA-MB-231 cells for 24 h in a humidified 5% CO_2 atmosphere at 37 °C. Subsequently, cells were washed twice with PBS and fixed with 4% paraformaldehyde for 20 min. Aliquots (5 µL) of the cell suspension were placed in clear microscope slides, covered with a drop of FluorSave™ Reagent (Invitrogen) and mounted with a coverslip. Images, including z-axis projection images, were taken using a Nikon A1R (Nikon instruments, Melville, NY, USA) confocal laser scanning microscope. The uptake of the NN/NKEXO cocktail by CHLA-255 cells was also imaged following similar steps after incubating for 12 and 24 h.

4.4. Flow Cytometry

FAM-labeled let-7a loaded PAMAM and PKH26-labeled NKEXOs were coupled to fabricate the nanoparticle cocktail as indicated before. To quantify the cellular uptake of the cocktail by tumor cells, CHLA-255 cells (10^5 cells per well) were cultured with the NN/NKEXO cocktail made of let-7a (0.5 µg) and NKEXOs (50 µg), PBS or equivalent 293N/293Exo cocktail between 12 to 48 h, harvested, and washed twice with PBS. Then, the samples were centrifuged and the supernatants decanted. Cells were resuspended and collected before analysis with a Cytoflex flow cytometer (Beckman Coulter, Life Science, Indianapolis, IN, USA).

4.5. Preparation of the NN/NKEXO Cocktail

To prepare NN/NKEXO cocktails in this study, 0.05/0.5/5.28 µg let-7a mimics (Genepharma) were added to dendrimers following manufacturer's instructions (SL100568, SignaGen Laboratories, Rockville, MD, USA) and mixed thoroughly to react at 4 °C for 15 min. The resulting let-7a loaded PAMAM were precipitated at high-speed (10,000 rpm) for 30 min to remove excess let-7a. Subsequently, 40/50/100 µg of NKEXOs suspension were added to the precipitated let-7a loaded PAMAM respectively and the mixture incubated for 24 hours at 4 °C. To obtain NNs, the NN/NKEXO cocktail was precipitated at high-speed (10,000 rpm) for 30 min and resuspended in PBS. The supernatants with excess NKEXOs were used for TEM and the precipitated NNs for both Western blotting analysis and TEM. The same procedure was used in fabricating another cocktail in this study.

Confocal laser scanning microscopy (Nikon A1R) was used to validate whether NKEXOs were successfully fused with the let-7a loaded-PMAM. Exosomes and let-7a mimics were fluorescently labeled by PKH26 and FAM, respectively. Laser excitation of PKH67 and FAM was done sequentially using 586- and 488-nm lasers.

4.6. In Vitro Cytotoxicity

To evaluate NKEXO cytotoxicity, MDA-MB-231 breast cancer cells and CHLA-255 neuroblastoma cells were transfected with the firefly luciferase gene to quantify target cell survival using bioluminescence. MDA-MB-231-luc and CHLA-255-luc cells (10^4 cells per well) were cultured with different quantities of NKEXOs (10, 20 and 40 µg) in clear-bottomed 96-well plates for 24 h. The culture medium was discarded and cells washed with PBS three times, followed by the addition of 120 µL of cell lysis buffer from a luciferase reporter Gene Assay kit (Yisheng, Shanghai, China). The 96-well plates were then shaken in a micro-shaker at room temperature for 15 min to fully lyse the cells. Next, the pyrolyzed lysates were centrifuged at 10,000 rpm for 3–5 minutes. After centrifugation, 100 µL of the supernatants from each well were transferred to a clear-bottomed 96-well plate, and 100 µL of firefly luciferase assay reagent added. Bioluminescent signals of the mixture were measured by the IVIS® Lumina III imaging system (PerkinElmer, Santa Clara, CA, USA) and expressed as photon flux (photons/s). All experiments were done in triplicate from independent cell cultures.

To evaluate the cytotoxicity of cocktail-let-7a against the neuroblastoma cells in vitro, CHLA-255-luc cells (10^4 cells per well) were treated with NKEXOs, let-7a alone or cocktail-let-7a containing 40 µg NKEXOs and 0.05 µg let-7a. Bioluminescent signals of the mixture were measured by an automatic ELISA plate reader and the relative light unit read at 562 nm.

4.7. In Vivo Animal Experiments

In vivo analysis was performed using specific pathogen-free, 6-week-old, female NOD/SCID mice (Slaccas, Shanghai, China). All animal experimental protocols were conducted in accordance with all national guidelines and regulations, and approved by the Animal Ethics Committee (NO. 2018R03042).

4.7.1. In Vivo Targeting Capability of the Nanoparticle Cocktail

The cocktail was labeled with Cy5-let-7a loaded PAMAM or DiR-NKEXOs. Then, 5×10^6 CHLA255 cells were intravenously injected into mice, which were randomly separated into four groups after 21 days in captivity. Animals in one group received intravenous injections containing 400 µL of labeled cocktail with identical amounts of let-7a (5.28 µg) and NKEXOs (100 µg). A second group received let-7a loaded PAMAM and the third group received let-7a only. At the end of the experiment (6 h after injection), the mice were euthanized and dissected tissues (heart, lung, liver, kidneys, spleen, livers and tumors) were imaged immediately. Fluorescence imaging was performed using the IVIS® Lumina III imaging system. Background fluorescence was measured and subtracted by setting up a background measurement at time of data acquisition. A separate in vivo biodistribution study was performed using the following procedure. CHLA-255-luc cells (2×10^7 cells/200 µL) were subcutaneously injected into the forward thighs of NOD/SCID mice. After 14 days, the mice were anesthetized and the subcutaneous tumor tissue was carefully exposed using surgical scissors. Mice were injected intravenously with 400 µL of a cocktail made of FAM-labeled miRNA let7a (5.28 µg) and PKH26-labeled NKEXOs (100 µg). After 20 min, in vivo two-photon confocal microscopy (Olympus BX61, Olympus America, Center Valley, PA, USA) was performed to detect each fluorescence signal from the subcutaneous tumor.

4.7.2. In Vivo Antitumor Assay

The ability of the cocktail to inhibit tumor growth was evaluated in a neuroblastoma tumor-bearing mouse model. Fifteen mice were used in this experiment. Briefly, CHLA-255-luc cells (10^7 cells/500 µL) were i.v. injected into the NOD/SCID mice. Mice were randomly separated into five groups ($n = 3$) 14 days later, and intravenously injected with different cocktail formulations: NKEXOs, cocktail-let-7a, PAMAM, let7a or with PBS as control group at let-7a dose of 5.28 µg and NKEXO dose of 100 µg. The same treatments were repeated after three days. After treatment, bioluminescence imaging (BLI) was performed with the IVIS® Lumina III imaging system to analyze the cocktail's therapeutic effect.

4.8. Statistics

Data are expressed as mean ± SD. SPSS Statistics 24 software (IBM, Armonk, NY, USA) and GraphPad Prism 5 software (GraphPad Software, Inc., San Diego, CA, USA) were used to perform data analysis using the analysis of variance (ANOVA) function. $p < 0.05$ values were considered statistically significant.

5. Conclusions

In summary, we reported the novel strategy for tumor targeting therapy based on NN/NKEXO cocktail. As displayed in Figure 5, the NNs constituted a novel biomimetic core–shell polymer, formed by the self-assembly of two components: (1) A PAMAM dendrimer-based inner core part for loading gene therapeutic agents and (2) the NKEXO based outer shell facilitating tumor targeting and acting as a direct antitumor agent. The NKEXOs coating guided NNs to the tumor and interacted with the plasma membrane of the target cells via endocytosis/fusion or via FasL/Fas. Finally, the therapeutic miRNA was released and regulated the transcriptome batch or gene of the cell, which performed a combined anti-tumoral effect with NKEXOs.

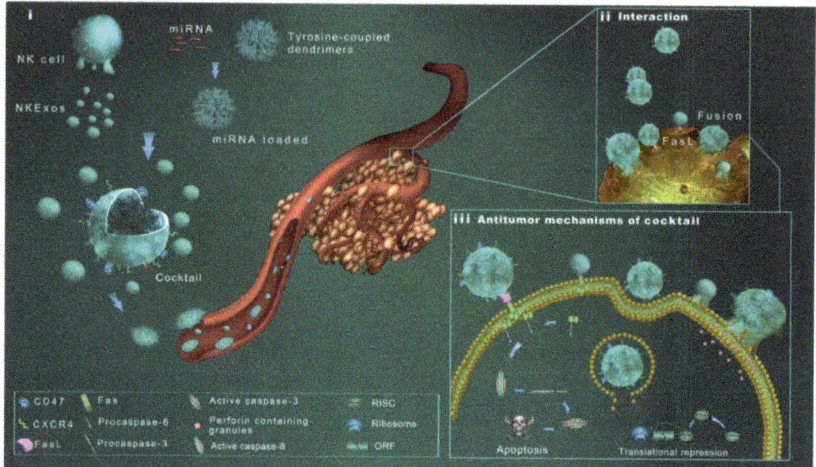

Figure 5. Schematic design of the NN/NKEXO cocktail for tumor targeting and drug delivery. (i) Main components of the cocktail: exosomes derived from NK cells (NKEXOs); exosome camouflaged core–shell nanoparticles (NNs). CD47 and CXCR4 facilitate a more accurate and active delivery of NNs. (ii) Interaction of the nanoparticle cocktail with target cells. Both NKEXOs and NNs are involved in exosome-to-membrane fusion and receptor-ligand interaction. (iii) Mechanisms of cocktail antitumor effect include perforin/granzyme mediated apoptosis, FasL/Fas mediated apoptosis and the effect of released therapeutic miRNA.

Supplementary Materials: The following are available online at http://www.mdpi.com/2072-6694/11/10/1560/s1, Figure S1: Confocal laser scanning microscopy examination of MDA-MB-231 cellular uptake of NKEXOs; Table S1: Parameters of high-content screening (HCS) analysis; Video S1: A rotating 3D rendering of z-stack images showing the internalization of NKEXOs into MDA-MB-231-luc cells; Video S2: Fluorescence signal of NN/NKEXO cocktail detected in the tumor tissues using TPEFI.

Author Contributions: Conceptualization, G.W. and Y.X.; methodology, G.W., W.H. and H.C.; software, T.Y.; validation, G.W., W.H., H.C., X.S., T.Y. and Y.X.; formal analysis, G.W., W.H. and H.C.; investigation, G.W., W.H., H.C and X.S.; resources, Y.X.; data curation, G.W., W.H., X.S. and T.Y.; writing—original draft preparation, G.W.; writing—review and editing, W.H. and Y.X.; visualization, G.W. and W.H.

Funding: This research was funded by the Startup Foundation for Talented Scholars of Zhejiang University, grant number 119000-193820101.

Acknowledgments: We acknowledge the technical support by the Core Facilities, Zhejiang University School of Medicine.

Conflicts of Interest: The authors declare no conflict of interest.

References

1. Langer, R. Drug delivery and targeting. *Nature* **1998**, *392*, 5–10.
2. Allen, T.M.; Cullis, P.R. Drug delivery systems: Entering the mainstream. *Science* **2004**, *303*, 1818–1822. [CrossRef] [PubMed]
3. Mura, S.; Nicolas, J.; Couvreur, P. Stimuli-responsive nanocarriers for drug delivery. *Nat. Mater.* **2013**, *12*, 991–1003. [CrossRef] [PubMed]

4. Tomalia, D.A.; Baker, H.; Dewald, J.; Hall, M.; Kallos, G.; Martin, S.; Roeck, J.; Ryder, J.; Smith, P. A new class of polymers: Starburst-dendritic macromolecules. *Polym. J.* **1985**, *17*, 117. [CrossRef]
5. Wagner, E. Strategies to improve DNA polyplexes for in vivo gene transfer: Will "artificial viruses" be the answer? *Pharm. Res.* **2004**, *21*, 8–14. [CrossRef]
6. Tang, M.X.; Redemann, C.T.; Szoka, F.C., Jr. In vitro gene delivery by degraded polyamidoamine dendrimers. *Bioconjug. Chem.* **1996**, *7*, 703–714. [CrossRef]
7. Fox, L.J.; Richardson, R.M.; Briscoe, W.H. PAMAM dendrimer-cell membrane interactions. *Adv. Colloid Interface Sci.* **2018**, *257*, 1–18. [CrossRef]
8. Li, J.; Liang, H.; Liu, J.; Wang, Z. Poly (amidoamine) (PAMAM) dendrimer mediated delivery of drug and pDNA/siRNA for cancer therapy. *Int. J. Pharm.* **2018**, *546*, 215–225. [CrossRef]
9. Luong, D.; Kesharwani, P.; Deshmukh, R.; Mohd Amin, M.C.I.; Gupta, U.; Greish, K.; Iyer, A.K. PEGylated PAMAM dendrimers: Enhancing efficacy and mitigating toxicity for effective anticancer drug and gene delivery. *Acta Biomater.* **2016**, *43*, 14–29. [CrossRef]
10. Fang, R.H.; Hu, C.M.; Luk, B.T.; Gao, W.; Copp, J.A.; Tai, Y.; O'Connor, D.E.; Zhang, L. Cancer cell membrane-coated nanoparticles for anticancer vaccination and drug delivery. *Nano Lett.* **2014**, *14*, 2181–2188. [CrossRef]
11. Parodi, A.; Quattrocchi, N.; van de Ven, A.L.; Chiappini, C.; Evangelopoulos, M.; Martinez, J.O.; Brown, B.S.; Khaled, S.Z.; Yazdi, I.K.; Enzo, M.V.; et al. Synthetic nanoparticles functionalized with biomimetic leukocyte membranes possess cell-like functions. *Nat. Nanotechnol.* **2013**, *8*, 61–68. [CrossRef] [PubMed]
12. Hu, C.M.; Fang, R.H.; Copp, J.; Luk, B.T.; Zhang, L. A biomimetic nanosponge that absorbs pore-forming toxins. *Nat. Nanotechnol.* **2013**, *8*, 336–340. [CrossRef] [PubMed]
13. Hu, Q.; Sun, W.; Qian, C.; Wang, C.; Bomba, H.N.; Gu, Z. Anticancer Platelet-Mimicking Nanovehicles. *Adv. Mater.* **2015**, *27*, 7043–7050. [CrossRef] [PubMed]
14. Zhang, Y.; Chen, Y.; Lo, C.; Zhuang, J.; Angsantikul, P.; Zhang, Q.; Wei, X.; Zhou, Z.; Obonyo, M.; Fang, R.H.; et al. Inhibition of pathogen adhesion by bacterial outer membrane-coated nanoparticles. *Angew. Chem. Int. Ed. (English)* **2019**, *58*, 11404–11408. [CrossRef]
15. Chen, Y.; Zhang, Y.; Chen, M.; Zhuang, J.; Fang, R.H.; Gao, W.; Zhang, L. Biomimetic nanosponges suppress in vivo lethality induced by the whole secreted proteins of pathogenic bacteria. *Small* **2019**, *15*, e1804994. [CrossRef]
16. Molinaro, R.; Evangelopoulos, M.; Hoffman, J.R.; Corbo, C.; Taraballi, F.; Martinez, J.O.; Hartman, K.A.; Cosco, D.; Costa, G.; Romeo, I.; et al. Design and development of biomimetic nanovesicles using a microfluidic approach. *Adv. Mater.* **2018**, *30*, e1702749. [CrossRef]
17. Corbo, C.; Cromer, W.E.; Molinaro, R.; Toledano Furman, N.E.; Hartman, K.A.; De Rosa, E.; Boada, C.; Wang, X.; Zawieja, D.C.; Agostini, M.; et al. Engineered biomimetic nanovesicles show intrinsic anti-inflammatory properties for the treatment of inflammatory bowel diseases. *Nanoscale* **2017**, *9*, 14581–14591. [CrossRef]
18. Molinaro, R.; Pasto, A.; Corbo, C.; Taraballi, F.; Giordano, F.; Martinez, J.O.; Zhao, P.; Wang, X.; Zinger, A.; Boada, C.; et al. Macrophage-derived nanovesicles exert intrinsic anti-inflammatory properties and prolong survival in sepsis through a direct interaction with macrophages. *Nanoscale* **2019**, *11*, 13576–13586. [CrossRef]
19. Zhai, Y.; Su, J.; Ran, W.; Zhang, P.; Yin, Q.; Zhang, Z.; Yu, H.; Li, Y. Preparation and application of cell membrane-camouflaged nanoparticles for cancer therapy. *Theranostics* **2017**, *7*, 2575–2592. [CrossRef]
20. O'Sullivan, T.E.; Sun, J.C.; Lanier, L.L. Natural killer cell memory. *Immunity* **2015**, *43*, 634–645. [CrossRef]
21. Vivier, E.; Raulet, D.H.; Moretta, A.; Caligiuri, M.A.; Zitvogel, L.; Lanier, L.L.; Yokoyama, W.M.; Ugolini, S. Innate or adaptive immunity? The example of natural killer cells. *Science* **2011**, *331*, 44–49. [CrossRef] [PubMed]
22. Zhu, L.; Oh, J.M.; Gangadaran, P.; Kalimuthu, S.; Baek, S.H.; Jeong, S.Y.; Lee, S.-W.; Lee, J.; Ahn, B.-C. Targeting and therapy of glioblastoma in a mouse model using exosomes derived from natural killer cells. *Front. Immunol.* **2018**, *9*, 824. [CrossRef] [PubMed]
23. Lugini, L.; Cecchetti, S.; Huber, V.; Luciani, F.; Macchia, G.; Spadaro, F.; Paris, L.; Abalsamo, L.; Colone, M.; Molinari, A.; et al. Immune surveillance properties of human NK cell-derived exosomes. *J. Immunol.* **2012**, *189*, 2833–2842. [CrossRef] [PubMed]
24. Zhu, L.; Kalimuthu, S.; Gangadaran, P.; Oh, J.M.; Lee, H.W.; Baek, S.H.; Jeong, S.Y.; Lee, S.W.; Lee, J.; Ahn, B.C. Exosomes derived from natural killer cells exert therapeutic effect in melanoma. *Theranostics* **2017**, *7*, 2732–2745. [CrossRef] [PubMed]
25. Jong, A.Y.; Wu, C.H.; Li, J.; Sun, J.; Fabbri, M.; Wayne, A.S.; Seeger, R.C. Large-scale isolation and cytotoxicity of extracellular vesicles derived from activated human natural killer cells. *J. Extracell. Vesicles* **2017**, *6*, 1294368. [CrossRef]

26. Parolini, I.; Federici, C.; Raggi, C.; Lugini, L.; Palleschi, S.; De Milito, A.; Coscia, C.; Iessi, E.; Logozzi, M.; Molinari, A.; et al. Microenvironmental pH is a key factor for exosome traffic in tumor cells. *J. Biol. Chem.* **2009**, *284*, 34211–34222. [CrossRef] [PubMed]
27. Oberschmidt, O.; Kloess, S.; Koehl, U. Redirected primary human chimeric antigen receptor natural killer cells as an "off-the-shelf immunotherapy" for improvement in cancer treatment. *Front. Immunol.* **2017**, *8*, 654. [CrossRef]
28. Fujisaki, H.; Kakuda, H.; Shimasaki, N.; Imai, C.; Ma, J.; Lockey, T.; Eldridge, P.; Leung, W.H.; Campana, D. Expansion of highly cytotoxic human natural killer cells for cancer cell therapy. *Cancer Res.* **2009**, *69*, 4010–4017. [CrossRef]
29. Théry, C.; Amigorena, S.; Raposo, G.; Clayton, A. Isolation and characterization of exosomes from cell culture supernatants and biological fluids. *Curr. Protoc. Cell Biol.* **2006**, *30*, 3–22. [CrossRef]
30. Lotvall, J.; Hill, A.F.; Hochberg, F.; Buzas, E.I.; Di Vizio, D.; Gardiner, C.; Gho, Y.S.; Kurochkin, I.V.; Mathivanan, S.; Quesenberry, P.; et al. Minimal experimental requirements for definition of extracellular vesicles and their functions: A position statement from the International Society for Extracellular Vesicles. *J. Extracell. Vesicles* **2014**, *3*, 26913. [CrossRef]
31. Fonseca, A.C.; Frias, M.A.; Bouchet, A.M.; Jarmelo, S.; Simoes, P.N.; Fausto, R.; Gil, M.H.; Lairion, F.; Disalvo, E.A. Role of guanidyl moiety in the insertion of arginine and Nalpha-benzoyl-L-argininate ethyl ester chloride in lipid membranes. *J. Phys. Chem. B* **2010**, *114*, 5946–5952. [CrossRef] [PubMed]
32. Zeng, H.; Little, H.C.; Tiambeng, T.N.; Williams, G.A.; Guan, Z. Multifunctional dendronized peptide polymer platform for safe and effective siRNA delivery. *J. Am. Chem. Soc.* **2013**, *135*, 4962–4965. [CrossRef] [PubMed]
33. Wang, F.; Wang, Y.; Wang, H.; Shao, N.; Chen, Y.; Cheng, Y. Synergistic effect of amino acids modified on dendrimer surface in gene delivery. *Biomaterials* **2014**, *35*, 9187–9198. [CrossRef] [PubMed]
34. Powers, J.T.; Tsanov, K.M.; Pearson, D.S.; Roels, F.; Spina, C.S.; Ebright, R.; Seligson, M.; de Soysa, Y.; Cahan, P.; Theissen, J.; et al. Multiple mechanisms disrupt the let-7 microRNA family in neuroblastoma. *Nature* **2016**, *535*, 246–251. [CrossRef]
35. Molenaar, J.J.; Domingo-Fernandez, R.; Ebus, M.E.; Lindner, S.; Koster, J.; Drabek, K.; Mestdagh, P.; van Sluis, P.; Valentijn, L.J.; van Nes, J.; et al. LIN28B induces neuroblastoma and enhances MYCN levels via let-7 suppression. *Nat. Genet.* **2012**, *44*, 1199–1206. [CrossRef]
36. Li, Y.M.; Pan, Y.; Wei, Y.; Cheng, X.; Zhou, B.P.; Tan, M.; Zhou, X.; Xia, W.; Hortobagyi, G.N.; Yu, D.; et al. Upregulation of CXCR4 is essential for HER2-mediated tumor metastasis. *Cancer Cell* **2004**, *6*, 459–469. [CrossRef]
37. Bajetto, A.; Barbieri, F.; Dorcaratto, A.; Barbero, S.; Daga, A.; Porcile, C.; Ravetti, J.L.; Zona, G.; Spaziante, R.; Corte, G.; et al. Expression of CXC chemokine receptors 1-5 and their ligands in human glioma tissues: Role of CXCR4 and SDF1 in glioma cell proliferation and migration. *Neurochem. Int.* **2006**, *49*, 423–432. [CrossRef]
38. Jaiswal, S.; Jamieson, C.H.; Pang, W.W.; Park, C.Y.; Chao, M.P.; Majeti, R.; Traver, D.; van Rooijen, N.; Weissman, I.L. CD47 is upregulated on circulating hematopoietic stem cells and leukemia cells to avoid phagocytosis. *Cell* **2009**, *138*, 271–285. [CrossRef]
39. Fais, S.; Logozzi, M.; Lugini, L.; Federici, C.; Azzarito, T.; Zarovni, N.; Chiesi, A. Exosomes: The ideal nanovectors for biodelivery. *Biol. Chem.* **2013**, *394*, 1–15. [CrossRef]
40. Hernandez, P.A.; Gorlin, R.J.; Lukens, J.N.; Taniuchi, S.; Bohinjec, J.; Francois, F.; Klotman, M.E.; Diaz, G.A. Mutations in the chemokine receptor gene CXCR4 are associated with WHIM syndrome, a combined immunodeficiency disease. *Nat. Genet.* **2003**, *34*, 70–74. [CrossRef]
41. Liotta, L.A. An attractive force in metastasis. *Nature* **2001**, *410*, 24–25. [CrossRef] [PubMed]
42. Muller, A.; Homey, B.; Soto, H.; Ge, N.; Catron, D.; Buchanan, M.E.; McClanahan, T.; Murphy, E.; Yuan, W.; Wagner, S.N.; et al. Involvement of chemokine receptors in breast cancer metastasis. *Nature* **2001**, *410*, 50–56. [CrossRef] [PubMed]

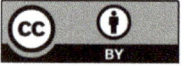

© 2019 by the authors. Licensee MDPI, Basel, Switzerland. This article is an open access article distributed under the terms and conditions of the Creative Commons Attribution (CC BY) license (http://creativecommons.org/licenses/by/4.0/).

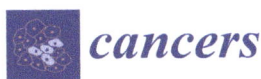

Article

Matryoshka-Type Liposomes Offer the Improved Delivery of Temoporfin to Tumor Spheroids

Ilya Yakavets [1,2,3], Marie Millard [1,2], Laureline Lamy [1,2], Aurelie Francois [1,2], Dietrich Scheglmann [4], Arno Wiehe [4], Henri-Pierre Lassalle [1,2], Vladimir Zorin [3,5] and Lina Bezdetnaya [1,2,*]

1. Centre de Recherche en Automatique de Nancy, Centre National de la Recherche Scientifique UMR 7039, Université de Lorraine, Campus Sciences, Boulevard des Aiguillette, 54506 Vandoeuvre-lès-Nancy, France
2. Research Department, Institut de Cancérologie de Lorraine, 6 avenue de Bourgogne, 54519 Vandoeuvre-lès-Nancy, France
3. Laboratory of Biophysics and Biotechnology, Belarusian State University, 4 Nezavisimosti Avenue, 220030 Minsk, Belarus
4. Biolitec research GmbH, Otto-Schott-Strasse 15, 07745 Jena, Germany
5. International Sakharov Environmental Institute, Belarusian State University, Dauhabrodskaja 23, 220030 Minsk, Belarus
* Correspondence: l.bolotine@nancy.unicancer.fr; Tel.: +33-(0)3-0859-8353

Received: 23 August 2019; Accepted: 12 September 2019; Published: 13 September 2019

Abstract: The balance between the amount of drug delivered to tumor tissue and the homogeneity of its distribution is a challenge in the efficient delivery of photosensitizers (PSs) in photodynamic therapy (PDT) of cancer. To date, many efforts have been made using various nanomaterials to efficiently deliver temoporfin (mTHPC), one of the most potent photosensitizers. The present study aimed to develop double-loaded matryoshka-type hybrid nanoparticles encapsulating mTHPC/cyclodextrin inclusion complexes in mTHPC-loaded liposomes. This system was expected to improve the transport of mTHPC to target tissues and to strengthen its accumulation in the tumor tissue. Double-loaded hybrid nanoparticles (DL-DCL) were prepared, characterized, and tested in 2D and 3D in vitro models and in xenografted mice in vivo. Our studies indicated that DL-DCL provided deep penetration of mTHPC into the multicellular tumor spheroids via cyclodextrin nanoshuttles once the liposomes had been destabilized by serum proteins. Unexpectedly, we observed similar PDT efficiency in xenografted HT29 tumors for liposomal mTHPC formulation (Foslip®) and DL-DCL.

Keywords: temoporfin; drug-in-cyclodextrin-in-liposome; hybrid nanoparticles; multicellular tumor spheroids; cyclodextrins; photodynamic therapy article; yet reasonably common within the subject discipline

1. Introduction

Nanomaterials are the cornerstone in the rapidly advancing field of nanotechnology, playing a crucial role in successful drug delivery at diseased sites [1]. To date, many nanoplatforms have been applied for the delivery of temoporfin (5,10,15,20-tetra(m-hydroxyphenyl)chlorin, mTHPC), one of the most promising photosensitizers (PSs) used in the photodynamic therapy (PDT) of solid cancers. Temoporfin has been marketed in the European Union since 2001 under the trade name Foscan® (biolitec pharma Ltd., Jena, Germany), and is indicated for the palliative treatment of head and neck squamous cell carcinoma [2]. Nanodelivery systems were supposed to overcome or improve the major constraints of mTHPC, such as low solubility, unfavorable pharmacokinetic profiles, and side effects (pain upon injection, skin photosensitivity) [3]. However, due to the complexity of drug distribution processes, the use of individual NPs offered neither optimal, leakage-free delivery of mTHPC to the tumor nor the local release of large amounts of mTHPC. At the same time, multifunctional nanomedicines featuring high drug loading capacity, controllable drug release, and real-time self-monitoring are attracting immense interest due to their potential to improve cancer therapy efficacy [4–6].

In the present study, we have suggested combining NPs into one nanoplatform as an advanced alternative strategy for mTHPC delivery. Recently, we reported the encapsulation of mTHPC-cyclodextrin (CD) supramolecular complex into liposomes, namely drug-in-cyclodextrin-in-liposome (DCL), as a prospective nanodelivery system for mTHPC [7]. The upgraded double-loaded mTHPC-DCLs (DL-DCL) contained mTHPC in both lipid and aqueous compartments of lipid vesicles. We hypothesized that such "matryoshka-type" hybrid liposomes would combine the advantages of each delivery system (Figure 1). Liposomes are effective containers for selective mTHPC delivery to target sites [8]. However, liposomes have limited penetration into deep tissue layers [9,10]. Alternatively, mTHPC/CDs inclusion complexes easily penetrate tumor tissue, thereby significantly increasing PS accumulation [11]. However, these supramolecular complexes are prone to dissociation in vivo, once diluted in the bloodstream [12]. Thus, we suggested that the coupling of both delivery systems intp one DL-DCL could restrain the dissociation of drug–mTHPC complexes, avoid rapid drug release, and favorably alter PS penetration into tumor tissues.

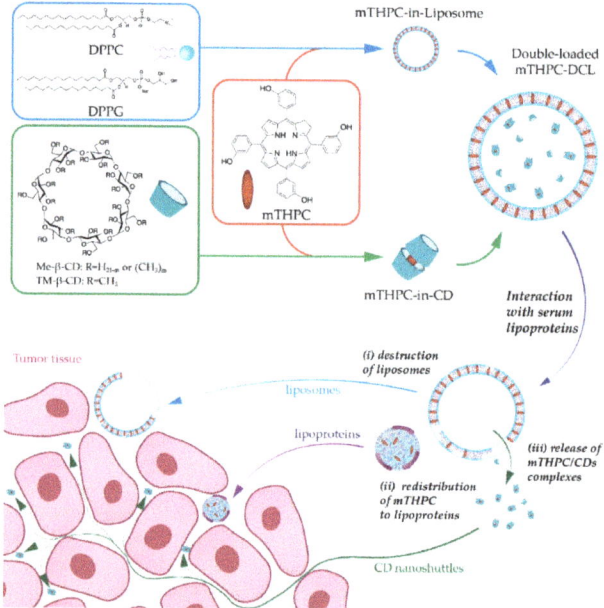

Figure 1. Double-loaded matryoshka-typemTHPC drug-in-cyclodextrin-in-liposomes (mTHPC-DCLs). Schematic illustration of the serum-mediated mTHPC release and penetration into the tumor tissue: (*i*) serum proteins disintegrate liposomal bilayer resulting in (*ii*) redistribution of lipid bilayer components (lipids and mTHPC) to serum lipoproteins (*iii*) as well as the release of water-soluble mTHPC/CD (cyclodextrin) inclusion complexes. Liposomes (blue arrow, Foslip®) and serum lipoproteins (purple arrow) interact only with outer layer cells, while CDs (green arrow) can penetrate the tumor tissue and deliver PS.

In the present work, we prepared and characterized DL-DCLs and tested these complexes in 2D and 3D tumor cell cultures. We focused on the study of double-loaded mTHPC-DCLs in 3D multicellular tumor spheroids in terms of PS penetration and accumulation. Finally, we conducted a preliminary study on double-loaded mTHPC-DCL efficacy in vivo in tumor-xenografted mice.

2. Results

2.1. Characterization

We prepared DL-DCLs with mTHPC encapsulated in the lipid membrane as well as in the aqueous core in the soluble form of inclusion complexes with β-CDs. Abbreviations MD and TD stand for DL-DCL with encapsulated mTHPC-Methyl-β-CD or mTHPC-Trimethyl-β-CD complexes, respectively. The hydrodynamic size, polydispersity index (PDI), and Zeta-potential of MD and TD were measured by dynamic light scattering. Both DL-DCLs had a narrow size distribution with a mean hydrodynamic diameter of 143.2 ± 1.5 nm for MD (PDI = 0.055 ± 0.033) and 122.9 ± 1.1 nm for TD (PDI = 0.040 ± 0.013) (Figure 2). The surface charge of MD and TD was negative, with Zeta potentials of −36.2 ± 4.3 mV and −37.5 ± 1.6 mV, respectively. It is worth noting that DL-DCLs have high colloidal stability (>3 months) (data not shown). The encapsulation efficiencies (EE) of mTHPC in MD and TD were estimated as 11% and 16%. As control NPs, we used a conventional liposomal mTHPC formulation (Foslip®) with a hydrodynamic size of 114.2 ± 1.0 nm (PDI = 0.110 ± 0.015) and a Zeta potential of −34.4 ± 4.3 mV.

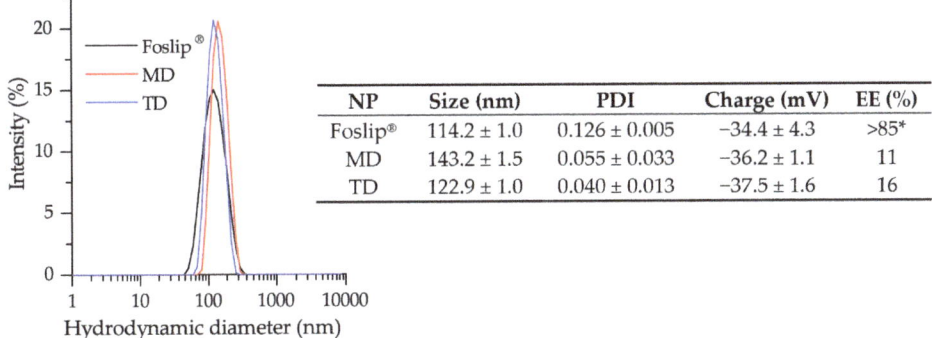

Figure 2. The hydrodynamic size of Foslip® (black) and DL-DCLs: MD (red) and TD (blue). Insert shows the physico-chemical characteristics of the NPs of hydrodynamic diameter (nm), polydispersity index (PDI), Z-potential (mV), and encapsulation efficiency (EE,%). *—taken from Reference [13]. Abbreviations MD and TD stand for DL-DCL with encapsulated mTHPC-Methyl-β-CD or mTHPC-Trimethyl-β-CD complexes, respectively.

Spectral characteristics of mTHPC-based nanoformulations in PBS are presented in Figure 3. All mTHPC formulations exhibited narrow spectral bands, indicating the monomeric state of mTHPC. The absorption spectra of Foslip®, MD, and TD in PBS were characterized by a Soret band (maximum at 416 nm) and four Q-bands with prominent peaks at 650 nm (Figure 3a). The extinction coefficients of mTHPC in DL-DCLs were slightly higher (35,400 $M^{-1}cm^{-1}$ and 37,200 $M^{-1}cm^{-1}$) than that of Foslip® (31,100 $M^{-1}cm^{-1}$). The mTHPC fluorescence was emitted at 652 nm for all NPs. The relative fluorescence quantum yield (FY) of mTHPC encapsulated in DL-DCLs was comparable with Foslip® and was only 20% lower than a standard mTHPC ethanol solution. Figure 3b exhibits the excitation fluorescence spectra of mTHPC in various NPs in the Soret band region, which is considered to be sensitive to the binding of mTHPC with β-CDs [14]. The relative fluorescence in a short wavelength shoulder was significantly increased in DL-DCLs compared with Foslip® due to the formation of inclusion complexes between mTHPC and β-CD derivatives. To assess the changes in the shape of spectral band, we calculated I_1/I_2, where I_1 and I_2 stand for the fluorescence intensities at 407 nm and 418 nm excitation, respectively. The calculated I_1/I_2 ratios for mTHPC in MD and TD were 0.88 and 1.00, while that of Foslip® was 0.80 (Figure 3b, insert). The microenvironment of mTHPC in NPs could also be characterized using fluorescence parameters such as fluorescence anisotropy and photoinduced fluorescence quenching (PIQ). Consistent with our previous report [13], the fluorescence anisotropy (r)

of mTHPC in Foslip® was 6.2 ± 0.4%, and the PIQ was 12 ± 2 % (Figure 3b, insert). In DL-DCL, both fluorescence anisotropy and PIQ values were increased, providing r = 7.3 ± 0.6% and PIQ = 21 ± 5% for MD, and r = 9.9 ± 0.7% and PIQ = 33 ± 5% for TD. Based on these values, we assessed that about 70% of mTHPC in the DL-DCLs was attached to the lipid bilayer, while 30% of PS was bound to CDs in the inner aqueous cores of the lipid vesicles.

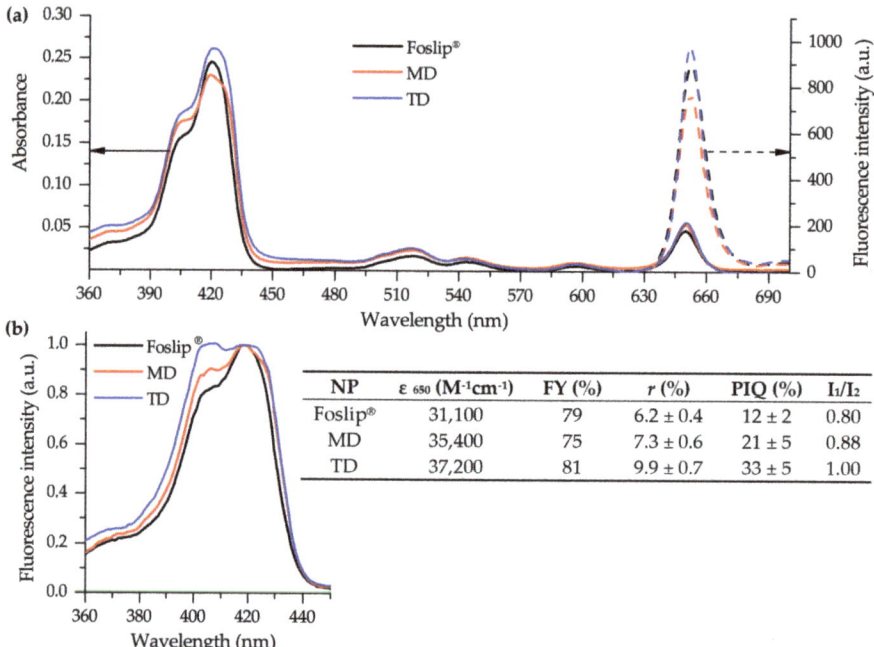

Figure 3. Spectral characteristics of Foslip® (black), MD (red), and TD (blue) in PBS. (**a**) Absorbance (solid line) and fluorescence emission (dotted line) spectra (λ_{ex} = 420 nm); (**b**) normalized fluorescence excitation spectra (λ_{em} = 652 nm). mTHPC concentration was 1.5 µM. Insert shows the main spectral characteristics of NPs, such as extinction coefficient at 650 nm (ε_{650}); FY—fluorescence yield, relative to the fluorescence of mTHPC in ethanol; r—the degree of fluorescence anisotropy; PIQ—the degree of photoinduced quenching; I_1/I_2—the ratio of Soret band components (I_1 and I_2 were measured under excitation at 407 nm and 418 nm, respectively, and emission at 652 nm).

2.2. Two-Dimensional (2D) Monolayer Cell Culture

The cellular uptake of mTHPC delivered by Foslip® or DL-DCLs was analyzed by flow cytometry. Flow cytometry histograms of HT29 human colon adenocarcinoma monolayer cells treated for 24 h with Foslip®, MD, and TD (1.5 µM) are presented in Figure 4a. All profiles had a narrow homogeneous distribution. The accumulation of mTHPC in HT29 monolayer was slightly lower for TD compared with MD and Foslip®. The estimated mean cellular fluorescent intensities for Foslip® and MD were 140 ± 14 a.u. and 149 ± 21 a.u. ($p > 0.05$), respectively, while that for TD was significantly lower (80 ± 9 a.u.; $p < 0.05$).

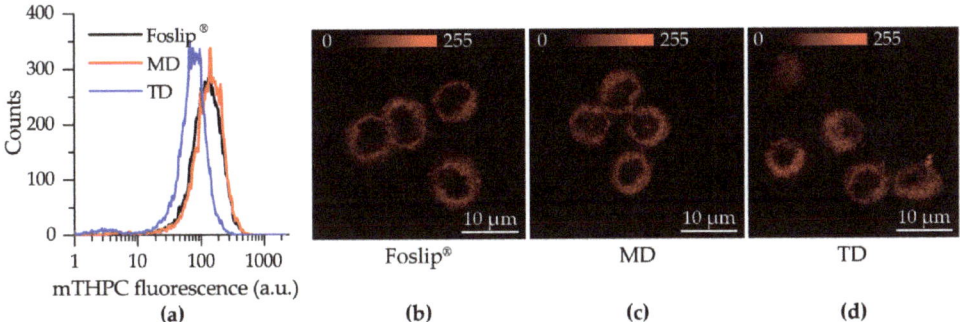

Figure 4. (a) Flow cytometry histograms of HT29 monolayer cells treated with Foslip® (black), MD, (red) and TD (blue) for 24 h; (b–d) Typical confocal images of mTHPC fluorescence in HT29 monolayer cells at 3 h post-incubation with (b) Foslip®, (c) MD, and (d) TD. Scale bar: 10 µm. The concentration of mTHPC was 1.5 µM. Serum concentration was 2%.

Intracellular localization of mTHPC in HT29 monolayer cells was evaluated using confocal microscopy after 3 h of incubation (Figure 4b–d). No remarkable difference in intracellular mTHPC localization between Foslip® and DL-DCLs was observed. All NPs exhibited a similar mTHPC fluorescence pattern in cells, characterized by diffuse fluorescence in the cytoplasm outside both the nucleus and outer plasma membrane. Similar localization patterns were observed in human pharynx squamous cell carcinoma (FaDu) (Figure S1).

2.3. Three-Dimensional (3D) Multicellular Tumor Spheroids

2.3.1. Accumulation and Distribution

We performed chemical extraction of mTHPC from HT29 spheroids after 3, 6, and 24 h incubation with Foslip® or DL-DCLs (4.5 µM) (Figure 5a). Accumulation of mTHPC in spheroids for all NPs increased continuously over 24 h. At short incubation times (3 and 6 h), mTHPC accumulation was slightly but significantly higher in TD-treated spheroids compared to those treated with Foslip® ($p > 0.05$). At 24 h incubation, the highest amount of mTHPC was observed in MD-treated spheroids (17.3 ± 2.9 ng/spheroid), although it was not significant compared with TD and Foslip® (14.6 ± 2.3 and 11.9 ± 2.6 ng/spheroid, respectively; $p > 0.05$).

Afterwards, we assessed the accumulation of mTHPC in individual cells in spheroids using flow cytometry analysis (Figure 5b–e and Figures S2 and S3). Figure 5b–d displays the kinetics of mTHPC uptake in HT29 spheroids treated with various nanoformulations. We observed that Foslip® continuously accumulated from 3 h incubation, but only in a small fraction of cells, thus resulting in a strongly heterogeneous distribution of mTHPC across the spheroids. On the other hand, spheroids treated with MD demonstrated a more homogeneous distribution, especially visible after 24 h of incubation (Figure 5e). Figure 5e displays a typical distribution of mTHPC in HT29 spheroids treated with nanoformulations, while the histograms from independent experiments are presented in Figure S2. Finally, the fluorescence in TD treated spheroids represented one narrow peak in the histogram irrespective of incubation time, indicating an almost homogeneous mTHPC distribution across spheroids. FaDu spheroids were assessed after 24 h incubation with nanoformulations (Figure S3). Foslip® and TD provided distribution profiles in FaDu spheroids similar to those in HT29 spheroids, while the MD distribution was more heterogenous compared with that in HT29.

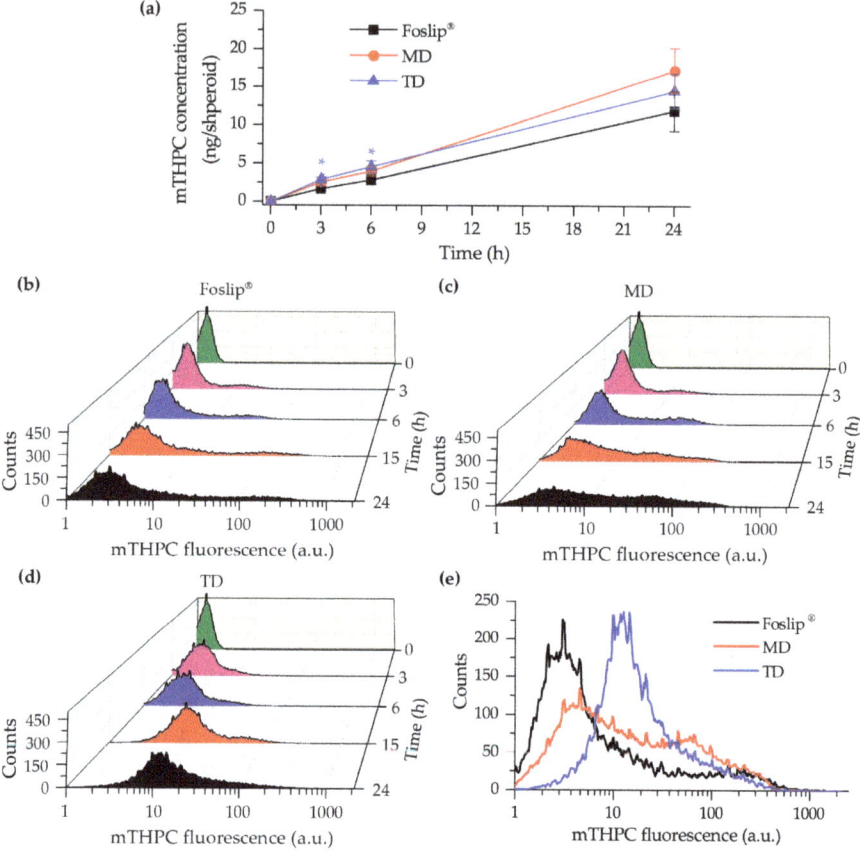

Figure 5. (a) Kinetics of mTHPC uptake in HT29 spheroids after incubation with Foslip® (black), MD (red), and TD (blue) using chemical extraction in absolute ethanol. The data are presented as mean ± standard deviation. * $p < 0.05$ compared to Foslip®; (b–e) Typical flow cytometry histograms of trypsinized spheroids treated with (b) Foslip®, (c) MD, and (d) TD at 3, 6, 15, and 24 h post-incubation. (e) Typical flow cytometry histograms of HT29 spheroids treated with Foslip® (black), MD (red), and TD (blue) for 24 h. mTHPC concentration was 4.5 µM. Serum concentration was 2%.

2.3.2. Penetration

To confirm the results of the flow cytometry-based distribution, we analyzed cryosections of spheroids treated with NPs for 24 h using laser scanning confocal microscopy (Figure 6a). For a better comparison of mTHPC distribution in spheroids, the images were completed with surface plots of fluorescence patterns (Figure 6b). As seen in Figure 6a,b, Foslip® and MD displayed strong mTHPC fluorescence only on the periphery of the spheroids, while for TD, mTHPC fluorescence was observed across the whole spheroid, demonstrating complete PS penetration. Similar patterns of mTHPC distribution were observed in FaDu spheroids treated with Foslip® and TD (Figure S4). The comparison of linear profiles demonstrated a slightly deeper penetration of MD in HT29 spheroids compared with Folsip®. However, the mTHPC fluorescence signal at 100 µm from the periphery of the spheroids was undetectable for both formulations. At the same time, the fluorescence of mTHPC delivered by TD was almost constant throughout the whole spheroid depth.

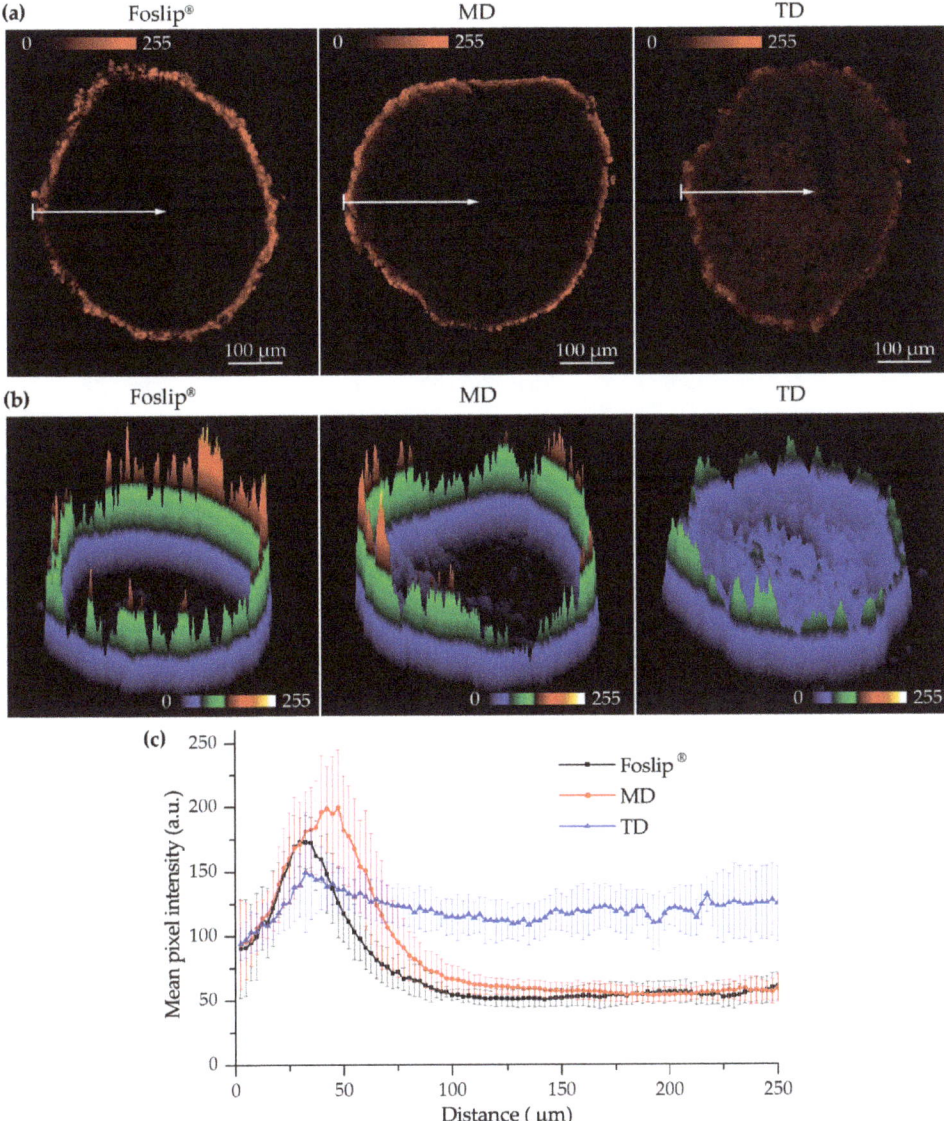

Figure 6. (**a**) Typical fluorescence images and corresponding (**b**) surface plots of mTHPC fluorescence in HT29 spheroids after 24 h incubation with various mTHPC formulations (Foslip®, MD, and TD); (**c**) penetration profiles of Foslip® (black), MD (red), and TD (blue) in HT29 spheroids after 24 h. The data are presented as mean ± standard deviation obtained from $n = 7$ spheroids. mTHPC concentration was 4.5 µM. Serum concentration was 2%. mTHPC fluorescence is displayed in red color (2D images) and in pseudo-colors (3D surface plots).

2.3.3. Serum-Induced Release of CDs

In order to confirm the release of CDs upon serum-induced destabilization of the liposomal vesicles, we analyzed mTHPC fluorescence intensities in the medium supplemented with serum at different concentrations (Figure 7a). After 24 h incubation of spheroids with NPs, the collected supernatant was centrifugated, filtered, and analyzed by gel exclusion chromatography. Figure 7b,c represents the distribution of mTHPC between eluted fractions. Based on the calibration experiment (data not shown), the elution range of liposomes and DL-DCLs was 30–45 mL, serum protein fractions were eluted at 50–90 mL, and mTHPC-CD complexes, as the smallest in size, were eluted only at 90–105 mL. The estimated percentage of mTHPC bound to each fraction is displayed in Figure 7d. According to these data, mTHPC was efficiently released from Foslip® and 50% of PS was bound to serum proteins in the medium enriched with 2% of serum. When the percentage of serum was increased up to 9%, only 15% of mTHPC was detected in liposomes. On the other hand, both DL-DCLs contained higher mTHPC concentrations after 24 h incubation with spheroids compared to Foslip®. The remaining fraction of mTHPC in MD and TD for 2% of serum was 79% and 76%, respectively, and 48% and 50% for 9% serum. Most importantly, we directly detected the presence of mTHPC-CD complexes in the medium after incubation of the spheroids with TD, and the fraction of mTHPC-CD complexes increased from 13% to 23% when the serum content in the medium increased from 2% to 9%. Alternatively, in the case of MD, the released mTHPC was bound to serum proteins only.

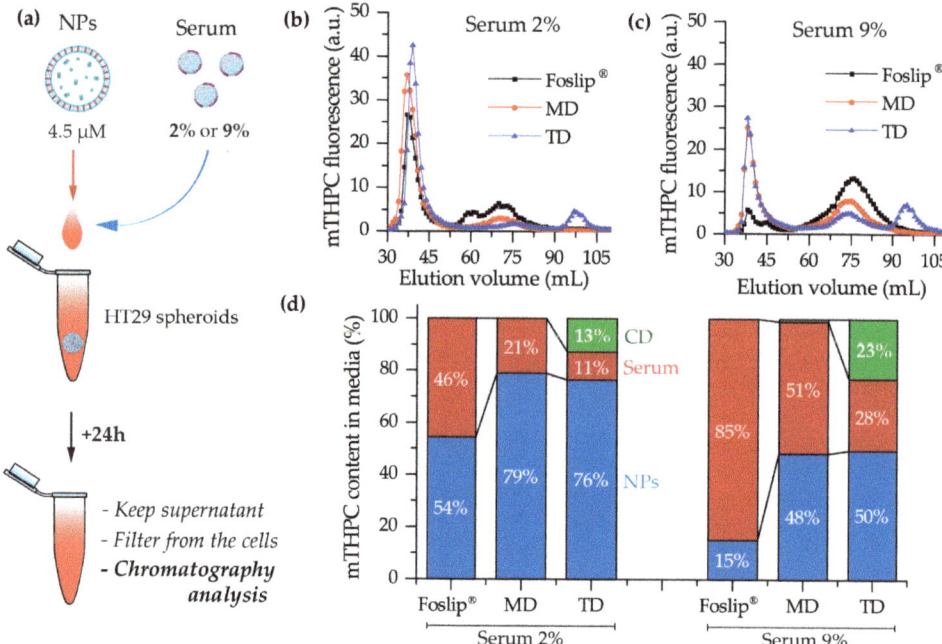

Figure 7. (a) Scheme of the experiment; (b,c) chromatography histograms of culture medium after 24 h incubation of HT29 spheroids with mTHPC (4.5 µM) in nanoformulations in the presence of (b) 2% and (c) 9% of serum; (d) the percentage of mTHPC bound with NPs (blue) or serum proteins (red) and in complexes with CDs (green).

2.4. PDT

Considering that better penetration and distribution of mTHPC delivered by DL-DCLs could improve PDT efficiency, we assessed the viability of HT29 spheroid cells using a propidium iodide fluorescent probe. Spheroids, treated with NPs for 24 h were irradiated at 40 J/cm^2 (90 mW/cm^2), trypsinated 6 h later, and analyzed by flow cytometry. Cell viability in control (no-drug, no-light) and (no-light) groups was about 82% for all NPs. PDT resulted in a significant decrease in cell viability, yielding about 40% necrotic cells. Surprisingly, photoinduced necrosis was similar for all types of NPs (39 ± 2% vs. 40 ± 4% vs. 41 ± 2% for Foslip®, MD, and TD, respectively; $p > 0.05$).

We further studied PDT tumor response in vivo in a xenografted mice model. Kaplan–Meier plots of tumor response to Foslip®- and TD–PDT are presented in Figure 8. The tumor growth delay was about 30.7 days for Foslip® and 26.6 days for TD ($p > 0.05$). For both NPs, the response was significantly different from the control no-light (n.l.) groups ($p < 0.05$).

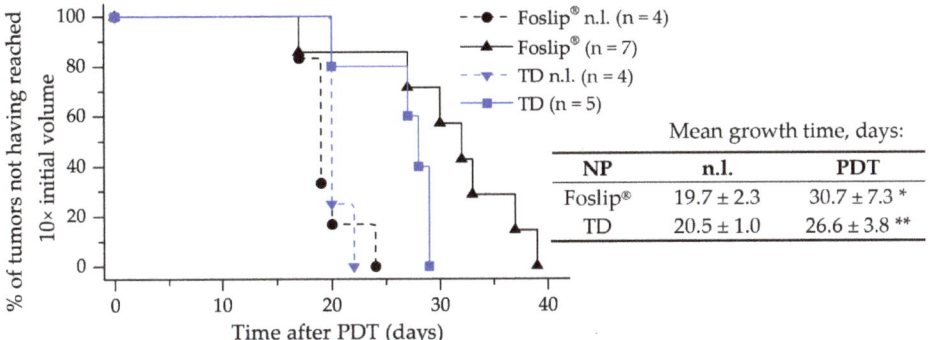

Figure 8. Kaplan–Meier plots of HT29 tumor growth delay and mean tumor growth time (time to reach 10× the initial tumor volume) of control no-light (n.l.) groups and mice after PDT with Foslip® and TD at 24 h of drug-light-interval. * statistically different from Foslip® n.l. control group, $p < 0.05$; ** statistically different from TD n.l. control group, $p < 0.05$.

3. Discussion

To date, hybrid NPs, combining several nanomaterials in one, have attracted increasing attention as anti-cancer delivery systems [15]. The careful selection of the combined nanomaterials could result in a considerable synergistic effect overcoming the individual nanostructures' limitations. In the case of mTHPC, a synergy could be achieved by a coupling of CD-based nanoshuttles and liposomes. mTHPC exhibits an extremely strong affinity to methylated β-CDs (10^6–10^7 M^{-1} for Me-β-CD and TM-β-CD, respectively [16]) leading to the unique possibility of altering mTHPC biodistribution via a nanoshuttle mechanism [11,17]. At the same time, liposomal formulations of mTHPC display selective delivery of PS to tumor tissue [8]. CDs could be regarded as an added value to mTHPC-based liposomes, and as such, could increase drug loading capacity, entrapment efficiency, prolong the circulation time of the drug in the bloodstream, reduce toxicity, and finally provide controlled release [18,19]. Thus, we supposed that such a "matryoshka-doll" nanostructure could be a potent delivery system, providing both passive tumor targeting by liposomes and deep penetration of mTHPC/CD complexes into the tumor tissue (Figure 1).

Recently, we optimized the composition of mTHPC-DCLs, selecting two of the most potent DCLs based on methylated β-CDs [7]. In the present study, the lipid bilayers of selected DCLs were additionally loaded with lipophilic mTHPC, achieving DL-DCLs. Physico-chemical characteristics (size, PDI, charge, and colloidal stability) of DL-DCLs were similar to those of single-loaded DCLs [7], and comparable with liposomal mTHPC formulation Foslip® (Figure 2). According to the preparation technique, the ratio between aqueous volume of liposomes and void volume during the liposome preparation was low, explaining the low EE values of mTHPC in DL-DCLs [7,20]. The complete monomerization of mTHPC in all NPs was confirmed by absorption spectra (Figure 3a), and double encapsulation of mTHPC in DCLs was established using fluorescence spectroscopy (Figure 3b). The presence of mTHPC/CD complexes led to the increase of I_1/I_2 ratio [14], demonstrating $I_1/I_2 = 0.88$ and 1.00 for MD and TD, respectively, while in the case of Foslip®, I_1/I_2 was 0.8 (Figure 3b). At the same time, the high loading of mTHPC in the lipid bilayer resulted in fluorescence quenching [13,21], causing the decrease of FY, PIQ, and r values (Figure 3b, insert). Overall, 30% of mTHPC was encapsulated in CD complexes, while the fraction of PS in the lipid bilayer was 70%.

We further tested DL-DCLs in 2D and 3D in vitro tumor models. In 2D monolayer cell cultures, the behavior of both double-loaded mTHPC-DCLs was similar to that of Foslip® (Figure 4 and Figure S1), while in 3D multicellular spheroids, we clearly demonstrated the benefits of matryoshka-type hybrid liposomes against conventional lipid vesicles. The 3D multicellular tumor spheroids more closely mimicked the native tumor environment, representing the tumor stroma tissue and offering better prediction potential when testing the penetration ability of nanomedicines [22]. The data of chemical extraction of mTHPC from spheroids demonstrated an almost similar amount of mTHPC at various incubation times (Figure 5a). However, detailed study using flow cytometry showed different profiles of mTHPC accumulation in the spheroid cells for DL-DCLs and Foslip®. The spheroids treated with TD displayed a homogeneous distribution between all cells at all time points for both HT29 (Figure 5d) and FaDu spheroids (Figure S2), while for MD and Foslip®, the accumulation of mTHPC was mainly associated with the PS uptake in a small fraction of cells (Figure 5b,c and Figure S2). At 24 h post-incubation, MD exhibited a slightly more homogeneous PS distribution in HT29 spheroids than Foslip® (Figure 6). The fluorescence imaging data of spheroid frozen-cut sections confirmed the almost homogeneous distribution of mTHPC delivered by TD in both types of spheroid cells (Figure 6 and Figure S3). In the case of TD, the mTHPC fluorescence signal was uniform for the whole spheroid, while for MD and Foslip®, a strong peripheral fluorescence signal dropped to background values at 50 and 100 μM from the spheroid periphery, respectively. In all probability, the observed effect was related to the presence of mTHPC/CDs in the media due to DL-DCL disintegration, as has been previously observed for Foslip® [10,23]. Indeed, in the case of TD, chromatography analysis of culture media after 24 h incubation of NPs with tumor spheroids demonstrated the presence of mTHPC/CD complexes. To confirm the serum-induced destruction of DL-DCLs, we demonstrated the increase of the mTHPC-TM-β-CD fraction in the medium supplemented with 9% of serum compared to 2% (Figure 7). It is worth noting that the MD-treated samples contained a similar amount of mTHPC in NPs, while all released mTHPC in the medium was localized only in serum proteins. Compared with TM-β-CD, Me-β-CDs possess less affinity to mTHPC [17]; thus, the equilibrium distribution of mTHPC is shifted to serum proteins [18]. Therefore, we suppose that the lifetime of mTHPC-Me-β-CDs was too short to penetrate the deep layers of spheroids, and mTHPC released from the MD was quickly redistributed to both serum proteins and the nearest tumor cells by Me-β-CDs, while long-living mTHPC-TM-β-CD complexes could easily penetrate to the deep tissue regions.

Finally, we assessed the PDT efficiency of TD and MD in 3D multicellular tumor spheroids in vitro, and of TD in xenografted mice in vivo. Despite the remarkable difference in penetration profiles, PDT-induced cell death in spheroids treated with TD and MD was similar to Foslip®. The same tendency was observed in the xenografted mice model: the difference in mean tumor growth delay for both TD and Foslip® was about 30 days (Figure 8). We likely did not achieve the desired balance between the accumulation and distribution of PS in the tumor. We suggest that increasing the TD concentration could be helpful in exceeding the threshold of intracellular PS accumulation needed for efficient DCL-PDT photokilling.

4. Materials and Methods

4.1. Materials

mTHPC and its liposomal formulation (Foslip®) were kindly provided by biolitec research GmbH (Jena, Germany). The stock solution of mTHPC (2 mM) was prepared in methanol and kept at 4 °C in the dark. Foslip®, based on dipalmitoylphosphatidylcholine (DPPC) and dipalmitoylphosphatidylglycerol (DPPG) liposomes with a mTHPC/lipid ratio of 1:12 (mol/mol), was prepared by solubilizing powder in ultrapure water (UPW, Milli-Q® Advantage A10® System, Millipore, Eschborn, Germany) to a final mTHPC concentration of 2 mM.

Random methyl-β-cyclodextrin (Me-β-CD; product code CY-2004.1,29; substitution degree of 12, average molecular weight 1135 Da) and heptakis(2,3,6-tri-O-methyl)-β-cyclodextrin (TM-β-CD;

product code CY-2003,34; molecular weight 1429.6 Da) were purchased from CYCLOLAB R&D. Ltd., (Budapest, Hungary). DPPC and DPPG were purchased from Sigma (USA).

4.2. DL-DCL Preparation

DCLs were prepared by the thin lipid film hydration method, as described previously [7]. Briefly, inclusion complexes of mTHPC with β-CDs were formed using the solvent co-evaporation method in UPW. DPPC/DPPG liposomes loaded with mTHPC were prepared by membrane extrusion technique according to the previously published procedure, yielding unilamellar liposomes [24]. These liposomes contained DPPC and DPPG at a molar ratio of 9:1, with a final lipid concentration of 15 mg/mL. To obtain DL-DCLs, mTHPC was added at the step of the preparation of lipid mixture at a molar drug/lipid ratio of 1:15, and mTHPC/β-CD inclusion complexes were encapsulated at the lipid film hydration step. The purification of DCLs from the non-encapsulated mTHPC/β-CDs in the medium was performed using a minicolumn chromatography technique [25].

4.3. Cell Lines

HT29 human colon adenocarcinoma cell line was purchased from ATCC (LGC Promochem, Molsheim, France). FaDu (human pharynx squamous cell carcinoma) cell line was purchased from ATCC (Cat. No: ATCC1 HTB-43™). Cells were cultured in phenol red-free Roswell Park Memorial Institute 1640 medium (RPMI-1640, Invitrogen™, Carlsbad, California, USA), supplemented with 9% (vol/vol) heat-inactivated fetal bovine serum (Sigma-Aldrich, St. Louis, MO, USA), penicillin (10,000 IU) streptomycin (10,000 mg/mL) and 1% (vol/vol) 0.2 M glutamine (Invitrogen™, Carlsbad, California, USA). Cells were kept as a monolayer culture in a humidified incubator (5% CO_2) at 37 °C. Cell culture was reseeded every week to ensure exponential growth.

4.4. Multicellular Tumor Spheroid Model

HT29 MCTSs were initiated as previously described [26]. Briefly, flasks coated with 1% L-agarose were seeded with 5×10^4 HT29 cells/mL. After three days, cellular aggregates were transferred into spinner flasks (Integra Biosciences, Cergy Pontoise, France) containing 125 mL RPMI-1640 medium supplemented with 9% FBS. Spinner flasks were placed under constant agitation at 75 rpm at 37 °C (5% CO_2, humidified atmosphere) for 15 days. Spheroids were filtered to approximatively 500 µm in diameter before conducting experiments.

MCTSs were generated from FaDu cells using the liquid overlay technique (LOT), as described previously [27]. Briefly, 100 µL of FaDu cells (5×10^4 cells/ml) and 100 µL of full RPMI medium were added to each well of a 96-well plate previously coated with 1% agarose (w/v in water), and cultured at 37 °C, 5% CO_2 for 5 days before being taken into experiments.

For dissociation, spheroids were transferred into a 12-well plate, washed twice with PBS and further incubated with 0.025% trypsin (GIBCO™, ThermoFisher, Waltham, MA, USA) and 0.01% ethylenediaminetetraacetic acid (GIBCO™, ThermoFisher, Waltham, MA, USA). For complete trypsinization, the plate with spheroids was placed on a rotatory shaker (60 rpm) for 30 min in subdued light. After dissociation, trypsin action was inhibited by the addition of 3 mL complete culture medium (9% FBS), and the cell suspension was centrifuged to a pellet and further re-suspended in a fresh medium.

4.5. Fluorescence Staining

For in vitro cell experiments, stock NP solutions were diluted in RPMI-1640 supplemented with 2% heat-inactivated fetal bovine serum (FBS, Life Technologies, Carlsbad, California, USA) to obtain the final mTHPC concentration of 1.5 µM for 2D monolayer cells and 4.5 µM for 3D tumor spheroid experimentation.

For the 2D monolayer cell culture, cells (5×10^4 cells/mL) were seeded in 24-well plates for 72 h and then incubated with Foslip®, MD, or TD (1.5 µM). In the case of 3D cell culture, before incubation with mTHPC NPs (4.5 µM), spheroids were washed with serum-free RPMI-1640 medium. PS incubation was performed in the dark at 37 °C in a humidified 5% CO_2 air atmosphere.

4.6. Animal Model

All experiments were performed in accordance with animal care guidelines from the European Union and were approved by the appropriate authority. The animal project registered under the number (#2438) received a favorable assessment from the Ethics Committee and was approved by the French Higher Education and Research Minister. All procedures involving animals were performed under general anesthesia with inhaled isoflurane (Vetflurane; Virbac, France) using a Univentor 400 anesthesia unit (Genestil, Royaucourt, France). Mice were housed in filtered air cabinets with a 12 h light/dark cycle at 22–24 °C and 50% humidity, provided with food and water ad libitum, and manipulated following aseptic procedures. Female NMRInu/nu mice (Janvier, St Berthevin, France) aged 9–10 weeks were used, with a mean bodyweight of 30 ± 3 g. Mice were inoculated subcutaneously in the left flank with 8×10^6 exponentially growing HT29 cells and the experiments were initiated 5–7 days after inoculation when the tumors reached 50 mm^3 in volume.

4.7. Analytical Techniques

4.7.1. Spectroscopy

Absorption measurements were recorded with a Lambda 35 spectrometer (Perkin Elmer, USA) and fluorescence measurements were conducted with a LS55B spectrofluorometer (PerkinElmer, USA) equipped with polarizers, thermostated cuvette compartments, and magnetic stirring for polarization experiments. The concentrations of mTHPC in DL-DCLs and Foslip® were estimated spectroscopically (λ_{em} = 652 nm) by dissolving nanoparticles in methanol. DL-DCLs were previously purified by minicolumn chromatography. Fluorescence quantum yield and photoinduced fluorescence quenching were measured as previously described (λ_{ex}: 416 nm; λ_{em}: 652 nm) [15]. The measurements of mTHPC fluorescence anisotropy were performed as described earlier (λ_{ex}: 430 nm; λ_{em}: 652 nm) [15]. EE of mTHPC in DCLs was measured spectroscopically (λ_{em}: 652 nm) immediately after extrusion and purification, as previously described [7].

The hydrodynamic diameter of NPs, polydispersity index, and Z-potential were determined using photon-correlated spectroscopy by a Zetasizer Nano ZS (Malvern Instruments, UK) as previously reported [7].

4.7.2. Flow Cytometry

Flow cytometry analysis was performed using a FACSCalibur (BD, Franklin Lakes, NJ, USA), equipped with lasers emitting at 488 nm and 633 nm. Flow cytometry histograms were obtained from the suspension of cells after dissociation of 50 NP-treated spheroids. The fluorescence of mTHPC was detected in the fluorescence channel FL4 with a 661 ± 16 nm filter under excitation at 633 nm. Propidium iodide (PI) fluorescence was detected in the FL2 channel with a 585 ± 42 nm filter (excitation at 488 nm). Data analysis was carried out using Flowing Software (Turku Centre for Biotechnology, Turku, Finland).

4.7.3. Fluorescence Microscopy

HT29 cells (3×10^4 cells/mL) were plated into Lab-Tek II chamber Slide (Roskilde, Denmark), incubated in the dark at 37 °C with 1.5 µM of mTHPC in different formulations for 3 h and then rinsed with PBS. mTHPC fluorescence was observed with a confocal laser-scanning microscope (Leica SP5 X AOBS LCSM, Leica microsystem, Wetzlar, Germany). For the 2D monolayer cell culture, fluorescence images were recorded using an oil immersion ×40 objective. The 3D tumor spheroids were embedded into a resin Shandon™ Cryomatrix™ (ThermoFisher, Waltham, MA, USA), frozen, cut, and 20 µm thick cryosections were further analyzed by confocal microscopy (×10 objective). Fluorescence of mTHPC in FaDu 2D monolayer cells and frozen-cut cryosections of FaDu spheroids was analyzed using an upright epifluorescence microscope (AX-70 Provis, Olympus, France). The fluorescence images were obtained using a filter set at 405–445 nm excitation associated with a 570 nm dichroic mirror and a 590 nm long-pass emission filter for fluorescence measurements.

Analysis of the images was performed with ImageJ (NIH, USA) software. To estimate the penetration profile of dye in the spheroids, special macros were proposed. Briefly, the spheroid area was divided into 100 concentric rims, with the diameter decreasing in a linear way. After that we calculated the mean intensity of pixels in each rim. The final profiles were plotted as mean ± standard deviation from different cryo-sections ($n = 7$).

4.7.4. Uptake in Spheroids

mTHPC uptake in spheroids was measured by chemical extraction of mTHPC. After 3, 6, and 24 h incubation with NPs (4.5 µM), spheroids were dissociated and individual cells were subjected to the extraction of mTHPC with ethanol (99.6%) as previously described [11]. Briefly, after sonication (15 min) and centrifugation (5 min, 1500 rpm), mTHPC fluorescence in the supernatant was assessed (λ_{ex}: 420 nm; λ_{em}: 652 nm).

4.7.5. Chromatography

Chromatographic experiments were performed on a Sigma 1.5 × 75 cm column filled with Sepharose CL-6B gel (GE Healthcare, USA) pre-equilibrated with PBS, with a total bed volume of 150 mL. HT29 tumor spheroids were incubated in RPMI-1640 media which was supplemented with 2% and 9% FBS. The NPs were added at final mTHPC concentration of 4.5 µM. After 24 h incubation, the supernatant was centrifuged (5 min, 1500 rpm), filtered using a 450 µm Millex® – HV syringe driven filter unit (Sigma-Aldrich, St. Louis, MO, USA), and injected into the column using a three-way connector. Fractions of 1 mL were collected by an automated fraction collector. The column was stored at room temperature and separation was carried out in a partially light-protected environment to avoid mTHPC photobleaching. Fractions with elution volumes from 25 to 120 mL were collected and analyzed for mTHPC content using a SAFAS Xenius XM (SAFAS, Monaco, France) spectrofluorometer, as previously reported [28]. The mTHPC content in the chromatographic fractions was estimated by measurements the fluorescence intensity after the addition of 0.2% Triton® X-100 to the samples. The analysis of chromatography histograms was performed using Origin software (OriginLab, Northampton, MA, USA).

4.8. Photoirradiation of Spheroids

HT29 spheroids were transferred from the spinner flask to 12-well plates and incubated with NPs for 24 h (4.5 µM). Spheroids were then washed and subjected to irradiation. Irradiation was performed at 652 nm with a Ceralas PDT diode laser (CeramOptec GmbH, Bonn, Germany) at 40 J/cm^2 (fluence rate of 90 mW/cm^2). Control spheroids were exposed to mTHPC only (drug, no light). The viability of the spheroid cells was assessed by propidium iodide probe. Spheroids were trypsinated 6 h post-PDT and the obtained cell suspension was stained with 1 µg/mL PI (Biolegend, San Diego, CA, USA) for 15 min in the dark at 37 °C, rinsed, and analyzed by flow cytometry.

4.9. Animal Experiments

NPs were administered intravenously by a tail vein injection at a dose of 0.15 mg/kg of mTHPC. Following the injection, mice were kept in the dark, and experiments were undertaken with minimal ambient light. Tumor irradiation was performed at 652 nm with a Ceralas PDT diode laser. The mice were treated 24 h post-administration at a fluence of 10 J/cm^2 and the fluence rate of 100 mW/cm^2. Just after PDT and 24 h later, mice received analgesia by subcutaneous injection of a mixture of 0.08 mg/kg buprenorphine (Axience, Pantin, France) and 1 mg/kg of the non-steroid anti-inflammatory Metacam (Boehringer Ingelhein, Ingelheim, Germany) Mice were kept in the dark for 7 days after PDT. Three times per week, the perpendicular diameters of the tumors were measured to document tumor growth. Tumor volume (V) was calculated using the equation: $V = W^2 \times Y/2$, where (W) and (Y) are the smaller and larger diameters. Mice were sacrificed when tumor volume reached the ethical size of 1000 mm^3.

4.10. Statistics

The data from at least three independent experiments are presented as mean ± standard deviation. The data were evaluated using nonparametric Mann–Whitney U test (StatView^{TM} software) with a significance level of $p < 0.05$.

5. Conclusions

The complexity of drug distribution processes requires innovative approaches in designing drug delivery platforms. Hybrid delivery systems have proven to be a powerful tool capable of combining the benefits of individual NPs intp one nanoplatform. Our study confirmed the advantage of double-loaded mTHPC-DCLs over a conventional mTHPC liposomal formulation (Foslip®) in terms of tumor tissue penetration. Altogether, the proposed matryoshka-type lipid vesicles releasing mTHPC/CD complexes illustrated an optimal PS distribution in in vitro 3D models of tumor tissue.

Unexpectedly, we did not find phototoxic benefits of matryoshka-type liposomes over Foslip® in multicellular spheroids in vitro or in an animal experiment in vivo, at least under our experimental conditions. Our ongoing studies address different experimental settings, aiming for matryoshka system optimization in preclinical models. One of the possible solutions is the incorporation of stimulus-response moieties in liposomes to promote the release of CD nanoshuttles at the target site.

Supplementary Materials: The following are available online at http://www.mdpi.com/2072-6694/11/9/1366/s1, Figure S1: Typical epifluorescence images of mTHPC fluorescence in FaDu monolayer cells at 3 h post-incubation with Foslip®, MD, and TD; Figure S2: Flow cytometry histograms of HT29 spheroids treated with Foslip®, MD, and TD for 24 h. Figure S3: Typical flow cytometry histograms of FaDu spheroids treated with Foslip®, MD, and TD for 24 h; Figure S4: Typical brightfield/fluorescence overlay images of mTHPC in FaDu spheroid cryosections after 24 h incubation with various mTHPC formulations (Foslip®, MD, and TD).

Author Contributions: I.Y. designed and performed the experiments and drafted the manuscript, M.M., L.L. and A.F. performed the experiments; H.-P.L. contributed to manuscript editing, D.S. and A.W. contributed to manuscript editing and validated the manuscript; V.Z. and L.B. participated in the conceptualization and supervision of the work. All authors read and approved the final manuscript.

Funding: This work was supported by the Institut de Cancérologie de Lorraine, French "Ligue Nationale contre le Cancer (CCIR-GE)", Belarusian Republican Foundation for Fundamental Research (BRFFR) [grant numbers: M17MC-028, M18MB-002] and the Ministry of Education of the Republic.

Acknowledgments: The authors are grateful to IBISA platform for the acquisition of confocal images and Platform of Biophysics and Structural Biology (UMS 2008 IBSLor, UL-CNRS-INSERM) for the access to photon correlation spectroscopy.

Conflicts of Interest: The authors declare no conflict of interest.

References

1. Patra, J.K.; Das, G.; Fraceto, L.F.; Campos, E.V.R.; del Pilar Rodriguez-Torres, M.; Acosta-Torres, L.S.; Diaz-Torres, L.A.; Grillo, R.; Swamy, M.K.; Sharma, S.; et al. Nano based drug delivery systems: Recent developments and future prospects. *J. Nanobiotechnol.* **2018**, *16*, 71. [CrossRef]
2. Senge, M.O.; Brandt, J.C. Temoporfin (Foscan®, 5,10,15,20-tetra(m-hydroxyphenyl)chlorin)—A second-generation photosensitizer. *Photochem. Photobiol.* **2011**, *87*, 1240–1296. [CrossRef] [PubMed]
3. Yakavets, I.; Millard, M.; Zorin, V.; Lassalle, H.-P.; Bezdetnaya, L. Current state of the nanoscale delivery systems for temoporfin-based photodynamic therapy: Advanced delivery strategies. *J. Control. Release* **2019**, *304*, 268–287. [CrossRef] [PubMed]
4. Genchi, G.G.; Marino, A.; Tapeinos, C.; Ciofani, G. Smart Materials Meet Multifunctional Biomedical Devices: Current and Prospective Implications for Nanomedicine. *Front. Bioeng. Biotechnol.* **2017**, *5*, 80. [CrossRef] [PubMed]

5. Fortuni, B.; Inose, T.; Ricci, M.; Fujita, Y.; Zundert, I.V.; Masuhara, A.; Fron, E.; Mizuno, H.; Latterini, L.; Rocha, S.; et al. Polymeric Engineering of Nanoparticles for Highly Efficient Multifunctional Drug Delivery Systems. *Sci. Rep.* **2019**, *9*, 1–13. [CrossRef] [PubMed]
6. Sarma, S.J.; Khan, A.A.; Goswami, L.N.; Jalisatgi, S.S.; Hawthorne, M.F. A Trimodal Closomer Drug-Delivery System Tailored with Tracing and Targeting Capabilities. *Chem. A Eur. J.* **2016**, *22*, 12715–12723. [CrossRef] [PubMed]
7. Yakavets, I.; Lassalle, H.-P.; Scheglmann, D.; Wiehe, A.; Zorin, V.; Bezdetnaya, L.; Yakavets, I.; Lassalle, H.-P.; Scheglmann, D.; Wiehe, A.; et al. Temoporfin-in-Cyclodextrin-in-Liposome—A New Approach for Anticancer Drug Delivery: The Optimization of Composition. *Nanomaterials* **2018**, *8*, 847. [CrossRef] [PubMed]
8. Reshetov, V.; Lassalle, H.-P.; François, A.; Dumas, D.; Hupont, S.; Gräfe, S.; Filipe, V.; Jiskoot, W.; Guillemin, F.; Zorin, V.; et al. Photodynamic therapy with conventional and PEGylated liposomal formulations of mTHPC (temoporfin): Comparison of treatment efficacy and distribution characteristics in vivo. *Int. J. Nanomed.* **2013**, *8*, 3817–3831. [CrossRef] [PubMed]
9. Gaio, E.; Scheglmann, D.; Reddi, E.; Moret, F. Uptake and photo-toxicity of Foscan®, Foslip® and Fospeg® in multicellular tumor spheroids. *J. Photochem. Photobiol. B* **2016**, *161*, 244–252. [CrossRef]
10. Millard, M.; Yakavets, I.; Piffoux, M.; Brun, A.; Gazeau, F.; Guigner, J.-M.; Jasniewski, J.; Lassalle, H.-P.; Wilhelm, C.; Bezdetnaya, L. mTHPC-loaded extracellular vesicles outperform liposomal and free mTHPC formulations by an increased stability, drug delivery efficiency and cytotoxic effect in tridimensional model of tumors. *Drug Deliv.* **2018**, *25*, 1790–1801. [CrossRef] [PubMed]
11. Yakavets, I.; Yankovsky, I.; Millard, M.; Lamy, L.; Lassalle, H.-P.; Wiehe, A.; Zorin, V.; Bezdetnaya, L. The alteration of temoporfin distribution in multicellular tumor spheroids by β-cyclodextrins. *Int. J. Pharm.* **2017**, *529*, 568–575. [CrossRef] [PubMed]
12. Stella, V.J.; He, Q. Cyclodextrins. *Toxicol. Pathol.* **2008**, *36*, 30–42. [CrossRef] [PubMed]
13. Reshetov, V.; Kachatkou, D.; Shmigol, T.; Zorin, V.; D'Hallewin, M.-A.; Guillemin, F.; Bezdetnaya, L. Redistribution of meta-tetra(hydroxyphenyl)chlorin (m-THPC) from conventional and PEGylated liposomes to biological substrates. *Photochem. Photobiol. Sci.* **2011**, *10*, 911–919. [CrossRef] [PubMed]
14. Yakavets, I.; Yankovsky, I.; Bezdetnaya, L.; Zorin, V. Soret band shape indicates mTHPC distribution between β-cyclodextrins and serum proteins. *Dyes Pigment.* **2017**, *137*, 299–306. [CrossRef]
15. Sailor, M.J.; Park, J.-H. Hybrid nanoparticles for detection and treatment of cancer. *Adv. Mater. Technol.* **2012**, *24*, 3779–3802. [CrossRef] [PubMed]
16. Yakavets, I.; Lassalle, H.-P.; Yankovsky, I.; Ingrosso, F.; Monari, A.; Bezdetnaya, L.; Zorin, V. Evaluation of temoporfin affinity to β-cyclodextrins assuming self-aggregation. *J. Photochem. Photobiol. A* **2018**, *367*, 13–21. [CrossRef]
17. Yankovsky, I.; Bastien, E.; Yakavets, I.; Khludeyev, I.; Lassalle, H.-P.; Gräfe, S.; Bezdetnaya, L.; Zorin, V. Inclusion complexation with β-cyclodextrin derivatives alters photodynamic activity and biodistribution of meta-tetra(hydroxyphenyl)chlorin. *Eur. J. Pharm. Sci.* **2016**, *91*, 172–182. [CrossRef] [PubMed]
18. Gharib, R.; Greige-Gerges, H.; Fourmentin, S.; Charcosset, C.; Auezova, L. Liposomes incorporating cyclodextrin-drug inclusion complexes: Current state of knowledge. *Carbohydr. Polym.* **2015**, *129*, 175–186. [CrossRef] [PubMed]
19. Chen, J.; Lu, W.-L.; Gu, W.; Lu, S.-S.; Chen, Z.-P.; Cai, B.-C.; Yang, X.-X. Drug-in-cyclodextrin-in-liposomes: A promising delivery system for hydrophobic drugs. *Expert Opin. Drug Deliv.* **2014**, *11*, 565–577. [CrossRef]
20. Akbarzadeh, A.; Rezaei-Sadabady, R.; Davaran, S.; Joo, S.W.; Zarghami, N.; Hanifehpour, Y.; Samiei, M.; Kouhi, M.; Nejati-Koshki, K. Liposome: Classification, preparation, and applications. *Nanoscale Res. Lett* **2013**, *8*, 102. [CrossRef]
21. Yakavets, I.V.; Yankovsky, I.V.; Khludeyev, I.I.; Lassalle, H.P.; Bezdetnaya, L.N.; Zorin, V.P. Optical Methods for the Analysis of the Temoporfin Photosensitizer Distribution Between Serum Proteins and Methyl-β-Cyclodextrin Nanocarriers in Blood Serum. *J. Appl. Spectrosc.* **2018**, *84*, 1030–1036. [CrossRef]
22. Millard, M.; Yakavets, I.; Zorin, V.; Kulmukhamedova, A.; Marchal, S.; Bezdetnaya, L. Drug delivery to solid tumors: The predictive value of the multicellular tumor spheroid model for nanomedicine screening. *Int. J. Nanomed.* **2017**, *12*, 7993–8007. [CrossRef]
23. Reshetov, V.; Zorin, V.; Siupa, A.; D'Hallewin, M.-A.; Guillemin, F.; Bezdetnaya, L. Interaction of liposomal formulations of meta-tetra(hydroxyphenyl)chlorin (temoporfin) with serum proteins: Protein binding and liposome destruction. *Photochem. Photobiol.* **2012**, *88*, 1256–1264. [CrossRef] [PubMed]

24. Kuntsche, J.; Freisleben, I.; Steiniger, F.; Fahr, A. Temoporfin-loaded liposomes: Physicochemical characterization. *Eur. J. Pharm. Sci.* **2010**, *40*, 305–315. [CrossRef] [PubMed]
25. Torchilin, V.; Weissig, V. *Liposomes: A Practical Approach*; Oxford University Press: Oxford, UK, 2003; ISBN 978-0-19-963654-9.
26. Marchal, S.; Fadloun, A.; Maugain, E.; D'Hallewin, M.-A.; Guillemin, F.; Bezdetnaya, L. Necrotic and apoptotic features of cell death in response to Foscan photosensitization of HT29 monolayer and multicell spheroids. *Biochem. Pharm.* **2005**, *69*, 1167–1176. [CrossRef]
27. Colley, H.E.; Hearnden, V.; Jones, A.V.; Weinreb, P.H.; Violette, S.M.; Macneil, S.; Thornhill, M.H.; Murdoch, C. Development of tissue-engineered models of oral dysplasia and early invasive oral squamous cell carcinoma. *Br. J. Cancer* **2011**, *105*, 1582–1592. [CrossRef]
28. Yakavets, I.; Lassalle, H.-P.; Zorin, V.; Bezdetnaya, L. Cyclodextrin-based photoactive liposomal nanoparticles for tumor targeting. In Proceedings of the 17th International Photodynamic Association World Congress SPIE, Boston, MA, USA, 28 June–4 July 2019; Volume 11070, p. 110701P.

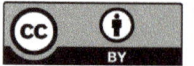

© 2019 by the authors. Licensee MDPI, Basel, Switzerland. This article is an open access article distributed under the terms and conditions of the Creative Commons Attribution (CC BY) license (http://creativecommons.org/licenses/by/4.0/).

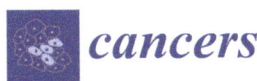

Article

Hybrid Clustered Nanoparticles for Chemo-Antibacterial Combinatorial Cancer Therapy

Barbara Cortese [1], Stefania D'Amone [2], Mariangela Testini [2], Patrizia Ratano [1] and Ilaria Elena Palamà [2],*

[1] Nanotechnology Institute, CNR-NANOTEC, University La Sapienza, P.zle A. Moro, 00185 Rome, Italy
[2] Nanotechnology Institute, CNR-NANOTEC, via Monteroni, 73100 Lecce, Italy
* Correspondence: ilaria.palama@nanotec.cnr.it

Received: 6 August 2019; Accepted: 5 September 2019; Published: 10 September 2019

Abstract: *Background*: A great number of therapeutic limitations, such as chemoresistance, high dosage, and long treatments, are still present in cancer therapy, and are often followed by side effects such as infections, which represent the primary cause of death among patients. *Methods*: We report pH- and enzymatic-responsive hybrid clustered nanoparticles (HC-NPs), composed of a PCL polymeric core loaded with an anticancer drug, such as Imatinib Mesylate (IM), and coated with biodegradable multilayers embedded with antibacterial and anticancer baby-ship silver NPs, as well as a monoclonal antibody for specific targeting of cancer cells conjugated on the surface. *Results*: The HC-NPs presented an onion-like structure that serially responded to endogenous stimuli. After internalization into targeted cancer cells, the clustered nanoparticles were able to break up, thanks to intracellular proteases which degraded the biodegradable multilayers and allowed the release of the baby-ship NPs and the IM loaded within the pH-sensible polymer present inside the mothership core. In vitro studies validated the efficiency of HC-NPs in human chronic leukemic cells. This cellular model allowed us to demonstrate specificity and molecular targeting sensitivity, achieved by using a combinatorial approach inside a single nano-platform, instead of free administrations. The combinatory effect of chemotherapic drug and AgNPs in one single nanosystem showed an improved cell death efficacy. In addition, HC-NPs showed a good antibacterial capacity on Gram-negative and Gram-positive bacteria. *Conclusions*: This study shows an important combinatorial anticancer and antimicrobial effect in vitro.

Keywords: nanoparticles; combinatorial therapy; anticancer and antibacterial activity

1. Introduction

Cancer represents one of the most formidable reasons of death in the world, despite important advances in oncology. Clinical practice indicates that cytotoxic therapeutic molecules are most effective when provided in combination, in order to realize synergistic or additive outcomes [1,2], even though important side effects [3], such as cardiotoxicity and bone marrow suppression [4,5], are reported. An underestimated important consequence of chemotherapy is represented by infections after treatment that remain the main cause of hospitalization and death amongst most patients [6]. Combinatorial cancer therapy, with the aim to prevent infection and to specifically kill cancer cells, can result in important cutbacks in morbidity and mortality for cancer patients. Recent progress in nano-cancer therapy represents an important oncological challenge [7]. Nanomedical materials have improved the gold standard in drug delivery with regards to biodistribution, intracellular uptake, and dosing efficacy, thanks to the use of nanoparticles (NPs) that are able to load therapeutic agents and specifically target the disease [8]. Currently, different liposome- and polymer-based NPs have been approved by the Food and Drug Administration (FDA) for clinical use [7].

In addition, the development of multifunctional materials for combination therapy via nanoparticles has emerged as an innovative therapeutic stratagem to attain synergistic combination effects for cancer therapy [9]. Multifunctional NPs have the ability to deliver different therapeutic agents and to improve drug efficiency within single administrations, releasing drug at the action site and reducing side effects [7,10–12]. Recent work has reported that the use of NPs with anti-cancer properties and chemotherapic drugs for combinatorial cancer therapy have shown an improved efficacy of chemotherapy, minimizing toxic side effects [13–15].

In this context, inorganic nanoparticles [15], such as silver nanoparticles (AgNPs), have shown important cancer activity [14,16,17], and numerous studies have described the cytotoxicity of AgNPs as being accredited to their ability to release Ag ions in the lysosome acid environment, inducing reactive oxygen species (ROS) production, leading to DNA damage and cell death [18–20]. In addition, the use of AgNPs as an antimicrobial agent in humans, has been approved by the FDA in situations such as in burns and wound healing [21].

Recently, we have shown how a combination of two different drugs loaded inside one nanosystem, such as Poly-caprolactone (PCL) NPs, can be used to overcome the problem of drug resistance, with low concentrations and showing a synergic effect [10].

In this paper, we move forward from our previous results, proposing to overcome actual clinical therapeutic problems associated with a high dose of chemotherapic drugs and infections, by developing hybrid clustered nanoparticles (HC-NPs), which can show combined chemo/antibacterial potential and therapeutic advantages in order to reach a cancer cure, and in reducing adverse effects such as infections. The chemo/antibacterial potential of our HC-NPs were investigated on chronic myeloid leukemia (CML), used as a model of cancer. CML is a stem cell-derived disorder [22], generated by a BCR-ABL oncoprotein. The current gold standard therapy is represented by tyrosine kinase inhibitors (TKIs), such as imatinib mesylate (IM). In addition, leukemia stops the bone marrow from producing enough healthy white blood cells, thus the CML patient is subject to infections.

Our HC-NPs presented an onion-like structure which was composed of compartmentalized loaded payload polymeric nanovectors functionalized with specific monoclonal antibody (mAb), in order to specifically target cancer and simultaneously prevent bacterial infections.

Specifically, our nanosystem was composed of two different nanoparticles: a mothership nanocarrier (size of approximately 200 nm) which represented the inner core, and 30 nm-sized babyship nanocarriers attached to the surface of the mothership. The mothership nanocarrier was produced using FDA-approved PCL polymer and was loaded with IM [10] in order to kill leukemia cells. Babyship nanoparticles were composed of silver in order to induce anticancer and antibacterial effects.

In vitro studies showed excellent anti-leukemic activity of our HC-NPs, thanks to the combinatory effect of IM and AgNPs that improved cell death efficacy. In addition, our HC-NPs showed a good antibacterial capacity on Gram-negative and Gram-positive bacteria.

To the best of the authors' knowledge, this is the first time that a chemo-antibacterial combinatorial therapy strategy has been developed, which potentiates single drugs and elicits an antibacterial response. Our strategy may have important therapeutic and pharmacological applications in cancer therapy, in order to simultaneously kill cancer cells and prevent infections.

2. Results

2.1. Synthesis and Characterization of Hybrid Cluster NPs

Our HC-NPs presented an onion-like structure (Figure 1) in which two different types of NPs were combined in order to improve the therapeutic efficacy. HC-NPs were composed of (i) a mothership biodegradable polymeric inner core (PCL), loaded with IM; (ii) an intermediate layer (capsosoma) composed of pH-sensible chitosan (CH) filled with babyship AgNPs; and (iii) a final outer layer (enzyme sensible protamine, PRM) functionalized with a specific monoclonal antibody, an anti-CD38 [23] antibody (Ab), for cell targeting. The synthesis of hybrid cluster NPs (HC-NPs) are illustrated in Figure 1.

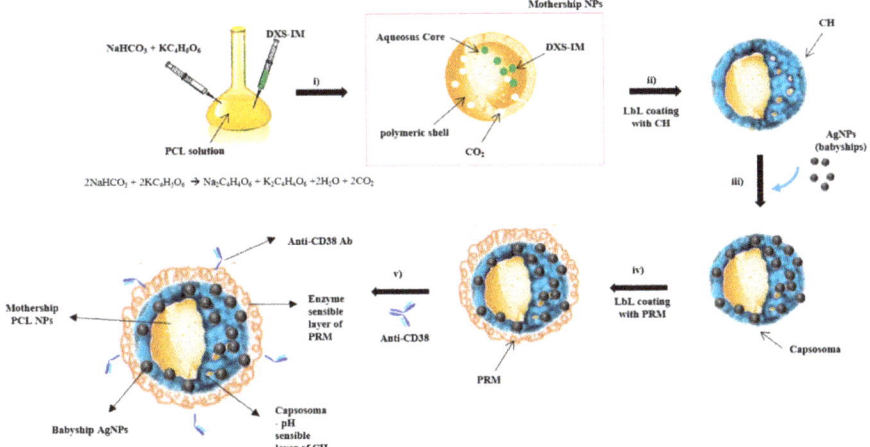

Figure 1. Illustration of the production of HC-NPs. AgNPs: silver nanoparticles, PRM: enzyme sensible protamine, PCL: Poly-caprolactone polymer

Prior to assemblage of HC-NPs, the silver (babyship) and PCL NPs (mothership) were synthetized separately and characterized.

Colloidal suspension of silver nanoparticles (AgNPs) were prepared by reduction of an aqueous solution containing $AgNO_3$ with $NaBH_4$. The color change of solution from transparent to yellow indicated the formation of AgNPs, also confirmed by UV-VIS spectroscopy (Supplementary Figure S1). After the synthesis, AgNPs were centrifuged and resuspended in sodium citrate solution. AgNPs were shown to have a mean size of about 32 nm with a zeta potential of −27.9 mV (Table 1). Transmission electron microscopy (TEM) analysis of AgNPs (Supplementary Figure S2A) showed a spherical morphology and no aggregation.

Core-shell IM-loaded PCL NPs were prepared by an emulsion–diffusion–evaporation modified method [10], which allowed for the obtaining of NPs with a size of about 228 nm and with a ζ-potential of −11 mV (Table 1; Supplementary Figure S2B). Before the encapsulation of IM into the hydrophilic core of PCL NPs, these were complexed with dextran (DXS), an enzyme-sensible polymer [24] that permitted their controlled release after degradation by intracellular protease.

Hybrid IM-PCL/Ag cluster NPs (HC-NPs) were obtained following different steps (Figure 1). In order to assemble babyship and mothership NPs to form a capsosoma, the surface of IM-PCL NPs (mothership NPs) were coated with the layer-by-layer technique (LbL) using chitosan, a pH-sensible polymer, that allows the initial release of AgNPs in a cytoplasmic environment (Figure 1ii). Subsequently, a suspension of AgNPs (babyship NPs) was added, and an additional outer layer, due to the electrostatic interactions, was formed onto the surface of mothership NPs (Supplementary Figure S2C), obtaining a capsosoma. Size and zeta potential modifications in the mothership NPs after deposition of babyship NPs' layer were analyzed with Dynamic Light Scattering (DLS) (Table 1). Moreover, we measured using a DLS analysis the fixed aqueous layer thickness (FALT) [25,26] of our NPs (Table 1).

Table 1. Physicochemical characterization of different nanoparticle (NP) formulations. Representative measurements of three different sets of data have been reported (P-values < 0.05). HC-NPs: hybrid clustered nanoparticles, FALT: fixed aqueous layer thickness, PdI: Polydispersion Index.

Sample	ζ Potential (mV)	Size (nm)	PdI	FALT (nm)
Ag NPs	−27.9 ± 0.96	32.02 ± 0.69	0.6 ± 0.06	-
PCL NPs	−11.5 ± 0.24	228.1 ± 0.3	0.36 ± 0.03	-
PCL-Ag NPs	−25.4 ± 0.15	274.8 ± 0.25	0.57 ± 0.01	1.82 ± 0.02
HC-NPs	10.8 ± 0.88	286.5 ± 0.56	0.62 ± 0.05	2.55 ± 0.03

By adding a new layer on capsosoma, we observed an increase of the FALT value, showing that a fixed aqueous layer was formed on the surface of NPs. In addition, the assembly of HC-NPs was confirmed by FT-IR analysis (Supplementary Figure S3).

To provide the final outermost layer functionalized with anti-CD38 antibody, the capsosoma was coated with enzyme-sensible protamine (PRM) [24] solution (Supplementary Figure S2D) and a covalent binding of anti-CD38 antibody on the capsosoma surface was performed using EDC (1-ethyl-3-(3-dimethylaminopropyl)-carbodiimide). FACS (Fluorescence-activated cell sorting) analysis (Supplementary Figure S4A, red line) revealed that the HC-NPs were efficiently functionalized with the anti-CD38 antibody, and also that the integrity of the antibody was confirmed by SDS-PAGE, as shown in Supplementary Figure S4B.

The IM encapsulation efficiency (EE%) obtained in this study was of about 95% in PCL NPs and of 73% for AgNPs.

Release study of babyship AgNPs and IM loaded into the mothership core from HC-NPs was performed, mimicking the different intracellular compartments. In particular, HC-NPs were incubated in PBS at pH 5.8 and 7.4, in order to mimic the lyso/endosomal and cytoplasmatic environments, respectively. IM was released after degradation of protease-sensible DXS, and a release of about 42% was observed at pH 5.8 after 96 h (Supplementary Figure S5A).

For babyship AgNPs, we observed a biphasic release pattern (Supplementary Figure S5B). An initial burst release was followed by a sustained release at pH 5.8. A low release of about 5.5% was observed at pH 7.4 after 96 h. On the contrary, we observed an accelerated release of about 81% at pH 5.8, which seemed to be related to the presence of the combination of sodium bicarbonate and potassium tartrate in the core of the mothership NPs.

An IM release of about 23% and of about 32% for AgNps after 96 h at pH 5.8 was evident with control HC-NP formulations without the mixture of sodium bicarbonate and potassium tartrate in the mothership core, respectively (Supplementary Figure S5C,D).

In addition, HC-NPs maintained their hydrodynamic size and release profiles over a time window of 8 days when incubated in physiological conditions, and this evidence supports their stability.

2.2. Protein Corona Analysis

Our NPs (e.g., AgNPs, PCL NPs, and HC-NPs) were incubated with complete cell culture medium with 10% FBS or mouse blood plasma overnight in agitation at 37 °C. After the washing steps, the NPs' hard corona was analyzed with SDS-PAGE. As shown in Figure 2A,B, the quantity of hard protein corona by incubation of complete medium and blood plasma on the surface of AgNPs and PCL NPs appeared to be higher (lanes 1, 2) compared to HC-NPs (lanes 3). This was confirmed by the data from the bicinchoninic acid (BCA) assay (Figure 2C).

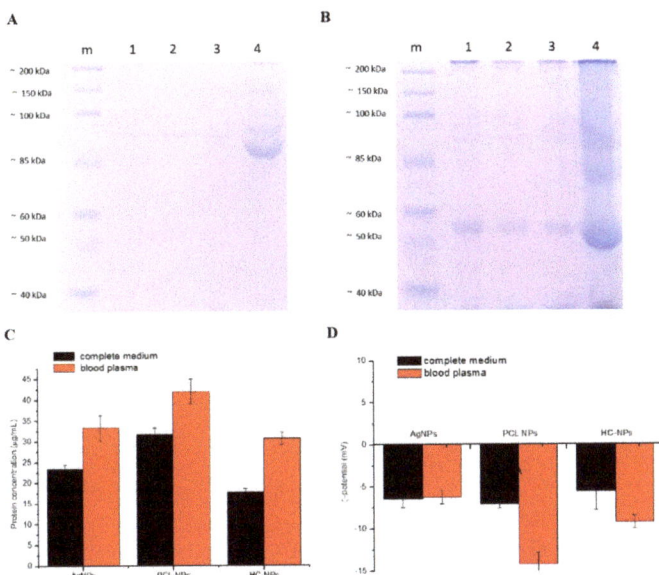

Figure 2. SDS-PAGE of hard protein corona after incubation with complete culture medium (**A**), and with mouse blood plasma (**B**) overnight at 37 °C with AgNPs (lane 1 of A and B); PCL NPs (lane 2 of A and B), HC-NPs (lane 3 of A and B), and control with only medium (lane 4 of A) and with solely mouse blood plasma (lane 4 of B). Quantification of adsorbed proteins on different NPs formulation by the bicinchoninic acid (BCA) assay (**C**). ζ-potential analysis of NPs after incubation with complete medium and blood plasma overnight (**D**). A representative result of three independent experiments is shown (P-values < 0.05).

In addition, zeta-potential analysis after incubation in complete medium or mouse blood plasma of different formulations of NPs suggested that the adsorption of serum proteins induced a change in their zeta potential (Figure 2D), confirming the formation of protein corona around the NPs.

Hemocompatibility of our formulation was analyzed performing a hemolysis assay. As shown in the Supplementary Figure S6, the HR% of AgNPs and HC-NPs was lower compared to the positive control (physiological solution and 2% blood), and in contrast, the HR% of PCL NPs was slightly higher, but still negligible.

2.3. Antibacterial Action

The antibacterial properties of the babyship AgNPs and HC-NPs were evaluated by measurement of bacteria growth in function of the optical density (OD, Figure 3B,D) and by the number of colony-forming units (CFU, Figure 3A,C) on Gram-negative *E. coli* DH5α and Gram-positive *S. aureus*. The antibacterial activity, reported in Figure 3, showed a good antibacterial capacity of the babyship AgNPs and HC-NPs on Gram-negative DH5α *E. coli*, and Gram-positive *S. aureus*, thus confirming that the babyship AgNPs inside the HC-NPs maintained the antibacterial efficacy, despite the assembly with the mothership NPs.

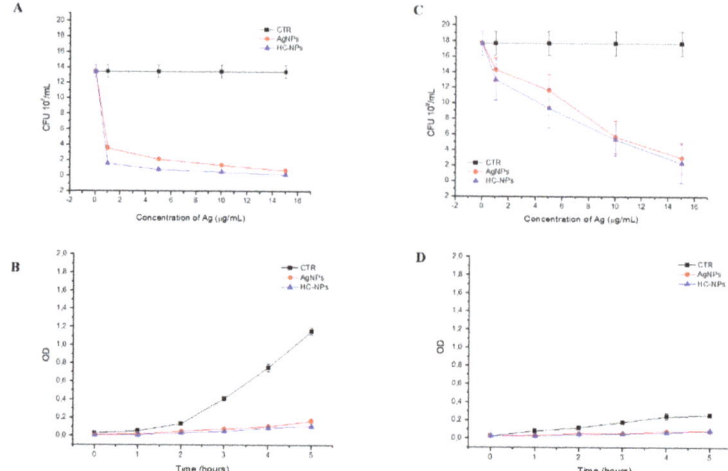

Figure 3. Antibacterial analysis on Gram-negative *E. coli* DH5α (**A,B**) and Gram-positive *S. aureus* (**C,D**) of AgNPs and HC-NPs by colony-forming units (CFU) counting on solid Luria–Bertani (LB) broth (**A,C**) as a function of Ag concentrations after 24 h. Measurement of optical density (OD) (**B,D**) as a function of time. Representative measurements of three different sets of data have been reported (P-values < 0.05).

2.4. Targeting and Cellular Uptake Analysis

Specific cell targeting of HC-NPs was analyzed in a co-culture of CD38-positive (KU812) and CD38-negative (C13895) cells after treatment with 500 ng/mL of Tetramethylrhodamine (TRITC)-conjugated anti-CD38 HC-NPs for 24 h. As shown in Figure 4, the antibody attached onto the HC-NPs surface can specifically target leukemia KU812 cells in a co-culture. The cellular uptake efficacy of HC-NPs was quantitatively evaluated by fluorimeter analysis, as shown in Figure 4E.

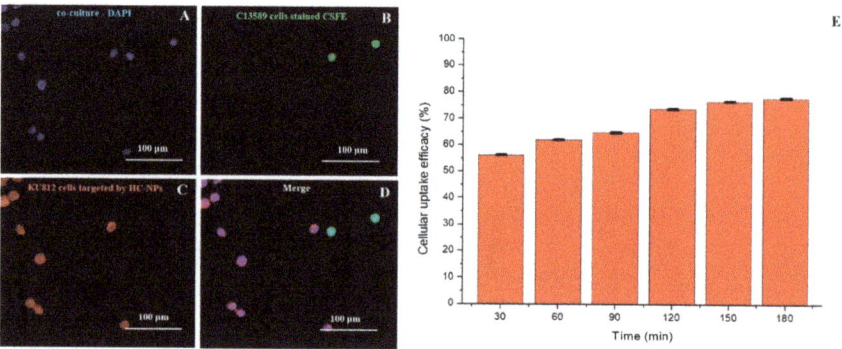

Figure 4. Confocal Laser Scanning Microscopy (CLSM) images of C13589 and KU812 cell co-culture. (**A**) Cell nuclei were counterstained with 4′,6-diamidino-2-phenylindole (DAPI,blue), (**B**) C13589 cells before of co-culture were stained with commercial CSFE (carboxyfluorescein diacetate, succinimidyl ester) fluorophore (green), (**C**) KU812 cells present in the co-culture were recognized by HC-NPs functionalized with anti-CD38 monoclonal antibody (red), (**D**) merged confocal images. Scale bars: 100 μm. Time-dependent cellular uptake efficiency of HC-NPs by KU812 cells (**E**). Representative measurements of three independent experiments have been reported (P-values < 0.05).

The cellular uptake was time-dependent, and surface functionalization of HC-NPs with anti CD38 antibody revealed an improved cellular uptake for leukemia compared with other NP formulations that do not present the antibody on their surface (Supplementary Figure S7).

2.5. Anti-Cancer Efficacy of HC-NPs

The anti-cancer effect of HC-NPs was studied in vitro using different NP formulations. Free IM and empty PCL NPs were used as controls. No cytotoxicity on healthy C13895 cells was noticed using the IC_{50} doses of all formulations (Supplementary Figure S8), confirmed by cell cycle analysis, as shown in Supplementary Figure S9. On KU812 leukemia cells, we observed a dose-dependent effect (Supplementary Figure S10A) when the leukemia cells were incubated with all NP formulations (IM-loaded PCL NPs, AgNPs, and HC-NPs). In particular, HC-NP formulation showed an improved cytotoxicity.

In Supplementary Figure S10B, the IC_{50} values of different formulations on KU812 leukemia cells are shown, and it is possible to observe an IC_{50} value much lower for HC-NPs due to the controlled release of the drug and the AgNPs. In addition, a combination index (CI) of 0.81 of IM and AgNPs on KU812 leukemia cells showed a synergistic effect.

Combinatorial effect on KU812 leukaemia cells was analyzed through FACS analysis using annexin V-FITC/PI staining. Flow cytometry plots of leukemia KU812 cells (Figure 5A) indicated an evident apoptosis when incubated with HC-NPs (about 72%). In addition, cell cycle blocking at G2/M phase (see Figure 5B) was evident with treatment with HC-NPs (~45%).

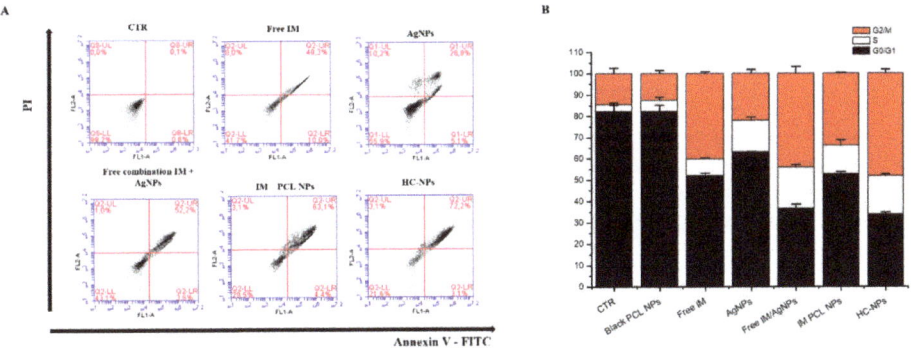

Figure 5. Analysis of cell apoptosis (**A**) and cell cycle (**B**) of KU812 leukaemia cells after 24 h of treatments with different formulations, compared with untreated control cells (CTR). Representative measurements of three independent experiments have been reported ($P < 0.05$).

The inhibition of tyrosine kinase activity of the oncoprotein BCR-ABL in leukemic cells KU812 was evaluated by western blotting analysis (Figure 6), after 7 days of incubation with the different formulations. Western blotting analysis was conducted using anti c-ABL antibody. As shown in Figure 6, a total inhibition of BCR-ABL was evident in treating the leukemia cells with HC-NPs.

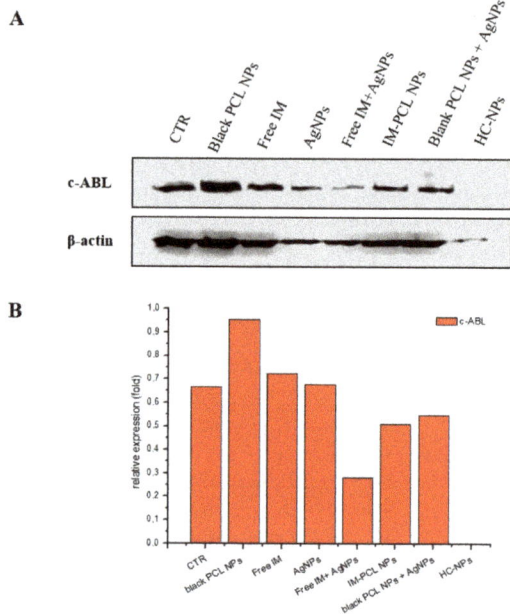

Figure 6. Inhibition of the oncoprotein BCR-ABL with western blotting after 7 days of treatment with different formulations (**A**) and densitometry analysis (**B**) of c-ABL levels normalized to the β-actin used as control. Representative measurements of three independent experiments have been reported.

In addition, we have validated the production of by reactive oxygen intermediates (ROI) metabolites that determinate cell death through the activity of superoxide dismutase (SOD). The inhibition rate of superoxide dismutase activity was significantly increased in HC-NP-treated KU812 cells at LD_{50} concentrations, compared with untreated control cells (CTR) and normal C13589 cell line, as show in Figure 7.

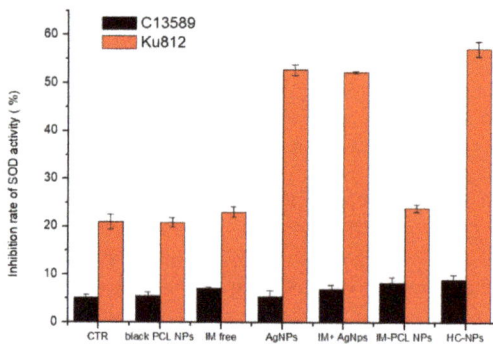

Figure 7. Inhibition rate of superoxide dismutase activity (SOD) in leukaemia KU812 and normal C13589 cell line after 6 h of treatment with black PCL NPs, free imatinib mesylate (IM), AgNPs, free IM/AgNP combination, IM-PCL NPs, and HC-NPs, compared with untreated control cells (CTR). Representative measurements of three independent experiments have been reported ($P < 0.05$).

3. Discussion

Side effects, such as infections, are often present after chemotherapy. However, this challenge can be overcome by performing targeted combination therapy, using a low dose of chemotherapic drugs and antimicrobial agents. Multifunctional nano-systems can be used to combine chemo and antibacterial agents in one single nano-system; in this way, is possible to specifically kill cancer cells and prevent infections.

Different studies have described the combination of different therapeutic agents inside one NP [13,14] to overcome the drug resistance of cancer cells [27,28]. No studies in the literature, however, report the combination in one single nanosystem of therapeutic agents with anticancer and antimicrobial properties.

In this work, we report a nano-platform in which a chemotherapic drug (IM) is combined with silver, showing good cancer action using a low dose and a good antibacterial effect.

Over the last few years, we have developed enzymatic [24,29] and pH-responsive polymeric [30] NPs for drug therapy in leukemia. Recently, we have reported [10] the effect of two different drugs combined into one single nanosystem, which showed the potentiality of overcoming drug resistance with low concentrations in a synergic effect.

In this paper, we adopted a different strategy by developing hybrid clustered nanoparticles (HC-NPs) to combine both the chemo/antibacterial potential of silver nanoparticles and therapeutic advantages of IM drugs in order to reduce adverse effects, such infections, and to achieve a cancer cure.

The onion-like structure of our HC-NPs was formed specifically by two different nanoparticles. The inner core structure was characterized by a mothership nanocarrier (size of approximately 200 nm) with the role of compartmentalized loaded payload polymeric nanovector, functionalized with specific monoclonal antibody (mAb), in order to specifically target cancer. The external surface of the mothership was covered with 30 nm-sized babyship silver nanocarriers to induce anticancer and antibacterial effects. With this HC-NP configuration, we expected a multistep release mechanism (see scheme in Supplementary Figure S11) in which (i) HC-NPs were internalized by target cells thanks to the specific antibody and degradation of enzyme-sensible layer of PRM by intracellular proteases; (ii) the acidification of the capsosoma environment allowed the release of babyship NPs complexed with pH-sensible polymers (first release) into the cytoplasm. In particular, an initial babyship AgNP release started in the cytoplasm, thanks to the acidification of the capsosoma environment, and their complete release occurred in the endosome/lysosome compartment; and (iii) and (iv) babyship NPs and mothership NPs (inner core) were carried into the lysosomal compartment. In this environment (pH 5.0) the generation of CO_2 bubbles and the cationization of the mothership NPs led to their escape into the cytoplasmic compartment and the release of IM (second release); on the other hand, babyship AgNPs released Ag^+ ions and allowed ROS production. The release of IM and ROS production by Ag^+ ions facilitated the killing of leukemia cells (cancer therapy) and, at the same time, the release by dying cells (see schema in Supplementary Figure S11, point (v) of AgNPs and Ag^+ ions, which allowed for antibacterial activity external of the cancer cell.

A good nanosystem for cancer therapy should have a high loading efficiency. In our study, the IM encapsulation efficiency (EE%) obtained was about 95% in PCL NPs and 73% for AgNPs. The build-up of different layers on the mothership NPs did not influence the IM EE%.

In addition, the release study (Supplementary Figure S5) of babyship AgNPs and IM by HC-NPs showed a different release when the HC-NPs were incubated in a solution of PBS with different pH values (5.8 and 7.4) that mimicked lysosomal and cytoplasmatic milieus. The release of IM was subjected at the protease degradation of DXS, and the release was different pH values after 96 h (about 42%). On the contrary, we detected an initial rapid release in the first hours and a gradual and sustained release in the late time of AgNPs at pH 5.8 (about 81%). At pH 7.4, we observed a low release for AgNPs (only 5%). This dissimilar behavior can be due to the fact that during synthesis process, in the NP core, a mixture of sodium bicarbonate and potassium tartrate was added, which swiftly produced CO_2 bubbles in the acidic pH in order to produce holes in the NP's shell and support IM release [10].

In an acid compartment of lyso/endosomal (pH 5.8) the sodium bicarbonate and potassium tartrate combination rapidly produced CO_2 bubbles, allowing the formation of big pores in the NP wall, which allowed the release of payloads, as demonstrated in our previous work [10]. The release profiles of IM and AgNPs showed that our HC-NPs responded specifically to the environmental conditions (pH and proteases) for which they were produced. In addition, as we have demonstrated, the inner core presented a negative charge in physiological pH, which was reverted to a positive charge in the acidic pH of endo-lysosomal vesicles [10,31], determining NPs endo-lysosomal escape.

Another important aspect to consider is the fact that in a physiological environment, NPs interact with different biomolecules and form a protein corona [32,33], which affects the cellular response and the recognition by mononuclear phagocyte system. It is reported that a low quantity of proteins that form the protein corona around nanoparticles induce a reduction of macrophages uptake [34]. We have observed that AgNPs and PCL NPs present a high quantity of protein corona after incubation with complete medium or mouse blood plasma (Figure 2) when compared with HC-NPs. This dissimilar protein absorption was attributed to the modified surface of HC-NPs that reduced the protein corona. A lower protein corona arrangement can influence the in vivo destiny of HC-NPs via immune elusion and short uptake by mononuclear phagocytic system.

An additional key parameter that can influence the possibility of use of NPs in vivo is hemocompatibility. After incubation with mouse blood (Supplementary Figure S6), the HC-NPs' hemolytic rate was lower compared to the positive control (physiological solution and blood). Our results confirmed that our HC-NPs were hemocompatible with mouse erythrocytes, and that they can be administrated intravenously.

The key point of this study was the combination of organic and inorganic NPs inside one single nano-platform. Inorganic NPs [15], such as AgNPs with significant cancer [14,16,17] and antimicrobial properties [21], were combined in our HC-NP platform. In particular, the FDA has approved the human use of AgNPs as an antimicrobial agent [21], and their antibacterial properties have been studied extensively [35,36]. In this context, we have designed our HC-NPs in order to prevent the infections in patients after chemotherapy treatments, and AgNPs result as a powerful broad-spectrum antibacterial agent. AgNPs and HC-NPs have shown a good antibacterial capacity on Gram-negative *E. coli*, DH5α *E. coli*, and Gram-positive *S. aureus* (Figure 3), confirming the antibacterial efficacy of the babyship AgNPs inside the HC-NPs, which also can be used as a prophylaxis tool.

In this study, we chose chronic myeloid leukemia cells as a disease model for validation of our HC-NPs. Clinical treatment of this disease makes use of tyrosin kinase inhibitors, such as IM. This drug is active against BCR-ABL oncoprotein expressed by this cell population. It is renown, in fact, that IM is cytostatic and not cytotoxic in the CML stem cell compartment, and for this reason, we loaded the IM into NPs along with AgNPs with anticancer properties, as the use IM alone is unable to remove leukemic stem cells.

Cell targeting is a crucial step for specific delivery of active molecules to cancer cells, in order to avoid an adverse effect on healthy cells. For this aim, we have functionalized our HC-NPs with an antibody against CD38 specific for leukemia cells. We investigated HC-NP-specific cell targeting using a co-culture of CD38-positive (KU812) and CD38-negative (C13895) cells for 24 h. Confocal analysis confirmed that HC-NPs can specifically target leukemia KU812 cells in a co-culture (Figure 4) and the specific targeting established the importance of the antibody anti-CD38 functionalization of our HC-NPs, in order to improve the efficacy of therapy and to reduce side effects.

Combinatorial cancer therapy using a combination of drugs inside one nanosystem has revealed an enhanced chemotherapy efficacy, reducing toxic side effects [10,13,14]. In addition, AgNPs have important cancer activity [14,16,17] and no adverse effect on healthy cells [17,37]. In our HC-NPs, we combined the specific anticancer activity of IM that binds specifically to the BCR-ABL oncoprotein present only in the CML cells, and the anticancer property of AgNPs, thanks to the production of ROS, in order to improve their efficacy on cancer cells only.

Using different NP formulations, we investigated the anti-cancer effects of HC-NPs in vitro. No cytotoxic effects were observed on healthy C13895 cells using all formulations of the IC$_{50}$ doses (Supplementary Figure S8). Healthy cells did not respond to IM because of the absence of the oncoprotein BCR-ABL. In addition, in healthy cells, the AgNPs did not induce cytotoxicity because these present a functional antioxidant system. A dose-dependent effect (Supplementary Figure S10A) was observed when leukemia cells were incubated with all NP formulations (IM loaded PCL NPs, AgNPs, and HC-NPs). Specifically, HC-NP formulation with a lower IC$_{50}$ value showed an enhanced cytotoxic effect for HC-NPs due the controlled release of the drug and the AgNPs. Moreover, an advanced synergistic effect with a combination index (CI) of 0.81 of IM and AgNPs on KU812 leukemia cells was observed. In vitro cytotoxicity showed that the combination of IM and AgNPs induced an improved anti-leukemia effect at low concentrations.

The combinatorial effect on leukemia cells (Figure 5A) was more evident when incubated with HC-NPs (about 72%) with high apoptosis. Also, cell cycle blocking at the G2/M phase (see Figure 5B) was noticed when treated with HC-NPs (~45%). In vitro studies indicated that the combinatory effect of our HC-NPs exhibited an excellent anti-leukemic activity, improving cell death efficiency.

The long-time inhibition of tyrosine kinase activity of BCR-ABL in leukemic cells KU812 was evaluated by western blotting analysis after 7 days, using different formulations. As shown in Figure 6, a sustained and total inhibition of BCR-ABL was evident when leukemia cells were treated with HC-NPs. It is important to note that BCR-ABL tyrosine phosphorylation was only prevented using free IM or in free combination with AgNPs, whereas the co-encapsulation of the IM and AgNPs in HC-NPs achieved an effective in vitro inhibition. Improving the inhibition BCR-ABL tyrosine activity for a long-time window will possibly allow an extended block of BCR-ABL autokinase action that is decisive in endorsing cell apoptosis.

Moreover, the production of reactive oxygen intermediate (ROI) metabolites inducted by AgNPs, which determinate cell death, was investigated through the activity of superoxide dismutase (SOD), showing a significant increase of the inhibition rate of superoxide dismutase activity in KU812 cells treated with HC-NPs at LD$_{50}$ concentrations, as shown in Figure 7. In healthy C13895 cells with an efficient antioxidant system, no increasing of SOD was observed.

The toxic effect of different formulation of NPs on the appearance and the general behavioral pattern of healthy mice was evaluated in preliminary experiments. No toxic symptoms or mortality were observed in any animal. Similarly, at a general observation, no changes in behavioral pattern, clinical signs, or food consumption were noticed in both control and treated mice (data not shown). In vivo experiments treating leukemia xenograft mice are the subject of future work.

In this work, a chemo-antibacterial combinatorial therapy strategy was developed, which potentiated single drugs and elicited an antibacterial response. Our strategy may have important therapeutic and pharmacological applications in cancer therapy, in order to simultaneously kill cancer cells and prevent infections.

4. Materials and Methods

Media for cell culture and chemicals were acquired from Sigma-Aldrich. Human chronic myeloid leukaemia cells (KU812), human normal B lymphoblast (C13589), and Gram-negative DH5-Alpha *E. coli* were acquired from the American Tissue Type Collection (ATTC). Gram-positive *S. aureus* was obtained from Dr. Federica Paladini. Annexin V-PI kit and nitrocellulose membrane were obtained from Abcam; Coomassie brilliant blue staining and Clarity—Western ECL Substrate were obtained from BioRad; anti-c-ABL antibody was obtained from Santa Cruz Biotechnology Inc.; HRP-conjugated antibody was obtained from Cell Signaling.

Blood for protein corona analysis and hemolytic activity was collected from male adult C57BL/6j mice, weighting 20–30 g. For protein corona analysis, blood was collected in tubes with heparin and centrifugated in order to obtain the plasma. All procedures involving animal care were approved by the ethics committee of La Sapienza University (Rome), the Animal Care and Use Committee of the Italian Ministry of Health, and performed in compliance with the guidelines of the European Community Council (2010/63/UE) and the decree law (D.L.) 26/2014 of Italian Ministry of Health. All efforts were made to minimize animal suffering and to reduce the number of animals used.

4.1. Synthesis and Characterization of AgNPs

A 50 mL aqueous solution containing $AgNO_3$ (1 mM) was kept under constant agitation on a magnetic stirrer at 1500 rpm in ice and mixed with an equal volume of an aqueous solution of sodium citrate (50 mM). Subsequently, 75 mL of $NaBH_4$ (20 mM) was added drop by drop into this solution until it became yellow. Next, the AgNP suspension was washed three times with water by centrifugation at 12,500 rpm for 20 min and then resuspended in sodium citrate and stored at 4 °C until use.

4.2. Synthesis of HC-NPs

4.2.1. Synthesis of IM Loaded PCL NPs

Poly ε- caprolactone (PCL) NPs loaded with IM were synthetized, as according to our previous works [10]. A homogenous size of NPs, density gradient centrifugation was applied using 5, 10, 15, 20, and 25% w/v sucrose dissolved in PBS 1×. In an Eppendorf tube, 200 µL of each sucrose solution were layered one on the top of each other. One-hundred microliters of NPs solution was layered on the top of the sucrose layer and was centrifuged at 14,000 rpm for 60 min. After centrifugation, 10 µL from each layer was analyzed by DLS.

4.2.2. Synthesis of HC-NPs

Hybrid IM-PCL/Ag cluster NPs (HC-NPs) were obtained by coating with the layer-by-layer technique (LbL), with the IM loaded PCL NPs (1 mg) using 1 mL of chitosan medium molecular weight (CH, 3 mg/mL in NaCl 0.1M). The dispersion was continuously shaken for 10 min. The excess of CH was removed by three centrifugation/washing steps with a 0.1 M NaCl solution. Thereafter, 1 mL of AgNPs (0.1 to 10 ppm) was added, and the dispersion was continuously shaken for 2 h, followed again by three centrifugations (12,500 rpm for 20 min) and washing steps. Subsequently, 1 mL of a 0.1 M NaCl solution containing the polycation protamine (PRM, 2 mg/mL) was added, and the dispersion was continuously shaken for 10 min, followed again by three centrifugation/washing steps. The mixture was then dialyzed with pure water for 8 h. For fluorescent HC-NPs, a 0.05 mg/mL of $DiOC_{18}(3)$(3,3'-Dioctadecyloxacarbocyanine Perchlorate), DiO, in chloroform was added to the PCL solution and the preparation was carried out as described previously [10]. The labelled HC-NPs were stored in the dark at 4 °C until use.

4.2.3. HC-NPs Functionalization with Anti-CD38 Antibody

For covalent binding of monoclonal anti-CD38 antibody onto HC-NPs, 5 µg of EDC (1-ethyl-3-(3-dimethylaminopropyl)-carbodiimide) was mixed with 400 µL of a solution containing 450 µL of HC-NPs and 450 µL of antibody; in this way, the molar ratio between EDC and antibody was about 9. The mixed solution was stirred under constant agitation on a magnetic stirrer at 500 rpm for 2 h at room temperature (RT). After incubation, the sample was centrifuged at 12,500 rpm for 20 min, and the pellet was washed three times with 1 mL of blocking and storage buffer (0.1 M boric acid and 0.1% Bovine Serum Albumin (BSA), pH 7.5) containing 2 µL of TRITC-conjugated secondary antibody (1:250). The sample was stirred gently for 1 h at RT and was then centrifuged, and the pellet of the HC-NP antibody conjugate was suspended in 1 mL of blocking and storage buffer and kept in the dark at 4 °C until use.

4.3. Characterization of NPs

4.3.1. Dynamic Light Scattering

Hydrodynamic size and zeta potential of AgNPs, IM-PCL NPs, and HC-NPs were evaluated by a Zetasizer Nano ZS90 (Malvern Instruments Ltd, USA). Stability of HC-NPs over time (8 days) in complete Roswell Park Memorial Institute (RPMI) 1640 medium was verified by DLS analysis (three independent experiments).

Fixed aqueous layer thickness (FALT) was calculated on the basis of zeta potential of NP solutions with a serial dilution with an isotonic solution of 10 mM lactate buffer (pH 4) with various concentration of NaCl and sucrose. The ln zeta potential ζ (V) was plotted against the Debye Hückel parameter (k). k represents $3.3\nu C$, where C is the concentration of electrolytes in the solution. The slope of the obtained plots indicated the thickness of the fixed aqueous layer in nm.

4.3.2. UV-VIS Spectroscopy

UV-visible spectra were acquired with a UV-visible spectrophotometer (Varian Cary 300 Scan; Varian Instruments, CA, USA) at RT, and spectral analysis was performed in the 300–800 nm range.

4.3.3. Scanning and Transmission Electron Microscopy

The external morphology of AgNPs, IM-PCL NPs, and HC-NPs was examined by scanning electron microscopy (SEM) and transmission electron microscopy (TEM). Prior to SEM analysis, the samples were coated with a 10 nm gold layer. SEM analyses were taken with a Carl Zeiss Merlin SEM supplied with a Gemini II column and a field emission gun (FEG). In addition, AgNPs were analyzed using a JEOL Jem 1011 TEM microscope (Japan).

4.3.4. FT-IR Spectroscopy

FT-IR analysis was performed using a VERTEX 70v FT-IR Spectrometer (Bruker) in order to assess the secondary structure of AgNPs, PCL NPs, and HC-NPs. Infrared (IR) spectra were acquired in absorbance mode, and each spectrum was obtained by the 60 scans with the wavenumber ranging from 0 to 4000 cm^{-1}.

4.3.5. Flow Cytometry and SDS-PAGE Assay

To confirm the antibody functionalization on the HC-NPs' surface, we performed a flow cytometry analysis. One milliliter of HC-NPs conjugated with anti-CD38 antibody labelled with TRITC anti-mouse secondary antibody was introduced into a flow cytometer and analyzed using a C6 Flow Cytometer (Accuri, USA). As a control, non-conjugated HC-NPs were used. The antibody content onto HC-NPs was determined by bicinchoninic acid (BCA) protein assay according to the manufacturer's instructions (Sigma-Aldrich, USA). The BSA was used as a standard and the antibody conjugated was quantified using a UV-visible spectrophotometer (Varian Cary 300 Scan; Varian Instruments, CA, USA) at a wavelength of 562 nm. In addition, to control the integrity of antibody after conjugation, HC-NPs were subjected to 4%–12% SDS-polyacrylamide gel electrophoresis (SDS-PAGE). The resolved protein bands were visualized by Coomassie brilliant blue staining (BioRad), according to the manufacturer's instructions. Representative results of three independent experiments were reported.

4.3.6. Protein Corona

Protein corona analyses were achieved by SDS-PAGE. First, 500 ng/mL of AgNPs, PCL NPs, and HC-NPs were raised in complete RPMI medium supplemented with 10% FBS or with 2% of mice blood plasma at 37 °C overnight in a shaker. Afterward, NPs were centrifuged in order to remove hard corona and resuspended in PBS 1×. Washing procedure was repeated three times prior to SDS-PAGE. Protein concentration on NPs was determined by using bicinchoninic acid (BCA, Sigma-Aldrich) at

562 nm. Eluted hard corona proteins from all samples were mixed with SDS sample buffer and boiled at 100 °C for 10 min. The samples were subjected to 4–12% SDS-PAGE for 90 min at 120 V. Coomassie blue staining was used for detection protein bands.

In addition, zeta potential was measured by DLS analysis.

Representative results of three independent experiments have been reported.

4.3.7. Hemolytic Activity

Hemolysis assays were performed incubating the HC-NPs with 2% mouse blood suspension for 24 h at 37 °C. After the suspension, it was centrifuged at 15,000 rpm for 20 min at 4 °C, and the supernatant adsorption (A) was analyzed by UV-visible spectrophotometer (Varian Cary 300 Scan; Varian Instruments, CA, USA) at a wavelength of 540 nm. Hemolytic rate was calculated using the following equation:

$$\text{Hemolytic rate (\%)} = \frac{A(\text{material}) - A(\text{negative control})}{A(\text{positive control}) - A(\text{negative control})} \times 100$$

where negative control was composed of saline solution and blood without NPs, while positive control was saline solution. Representative results of three independent experiments were reported.

Antibacterial activity. Gram-negative DH5-Alpha *E. coli* and Gram-positive *S. aureus* were grown in a Luria–Bertani (LB) broth. For antibacterial assay, growth bacterial inoculum (10^4 cells/mL) was incubated with different formulation of NPs, such as AgNPs and HC-NPs. Optical density (OD) at a wavelength of 600 nm using a UV-visible spectrophotometer (Varian Cary 300 Scan; Varian Instruments, CA, USA) every 1 h to measure the bacteria growth. In addition, Gram-negative DH5-Alpha *E. coli* and Gram-positive *S. aureus* treated with different NP formulation were spread on solid LB plates, and the colony forming unit number (CFU) was counted using a Miles–Misra method after 24 h at 37 °C. Representative measurements of three different sets of data were reported.

Entrapment efficacy and in vitro release. The IM entrapment efficacy of mothership PCL NPs and babyship AgNPs into HC-NPs was evaluated as described in [10], through analysis of the supernatant after the NPs' centrifugation.

4.4. Targeting and HC-NP Cellular Uptake

KU812 leukemia cells and C13589 normal lymphoblasts were maintained in culture using RPMI 1640 medium with 10% FBS. To study the ability of mAb-conjugated HC-NPs to target specific cells, a co-culture of CD38-positive (KU812) and CD38-negative (C13895) cells was prepared by seeding 10^4 CSFE labelled C13589 with 10^4 KU812 cells and treated with 500 ng/mL of TRITC-conjugated anti-CD38 HC-NPs for 24 h. For fluorescence confocal analysis, cells were fixed for 5 min in 3.7% formaldehyde and mounted.

Cellular uptake efficiency (%) of HC-NPs was evaluated in accordance with [10]. Representative measurements of three distinct sets of data have been reported.

4.5. In Vitro Cancer Efficacy

In vitro cytotoxicity of different formulations was analyzed using an MTT test after 2 days of treatment, and the IC_{50} was calculated.

IM and AgNPs' synergistic effect were calculated using a combination index (CI) [38].

4.5.1. Apoptosis and Cell Cycle Analysis

Apoptosis and cell cycle were examined with annexin V-FITC/PI assay, and 10,000 ungated cells were evaluated with a Flow Cytometer (C6, Accuri, USA). In particular, KU812 cells (10^5 cells/mL) were incubated with the different formulations, such as 500 ng/mL of empty PCL NPs, 150 nM of IM,

250 nM of AgNPs, 100 nM of IM/AgNPs free combination in the medium, 100 nM of IM-PCL NPs, and 50 nM of HC-NPs for 24 h. All experiments were performed in triplicate.

4.5.2. Western Blotting for BCR-ABL Inhibition Analysis

KU812 leukemia cells (10^6 cells/mL) were incubated with 500 ng/mL of empty PCL NPs, 150 nM of IM, 250 nM of AgNPs, 100 nM of IM/AgNPs free combination in the medium, 100 nM of IM-PCL NPs, and 50 nM of HC-NPs. After 7 days of incubations with the different formulations, the samples were washed in PBS 1× at 4 °C and resuspended in lysis buffer containing a protease inhibitor cocktail on ice for 30 min. Protein concentration was determined using the BCA protein assay (Sigma-Aldrich). Protein bands were separated on 10% (w/v) SDS-polyacrylamide gels, and immunoblotting was performed using nitrocellulose membrane (Amersham Hybond ECL Nitrocellulose Membrane-GE, Abcam). Primary incubations with specific primary antibody directed against anti-c-ABL 1:1000 (clone K-12, Santa Cruz Biotechnology Inc., CA, USA) and anti-βactin 1:5000 (Sigma-Aldrich) were performed overnight. Secondary incubations were for 1 h with HRP-conjugated anti-mouse antibody (Cell Signaling). Proteins were visualized by chemiluminescence (Clarity—Western ECL Substrate, BioRad) using the C-DiGit blot scanner (LI-COR, Cornaredo Milano, Italy). Densitometric analysis was performed using Image J software on the western blots, normalizing to β-actin used as control.

4.5.3. Superoxide Dismutase (SOD) Assay

Cell death can be produced by reactive oxygen intermediates (ROI). Superoxide dismutase (SOD), which catalyzes the dismutation of the superoxide anion (O_2) into hydrogen peroxide and molecular oxygen, is one of the most important antioxidative enzymes. Antioxidant production was measured using a superoxide dismutase (SOD) assay kit (Sigma-Aldrich, USA) according to the manufacturer's instructions. Briefly, to determine the activity of SOD, human chronic leukemia cells (KU812) and normal human B lymphocyte cells (C13589) were incubated with blank PCL NPs (500 ng/mL), free IM (150 nM), AgNPs (250 nM), free combination of IM/AgNPs (100 nM), IM-PCL NPs (100 nM), and HC-NPs (50 nM) for 6 h. Cells were then washed three times with PBS and sonicated on ice in an ultrasonicator (80 watts outpower) for 15 s periods for a total of 4 min. The solution was then centrifuged at 1500 rpm for 5 min at 4°C. The resulting supernatants were used to determine intracellular antioxidants using a spectrophotometer at 440 nm. Each assay was performed in triplicate.

4.6. Statistical Analysis

Three independent experiments were performed, and the results are expressed as mean ± standard deviation. Statistical analysis was achieved by one-way ANOVA.

5. Conclusions

In this study, a hybrid clustered nanoparticle that serially responds to endogenous stimuli was developed for chemo-antibacterial combinatorial cancer therapy.

In vitro studies showed an excellent anti-cancer activity of HC-NPs on chronic myeloid leukemia (CML), used as a model of cancer, improving the cell death efficacy thanks to the combinatory effect of chemotherapic drug and AgNPs. In addition, our HC-NPs showed a good antibacterial capacity on Gram-negative and Gram-positive bacteria.

The chemo-antibacterial combinatorial therapy strategy developed in this study, which potentiates the presence of single drugs and elicits an antibacterial response, paves the way for developing new multifunctional nanoplatforms in cancer therapy.

Supplementary Materials: The following are available online at http://www.mdpi.com/2072-6694/11/9/1338/s1, Figure S1. Absorption spectra of AgNPs. Figure S2. TEM image of AgNPs and SEM images of black PCL NPs, PCL-Ag NPs, and HC-NPs. Figure S3. FT-IR analysis of AgNPs, PCL NPs, and HC-NPs. Figure S4. FACS analysis and SDS-PAGE of non-conjugated and mAb-coated HC-NPs. Figure S5. In vitro IM and AgNPs' cumulative release from HC-NPs. Figure S6. Hemolysis assay (HR %) of AgNPs, PCL NPs, and HC-NPs after 24 h. Figure S7. Time-dependent cellular uptake efficiency of not conjugated HC-NPs with antibody. Figure S8. Cytotoxicity of free IM, AgNPs, free IM/AgNPs combination, IM-PCL NPs, and HC-NPs after 48 h toward C13895 healthy cells. Figure S9. Analysis of cell apoptosis and cell cycle of C13895 healthy cells after 24 h of treatment with different formulations. Figure S10. Cytotoxicity assay using different NP formulations in KU812 cells after 48 h of treatment. IC_{50} values of NPs in KU812 leukemia cells. Figure S11. Illustration of multistep release mechanism.

Author Contributions: All authors collected and discussed the material, providing experimental data. I.E.P. conceived the research and supervision of the work. I.E.P., B.C., and S.D. performed the synthesis and physical chemical characterization of all nanomaterials used in the work and performed the in vitro validations. M.T. performed the western blot analysis. P.R. collected the blood of the mice. I.E.P. and B.C. undertook the writing, review, and editing.

Funding: This study was supported partially by Fondo Integrativo Speciale per la Ricerca(FISR) project—CNR "Tecnopolo di Nanotecnologia e Fotonica per la Medicina di Precisione"—CUP B83B17000010001 Tecnomed and Italian Association for Cancer Research (AIRC) through the grant My First AIRC Grant (MFAG) n. 16803.

Conflicts of Interest: The authors declare no conflict of interest.

References

1. Yap, T.A.; Omlin, A.; Bono, J.S.D. Development of Therapeutic Combinations Targeting Major Cancer Signaling Pathways. *J. Clin. Oncol.* **2013**, *31*, 1592–1605. [CrossRef] [PubMed]
2. Chabner, B.A.; Roberts, T.G. Chemotherapy and the war on cancer. *Nat. Rev. Cancer* **2005**, *5*, 65–72. [CrossRef] [PubMed]
3. Partridge, A.H.; Winer, E.P.; Burstein, H.J. Side Effects of Chemotherapy and Combined Chemohormonal Therapy in Women with Early-Stage Breast Cancer. *JNCI Monogr.* **2001**, *2001*, 135–142. [CrossRef] [PubMed]
4. Gianni, L.; Salvatorelli, E.; Minotti, G. Anthracycline cardiotoxicity in breast cancer patients: Synergism with trastuzumab and taxanes. *Cardiovasc. Toxicol.* **2007**, *7*, 67–71. [CrossRef] [PubMed]
5. Kaye, S.; Merry, S. Tumor-Cell Resistance to Anthracyclines—A Review. *Cancer Chemother. Pharmacol.* **1985**, *14*, 96–103. [CrossRef] [PubMed]
6. Dunbar, A.; Tai, E.; Nielsen, D.B.; Shropshire, S.; Richardson, L.C. Preventing Infections During Cancer Treatment: Development of an Interactive Patient Education Website. *Clin. J. Oncol. Nurs.* **2014**, *18*, 426–431. [CrossRef] [PubMed]
7. Sanna, V.; Pala, N.; Sechi, M. Targeted therapy using nanotechnology: Focus on cancer. *Int. J. Nanomed.* **2014**, *9*, 467–483. [CrossRef]
8. Farokhzad, O.C.; Langer, R. Impact of Nanotechnology on Drug Delivery. *ACS Nano* **2009**, *3*, 16–20. [CrossRef]
9. Davis, M.E.; Chen, Z.; Shin, D.M. Nanoparticle therapeutics: An emerging treatment modality for cancer. *Nat. Rev. Drug Discov.* **2008**, *7*, 771. [CrossRef]
10. Cortese, B.; D'Amone, S.; Palama, I.E. Wool-Like Hollow Polymeric Nanoparticles for CML Chemo-Combinatorial Therapy. *Pharmaceutics* **2018**, *10*, 52. [CrossRef]
11. Nam, J.; La, W.-G.; Hwang, S.; Ha, Y.S.; Park, N.; Won, N.; Jung, S.; Bhang, S.H.; Ma, Y.-J.; Cho, Y.-M.; et al. pH-Responsive Assembly of Gold Nanoparticles and "Spatiotemporally Concerted" Drug Release for Synergistic Cancer Therapy. *ACS Nano* **2013**, *7*, 3388–3402. [CrossRef] [PubMed]
12. Wang, C.; Li, Z.; Cao, D.; Zhao, Y.-L.; Gaines, J.W.; Bozdemir, O.A.; Ambrogio, M.W.; Frasconi, M.; Botros, Y.Y.; Zink, J.I.; et al. Stimulated Release of Size-Selected Cargos in Succession from Mesoporous Silica Nanoparticles. *Angew. Chem. Int. Ed.* **2012**, *51*, 5460–5465. [CrossRef] [PubMed]
13. Moorthi, C.; Manavalan, R.; Kathiresan, K. Nanotherapeutics to Overcome Conventional Cancer Chemotherapy Limitations. *J. Pharm. Pharm. Sci.* **2011**, *14*, 67–77. [CrossRef]
14. Ostad, S.N.; Dehnad, S.; Nazari, Z.E.; Fini, S.T.; Mokhtari, N.; Shakibaie, M.; Shahverdi, A.R. Cytotoxic Activities of Silver Nanoparticles and Silver Ions in Parent and Tamoxifen-Resistant T47D Human Breast Cancer Cells and Their Combination Effects with Tamoxifen against Resistant Cells. *Avicenna J. Med. Biotechnol.* **2010**, *2*, 187–196. [PubMed]
15. Bhattacharyya, S.; Kudgus, R.A.; Bhattacharya, R.; Mukherjee, P. Inorganic Nanoparticles in Cancer Therapy. *Pharm. Res.* **2011**, *28*, 237–259. [CrossRef]

16. Elbaz, N.M.; Ziko, L.; Siam, R.; Mamdouh, W. Core-Shell Silver/Polymeric Nanoparticles-Based Combinatorial Therapy against Breast Cancer In-vitro. *Sci. Rep.* **2016**, *6*, 30729. [CrossRef] [PubMed]
17. Palama, I.E.; Pollini, M.; Paladini, F.; Accorsi, G.; Sannino, A.; Gigli, G.; Palama, I. Inhibiting Growth or Proliferation of a Cancer Cell e.g., Myeloid Leukemia Cell, Comprises Contacting the Cancer Cell with Silver Nanoparticles. WO2015015301-A2 WOIB001895, 5 February 2015. 31 July 2014.
18. Guo, D.; Zhu, L.; Huang, Z.; Zhou, H.; Ge, Y.; Ma, W.; Wu, J.; Zhang, X.; Zhou, X.; Zhang, Y.; et al. Anti-leukemia activity of PVP-coated silver nanoparticles via generation of reactive oxygen species and release of silver ions. *Biomaterials* **2013**, *34*, 7884–7894. [CrossRef]
19. Heravi, R.E.; Zakeri, S.; Nazari, P. Anticancer activity evaluation of green synthesised gold-silver alloy nanoparticles on colourectal HT-29 and prostate DU-145 carcinoma cell lines. *Micro Nano Lett.* **2018**, *13*, 1475–1479. [CrossRef]
20. De Matteis, V.; Malvindi, M.A.; Galeone, A.; Brunetti, V.; De Luca, E.; Kote, S.; Kshirsagar, P.; Sabella, S.; Bardi, G.; Pompa, P.P. Negligible particle-specific toxicity mechanism of silver nanoparticles: The role of Ag+ ion release in the cytosol. *Nanomed. Nanotechnol. Biol. Med.* **2015**, *11*, 731–739. [CrossRef]
21. Richa, S.; Dimple, S.C. Regulatory Approval of Silver Nanoparticles. *Appl. Clin. Res. Clin. Trials Regul. Aff.* **2018**, *5*, 74–79. [CrossRef]
22. Vardiman, J.W. Chronic Myelogenous Leukemia, BCR-ABL1+. *Am. J. Clin. Pathol.* **2009**, *132*, 250–260. [CrossRef] [PubMed]
23. Yalcintepe, L.; Halis, E.; Ulku, S. Effect of CD38 on the multidrug resistance of human chronic myelogenous leukemia K562 cells to doxorubicin. *Oncol. Lett.* **2016**, *11*, 2290–2296. [CrossRef] [PubMed]
24. Palamà, I.E.; Leporatti, S.; Luca, E.D.; Renzo, N.D.; Maffia, M.; Gambacorti-Passerini, C.; Rinaldi, R.; Gigli, G.; Cingolani, R.; Coluccia, A.M. Imatinib-loaded polyelectrolyte microcapsules for sustained targeting of BCR-ABL+ leukemia stem cells. *Nanomedicine* **2010**, *5*, 419–431. [CrossRef] [PubMed]
25. Abdelbary, A.A.; Li, X.L.; El-Nabarawi, M.; Elassasy, A.; Jasti, B. Effect of fixed aqueous layer thickness of polymeric stabilizers on zeta potential and stability of aripiprazole nanosuspensions. *Pharm. Dev. Technol.* **2013**, *18*, 730–735. [CrossRef] [PubMed]
26. Sadzuka, Y.; Nakade, A.; Hirama, R.; Miyagishima, A.; Nozawa, Y.; Hirota, S.; Sonobe, T. Effects of mixed polyethyleneglycol modification on fixed aqueous layer thickness and antitumor activity of doxorubicin containing liposome. *Int. J. Pharm.* **2002**, *238*, 171–180. [CrossRef]
27. Gurunathan, S.; Kang, M.-H.; Qasim, M.; Kim, J.-H. Nanoparticle-Mediated Combination Therapy: Two-in-One Approach for Cancer. *Int. J. Mol. Sci.* **2018**, *19*, 3264. [CrossRef] [PubMed]
28. Murugan, C.; Rayappan, K.; Thangam, R.; Bhanumathi, R.; Shanthi, K.; Vivek, R.; Thirumurugan, R.; Bhattacharyya, A.; Sivasubramanian, S.; Gunasekaran, P.; et al. Combinatorial nanocarrier based drug delivery approach for amalgamation of anti-tumor agents in breast cancer cells: An improved nanomedicine strategy. *Sci. Rep.* **2016**, *6*, 34053. [CrossRef] [PubMed]
29. Palamà, I.E.; Coluccia, A.M.; Gigli, G. Uptake of imatinib-loaded polyelectrolyte complexes by BCR-ABL+ cells: A long-acting drug-delivery strategy for targeting oncoprotein activity. *Nanomedicine* **2014**, *9*, 2087–2098. [CrossRef]
30. Cortese, B.; D'Amone, S.; Gigli, G.; Palama, I.E. Sustained anti-BCR-ABL activity with pH responsive imatinib mesylate loaded PCL nanoparticles in CML cells. *MedChemComm* **2015**, *6*, 212–221. [CrossRef]
31. Gujrati, M.; Malamas, A.; Shin, T.; Jin, E.; Sun, Y.; Lu, Z.-R. Multifunctional Cationic Lipid-Based Nanoparticles Facilitate Endosomal Escape and Reduction-Triggered Cytosolic siRNA Release. *Mol. Pharm.* **2014**, *11*, 2734–2744. [CrossRef]
32. Lynch, I.; Dawson, K.A. Protein-nanoparticle interactions. *Nano Today* **2008**, *3*, 40–47. [CrossRef]
33. Miceli, E.; Kar, M.; Calderón, M. Interactions of organic nanoparticles with proteins in physiological conditions. *J. Mater. Chem. B* **2017**, *5*, 4393–4405. [CrossRef]
34. Corbo, C.; Molinaro, R.; Taraballi, F.; Toledano Furman, N.E.; Hartman, K.A.; Sherman, M.B.; De Rosa, E.; Kirui, D.K.; Salvatore, F.; Tasciotti, E. Unveiling the in Vivo Protein Corona of Circulating Leukocyte-like Carriers. *ACS Nano* **2017**, *11*, 3262–3273. [CrossRef] [PubMed]
35. Le Ouay, B.; Stellacci, F. Antibacterial activity of silver nanoparticles: A surface science insight. *Nano Today* **2015**, *10*, 339–354. [CrossRef]

36. Lok, C.-N.; Ho, C.-M.; Chen, R.; He, Q.-Y.; Yu, W.-Y.; Sun, H.; Tam, P.K.-H.; Chiu, J.-F.; Che, C.-M. Proteomic Analysis of the Mode of Antibacterial Action of Silver Nanoparticles. *J. Proteome Res.* **2006**, *5*, 916–924. [CrossRef] [PubMed]
37. Azizi, M.; Ghourchian, H.; Yazdian, F.; Bagherifam, S.; Bekhradnia, S.; Nyström, B. Anti-cancerous effect of albumin coated silver nanoparticles on MDA-MB 231 human breast cancer cell line. *Sci. Rep.* **2017**, *7*, 5178. [CrossRef]
38. Chou, T.-C.; Talalay, P. Quantitative analysis of dose-effect relationships: The combined effects of multiple drugs or enzyme inhibitors. *Adv. Enzym. Regul.* **1984**, *22*, 27–55. [CrossRef]

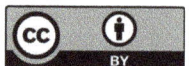

© 2019 by the authors. Licensee MDPI, Basel, Switzerland. This article is an open access article distributed under the terms and conditions of the Creative Commons Attribution (CC BY) license (http://creativecommons.org/licenses/by/4.0/).

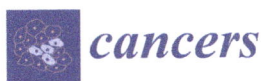

Article

A Tunable Nanoplatform of Nanogold Functionalised with Angiogenin Peptides for Anti-Angiogenic Therapy of Brain Tumours

Irina Naletova [1], Lorena Maria Cucci [2], Floriana D'Angeli [3], Carmelina Daniela Anfuso [3], Antonio Magrì [4], Diego La Mendola [1,5,*], Gabriella Lupo [3,*] and Cristina Satriano [1,2,*]

1. Consorzio Interuniversitario di Ricerca in Chimica dei Metalli nei Sistemi Biologici (CIRCMSB), Via Celso Ulpiani 27, I-70126 Bari, Italy; irina_naletova@yahoo.com
2. Hybrid NanobioInterfaces Lab (NHIL), Department of Chemical Sciences, University of Catania, Viale Andrea Doria 6, I-95125 Catania, Italy; lorena.cucci@unict.it
3. Department of Biomedical and Biotechnological Sciences, University of Catania, Via Santa Sofia 89, I-95123 Catania, Italy; fdangeli@unict.it (F.D.); daniela.anfuso@unict.it (C.D.A.)
4. Institute of Crystallography Catania, National Council of Research (IC-CNR), Via Paolo Gaifami 18, I-95126 Catania, Italy; leotony@unict.it
5. Department of Pharmacy, University of Pisa, via Bonanno Pisano 6, I-56126 Pisa, Italy
* Correspondence: lamendola@farm.unipi.it (D.L.M.); gabriella.lupo@unict.it (G.L.); csatriano@unict.it (C.S.); Tel.: +39-050-2219533 (D.L.M.); +39-095-4781158 (G.L.); +39-095-7385136 (C.S.)

Received: 9 August 2019; Accepted: 3 September 2019; Published: 6 September 2019

Abstract: Angiogenin (ANG), an endogenous protein that plays a key role in cell growth and survival, has been scrutinised here as promising nanomedicine tool for the modulation of pro-/anti-angiogenic processes in brain cancer therapy. Specifically, peptide fragments from the putative cell membrane binding domain (residues 60–68) of the protein were used in this study to obtain peptide-functionalised spherical gold nanoparticles (AuNPs) of about 10 nm and 30 nm in optical and hydrodynamic size, respectively. Different hybrid biointerfaces were fabricated by peptide physical adsorption (Ang$_{60-68}$) or chemisorption (the cysteine analogous Ang$_{60-68}$Cys) at the metal nanoparticle surface, and cellular assays were performed in the comparison with ANG-functionalised AuNPs. Cellular treatments were performed both in basal and in copper-supplemented cell culture medium, to scrutinise the synergic effect of the metal, which is another known angiogenic factor. Two brain cell lines were investigated in parallel, namely tumour glioblastoma (A172) and neuron-like differentiated neuroblastoma (d-SH-SY5Y). Results on cell viability/proliferation, cytoskeleton actin, angiogenin translocation and vascular endothelial growth factor (VEGF) release pointed to the promising potentialities of the developed systems as anti-angiogenic tunable nanoplaftforms in cancer cells treatment.

Keywords: plasmonics; nanomedicine; theranostics; copper; VEGF; glioblastoma; differentiated neuroblastoma; peptidomimetics; real-time quantitative polymerase chain reaction (qPCR); actin

1. Introduction

In recent decades, protein-nanoparticle and peptide-nanoparticle conjugates have emerged as powerful nanomedicine tools, enabling biomedical applications in the prevention, diagnosis and treatment of disease [1,2]. Unfunctionalised, bare nanoparticles (NPs), are often able to match several of the desired functions required by theranostic platforms, including the peculiar optical, electrical, magnetic properties of nanometer-sized materials [3], the tunable geometries and the tailored size and surface chemistry [4] and the intrinsic biological properties, such as anti-angiogenic nanogold [5,6] or antibacterial nanosilver [7,8]. Biological protein-based nanoparticles are advantageous in having biodegradability, bioavailability, and relatively low cost. Many protein nanoparticles, for instance naturally occurring protein cages such as ferritin, are easy to process and can be modified to achieve desired specifications such as size, morphology, and weight [9–11]. Natural product-based nanomedicine include, among the most common types of nanoparticles, polymeric micelles, solid lipid nanoparticles, liposomes, inorganic nanoparticles and dendrimers [3,12].

Each of these nanoparticles has its own advantages and disadvantages as drug delivery vehicle. Hybrid peptide- or protein-NP conjugates enable addressing many of the difficulties that arise as results of in vivo applications, replacing many materials that have a poor biocompatibility and have a negative impact on the environment. Specifically, both naturally derived and synthetic polypeptides may offer improved biocompatibility [13], targeted delivery [14] and prolonged lifetime before clearance, to ensure an efficient therapeutic action [1,15].

Angiogenin (ANG) is a secreted ribonuclease (also known as RNase 5), identified in media from cancer cells, but also present in normal tissues, such as plasma and amniotic fluid, and secreted from vascular endothelial cells, aortic smooth muscle cells, fibroblasts [16]. Angiogenin induces neovascularization by triggering cell migration, invasion, proliferation, and formation of tubular structures [16–19].

Physiologically, ANG is overexpressed during inflammation, exhibiting wound healing properties as well as microbicide activity and conferring host immunity [20]. However, uncontrolled activity of angiogenin is implicated in pathological processes.

The protein was isolated for the first time from medium conditioned by a human adenocarcinoma cell line (HT-29) [21]. A high expression of angiogenin has been described in different types of cancers and to their malignant transformation [16], including gliomas that are brain tumours fast-growing, aggressive and with a poor prognosis [22].

ANG expression has been identified also in neurons and acts as a part of the secretome of endothelial progenitor cells (EPCs) [23,24]; the modulation of ANG and EPCs as repair-associated factors has been found in stroke patients and mouse models of rehabilitation after cerebral ischemia [25]. Mutations in the ANG gene have been characterized in amyotrophic lateral sclerosis (ALS) [26] and Parkinson's disease (PD) [27]. Moreover, endogenous angiogenin levels are dramatically reduced in an alpha-synuclein mouse model of PD and exogenous angiogenin protects against cell loss in neurotoxin-based cellular models of PD [27]. Genetic studies revealed that angiogenin treatment delays motor dysfunction and motor neuron loss, also prolonging the survival in superoxide dismutase 1 (SOD1) mouse model of ALS [18].

In motor neurons, ANG can be upregulated by hypoxia thought the stimulation of ribosomal ribonucleic acid (rRNA) transcription of endothelial cells [28]. Such a process is critical for the cellular proliferation induced by other angiogenic proteins, including vascular endothelial growth factor (VEGF) [29]. While the predominant role of VEGF in the formation of new blood vessels is unquestioned, several recent studies demonstrate that VEGF also has trophic effects on neurons and glia in the central- (CNS) and peripheral- (PNS) nervous system, promoting neurogenesis, neuronal patterning, neuroprotection and glial growth [30]. Therefore, VEGF modulates neuronal health and nerve repair; and exogenous angiogenin delivery can be considered a promising tool of anti-angiogenic therapy for treating gliomas, where malignancy is highly related to angiogenesis.

Copper is an essential metal that plays a key role in the CNS development and function, and its dyshomeostasis is involved in many neurodegenerative diseases as Alzheimer's disease (AD), PD and ALS [31,32]. Furthermore, copper is known to be a strong angiogenic factor, with metal serum levels raising in a wide variety of human cancers [33,34]. Noteworthy, copper increases the expression of ANG and regulates its intracellular localization [35]. Moreover, ANG binds copper ions and the metal interaction largely influences its interaction with endothelial cells as well as its angiogenic activity [36–38]. Taking into account the correlations between angiogenin protein and copper in physiological and pathological conditions of the brain, a promising pharmacological approach in brain tumours therapy is the use of ANG as molecular target, whose activity may be modulated by the presence of copper ions.

As an alternative to protein-based drugs, peptides mimicking functional domains of the whole protein are becoming more relevant as drug candidates, to address problems exhibited by the protein in in vivo applications such as the additional effect or functions or binding sites for other ligands, the immunological clearance before reaching their target site [39,40].

Three domains of angiogenin have been demonstrated essential to the protein to explicate its biological activity, i.e.,: the catalytic site (involving His-13, Lys-40, and His-114 residues), the nuclear translocation sequence (encompassing residues 31–35, RRRGL); the putative cellular binding site (residues 60–68, KNGNPHREN) [41,42]. In previous works, peptide fragments encompassing such different domains of the protein have been synthesized and used as mimicking model of the whole protein [6,43,44]. In particular, hybrid nano-assemblies of gold nanoparticles (AuNPs) functionalized with different peptides encompassing the putative cellular binding site of the protein (Ang$_{60-68}$) have been demonstrated able to maintain their activity on cytoskeleton actin reorganization in a tumour cell line of human neuroblastoma [44].

Here, we report on the investigation of AuNPs functionalised with the peptide Ang$_{60-68}$ or its analogous having a cysteine residue in the C-terminus (Ang$_{60-68}$Cys), in the comparison with the whole ANG protein. Such systems have been scrutinised as potential nanomedicine platforms towards a brain cancer of human glioblastoma (A172 cell line). To compare the response of tumour and non-tumour brain cells, differentiated neuroblastoma (d-SH-SY5Y line) have been included in the study as model neuron-like cells.

Effects on cell proliferation, cytoskeleton actin changes, angiogenin translocation and VEGF expression upon the cell treatments with peptides- or protein-functionalized nanoparticles, in the absence or presence of copper ions, shed new light in the link between different factors involved in angiogenesis processes of non-tumour and tumour model brain cell cultures. Indeed, since ANG plays a key role in cell growth and survival, and the role of VEGF in brain tumour angiogenesis has been demonstrated [45], new perspectives in the therapeutic approaches may rely on the tiny modulation of the pro-/anti-angiogenic processes [46] for brain cancer treatment.

2. Results

2.1. Physicochemical Characterisation of Hybrid Peptides- and Protein-NP Conjugates

2.1.1. Optical (Plasmonic) Properties Changes of AuNP upon Interaction with Peptides/Protein

Peptide-functionalised NPs were fabricated by two different approaches, namely a purely physical adsorption and a prevalent covalent grafting, with the peptide sequences Ang$_{60-68}$ and Ang$_{60-68}$Cys, respectively. As positive control, samples of ANG-functionalised AuNPs were prepared by using the whole protein.

Figure 1 shows the Ultraviolet (UV)–visible spectra of gold nanoparticles, before and after the addition of Ang$_{60-68n}$, Ang$_{60-68}$Cys or ANG, respectively. The plasmon peak parameters, i.e., the wavelength at the maximum absorbance (λ_{max} = 519 nm) and the full width at half maximum (FWHM = 54 nm) point to the formation of a gold colloidal solution of spherical nanoparticles with an optical diameter of 11 nm [47].

The addition of 3×10^{-5} M Ang$_{60-68}$ (Figure 1a) or Ang$_{60-68}$Cys (Figure 1b) induced comparable red-shifts ($\Delta\lambda_{max}$ = 3 nm) and hyperchromic-shifts ($\Delta Abs \sim 0.07$), according to previous findings [44]. No significant changes in the width of the plasmon peak were detected. The addition of the 1×10^{-7} M ANG whole protein (Figure 1c), lead to a significantly larger red-shift in the plasmon peak ($\Delta\lambda_{max}$ = 4 nm) with respect to the bare nanoparticles than those found upon the addition of the peptides. Moreover, a hypochromic-shift ($\Delta Abs = -0.09$) in comparison to the bare AuNPs and a broadening of the plasmon band ($\Delta FWHM$ = 11 nm) with the appearance of a shoulder at around 600 nm, were found, likely due to a partial nanoparticle aggregation.

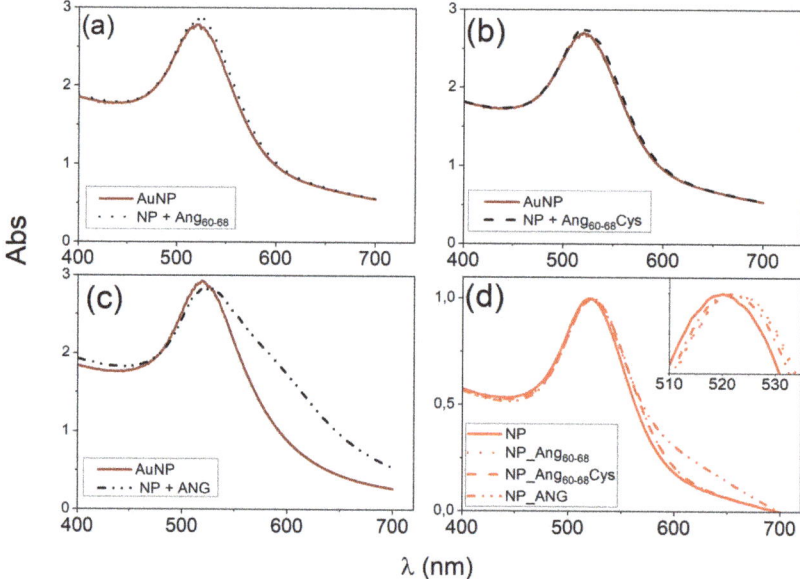

Figure 1. (**a–c**) Ultraviolet (UV)-visible spectra of gold nanopartilces (AuNPs) in the 1 mM 3-(N-morpholino)propanesulfonic acid)-Tris(2-carboxyethyl)phosphine hydrochloride (MOPS-TCEP) buffer (1:1 mol ratio) before and after the addition of: (**a**) 30 μM Ang_{60-68}, (**b**) 30 μM $Ang_{60-68}Cys$; (**c**) 100 nM angiogenin (ANG). (**d**) UV-visible spectra of the pellets collected after two rinsing steps by centrifugation (15 min at 6010 relative centrifugal force, RCF) and re-suspension in 1 mM MOPS-TCEP buffer.

As to the hybrid systems used for the cellular experiments, Figure 1d shows the UV-visible spectra of the protein/peptide-nanoparticle pellets samples after two washing steps, performed to remove unbound and/or weakly bound biomolecules.

The red-shift in the plasmon peak with respect to the bare AuNPs is still visible ($\Delta\lambda_{max}$~3 nm) for Ang_{60-68} and $Ang_{60-68}Cys$ peptides as well as for ANG protein). This finding confirms the irreversible adsorption of the peptides and protein molecules and hence the successful surface functionalisation of the gold nanoparticles by the used biomolecules.

2.1.2. Hydrodynamic Size and Conformational Features of Peptides- and Protein-Functionalised NPs in the Absence or Presence of Copper Ions

To gain insight into the actual hydrodynamic size of the angiogenin-functionalised nanoparticles, dynamic light scattering was used to take into account the dynamic soft shell made by the peptide/protein molecules at the AuNP surface, in contrast to the optical size that reflects merely the 'dry state' or internal 'core' of the functionalised particle. The hydrodynamic size of ~30 nm for the aqueous dispersion of gold nanoparticles (1.7×10^8 NP/mL) did not change significantly upon addition of the peptide solution (3×10^{-5} M), for both Ang_{60-68} and $Ang_{60-68}Cys$ fragments (Table 1). On the other hand, by addition of ANG (1×10^{-7} M), the nanoparticle size was largely increased in comparison to the bare AuNP, suggesting bridged interactions between the protein molecules immobilised at the nanoparticle surface that could also prompt a partial aggregation.

The Ang_{60-68}_NP and $Ang_{60-68}Cys$_NP pellets maintained a size range comparable to that of non-rinsed nanoparticles (both bare and functionalized), while a slight decrease in the size was found for ANG_NP, where a fraction of loosely bound proteins molecules was therefore likely rinsed off by the washing steps of the protein-nanoparticle hybrids.

Table 1. Hydrodynamic size of the different NPs either before or after the functionalisation with the peptides or the protein, and after the addition of 20 μM CuSO$_4$ aqueous solution.

Peptide/Protein	Hydrodynamic Size (nm)		
	Nanoparticle (NP) + Peptide/Protein [1]	Peptide/Protein_NP [2]	Peptide/Protein_NP + Cu(II) [3]
-	29 ± 3	30 ± 2	31 ± 5
Ang$_{60-68}$	28 ± 4	37 ± 4	175 ± 10
Ang$_{60-68}$Cys	30 ± 3	29 ± 5	281 ± 42
ANG	53 ± 4	41 ± 6	47 ± 5

[1] peptide/protein-added NP samples; [2] peptide/protein_NP samples after the centrifugation and rinsing steps; [3] same pellets as 2 added with copper ions.

Noteworthy, after the addition of copper ions, the average dimension of nanoparticles was still unchanged for bare AuNP, instead a dramatic increase in the hydrodynamic diameter was found for Ang$_{60-68}$_NP (to ~0.18 μm) and Ang$_{60-68}$Cys_NP (to ~0.3 μm), respectively.

The Ang$_{60-68}$ peptide is able to bind copper at physiological pH by the involvement of one imidazole, two deprotonated amide nitrogen and one carboxyl oxygen atoms, respectively [48]. The UV-vis parameters measured for the equimolar solutions at pH = 7.4 of copper(II) and Ang$_{60-68}$Cys (λ_{max} = 624 nm; ε = 100 M^{-1}cm^{-1}) were very similar to those of analogous complex formed with Ang$_{60-68}$ (λ_{max} = 630 nm; ε = 120 M^{-1}cm^{-1}).

Accordingly, the circular dichroism (CD) spectra of both Ang$_{60-68}$+Cu(II) and Ang$_{60-68}$Cys+Cu(II) (Figure 2) showed a minimum around 600 nm, assigned to copper d-d transition, and a broad band with a maximum approximately at 350 nm, assigned to charge transfer to the metal ion by the imidazole nitrogen (N$_{im}$→Cu(II)) and the deprotonated amide nitrogen (N$_{amide}$→Cu(II)).

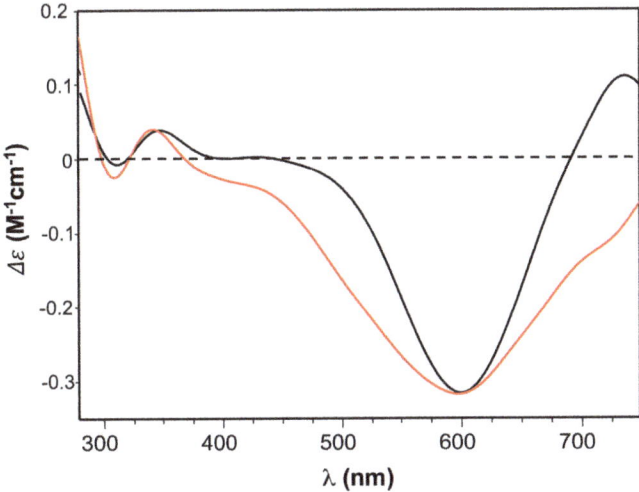

Figure 2. Circular dichroism (CD) spectra of Ang$_{60-68}$ + CuSO$_4$ (black line) and Ang$_{60-68}$Cys + CuSO$_4$ (red line) at pH = 7.4. Equimolar concentration of peptide and copper were used: [peptide] = [Cu(II)] = 1 × 10^{-3} M.

2.2. Biological Characterisation of the Interaction between Peptides- or Protein-NP Conjugates and Brain Tumour (A172 line) or Non-Tumour (d-SH-SY5Y) Cells

2.2.1. Determination of Angiogenin Expression in Glioblastoma (A172), Undifferentiated and Differentiated Neuroblastoma (SH-SY5Y) Cell Lines

To analyse the endogenous levels of ANG expression in the tested cancer cells (glioblastoma A172 and neuroblastoma SH-SY5Y) and neuronal-like cells (differentiated neuroblastoma, d-SH-SY5Y), we performed western blot analyses of protein extracts from crude cell lysates (Figure S1 in the Supplementary Material). Results confirmed that in tumour cells the expressed level of protein was significantly higher than in differentiated neuroblastoma (Figure S1a,b). Moreover, to control the specific interaction of anti-angiogenin antibody with Ang_{60-68} or $Ang_{60-68}Cys$ in the comparison with ANG, the peptides and protein samples were analysed by Western and dot blotting assays. The used anti-angiogenin antibody detected only the whole protein but did not interact with the two peptide fragments (Figure S1c,d).

2.2.2. Cell Viability

MTT (3-(4, 5-dimethylthiazolyl-2)-2, 5-diphenyltetrazolium bromide) assays were carried out to assess the effect on cell viability (Figure 3) of peptides- or protein-functionalised NPs, in the absence or presence of copper ions, for brain glioblastoma (A172 line) and differentiated neuroblastoma (d-SH-SY5Y), respectively.

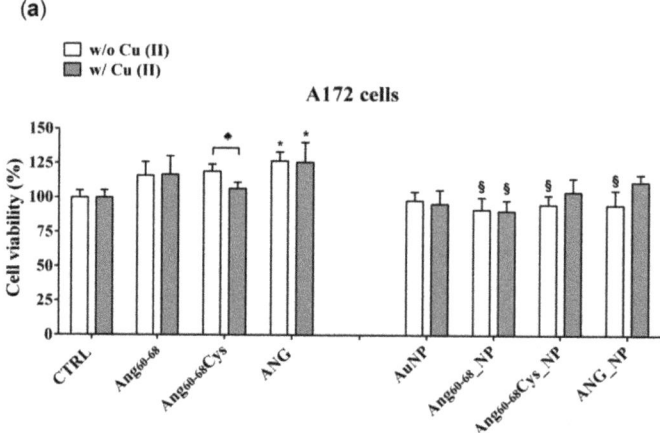

Figure 3. *Cont.*

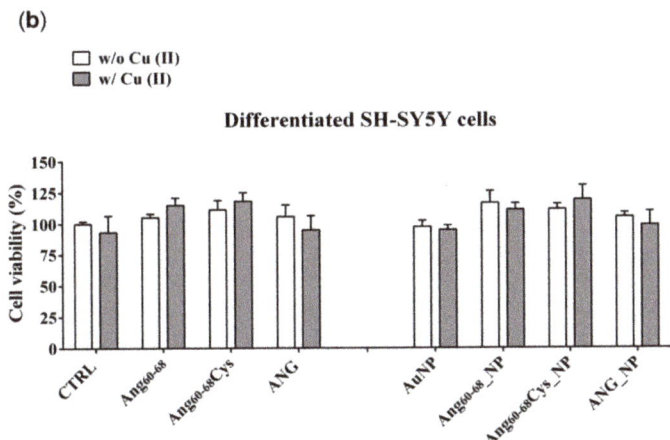

Figure 3. Cell viability determined by 3-(4, 5-dimethylthiazolyl-2)-2, 5-diphenyltetrazolium bromide (MTT) assay of A172 (**a**) and d-SH-SY5Y (**b**) cell lines. Cells were grown in basal culture medium (control: CTRL) and in culture medium supplemented with: Ang_{60-68} (30 µM), $Ang_{60-68}Cys$ (30 µM); ANG (100 nM), AuNP (9.4 nM = 1.4×10^8 NP/mL), Ang_{60-68}_NP (1.4 nM = 4.0×10^6 NP/mL, [Ang_{60-68}] = 2.8×10^{-12} M), $Ang_{60-68}Cys$_NP (1.4 nM = 4.0×10^6 NP/mL, [$Ang_{60-68}Cys$] = 2.6×10^{-12} M), ANG_NP (1.2 nM = 3.4×10^6 NP/mL, [ANG]= 0.2×10^{-12} M). All conditions were evaluated in presence or absence of metal ions (copper sulphate: Cu(II), 20 µM). The bars represent means ± SD of three independent experiments performed in triplicate (S.D. = standard deviation). Statistically significant differences, determined by one-way analysis of variance ANOVA are indicated: * $p \leq 0.05$ versus CTRL; § $p \leq 0.05$ versus the respective treatment with free peptides/protein; ♦ $p \leq 0.05$ versus the respective treatment w/o Cu(II).

In the tumour A172 cell line (Figure 3a), a significant increase on viability (+25%; $p \leq 0.05$ vs. control untreated cells) was found after the treatment with ANG, both in absence and in the presence of added Cu(II). The cells incubation either with free peptides of $Ang_{60-68}Cys$ or Ang_{60-68} did not induce any significant change on cell viability; similar results were found for cells treated with peptides in the presence of copper. As to nanoparticle-treated cells, the incubation with bare AuNP, both in the absence and with Cu(II), did not modify the cell viability in comparison with control cells. The incubation with Ang_{60-68}_NP reduced the cell viability by about 20–25% ($p \leq 0.05$ vs. the respective peptide and peptide + Cu(II) controls), both in the absence and in the presence of copper. As to $Ang_{60-68}Cys$_NP, a significant cell viability decrease in the absence of Cu(II) (−25%; $p \leq 0.05$ vs. the respective free peptide) was nullified by the incubation in presence of copper. A similar trend was found for the cells incubated with ANG_NP, where a reduced cell viability (−20%; $p \leq 0.05$ vs. the respective free protein) in the absence of copper but no significant difference in presence of copper were found.

In the non-tumour d-SH-SY5Y cell line (Figure 3b), none of the treatments used resulted in a statistically significant decrease of cell viability in comparison to untreated control cells. Trypan blue staining confirmed the above reported results (data not shown).

2.2.3. Cytoskeleton Actin Reorganisation and Intranuclear Angiogenin

Cell migration is a critical step in tumour invasion and metastasis; the regulation of this process is often monitored in therapies for treating cancer. Reorganization of the actin cytoskeleton is the primary mechanism of cell motility and is essential for most types of cell migration [49].

Confocal laser scanning microscopy (LSM) demonstrated substantial differences between the tumour A172 (Figure 4) and non-tumour d-SH-SY5Y (Figure 5) cell lines in the organization of the actin cytoskeleton, both before and after the treatments with the peptides/protein-conjugated nanoparticles, as well as the incubation in the copper-supplemented medium.

Combined staining for F-actin (green) and nuclei (blue) for untreated glioblastoma (Figure 4, panel 1, CTRL) clearly shows their polygonal shape along with different types of actin dorsal fibres and transverse arcs, typical for the lamellipodial actin meshwork [50]. The cell treatment with bare AuNP and/or the addition of Cu(II) (Figure 4, panels 2–4) increased actin stress fibres. In contrast to A172 cells, F-actin staining of untreated d-SH-SY5Y cells (Figure 5, panel 1, CTRL) analysed by Laser Scanning Confocal Microscopy (LSM) showed several distinct types of actin structures with broad leading edges, including a lamellipodium with a loose meshwork of actin filaments, an actin rich lamella, dorsal ruffles, transverse arcs and stress fibres, as expected for differentiated neuroblastoma [51].

A172 cells treated with the free peptides or protein showed a diffuse actin staining for several lamellipodia protruding from the cell body in all directions. The addition of copper did not change significantly the actin staining for Ang_{60-68} (Figure 4, see panels 1 and 3), instead visibly decreased the lamellipodia structures for $Ang_{60-68}Cys$ (Figure 4, panels 1 and 3) and ANG (Figure 4, panels 1 and 3), respectively. Both in absence and in the presence of copper, A172 cells treated with Ang_{60-68}_NP (Figure 4, panels 2 and 4) and ANG_NP (Figure 4, panels 2 and 4) still displayed a similar actin staining than those incubated with the free peptide or protein, respectively.

On the contrary, after incubation with $Ang_{60-68}Cys$_NP, both in the absence and presence of copper (Figure 4, panels 2 and 4), cells contained very few, if any, actin stress fibres in the central regions and lamellipodia structures.

For d-SH-SY5Y cells treated with the two peptides or the protein or their nanoparticle conjugates, irrespective of the incubation in copper-supplemented medium or not, the most notable change was a generally less dense meshwork of actin filaments after the treatment with Ang_{60-68} (Figure 5, panels 1–4) or $Ang_{60-68}Cys$ (Figure 5, panels 1–4). The central region of these cells contained neither ventral stress fibres nor dorsal ruffles or transverse arcs detectable by LSM. On the contrary, numerous and diffuse actin structures, as well as prominent actin stress fibres along the entire cell border were found for cells treated with ANG samples (Figure 5, panels 1–4).

LSM imaging of intracellular angiogenin in glioblastoma and differentiated neuroblastoma cells confirmed the western blot results (see Figure S1) that untreated non-tumour d-SHSY5Y cells (Figure 5, panel 5) showed lower levels of endogenous ANG in the cytoplasm and in the nucleus than untreated tumour A172 cells (Figure 4, panel 5).

Cells incubated with ANG for 2 hr exhibited a strong increase of the red staining, confirming the cellular uptake of exogenous angiogenin. In A172 cells the staining was especially enhanced in the presence of copper ions for the nuclear and perinuclear regions (Figure 4, panels 7,8). In d-SH-SY5Y cells, an increased red staining was visible in vesicles in the cytoplasm and in the neurites (Figure 5, panels 5–8), according to intracellular angiogenin localisation reported by Thiyagarajan et al. in similar neuronal cell lines [52]. We also observed the presence of intense punctuate structure of angiogenin in perinuclear and neurite regions, suggesting formation of resembling secretory granules.

Noteworthily, A172 cells treated with the peptide fragments Ang_{60-68} (Figure 4, panels 5–8) or $Ang_{60-68}Cys$ (Figure 4, panels 5–8) showed a diffuse cytoplasmic staining and a weak staining in the nucleus, neurites and cell membrane. A negligible staining of nuclear angiogenin was found after cell incubation with peptide-conjugated nanoparticles in the presence of copper ions.

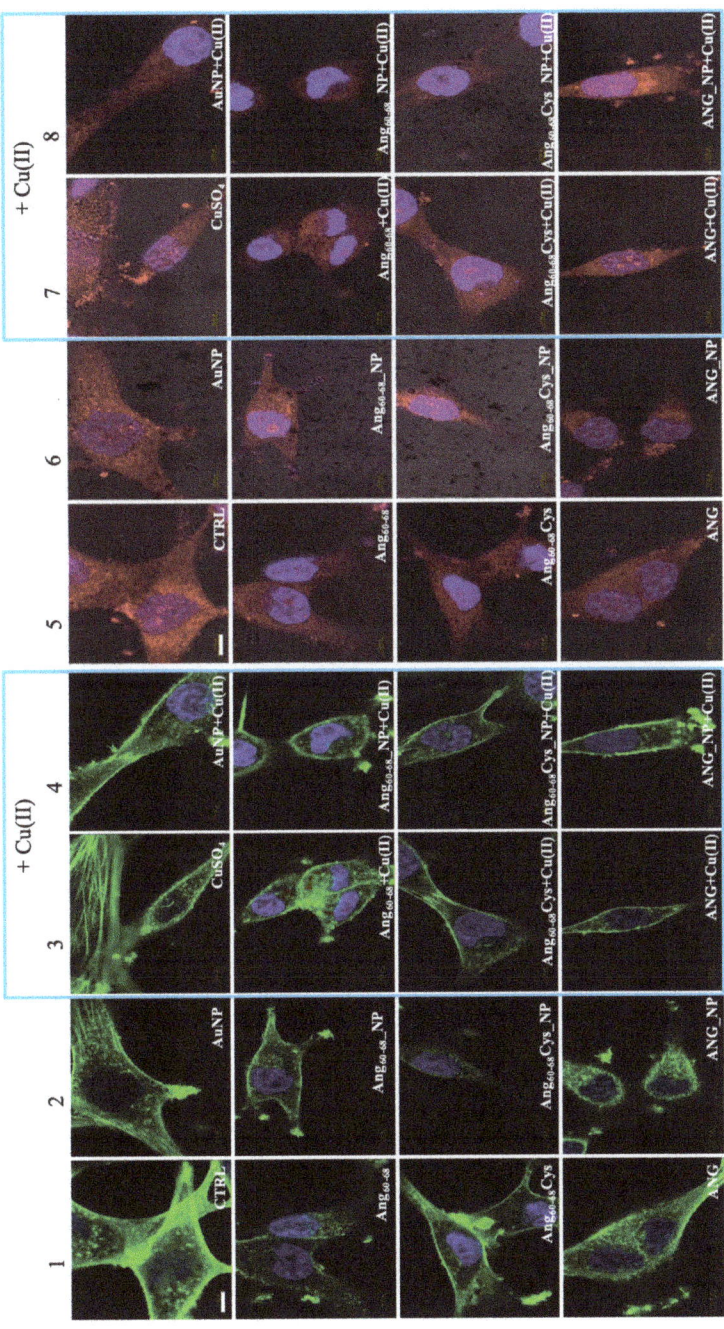

Figure 4. Confocal micrographs of A172 cells. Actin Green®488 (in green, ex/em= 488/500–530 nm) and Hoechst33342 (in blue, ex/em=405/425–475 nm) were used as F-actin and nuclear markers, respectively. Antibody against angiogenin shows angiogenin localisation in red (ex/em=543/560–700 nm) and micrographs are merged with optical bright field images (in grey). Before treatments, cell were rinsed with fresh culture medium and incubated for 2 h with basal culture medium (control: CTRL) and in culture medium supplemented with: Ang_{60-68} (30 µM), $Ang_{60-68}Cys$ (30 µM); ANG (100 nM), AuNP (9.4 nM = 1.4×10^8 NP/mL), Ang_{60-68}_NP (1.4 nM = 4.0×10^6 NP/mL, $[Ang_{60-68}] = 2.8 \times 10^{-12}$ M), $Ang_{60-68}Cys\_NP$ (1.4 nM = 4.0×10^6 NP/mL, $[Ang_{60-68}Cys] = 2.6 \times 10^{-12}$ M), ANG_NP (1.2 nM = 3.4×10^6 NP/mL, [ANG]= 0.2×10^{-12} M). Scale bar = 10 µm.

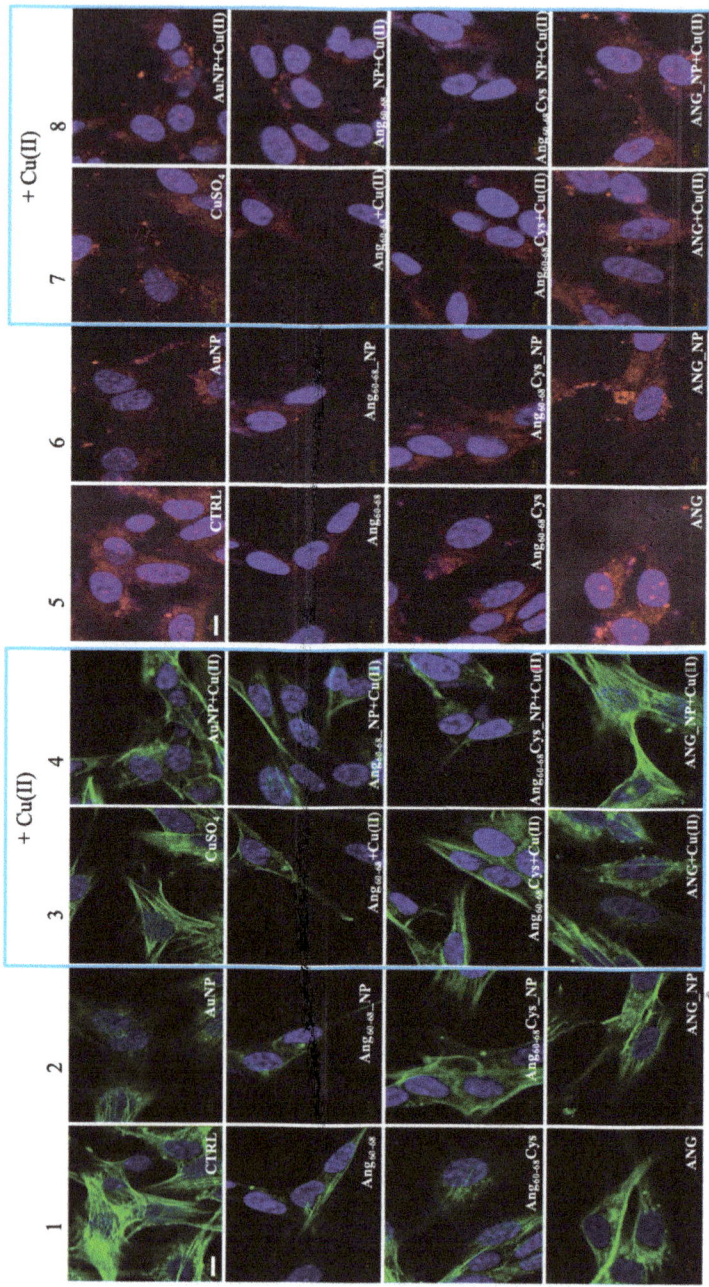

Figure 5. Confocal micrographs of d-SH-SY5Y cells Actin Green®488 (in green, ex/em = 488/500–530 nm) and Hoechst33342 (in blue, ex/em = 405/425–475 nm) were used as F-actin and nuclear markers, respectively. Antibody against angiogenin shows angiogenin localisation in red (ex/em=543/560–700 nm) and micrographs are merged with optical bright field images (in grey). Before treatments, cell were rinsed with fresh culture medium and incubated for 2 h with basal culture medium (control: CTRL) and in culture medium supplemented with: Ang_{60-63} (30 μM), $Ang_{60-68}Cys$ (30 μM); ANG (100 nM); AuNP (9.4 nM = 1.4×10^8 NP/mL), Ang_{60-68}_NP (1.4 nM = 4.0×10^6 NP/mL, $[Ang_{60-68}]$ = 2.8×10^{-12} M), $Ang_{60-63}Cys\_NP$ (1.4 nM = 4.0×10^6 NP/mL, $[Ang_{60-68}Cys]$ = 2.6×10^{-12} M), ANG_NP (1.2 nM = 3.4×10^6 NP/mL, [ANG]= 0.2×10^{-12} M). Scale bar = 10 μm.

2.2.4. VEGF Release and Synthesis

VEGF has been identified as the most important pro-angiogenic factor released by cancer cells and its concentration in the tissue of glioblastomas has been demonstrated significantly higher than that in normal brain [53]. Moreover, VEGF has a crucial role in neurogenesis, neuronal patterning, neuroprotection and glial growth [30,54]. Figure 6 shows the VEGF release after incubation for 24 h of tumour A172 cells and d-SH-SY5Y with peptides- or protein-conjugated NPs, in the absence or presence of copper ions.

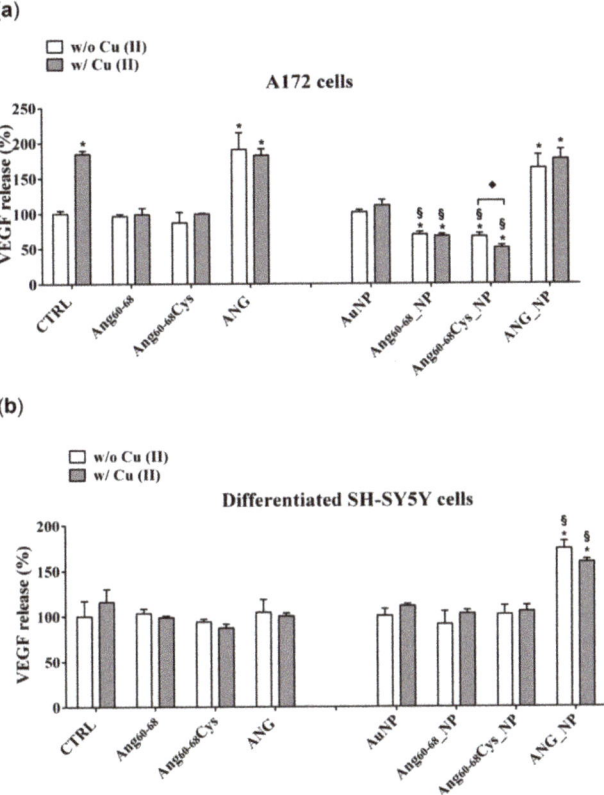

Figure 6. Vascular endothelial growth factor (VEGF) release in the medium of confluent cultures of A172 (**a**) and differentiated d-SH-SY5Y cells (**b**). Cells were grown in basal culture medium (control: CTRL) and in culture medium supplemented with: Ang_{60-68} (30 µM), $Ang_{60-68}Cys$ (30 µM); ANG (100 nM), AuNP (9.4 nM = 1.4×10^8 NP/mL, Ang_{60-68}_NP (1.4 nM = 4.0×10^6 NP/mL, $[Ang_{60-68}]$ = 2.8×10^{-12} M), $Ang_{60-68}Cys$_NP (1.4 nM = 4.0×10^6 NP/mL, $[Ang_{60-68}Cys]$ = 2.6×10^{-12} M), ANG_NP (1.2 nM = 3.4×10^6 NP/mL, [ANG]= 0.2×10^{-12} M). All conditions were evaluated in presence or absence of metal ions (copper sulphate: Cu(II), 20 µM). Sandwich enzyme-linked immunosorbent assay (ELISA) with monoclonal anti-VEGF antibody was used. The bars represent means ± SD of three independent experiments performed in triplicate (S.D. = standard deviation). Statistically significant differences, determined by one-way analysis of variance ANOVA are indicated: * $p \leq 0.05$ versus CTRL; § $p \leq 0.05$ versus the respective treatment with free peptides/protein; ♦ $p \leq 0.05$ versus the same treatment w/o Cu (II).

In A172 cells (Figure 6a) the treatments with copper alone increased the VEGF release by about 2.0 folds ($p \leq 0.05$ vs. control untreated cells), confirming the relevant role of this cation in cancer progression [55].

The incubation of the cells with $Ang_{60-68}Cys$ or with Ang_{60-68} did not modify the VEGF release in comparison to control cells, both in the absence and in the presence of Cu(II) whereas the treatments with ANG or ANG + Cu(II) increased the VEGF release by about 2.3-fold ($p \leq 0.05$ vs. control untreated cells).

The treatments with bare AuNP, both in the absence and in the presence of copper ions, did not significantly modify the VEGF release in comparison to control cells. Surprisingly, the incubation with AuNPs functionalized with peptide fragment $Ang_{60-68}Cys$ and Ang_{60-68}, induced a significant reduction of VEGF release respectively by 27% and by 30%, in comparison to the corresponding control (free $Ang_{60-68}Cys$ and free Ang_{60-68}). Moreover, further reduction of the release was found when the incubation with peptide fragment $Ang_{60-68}Cys$ was performed in presence of copper. No difference was found in VEGF release after treatment of A172 cells with ANG_NP in comparison to cells treated with free ANG.

The incubation of d-SH-SY5Y cells with ANG did not modulate the VEGF release, as well as with Ang_{60-68} and $Ang_{60-68}Cys$, both in absence and in presence of copper, in comparison to the respective controls.

Differently from A172 cells, in non-tumour d-SH-SY5Y cells (Figure 6b), only the treatment with AuNP functionalized with ANG, both in the absence and in presence of copper, induced an increase of the VEGF release in comparison to untreated control cells. The incubation of control cells with copper did not modulate the VEGF release. The concentration of VEGF released by A172 and d-SH-SY5Y was 133 pg/mL ± 10.1 and 58 pg/mL ± 4.3, respectively.

These results were confirmed by determination of VEGF messenger RNA (mRNA) levels (Figure 7). In A172 cells (Figure 7a) the treatments with ANG significantly increased mRNA transcription, whereas ANG_NP induced a significant reduction of transcription in comparison with free ANG but with values higher than control cells. No differences were found after treatment with free Ang_{60-68}, free $Ang_{60-68}Cys$ as well as bare NPs. On the other hand, the incubation with Ang_{60-68}_NP and $Ang_{60-68}Cys$_NP induced a significant reduction of mRNA transcription by about 2.2 and 2.7 folds, respectively, in comparison to the respective control (free Ang_{60-68} and free Ang_{60-68} Cys). Moreover, further reduction of the transcription was found after incubation in the presence of copper.

In non-tumour d-SH-SY5Y cells (Figure 7b), only the treatment with AuNP functionalized with ANG, both in the absence and in presence of copper, induced an increase of the VEGF mRNA transcription in comparison to the respective control (free ANG).

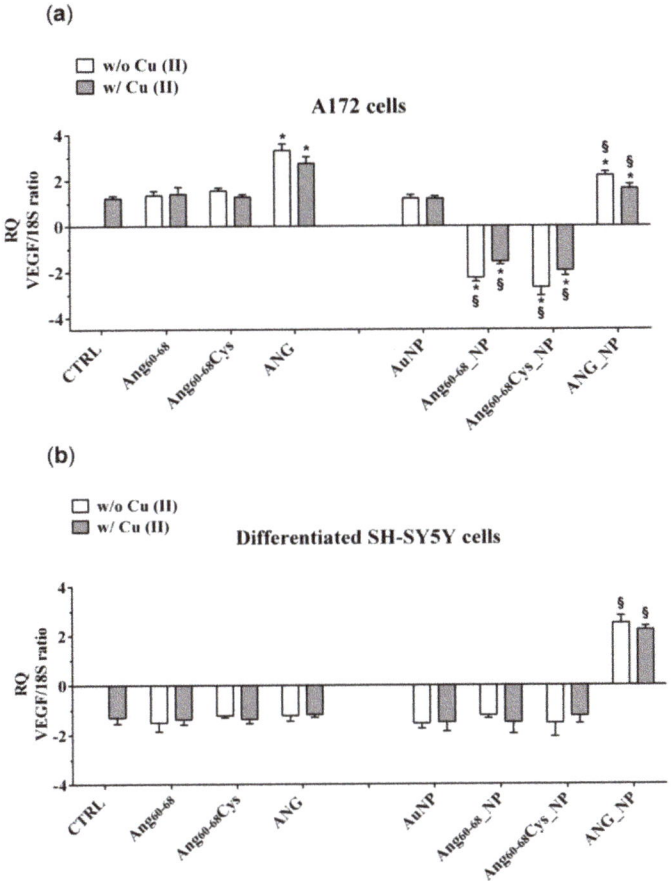

Figure 7. Vascular endothelial growth factor (VEGF) mRNA levels determination by qPCR in A172 (**a**) and differentiated d-SH-SY5Y cells (**b**). Cells were grown in basal culture medium (control: CTRL) and in culture medium supplemented with: Ang_{60-68} (30 µM), $Ang_{60-68}Cys$ (30 µM); ANG (100 nM), AuNP (9.4 nM = 1.4×10^8 NP/mL), Ang_{60-68}_NP (1.4 nM = 4.0×10^6 NP/mL, [Ang_{60-68}] = 2.8×10^{-12} M), $Ang_{60-68}Cys$_NP (1.4 nM = 4.0×10^6 NP/mL, [$Ang_{60-68}Cys$] = 2.6×10^{-12} M), ANG_NP (1.2 nM = 3.4×10^6 NP/mL, [ANG]= 0.2×10^{-12} M). All conditions were evaluated in presence or absence of metal ions (copper sulphate: Cu(II), 20 µM). Relative quantification is referred to untreated cells (CTRL). Data normalized with respect to the expression level of S18 mRNA. The bars represent means ± standard deviation (SD) of three independent experiments performed in triplicate. Statistically significant differences, determined by one-way analysis of variance (ANOVA) are indicated: * $p \leq 0.05$ versus control; § $p \leq 0.05$ versus the respective treatment with free peptides/protein.

3. Discussion

In this study, two brain cell lines, namely tumour glioblastoma (A172) and differentiated neuroblastoma (d- SH-SY5Y) neuron-like cells, were scrutinised after incubation with hybrid nanoassemblies made of gold nanoparticles functionalised with angiogenin protein or with two different angiogenin-mimicking peptides (Ang_{60-68} and its cysteine derivative at the C-terminus, $Ang_{60-68}Cys$) containing the ANG residues from 60 to 68, which is the the exposed protein loop region that is part of a cell-surface receptor binding site [56].

The Ang$_{60-68}$ peptide has been demonstrated to specifically interact with cytoskeleton actin [6], whereas the Ang$_{60-68}$Cys peptide has been successfully used to tailor gold nanoparticles by chemical grafting [44]. Gold, indeed, being a soft acid, binds to soft bases like thiols, to form stable Au-S bonds (40–50 kcal/mol) that are able to replace the citrate shell on the nanoparticle surface due to the strong affinity binding of the thiol groups with the metal [57].

In a previous study, we scrutinised the actual immobilisation of Ang$_{60-68}$Cys and Ang$_{60-68}$ onto the surface of AuNPs upon the simple addition of the peptide solution to nanoparticles dispersed in water. Indeed, by a multitechnique characterisation approach, including UV-visible, attenuated total reflectance–Fourier transform infrared (ATR/FTIR) and circular dichroism (CD) spectroscopies as well as atomic force microscopy(AFM), we could demonstrate an irreversible strong interaction between the peptide molecules and the gold nanoparticles resulting into the biomolecule-coated nanoparticles [44]. In the present work, to functionalize the gold nanoparticles with Ang$_{60-68}$, Ang$_{60-68}$Cys or ANG, the biomolecules were added to the colloidal dispersion (1.7×10^8 AuNP/mL) at the concentration respectively of 3×10^{-5} M for the peptides and 1×10^{-7} M for the protein, and the shifts in the plasmon band were monitored (Figure 1).

The optical interface established between the biomolecules and the metal nanoparticle surface, as investigated by UV–visible spectroscopy, clearly evidenced an irreversible immobilisation of the peptides and protein molecules onto AuNPs (Figure 1d).

Noteworthy, a red-shift in the wavelength of maximum absorption (λ_{max}) as well as a broadening in the FWHM of the plasmon peak were found for both peptides- and protein-added nanoparticles in comparison to bare AuNPs. These spectral changes point to an increase in the nanoparticle optical size, which is dependent on the following two concomitant processes: (i) nanoparticle surface decoration by biomolecules adsorption; (ii) nanoparticles aggregation.

The latter contribution was most evident for the protein, as displayed by the plasmon peak broadening and the appearance of a shoulder approximately at 600 nm of wavelength. Hence, the NP functionalisation by the biomolecules immobilisation resulted in peptide-conjugated NPs with lower tendency to aggregation than the protein-conjugated NPs. To better understand these findings, the nanoparticle coverage (Γ, in molecule/NP) was calculated from the changes in λ_{max} by using equations (1), (2) and (3).

Theoretical predictions show how the local refractive index environment of a metal nanoparticle affects its absorption spectrum. By assuming the protein-coated nanoparticles as core-shell spheres with a metallic core of d diameter, corresponding to the uncoated nanoparticles, and a homogeneous spherical proteinaceous shell, the fraction of protein over the total particle, g, is related to the changes in the wavelength of maximum absorption for uncoated colloid ($\lambda_{max,0}$), as given by Equation (1):

$$g = (1 + \alpha_s)\left(\frac{\lambda_p^2(\varepsilon_s - \varepsilon_m)}{\Delta\lambda \cdot \lambda_{max,0}} + 2\alpha_s\right)^{-1}, \quad (1)$$

where λ_p is the free electron oscillation wavelength (which is 131 nm for gold [58]), ε is a dielectric constant or relative permittivity (equal to the squared refractive index); $\alpha_s = \frac{(\varepsilon_s - \varepsilon_m)}{(\varepsilon_s + 2\varepsilon_m)}$ is the polarizability of a sphere with shell dielectric constant ε_s in a surrounding medium of dielectric constant ε_m. According to Equation (2), which refers to the shell thickness (s):

$$s = \frac{d}{2}\left[\frac{1}{[1-g]^{1/3}} - 1\right], \quad (2)$$

and using the Feijter's formula in Equation (3):

$$\Gamma = s\frac{n_s - n_m}{dn/dc}, \quad (3)$$

where Γ is the coverage and dn/dc is the refractive index increment (typically 0.19 mL·g^{-1} for a protein [59]), the mass of protein absorbed per unit area can be calculated.

The estimated values from the experimental spectroscopic data as well as the theoretical coverage calculated by considering an ideal monolayer in the two limit configurations respectively of end-on or side-on, are given in Table 2.

Table 2. Protein fraction shell value (g) and peptide/protein coverage (Γ) calculated from the changes in the wavelength of maximum absorption (λ_{max}) of AuNP plasmon peak for peptide/protein added nanoparticles. The ideal monolayer coverage of the peptide/protein in the end-on and side-on limit configuration are given for comparison.

Sample	g [1]	Γ (ng/cm^2)	Γ [2] (molecules/NP)	Ideal Monolayer Coverage [3] (molecules/NP)	
				End-on	Side-on
Ang$_{60-68}$_NP	0.74	79	194	177	83
Ang$_{60-68}$Cys_NP	0.74	79	178	202	149
ANG_NP	0.90	165	32	23	10

[1] Values calculated from Equation (1) in Materials and Methods by considering the refractive index values (n) at 550 nm of 1.335 for water [60] and 1.38 for a pure protein [59], respectively. [2] Values calculated from Equation (3) in Materials and Methods, given the molecular weights (MW) of 1105.5 g/mol for Ang$_{60-68}$, 1209.3 g/mol for Ang$_{60-68}$Cys and 14,200 g/mol for ANG, respectively. [3] Calculated by using the average molecular dimensions (in nm^3) respectively of (1.7 × 1.5 × 3.2) for Ang$_{60-68}$, (1.6 × 1.4 × 1.9) for CysAng$_{60-68}$ [44], and (7 × 6.2 × 3.2) for ANG [61].

From Table 2 is evident that a multilayer coverage can be presumed for ANG_NP, while most likely a monolayer in end-on configuration and a sub-monolayer coverage can be assumed for Ang$_{60-68}$_NP and Ang$_{60-68}$Cys_NP, respectively. Hence, in the case of ANG, many protein molecules adsorbed at the nanoparticle surface and formed a 'thick' shell that could perturb the mechanism of electrostatic stabilisation for colloidal gold [3], thus explaining the partial aggregation measured in UV-visible spectra. As to the two peptide fragments, their smaller size lead to the formation of a thinner and stiffer shell around the nanoparticles than that formed by the protein molecules. This picture is further supported by the coverage calculated for the pellets recovered after the washing steps. Indeed, for ANG_Au pellet, a loss of unbound and/or weakly bound proteins of about 78% can be estimated by the protein fraction shell decrease to $g = 0.5$, which corresponds to coating thickness and absorbed protein mass of $s = 1.54$ nm and $\Gamma = 36$ ng/cm^2, respectively. On the other hand, for both Ang$_{60-68}$_NP and Ang$_{60-68}$ Cys_NP pellets, the calculated values for the peptide shell are still $g = 0.74$, $s = 3.36$ nm and $\Gamma = 79$ ng/cm^2. To note, even if the measured plasmon peak changes were comparable upon their approaching at the interface with the gold nanoparticles, the cysteine residue in Ang$_{60-68}$Cys is expected to drive, through the thiol-gold bonding [44], a more ordered and compact biomolecule gathering at the nanoparticle surface in comparison to Ang$_{60-68}$, which is in agreement with the estimation of a sub-monolayer coverage in Ang$_{60-68}$Cys_NP.

The DLS method is a reliable instrumental tool for non-perturbative and sensitive diagnostics of the aggregation processes of gold nanoparticle conjugates initiated by biospecific interactions on their surface [62]. Indeed, the nanoparticle hydrodynamic size determined by DLS (Table 1) showed the same trend of optical size change; moreover, also evidenced nanoparticles aggregation induced by the addition of copper ions to the peptides- or protein-functionalised NPs (i.e., hydrodynamic size increase approximately of 373%, 866% and 15% for Ang$_{60-68}$_NP, Ang$_{60-68}$Cys_NP and ANG_NP, respectively) but no size change for the bare AuNPs.

Transition metals, such as copper, can prompt the aggregation of proteins and peptides through the formation of metal complexes [63]. It is known that ANG is able to bind to copper ions [43] and bridged copper complexes can lead to the formation of nanoparticles clusters. This effect was more evident for the hybrids CysAng$_{60-68}$_NP, where the prevalent chemisorption process leads to a more ordered arrangement of the biomolecules around the nanoparticles.

The differences found in the presence of copper ions could also be due to different binding modes between the copper and the peptides- or the protein-functionalised nanoparticles. The UV-visible parameters of copper complexes formed by Ang_{60-68} and $Ang_{60-68}Cys$ were similar, suggesting that the metal ion experiences the same coordination environment with both peptides. However, the observed blue-shift ($\Delta\lambda = 6$ nm) and the parallel decrease of molar absorbance coefficient ($\Delta\varepsilon = 10$) for $Ang_{60-68}Cys + Cu(II)$ compared to $Ang_{60-68} + Cu(II)$, suggest a slight increase of ligand field strength and a more planar disposition of donor atoms bound to the metal ion [64,65].

The CD spectra (Figure 2) confirmed the involvement of imidazole and deprotonated amide nitrogen as donor atoms in metal binding for copper complexes formed by the two peptides [48]. The sharper peaks around 300 nm evidenced the slight increase of metal binding affinity of $Ang_{60-68}Cys$. Furthermore, the CD broad band in the d-d transition region suggested that the extra cysteine residue at C-terminus may affect peptide backbone conformation of $Ang_{60-68}Cys$ more than it happens for $Ang_{60-68}+Cu(II)$ system [66]. As for the protein, the main copper anchoring sites are the RNase catalytic sites His-13 and His-114 [38]; therefore ANG displays a different coordination mode compared to copper complexes formed by Ang_{60-68} and $Ang_{60-68}Cys$. However, it has been hypothesized that in the presence of excess copper a second metal ion can bind to the 60–68 region of ANG affecting protein binding with cell membrane [37]. The different metal coordination modes may potentially tune the biological response of functionalized nanoparticles.

The tests of cell viability/proliferation, cytoskeleton actin, angiogenin translocation and VEGF release were scrutinised both in basal and in copper-conditioned medium. Noteworthy, copper is another co-player of the angiogenesis process [33,34].

The cell response to nanoparticles is strongly dependent on the cell line, since, for instance, different cell models can overexpress different receptors at the membrane that may trigger the nanoparticle internalisation. ANG stimulates the expression of ANG receptors which mediate its nuclear translocation [16,28]; when nuclear translocation of ANG is inhibited, its angiogenic activity is abolished [67].

Neuroblastoma SH-SY5Y cells are used as a model of dopaminergic neurons as the cells possess similar biochemical functionalities of neurons. They are able to synthesize dopamine and also express dopamine transporter on the cell membrane [68]. On the other hand, SH-SY5Y cells have very low levels of the redox protein thioredoxin that together with glutathione redox cycle represents the major cellular redox buffer [69], acts as a growth factor and is found to be overexpressed in many human primary cancers including glioblastoma cells [70].

As to the cell viability effects measured on tumour glioblastoma (A172) and non-tumour differentiated neuroblastoma (d- SH-SY5Y) cell lines, our results (Figure 3) pointed to the very promising potentialities of peptide- and protein-functionalised gold nanoparticles to decrease the proliferation of tumour cells.

Indeed, after 24 h of A172 cells incubation with Ang_{60-68}_NP, $Ang_{60-68}Cys$_NP and ANG_NP a significantly decreased viability was found compared the cells treated with the free peptides or protein molecules as well as to the untreated control. Noteworthy, at the used experimental conditions, the bare AuNPs as well as the free peptides were found to not affect the cell viability, whereas the free protein increased the viability in comparison to untreated cells, both in the absence and in the presence of copper ions. Another interesting cue was found in the experiments performed in copper-supplemented medium, where cell treatments with $Ang_{60-68}Cys$_NP+Cu(II) and ANG_NP + Cu(II) nullified the abovementioned decrease of cell viability, whereas for cells treatments with Ang_{60-68}_NP+ Cu(II) no significant differences were found with respect to Ang_{60-68}_NP. These findings confirmed the higher capability in the copper binding for the $Ang_{60-68}Cys$- conjugated nanoparticles with respect to Ang_{60-68}-NP, as discussed above from CD results.

In contrast to A172 cells, no toxicity nor increase in viability was observed for any of the incubation conditions of differentiated neuroblastoma cells, as expected for not proliferating non-tumour cells.

These findings further support the good potentialities of our peptides- and protein-conjugated NPs as cell specific, anti-angiogenic nanomedicine tools.

Angiogenin is a protein with an extreme positive charge (pI >10.5), thus generally can avidly bind the cellular membrane [71]. Indeed, ANG binds to the membrane surface actin of vessel endothelial cells and activate the matrix protease cascades.

In the cytosol, angiogenin encounters an endogenous inhibitor protein, known as ribonuclease inhibitor (RI), which binds to angiogenin to form a complex with a dissociation constant value in the low femtomolar range, stabilized largely by favourable Coulombic interactions, as RI is highly anionic [72]. It has been demonstrated that upregulating RI suppresses tumour growth and tumour microvessel density through suppression of ANG function [73].

In order to explain the different response of two neural lines, we analysed via confocal microscopy the remodelling of actin filaments as well as the ANG translocation induced by the peptides- or protein-conjugated NPs, both in the absence and in the presence of Cu(II) (Figures 4 and 5).

Our results in tumour A172 cell line showed that the cell treatment with bare AuNPs and/or the addition of Cu(II) significantly increased actin stress fibres, while after incubation either with the free Ang_{60-68} peptide as well as its NP-conjugated derivative, an enhanced actin staining for several lamellipodia protruding from the cell body in all directions were found, with no significant changes observed in the presence of copper. A similar strong actin staining for lamellipodia in Ang_{60-68}Cys peptide-and ANG protein-treated cells was instead decreased by the presence of copper. Finally, after incubation with Ang_{60-68}Cys_NP, both in the absence and presence of copper, cells contained very few, if any, actin stress fibres in the central regions and lamellipodia structures.

As to the non-tumour d-SHSY5Y cell line, no significant changes in the cytoskeleton actin were found for cell incubation in the presence or not of copper ions, but only a generally less dense actin meshwork after the treatment with Ang_{60-68} or Ang_{60-68}Cys samples. Numerous and prominent actin stress fibres along the entire cell border were found for cells treated with ANG samples.

As migration and, thus, infiltration of glioma cells is largely governed by reshaping the cytoskeleton, it is no surprise that the composition and organization of the cytoskeleton in glioma cells differs strongly from that of healthy brain cells, such as the neuron-like differentiated neuroblastoma cells. In a study on glioblastoma multiforme (GBM), the most lethal brain tumour, Memmel et al. found that inhibition of cell migration was associated with massive morphological changes and reorganization of the actin cytoskeleton [50].

ANG can interact with the actin, a protein able to form different polymeric structures inside the cells, which is essential to maintain the cell structure and motility [74]. The result of the binding to the actin is the inhibition of the polymerization with consequent changing of the cell cytoskeleton. These modifications play a fundamental role during proliferation of both endothelial and tumour cells [75]. The role of ANG in cell migration, necessary for tumour invasion and metastasis, has been confirmed by an important study which detected elevated levels of secreted and cell surface-bound ANG in highly invasive metastatic breast cancer cells. It has been indeed demonstrated that ANG interacts with the plasminogen activation system, thus increasing plasmin formation and cell migration of tumour cells [76].

Under physiologic conditions, ANG is present in the nucleus and in the cytoplasm, where is held in an inactive state through interaction with its known inhibitor Ribonuclease/Angiogenin Inhibitor 1 (RNH1), which prevents random cleavage of cellular RNA. A minor pool of ANG is secreted and is internalized by surrounding cells with a mechanism of endocytosis receptor mediated (reviewed by Shawn [71]. In stressed cells ANG dissociates from his inhibitor and becomes active. In this condition, nuclear ANG translocates from nuclear to the cytoplasmic compartment where cleaves mature transfer ribonucleic acid (tRNA), releasing two smaller RNA fragments, termed 5'- and 3' tRNA-derived Stress-induced RNAs (tiRNAs). The post-transcriptional tRNA processing is necessary to allow the tRNA to regulate in specific manner the transcription [77]. Moreover, tRNA fragments can bind to cytochrome c and block the apoptosoma assembling, thereby inhibiting caspase-3, with consequent increasing of cell viability and proliferation [78]. Noteworthy, the nuclear concentration of ANG increases in the endothelial cells under the stimulation with basic fibroblast growth factor (bFGF), VEGF, acidic fibroblast growth factor (aFGF), epidermal growth factor (EGF), and foetal bovine serum (FBS).

Authors hypothesized that the endogenous angiogenin participates in endothelial cell proliferation induced by other angiogenic factors [29]. Recombinant ANG plays an important role in neuroprotection against excitotoxic and endoplasmic reticulum (ER) stress in primary motor neuron cultures, and in SOD1G93A mice [18].

By LSM we were able to visualise the different intracellular localisation of endogenous angiogenin in A172 and d-SH-SY5Y cells, but similar effects on angiogenin translocation or uptake by the treatment with the peptides- or protein-conjugated nanoparticles, respectively.

For tumour glioblastoma, we found the endogenous angiogenin localised in the nucleus and in the cytosol, while neuron-like differentiated neuroblastoma displayed a weaker angiogenin staining (according to western blotting analysis, Figure S1), mainly localised in cytoplasm. Indeed, A172 cells treated with the free protein or the protein-conjugated NPs exhibited a strong angiogenin staining of the nuclear and perinuclear regions, especially for incubation in copper-supplemented medium. In d-SH-SY5Y cells, most of the protein was visible in the cytoplasm as large speckles but is also present in the nucleus, in the neurites and the membrane. In both cell lines, upon the treatment with bare AuNPs and/or the incubation in copper-supplemented medium, structural perturbation of intracellular angiogenin was observed, with an intense punctuate structure in perinuclear and neurite regions that suggested the formation of resembling secretory granules.

The treatment with peptides or peptide-conjugated nanoparticles was able to translocate angiogenin, with a diffuse cytoplasmic staining and a weak staining in the nucleus, neurites and cell membrane after the incubation with Ang_{60-68} or $Ang_{60-68}Cys$; in the presence of copper-supplemented medium, most of the protein remains in the cytoplasm and is absent from the neurites and membrane.

Nuclear angiogenin plays different roles. It is localised inside the nucleolus, centre of synthesis and assembly of the ribosomes, where stimulates rRNA production, required for cellular proliferation [79]. Moreover, ANG bind the histone protein and cause a modification which regulates mRNA transcription. The ability to bind the DNA allows to ANG to function as a adaptor protein which recruit other modifying enzymes with methyltransferase or acetyltransferase activity [16]. Moreover, ANG has a nuclear localization sequence (NLS), containing Arg 33, which equips the protein for nuclear import [28]. After entering the nucleus, ANG accumulates in the nucleolus, which is the site of ribosome biogenesis. Within the nucleolus, ANG stimulates ribosomal DNA (rDNA) transcription [80].

Our results demonstrate that ANG was able to enter glioma cells and to induce their proliferation. In A172 cancer cells, the mitogen activated protein kinase (MAPK)/extracellular-signal-regulated kinase (ERK) signalling pathway could be responsible of the ANG phosphorylation which prevent the binding with the RI. Consequently, free ANG could exercise his effect in the nucleus, promoting DNA transcription and cell proliferation [81]. The effect of ANG on A172 cells, but not of ANG_NP, was highlighted by the increase of VEGF transcription and release, after the ribonuclease activity of the protein in the nucleus.

The lower VEGF release after incubation of the cells with ANG_NP could be determined by the presence of NPs, which could prevent the phosphorylation of the protein, essential step for its nuclear translocation. A low concentration of phosphorylated protein could explain the reduction of VEGF release after incubation with ANG_NPs in comparison to free ANG.

The peptide fragments $Ang_{60-68}Cys$ and Ang_{60-68} were able to enter the cells but only few of them could cross nuclear membranes, because they are missing of the nucleolar targeting, specifically of Arg 33; the consequent effect is a level of release of VEGF very similar to control cells. Instead, $Ang_{60-68}Cys\_NP$ and Ang_{60-68}_NP entered the nucleus and successively they could bind rDNA. Probably, the fragments were not able to catalyse the digestion of the RNA on the promotor site, due to the lack of the catalytic sequence. Consequently, the dissociation of the transcription termination factor I-interacting protein (TIP5) from the rDNA promoter did not occur. The ensuing steric obstruction by the binding of $Ang_{60-68}Cys\_NP$ and Ang_{60-68}_NP to rDNA could block the binding of other native angiogenin molecules thereby significantly reducing rDNA transcription and VEGF production. The shield-effect of the NPs towards peptide fragments $Ang_{60-68}Cys$ and Ang_{60-68} could represent an interesting strategy to modulate VEGF release by glioma cells.

The different response of the SH-SY5Y cells to ANG could depend by the interaction of the peptide with his inhibitor, as the signalling pathway determining the phosphorylation are switch off in not tumour cells. In this condition, the protein could remain inactive in the cytosol, bound to its inhibitor.

In differentiated SH-SY5Y cells, the hybrid ANG_NP increased VEGF release in comparison to free ANG probably because in absence of NPs, after the adhesion to- and crossing- through plasma membrane, it binds its inhibitor inside the cells. The hybrid ANG_NP protects the protein by the bind with the inhibitor, thereby increasing VEGF mRNA transcription and VEGF release in comparison to free ANG probably because the presence of the NPs could protect the protein by the binding with the inhibitor, thereby increasing VEGF mRNA transcription and VEGF release.

4. Materials and Methods

4.1. Chemicals

Gold(III) chloride trihydrate (CAS Number 16961-25-4), trisodium citrate dihydrate (CAS Number: 6132-04-3), 3-(N-morpholino)propanesulfonic acid (MOPS, 1132-61-2), potassium chloride (7447-40-7), sodium chloride (7647-14-5), tris(2-carboxyethyl)phosphine (TCEP, 51805-45-9), hydrochloric acid (7647-01-0), nitric acid (7697-37-2), sodium hydroxide (1310-73-2), N,N-diisopropyl-ethylamine (DIEA, 7087-68-5), N,N-dimethylformamide (DMF, 68-12-2), 20% (v/v) piperidine (110-89-4) in DMF solution, N-hydroxybenzotriazole (HOBt, 123333-53-9), triisopropylsilane (TIS, 6485-79-6), trifluoroacetic acid (TFA, 76-05-1), isopropyl β-D-1-thiogalactopyranoside (IPTG, 367-93-1), Tris(hydroxymethyl)aminomethane hydrochloride (Tris-HCl buffer, 1185-53-1), ethylenediaminetetraacetic acid (EDTA, 60-00-4), guanidine hydrochloride (GdnHCl), 1,4-dithiothreitol (DTT, 3483-12-3), phosphate buffered saline (PBS) tablets and 3-(4,5-dimethyl-2-thiazolyl)-2,5-diphenyl-2H-tetrazolium bromide (MTT, 298-93-1), ethylene glycol-bis(2-aminoethylether)-N,N,N′,N′-tetraacetic acid (EGTA, 67-42-5), nonyl phenoxypolyethoxylethanol (NP40, 9016-45 -9), bovine serum albumin (BSA), 3,3′,5,5′-tetramethylbenzidine (TMB, 54827-17-7) sulphuric acid (7664-93-9) and Triton X-100 (9002-93-1) were purchased from Sigma-Aldrich (St. Louis, MO, USA). 2-(1-H-Benzotriazole-1-yl)-1,1,3,3-tetramethyluronium tetrafluoroborate (TBTU) was purchased from Novabiochem (Läufelfingen, Switzerland).

The designed primers for angiogenin (ANG) protein expression were purchased from Eurofins GWM (Ebersberg, Germany). The over-expression plasmid (pET22b(+)-ANG), including a codon-optimized gene for ANG, was obtained from Sloning BioTechnology (Puchheim, Germany). Terrific Broth (TB) liquid microbial growth medium, Dulbecco's modified eagle medium (DMEM), Ham's F-12 medium (F12), streptomycin, L-glutamine, foetal bovine serum (FBS) were provided by Lonza (Verviers, Belgium). DMEM high glucose 30-2002 was provided by ATCC (LGC Standards S.r.l., Sesto San Giovanni (MI), Italy). Ultrapure MilliQ water was used (18.2 mΩ·cm at 25 °C, Millipore, (Burlington, MA, USA).

4.2. Peptide Synthesis

The fragment Ang_{60-68} including the amino acid sequence Ac-KNGNPHSEN-NH$_2$ (molecular weight, MW, of 1105.5 g/mol, isoelectric point, PI, of 11.38), modified by N-terminal acetylation and the C-terminal amidation, was assembled by using the solid phase peptide synthesis strategy, on an initiator+ Alstra™ fully automated microwave peptide synthesizer (Biotage, Uppsala, Sweden). The synthesis was performed on TGR resin (0.25 mmol/g) on 0.11 mmol scale using a 30 mL reactor vial. The coupling reactions were carried out by using 5-fold excess of amino acid, 5 equivalents of hydroxybenzotriazol/2-(1H-benzotriazole-1-yl)-1,1,3,3-tetramethylaminiumtetrafluoroborate/N,N-diisopropylethylamine (HOBt/TBTU/DIEA) in N,N-dimethylformamide (DMF), under mixing for 10 min at room temperature. Fmoc deprotection steps were performed at room temperature by using 20% of piperidine in DMF for 15 min. The N-terminal amino group was acetylated using a DMF solution containing acetic anhydride (6% v/v) and DIEA (5% v/v). The resin was washed with dichloromethane and dried on synthesizer. The peptide was purified by preparative reversed-phase chromatography (rp)-HPLC using a PrepStar 200 (model SD-1, Varian, Palo Alto, CA, USA) equipped with a Prostar photodiode array detector, with a protocol previously reported [48]. The peptide Ac-KNGNPHRENC-NH$_2$ (Ang$_{60-68}$Cys) was purchased from CASLO (Lyngby, Denmark).

4.3. Protein Expression

The human angiogenin expression was carried out following the method reported by Holloway et al. (2001) [82]. Briefly, the *E. coli* (BL21(DE3)) expression strain was cultured at 37 °C under shaking (speed of 180 r.p.m.) in 5 mL of terrific broth (TB) (12 g peptone, 24 g granulated yeast extract, 4 mL glycerol 87%, 900 mL of distilled H$_2$O) supplemented with ampicillin (100 µg/mL). After 24 hrs of incubation the whole volume of the bacterial culture was inoculated in 1000 mL of fresh broth. When the density of the culture had reached the OD$_{600\,nm}$ value of 0.8, the Ang expression was induced by the addition of 1 mM IPTG and the incubation was continued for additional 2 h. Afterwards, the cell culture was harvested by centrifugation (15 min at 1503 RCF) and cells were lysed with 30 mL of lysis buffer (50 mM Tris-HCl, 2 mM EDTA, pH = 8) by using a high-pressure homogenizer (Emulsiflex, Ottawa, Canada) and a sonication step (Sonicator Q700, Qsonica, Newtown, CT, USA). Lysate was centrifuged (40 min at 15,871 RCF) and the pellet was re-suspended in 25 mL of lysis buffer supplemented with 1% (v/v) Triton X-100. Sonication and centrifugation steps were repeated twice and the final pellet was dissolved in 30 mL of denaturation buffer (0.24 M GdnHCl, 100 mM Tris-HCl, 1 mM EDTA, 4 mM NaCl, 0.4 mM DTT).

The expressed recombinant angiogenin (rANG) was refolded from inclusion bodies according to the procedure described by Jang et al. [83] and then purified by a cation exchange chromatography performed on an automated chromatographic workstation (Akta prime, GE Healthcare, Milan, Italy) equipped with a 15 × 1.6 cm column packed with SP Sepharose Fast Flow (GE Healthcare, Milan, Italy). After a washing step with 25 mM Tris-HCl (pH = 8.0), rAng was eluted with 25 mM Tris-HCl, 1 M NaCl (pH = 8.0) buffer solution. Sodium dodecyl sulphate-polyacrylamide gel electrophoresis (SDS-PAGE) (10% bis-tris, Invitrogen, Carlsbad, CA, USA, 1 mm × 15 well) was carried out to evaluate the presence of dimers.

To obtain wild-type angiogenin (ANG), rANG was incubated with 1 nM *Aeromonas* aminopeptidase, at the concentration of 1×10^{-5} M in 200 mM PBS (pH = 7.2) (overnight at 37 °C under gentle shaking). This procedure allows for the specific removal of the N-terminal methionine residue, Met(-1), in the primary sequence of rANG, thus obtaining the N-terminal glutamine residue, Glu1, that spontaneously cyclises to the pyroglutamate residue, PyrGlu1, which is characteristic of 'native' wtANG.

The reaction mixture was purified by dialysis (Spectra/por MWCO 6–8000) (Fisher Scientific, Hampton, NH, USA), which replaces PBS with 25 mM Tris-HCl (pH 7.4) buffer solution, followed by cation-exchange chromatography. The native folding of wtANG was evaluated by testing the ribonucleolytic activity of the protein, according to the procedure reported by Halloway et al. [82]. The protein concentration was determined by means of UV-visible spectroscopy (ε_{280nm} = 12,500 M^{-1} cm^{-1}) [38].

4.4. UV–Visible Spectroscopy, Circular Dichroism Spectroscopy and Dynamic Light Scattering (DLS) Analyses

UV-visible spectra of the aqueous dispersions were measured on a Lambda 2S spectrometer (Perkin Elmer, Waltham, MA, USA) using conventional quartz cells (light path 1 cm and 0.1 cm) under the following conditions: bandwidth, 1 nm; scan rate, 100 nm/min; response, medium; data interval, 0.5 nm. Circular dichroism (CD) spectra in the 290–750 nm UV-visible region were recorded at 25 °C in a constant nitrogen flow on a model 810 spectropolarimeter (Jasco, Cremella (LC), Italy) equipped with a Xe lamp. The following conditions were used: scan rate, 50 nm min^{-1}; bandwidth, 1 nm; scan rate, 50 nm/min; response, 4 s; accumulation, 3 times; data interval, 0.5 nm. Aqueous solution of (+)-ammonium camphorsulfonate-d$_{10}$ (0.06%) was used for a calibration of the spectrometer sensitivity and wavelength (θ = 190.4 mdeg at λ = 290.5 nm).

For the hydrodynamic size determination, a dynamic light scattering (DLS) nanoparticle size analyser (LB-550, Horiba, Rome, Italy) was used. The instrument, equipped with temperature controller in the range of 5–70 °C, could detect particle size in the range of 1 nm–6 µm; response time, about 30 s. The results are presented as the mean of at least three measurements.

4.5. Synthesis and Functionalisation of Gold Nanoparticles

Gold nanoparticles were synthesized modifying the method pioneered by Turkevich. This method uses the chemical reduction of the chloroauric acid by the action of trisodium citrate that acts as both reducing and capping agent [84]. The synthesis was carried out as follows. All glassware was cleaned with aqua-regia rinsing (HCl:HNO$_3$, 1:3 volume ratio) and then washed with MilliQ water immediately before starting the experiments. Gold(III) chloride dihydrate was dissolved in 20 mL of ultrapure Millipore water. The solution, at the final concentration of 1 mM, was heated to boiling on a hot plate while it is stirred in a 50 mL beaker. 2 mL of a 1% (m/v) solution of trisodium citrate dihydrate was quickly added to the rapidly-stirred auric solution. As soon as the solution turned from yellow to deep red, AuNPs were formed and the beaker was removed from the hot plate.

The concentration of synthesized AuNPs was typically of 16 nM, as estimated by the UV–visible spectra, according to the molar extinction coefficient ε (in M^{-1}cm^{-1},) calculated by the following equation [85]: $\varepsilon_{gold} = Ad^\gamma$, where d in (nm) is the core diameter of the nanoparticle, A and γ are constants (d $\leq$ 85 nm: $A = 4.7 \times 10^4$, $\gamma = 3.30$; d > 85 nm: $A = 1.6 \times 10^8$, $\gamma = 1.47$).

To calculate d, the UV-visible parameters of the plasmon peak were used, according to the following equation [47]: $d = \frac{\lambda_{max} - 515.04}{0.3647}$.

In order to remove the excess of sodium citrate, the citrate-capped gold nanoparticles were washed through two centrifugation steps (15 min at 6010 RCF), with rinsing in between and at the end with 3-(N-morpholino)propanesulfonic acid) -Tris(2-carboxyethyl)phosphine hydrochloride MOPS-TCEP buffer. To prepare the MOPS-TCEP buffer, 1 mM MOPS buffer solution (added with 0.27 mM KCl and 13.7 mM NaCl) was mixed to TCEP at 1:1 molar ratio, and the pH corrected to 7.4 (25 °C) by the addition of concentrated NaOH.

The pellets of the rinsed citrate-capped gold nanoparticles were resuspended in 1 mM MOPS-TCEP at the concentration of 1.5$\times$10^{-8} M, corresponding to 1.7 $\times$ 10^8 AuNP/mL, as determined by the absorbance of the plasmon peak, and functionalized by physical adsorption (for Ang$_{60-68}$ and ANG), and prevalent chemisorption (for Ang$_{60-68}$Cys). The functionalization was carried out through the gradual addition, in a concentration range from 5 $\times$ 10^{-6} M up to 3 $\times$ 10^{-5} M, of the two different peptides (Ang$_{60-68}$ and Ang$_{60-68}$Cys) and through the one step addition of the whole protein (ANG) at the concentration of 1 $\times$ 10^{-7} M, to 1.5 $\times$ 10^{-8} M aqueous dispersion of AuNP and analysed by UV–visible spectroscopy titrations. Eventually, to rinse off unbounded or weakly bound biomolecules, the peptide-AuNP hybrid systems were purified by two centrifugation steps (15 min at 6010 RCF), with rinsing in between and at the end with MOPS-TCEP buffer.

4.6. Cellular Experiments

Human neuroblastoma cells (SH-SY5Y cell line) were cultivated in full medium, i.e., DMEM/F12 supplemented with 10% FBS, 2 mM L-glutamine and 100 µg mL^{-1} streptomycin. For differentiation, cells were seeded at a density of 2.3 $\times$ 10^5 cells/mL in full medium for 24 hrs and then neuronal differentiation of SH-SY5Y was induced by treatment for 5 days in vitro (DIV) with 10 µM of retinoic acid (RA) for 5 days in Dulbecco's Modified Eagle Medium (DMEM) high glucose medium supplemented with 0.5% of FBS.

Human glioblastoma cell line (A172) was cultivated in DMEM (n. 30–2002) supplemented with 10% FBS and 100 µg·mL^{-1} streptomycin. The cell cultures were grown in tissue-culture treated Corning® flasks (Sigma-Aldrich) in humidified atmosphere (5% CO_2) at 37 °C (HeraCell 150C incubator, Heraeus, Hanau, Germany). For the cellular treatments, the day before the experiment glioblastoma cells were seeded at a density of 2×10^5 cells/mL in full medium.

4.6.1. Cellular Experiments

Corning® 48 well multiwell plates were used for cytotoxicity assays (Sigma-Aldrich). The effect of AuNPs with ANG protein and Ang peptides on cell viability was tested at 50–60% of cell confluence by incubation with the compounds with concentrations 5 and 10 nM with or without 20 uM of copper for 24 hrs in DMEM medium supplemented with 0.5% of FBS. The viable cells were quantified by the reaction with MTT. After 90 min, the reaction was stopped by adding DMSO, and absorbance was measured at 570 nm (Varioskan® Flash Spectral Scanning Multimode Readers, Thermo Scientific, Waltham, MA, USA). Results were expressed as % of viable cells over the concentration of each compound. The experiments were repeated at least five times in triplicate and results expressed as mean ± standard error of the mean (SEM). The statistical analysis was performed with a one-way Analysis of Variance (ANOVA test, by using the Origin software, version 8.6, Microcal, Northampton, MA, USA).

4.6.2. Western Blot (WB) Analysis

For the determination of protein amount by WB, cells were cultivated at 37 °C (in 5% CO_2 atmosphere) on Corning® tissue-culture treated culture dishes 60 mm × 15 mm (D × H) (Sigma-Aldrich) at 80% of confluence. Cells lysates were prepared by cells treatment with RIPA lysis buffer (50 mM Tris-HCl, pH 8.0, 150 mM NaCl, 0.5 mM EDTA, 1% Triton X-100, 0.5 mM EGTA, 1% NP40) containing an inhibitor of the protease and phosphatase cocktail. Immediately after the addition of the buffer, cells were collected by the scratch method and transferred to Eppendorf tubes (1.5 mL of size, purchased from Sigma-Aldrich) for incubation on ice for 30 min. After a centrifugation step (10 min at 18,407 RCF) the supernatants were collected and the protein concentration was measured by Bradford's method using BSA as the standard curve. SDS-PAGE with precast gel (4–20%, mini-PROTEAN, BioRad, Hercules, CA, USA) was used to separate proteins lysates or Ang protein and peptides. Nitrocellulose membranes (Sigma-Aldrich) were used to transfer proteins from the gel. Membranes were incubated with blocking buffer (0.1% Tween20 in tris-buffered saline added with either 5% non-fat milk) at room temperature for 1 h, and then incubated with primary anti-angiogenin or anti-GAPDH antibody (code: sc-9044, 1:500 dilution, Santa Cruz Biotechnology (Dallas, TX, USA) or code: ab8245, 1:2000 dilution, Abcam (Cambridge, UK), respectively) overnight at 4 °C. After that, 1 h treatment with goat anti-rabbit or anti-mouse IgG horseradish peroxidase-conjugated secondary antibodies (code: AP307P and AP181P, respectively, 1:3000 dilution, MD Millipore Bioscience (Burlington, MA, USA). Measurements were performed by a ChemiDoc MP Imaging System (BioRad, Hercules, CA, USA) using enhanced Western Lighting Chemiluminescence Reagent Plus (PerkinElmer, Waltham, MA, USA).

4.6.3. Dot Blot Analysis

Peptides or whole protein were dissolved in phosphate buffer saline solution (PBS, pH = 7.4) at 0.2 mg/mL. Using narrow-mouth pipette tip, 2 µL of samples were spotted onto the nitrocellulose membrane. To block the non-specific sites membrane was incubated in 5% non-fat milk in 0.1% Tween20 in tris-buffered (30 min, room temperature). After that, membranes were incubated with primary anti-angiogenin antibody (code: sc-9044, 1:500 dilution, from Santa Cruz Biotechnology, Dallas, TX, USA) overnight at 4 °C. Than membranes were incubated with secondary antibody conjugated with horseradish peroxidase (HRP) enzyme (code: AP307P, 1:3000 dilution, MD Millipore Bioscience, Burlington, MA, USA) for 1 h. Measurements were performed by a ChemiDoc MP Imaging System

(BioRad, Hercules, CA, USA) using enhanced Western Lighting Chemiluminescence Reagent Plus (PerkinElmer, Waltham, MA, USA).

4.6.4. Quantitative qPCR

For qPCR experiments, cells were cultivated at 37 °C (in 5% CO_2 atmosphere) on Corning® tissue-culture treated culture dishes 60 mm × 15 mm (D × H) (Sigma-Aldrich) at 80% of confluence. Total RNA was extracted with TRIzol (Life Technologies, Foster City, CA, USA), according to the manufacturer's instructions. RNA quantification was performed by Epoch™ Microplate Spectrophotometer (BioTek®, Winooski, VT, USA). Extracted RNA was reverse transcribed by using a High Capacity RNA-to-cDNA Kit (Life Technologies), according to the manufacturer's instructions. Resulting cDNAs (30 ng per sample) were amplified through a LightCycler® 480 System (Roche, Pleasanton, CA, USA). Single-gene specific assays were performed through real-time PCR by using Fast SYBR Green Master Mix (Life Technologies, Carlsbad, CA, USA) according to the manufacturer's instruction. To allow statistical analysis, PCRs were performed in three independent biological replicates. 18S was used as housekeeping gene to normalize PCR data. Primer sequences are listed in Table 3.

Table 3. Primer sequences for vascular endothelial growth factor A (VEGFA) and 18S ribosomal RNA (18S) genes.

Gene Symbol	Forward	Reverse
Human VEGFA	5′-ATCTTCAAGCCATCCTGTGTGC-3′	5′- GAGGTTTGATCCGCATAATCTG-3′
18S	5′-AGTCCCTGCCCTTTGTACACA-3′	5′-GATCCGAGGGCCTCACTAAAC-3′

4.6.5. Sandwich ELISA Assay

Medium samples were collected after a 24-h treatment exposure with AuNPs, ANG and peptides, and hybrids Ang_{60-68}_NP, Ang_{60-68}Cys_NP and ANG_NP in DMEM medium supplemented with 0.5% of FBS and centrifuged (14,000× g, 10 min), the supernatants were transferred into clean microtubes and stored at −80 °C until analysed. The concentration of VEGF release was determined from the cell culture media samples using ELISA sandwich assay. Polyvinyl chloride (PVC) microtiter plates were coated overnight at 4 °C with 5 µg/mL of capture antibody (anti-VEGF, code: PAB12284) in carbonate/bicarbonate buffer (pH 9.6). Then plates were washed twice with PBS, blocked by blocking buffer (5% non-fat dry milk/PBS) for 2 hrs at room temperature, washed with PBS and incubated with cell culture media samples for 90 min at 37 °C. After plates were washed with PBS, incubated for 2 hrs with 1 µg/mL of detection antibody (anti-VEGF, code: H00007422-M05), washed again, then incubated for 2 hrs with HRP-conjugated secondary antibody and washed with PBS. Result was detected by 3,3′,5,5′-tetramethylbenzidine (TMB) solution after the incubation for 15 min. The reaction was stopped by stopping solution (2 M H_2SO_4) and the optical density was measured at 450 nm by a plate reader (Varioskan® Flash Spectral Scanning Multimode Reader, Waltham, MA, USA).

4.6.6. Laser Scanning Confocal Microscopy (LSM)

SH-SY5Y cells were seeded (30×10^3 cells per dish) and differentiated (see 2.6.1) in glass bottom dishes with 22 mm of glass diameter (WillCo-dish®, Willco Wells, B.V., Amsterdam Netherlands). Glioblastoma cells were seeded at the density 30×10^3 cells per dish in glass bottom dishes with complete medium for 24 hrs until cellular adhesion with a minimal cell confluence of 50% was attained. Thereafter, cells were treated with AuNPs (5 nM) or ANG (100 nM) or angiogenin peptides (30 µM) and their hybrids in the presence or absence of copper for 2 hrs in DMEM high glucose medium without FBS. After the incubation time, cells were stained with nuclear dye Hoechst33342, washed with PBS, and fixed with high purity 2% paraformaldehyde in PBS (pH = 7.3). Afterwards, cells were permeabilized with 0.5% Triton X-100 with 0.1% BSA and stained firstly with a high-affinity

F-actin probe (Actin Green 488 Ready Probes Reagent, ThermoFisher), conjugated to green-fluorescent Alexa Fluor® 488 dye for 30 min, washed with PBS and then with anti-angiogenin antibody (code: sc-9044, 1:50 dilution, Santa Cruz Biotechnology, Dallas, TX, USA) overnight at 4 °C. After that, 1 h treatment with donkey anti-rabbit IgG H&L (Alexa Fluor® 568) pre-adsorbed secondary antibodies (code: ab175692, 1:1000 dilution, MD Millipore Bioscience, Burlington, MA, USA).

For multichannel imaging, fluorescent dyes were imaged sequentially to eliminate cross talk between the channels, namely: (i) the blue (ex405/em 425–475), for the emission of the Hoechst33342-stained nuclei, (ii) the green (ex488/em 500–530), for the emission of the Actin Green 488 Ready Probes Reagent, (iii) the red (ex543/em 560–700), for Alexa Fluor® 568 of secondary antibody.

Confocal imaging microscopy was performed with a FV1000 confocal laser scanning microscope (LSM, Olympus, Tokyo, Japan), equipped with diode UV (405 nm, 50 mW), multiline Argon (457 nm, 488 nm, 515 nm, total 30 mW), HeNe(G) (543 nm, 1 mW) and HeNe(R) (633 nm, 1 mW) lasers. An oil immersion objective (60xO PLAPO) and spectral filtering system were used. The detector gain was fixed at a constant value and images were taken, in sequential mode, for all the samples at random locations throughout the area of the well. The image analysis was carried out using Huygens Essential software (by Scientific Volume Imaging B.V., Hilversum, The Netherlands).

5. Conclusions

The results obtained from experiment performed on A172 cells indicate that $Ang_{60-68}Cys$ and Ang_{60-68} anchored on AuNPs could be considered as effective inhibitors of glioblastoma tumour cell proliferation and VEGF release. However, the mechanism of action and potential side effects need to be elucidated further. Moreover, exogenous delivery of angiogenin by gold nanoparticles could represent a strategic approach to re-establish the physiological concentrations of angiogenin in the course of diseases in which the protein levels are strongly reduced and suggests that further studies are required to translate these effects into meaningful therapies.

Our results demonstrated that copper induced a decrease of VEGF mRNA transcription on d-SH-SY5Y cells. These data confirmed those of other studies, demonstrating the toxic effect of the copper on SH-SY5Y cells, particularly on the mitochondria, with decreased levels of mitochondrial proteins [86]. On the other hand, the treatment of A172 cancer cells with Cu(II) induced an increase of VEGF release, demonstrating the different role of the copper in both tumoral and non-tumoral cells. It has been demonstrated that copper induces the expression of VEGF in breast and hepatic cancer cells through the activation of the epidermal growth factor receptor/extracellular signal-regulated protein kinases (EGFR/ERK)/c-fos transduction pathway [87]. Surprisingly, the incubation of A172 cells with copper in presence of $Ang_{60-68}Cys\_NP$ potentiated the inhibitory effect of the protein fragment on VEGF release, demonstrating the therapeutic potential of copper chelating agents against tumour progression. However, the mechanism of action and potential side effects need to be elucidated further.

Supplementary Materials: The following are available online at http://www.mdpi.com/2072-6694/11/9/1322/s1, Figure S1: Densitometric analyses (a) and representative Western blot (b) of SH-SY5Y, differentiated SH-SY5Y and A172 cell lysates.

Author Contributions: Conceptualization, D.L.M. and C.S.; methodology, G.L. and C.S.; validation and formal analysis, C.D.A. and D.L.M.; investigation, I.N., L.M.C., F.D. and A.M.; data curation, L.M.C. and F.D.; writing—original draft preparation, I.N., L.M.C. and F.D.; writing—review and editing, D.L.M., G.L. and C.S.

Funding: This research was partially funded by MIUR under Grant PRIN 2015 (20152EKS4Y project) and University of Catania (Piano della Ricerca di Ateneo, Linea di Intervento 2, 2018–2020). D.L.M. acknowledges University of Pisa (PRA_2017_51).

Acknowledgments: Örjan Hansson (Gothenburg University, Sweden) is kindly acknowledged for the scientific and technical support in the expression of wild type angiogenin.

Conflicts of Interest: The authors declare no conflict of interest. The funders had no role in the design of the study; in the collection, analyses, or interpretation of data; in the writing of the manuscript, or in the decision to publish the results.

References

1. Spicer, C.D.; Jumeaux, C.; Gupta, B.; Stevens, M.M. Peptide and protein nanoparticle conjugates: Versatile platforms for biomedical applications. *Chem. Soc. Rev.* **2018**, *47*, 3574–3620. [CrossRef]
2. Cucci, L.; Naletova, I.; Consiglio, G.; Satriano, C. A Hybrid Nanoplatform of Graphene Oxide/Nanogold for Plasmonic Sensing and Cellular Applications at the Nanobiointerface. *Appl. Sci.* **2019**, *9*, 676. [CrossRef]
3. Di Pietro, P.; Strano, G.; Zuccarello, L.; Satriano, C. Gold and Silver Nanoparticles for Applications in Theranostics. *Curr. Top. Med. Chem.* **2016**, *16*, 3069–3102. [CrossRef]
4. Xu, R.; Xu, Y. *Modern Inorganic Synthetic Chemistry*, 2nd ed.; Elsevier: Amsterdam, The Netherlands, 2017; p. xxii, 785 Seiten.
5. Singh, P.; Pandit, S.; Mokkapati, V.; Garg, A.; Ravikumar, V.; Mijakovic, I. Gold Nanoparticles in Diagnostics and Therapeutics for Human Cancer. *Int. J. Mol. Sci.* **2018**, *19*, 1979. [CrossRef] [PubMed]
6. Satriano, C.; Munzone, A.; Cucci, L.M.; Giacomelli, C.; Trincavelli, M.L.; Martini, C.; Rizzarelli, E.; La Mendola, D. Angiogenin-mimetic peptide functionalised gold nanoparticles for cancer therapy applications. *Microchem. J.* **2018**, *136*, 157–163. [CrossRef]
7. Qing, Y.; Cheng, L.; Li, R.; Liu, G.; Zhang, Y.; Tang, X.; Wang, J.; Liu, H.; Qin, Y. Potential antibacterial mechanism of silver nanoparticles and the optimization of orthopedic implants by advanced modification technologies. *Int. J. Nanomed.* **2018**, *13*, 3311–3327. [CrossRef]
8. Di Pietro, P.; Zaccaro, L.; Comegna, D.; Del Gatto, A.; Saviano, M.; Snyders, R.; Cossement, D.; Satriano, C.; Rizzarelli, E. Silver nanoparticles functionalized with a fluorescent cyclic RGD peptide: A versatile integrin targeting platform for cells and bacteria. *RSC Adv.* **2016**, *6*, 112381–112392. [CrossRef]
9. DeFrates, K.; Markiewicz, T.; Gallo, P.; Rack, A.; Weyhmiller, A.; Jarmusik, B.; Hu, X. Protein Polymer-Based Nanoparticles: Fabrication and Medical Applications. *Int. J. Mol. Sci.* **2018**, *19*, 1717. [CrossRef]
10. Muñoz-Juan, A.; Carreño, A.; Mendoza, R.; Corchero, J.L. Latest Advances in the Development of Eukaryotic Vaults as Targeted Drug Delivery Systems. *Pharmaceutics* **2019**, *11*, 300. [CrossRef]
11. Satriano, C.; Lupo, G.; Motta, C.; Anfuso, C.D.; Di Pietro, P.; Kasemo, B. Ferritin-supported lipid bilayers for triggering the endothelial cell response. *Colloids Surf. B Biointerfaces* **2017**, *149*, 48–55. [CrossRef]
12. Watkins, R.; Wu, L.; Zhang, C.; Davis, R.; Xu, B. Natural product-based nanomedicine: Recent advances and issues. *Int. J. Nanomed.* **2015**, *10*, 6055–6074. [CrossRef]
13. Chan, K.H.; Lee, W.H.; Zhuo, S.; Ni, M. Harnessing supramolecular peptide nanotechnology in biomedical applications. *Int. J. Nanomed.* **2017**, *12*, 1171–1182. [CrossRef]
14. Chen, G.; Xie, Y.; Peltier, R.; Lei, H.; Wang, P.; Chen, J.; Hu, Y.; Wang, F.; Yao, X.; Sun, H. Peptide-Decorated Gold Nanoparticles as Functional Nano-Capping Agent of Mesoporous Silica Container for Targeting Drug Delivery. *ACS Appl. Mater. Interfaces* **2016**, *8*, 11204–11209. [CrossRef]
15. Silva, S.; Almeida, A.J.; Vale, N. Combination of Cell-Penetrating Peptides with Nanoparticles for Therapeutic Application: A Review. *Biomolecules* **2019**, *9*, 22. [CrossRef]
16. Sheng, J.; Xu, Z. Three decades of research on angiogenin: A review and perspective. *Acta Biochim. Biophys. Sin. (Shanghai)* **2016**, *48*, 399–410. [CrossRef]
17. Tsuji, T.; Sun, Y.; Kishimoto, K.; Olson, K.A.; Liu, S.; Hirukawa, S.; Hu, G.-f. Angiogenin Is Translocated to the Nucleus of HeLa Cells and Is Involved in Ribosomal RNA Transcription and Cell Proliferation. *Cancer Res.* **2005**, *65*, 1352–1360. [CrossRef]
18. Kieran, D.; Sebastia, J.; Greenway, M.J.; King, M.A.; Connaughton, D.; Concannon, C.G.; Fenner, B.; Hardiman, O.; Prehn, J.H. Control of motoneuron survival by angiogenin. *J. Neurosci.* **2008**, *28*, 14056–14061. [CrossRef]
19. Koutroubakis, I.E.; Xidakis, C.; Karmiris, K.; Sfiridaki, A.; Kandidaki, E.; Kouroumalis, E.A. Serum Angiogenin in Inflammatory Bowel Disease. *Dig. Dis. Sci.* **2004**, *49*, 1758–1762. [CrossRef]
20. Tello-Montoliu, A.; Patel, J.V.; Lip, G.Y. Angiogenin: A review of the pathophysiology and potential clinical applications. *J. Thromb. Haemost.* **2006**, *4*, 1864–1874. [CrossRef]
21. Strydom, D.J.; Fett, J.W.; Lobb, R.R.; Alderman, E.M.; Bethune, J.L.; Riordan, J.F.; Vallee, B.L. Amino acid sequence of human tumor derived angiogenin. *Biochemistry* **1985**, *24*, 5486–5494. [CrossRef]
22. Eberle, K.; Oberpichler, A.; Trantakis, C.; Krupp, W.; Knupfer, M.; Tschesche, H.; Seifert, V. The expression of angiogenin in tissue samples of different brain tumours and cultured glioma cells. *Anticancer Res.* **2000**, *20*, 1679–1684.

23. Huang, L.; Huang, Y.; Guo, H. Dominant expression of angiogenin in NeuN positive cells in the focal ischemic rat brain. *J. Neurol. Sci.* **2009**, *285*, 220–223. [CrossRef]
24. Maki, T.; Morancho, A.; Martinez-San Segundo, P.; Hayakawa, K.; Takase, H.; Liang, A.C.; Gabriel-Salazar, M.; Medina-Gutiérrez, E.; Washida, K.; Montaner, J.; et al. Endothelial Progenitor Cell Secretome and Oligovascular Repair in a Mouse Model of Prolonged Cerebral Hypoperfusion. *Stroke* **2018**, *49*, 1003–1010. [CrossRef]
25. Gabriel-Salazar, M.; Morancho, A.; Rodriguez, S.; Buxo, X.; Garcia-Rodriguez, N.; Colell, G.; Fernandez, A.; Giralt, D.; Bustamante, A.; Montaner, J.; et al. Importance of Angiogenin and Endothelial Progenitor Cells After Rehabilitation Both in Ischemic Stroke Patients and in a Mouse Model of Cerebral Ischemia. *Front. Neurol.* **2018**, *9*, 508. [CrossRef]
26. Sebastia, J.; Kieran, D.; Breen, B.; King, M.A.; Netteland, D.F.; Joyce, D.; Fitzpatrick, S.F.; Taylor, C.T.; Prehn, J.H. Angiogenin protects motoneurons against hypoxic injury. *Cell Death Differ.* **2009**, *16*, 1238–1247. [CrossRef]
27. Steidinger, T.U.; Slone, S.R.; Ding, H.; Standaert, D.G.; Yacoubian, T.A. Angiogenin in Parkinson disease models: Role of Akt phosphorylation and evaluation of AAV-mediated angiogenin expression in MPTP treated mice. *PLoS ONE* **2013**, *8*, e56092. [CrossRef]
28. Moroianu, J.; Riordan, J.F. Nuclear translocation of angiogenin in proliferating endothelial cells is essential to its angiogenic activity. *Proc. Natl. Acad. Sci. USA* **1994**, *91*, 1677–1681. [CrossRef]
29. Kishimoto, K.; Liu, S.; Tsuji, T.; Olson, K.A.; Hu, G.-f. Endogenous angiogenin in endothelial cells is a general requirement for cell proliferation and angiogenesis. *Oncogene* **2004**, *24*, 445–456. [CrossRef]
30. Rosenstein, J.M.; Krum, J.M.; Ruhrberg, C. VEGF in the nervous system. *Organogenesis* **2010**, *6*, 107–114. [CrossRef]
31. Bush, A.I. The metal theory of Alzheimer's disease. *J. Alzheimers Dis.* **2013**, *33* (Suppl. S1), S277–S281. [CrossRef]
32. Opazo, C.M.; Greenough, M.A.; Bush, A.I. Copper: From neurotransmission to neuroproteostasis. *Front. Aging Neurosci.* **2014**, *6*, 143. [CrossRef]
33. Urso, E.; Maffia, M. Behind the Link between Copper and Angiogenesis: Established Mechanisms and an Overview on the Role of Vascular Copper Transport Systems. *J. Vasc. Res.* **2015**, *52*, 172–196. [CrossRef]
34. Denoyer, D.; Masaldan, S.; La Fontaine, S.; Cater, M.A. Targeting copper in cancer therapy: 'Copper That Cancer'. *Metallomics* **2015**, *7*, 1459–1476. [CrossRef]
35. Giacomelli, C.; Trincavelli, M.L.; Satriano, C.; Hansson, O.; La Mendola, D.; Rizzarelli, E.; Martini, C. diamondCopper (II) ions modulate Angiogenin activity in human endothelial cells. *Int. J. Biochem. Cell Biol.* **2015**, *60*, 185–196. [CrossRef]
36. Badet, J.; Soncin, F.; Guitton, J.D.; Lamare, O.; Cartwright, T.; Barritault, D. Specific binding of angiogenin to calf pulmonary artery endothelial cells. *Proc. Natl. Acad. Sci. USA* **1989**, *86*, 8427–8431. [CrossRef]
37. Soncin, F.; Guitton, J.D.; Cartwright, T.; Badet, J. Interaction of human angiogenin with copper modulates angiogenin binding to endothelial cells. *Biochem. Biophys. Res. Commun.* **1997**, *236*, 604–610. [CrossRef]
38. La Mendola, D.; Arnesano, F.; Hansson, O.; Giacomelli, C.; Calo, V.; Mangini, V.; Magri, A.; Bellia, F.; Trincavelli, M.L.; Martini, C.; et al. Copper binding to naturally occurring, lactam form of angiogenin differs from that to recombinant protein, affecting their activity. *Metallomics* **2016**, *8*, 118–124. [CrossRef]
39. Gross, A.; Hashimoto, C.; Sticht, H.; Eichler, J. Synthetic Peptides as Protein Mimics. *Front. Bioeng. Biotechnol.* **2015**, *3*, 211. [CrossRef]
40. Trapani, G.; Satriano, C.; La Mendola, D. Peptides and their Metal Complexes in Neurodegenerative Diseases: From Structural Studies to Nanomedicine Prospects. *Curr. Med. Chem.* **2018**, *25*, 715–747. [CrossRef]
41. Strydom, D.J. The angiogenins. *Cell. Mol. Life Sci.* **1998**, *54*, 811–824. [CrossRef]
42. Gao, X.; Xu, Z. Mechanisms of action of angiogenin. *Acta Biochim. Biophys. Sin. (Shanghai)* **2008**, *40*, 619–624. [CrossRef]
43. Magri, A.; Munzone, A.; Peana, M.; Medici, S.; Zoroddu, M.A.; Hansson, O.; Satriano, C.; Rizzarelli, E.; La Mendola, D. Coordination Environment of Cu(II) Ions Bound to N-Terminal Peptide Fragments of Angiogenin Protein. *Int. J. Mol. Sci.* **2016**, *17*, 1240. [CrossRef]
44. Cucci, L.M.; Munzone, A.; Naletova, I.; Magri, A.; La Mendola, D.; Satriano, C. Gold nanoparticles functionalized with angiogenin-mimicking peptides modulate cell membrane interactions. *Biointerphases* **2018**, *13*, 03C401. [CrossRef] [PubMed]

45. Plate, K.H. Mechanisms of angiogenesis in the brain. *J. Neuropathol. Exp. Neurol.* **1999**, *58*, 313–320. [CrossRef] [PubMed]
46. Lupo, G.; Caporarello, N.; Olivieri, M.; Cristaldi, M.; Motta, C.; Bramanti, V.; Avola, R.; Salmeri, M.; Nicoletti, F.; Anfuso, C.D. Anti-angiogenic Therapy in Cancer: Downsides and New Pivots for Precision Medicine. *Front. Pharmacol.* **2016**, *7*, 519. [CrossRef]
47. He, Y.Q.; Liu, S.P.; Kong, L.; Liu, Z.F. A study on the sizes and concentrations of gold nanoparticles by spectra of absorption, resonance Rayleigh scattering and resonance non-linear scattering. *Spectrochim. Acta A Mol. Biomol. Spectrosc.* **2005**, *61*, 2861–2866. [CrossRef] [PubMed]
48. La Mendola, D.; Magrì, A.; Vagliasindi, L.I.; Hansson, O.; Bonomo, R.P.; Rizzarelli, E. Copper(II) complex formation with a linear peptide encompassing the putative cell binding site of angiogenin. *Dalton Trans.* **2010**, *39*, 10678–10684. [CrossRef]
49. Yamazaki, D.; Kurisu, S.; Takenawa, T. Regulation of cancer cell motility through actin reorganization. *Cancer Sci.* **2005**, *96*, 379–386. [CrossRef] [PubMed]
50. Hohmann, T.; Dehghani, F. The Cytoskeleton-A Complex Interacting Meshwork. *Cells* **2019**, *8*, 362. [CrossRef]
51. Xu, X.; Harder, J.; Flynn, D.C.; Lanier, L.M. AFAP120 regulates actin organization during neuronal differentiation. *Differentiation* **2009**, *77*, 38–47. [CrossRef]
52. Thiyagarajan, N.; Ferguson, R.; Subramanian, V.; Acharya, K.R. Structural and molecular insights into the mechanism of action of human angiogenin-ALS variants in neurons. *Nat. Commun.* **2012**, *3*, 1121. [CrossRef]
53. Takano, S.; Yoshii, Y.; Kondo, S.; Suzuki, H.; Maruno, T.; Shirai, S.; Nose, T. Concentration of vascular endothelial growth factor in the serum and tumor tissue of brain tumor patients. *Cancer Res.* **1996**, *56*, 2185–2190.
54. Schiera, G.; Proia, P.; Alberti, C.; Mineo, M.; Savettieri, G.; Di Liegro, I. Neurons produce FGF2 and VEGF and secrete them at least in part by shedding extracellular vesicles. *J. Cell. Mol. Med.* **2007**, *11*, 1384–1394. [CrossRef]
55. Finney, L.; Vogt, S.; Fukai, T.; Glesne, D. Copper and angiogenesis: Unravelling a relationship key to cancer progression. *Clin. Exp. Pharmacol. Physiol.* **2009**, *36*, 88–94. [CrossRef]
56. Hu, G.F.; Riordan, J.F.; Vallee, B.L. A putative angiogenin receptor in angiogenin-responsive human endothelial cells. *Proc. Natl. Acad. Sci. USA* **1997**, *94*, 2204–2209. [CrossRef]
57. Vericat, C.; Vela, M.E.; Corthey, G.; Pensa, E.; Cortés, E.; Fonticelli, M.H.; Ibañez, F.; Benitez, G.E.; Carro, P.; Salvarezza, R.C. Self-assembled monolayers of thiolates on metals: A review article on sulfur-metal chemistry and surface structures. *RSC Adv.* **2014**, *4*, 27730–27754. [CrossRef]
58. Miller, M.M.; Lazarides, A.A. Sensitivity of Metal Nanoparticle Surface Plasmon Resonance to the Dielectric Environment. *J. Phys. Chem. B* **2005**, *109*, 21556–21565. [CrossRef]
59. Zhou, C.; Friedt, J.-M.; Angelova, A.; Choi, K.-H.; Laureyn, W.; Frederix, F.; Francis, L.A.; Campitelli, A.; Engelborghs, Y.; Borghs, G. Human Immunoglobulin Adsorption Investigated by Means of Quartz Crystal Microbalance Dissipation, Atomic Force Microscopy, Surface Acoustic Wave, and Surface Plasmon Resonance Techniques. *Langmuir* **2004**, *20*, 5870–5878. [CrossRef]
60. Díaz-Herrera, N.; González-Cano, A.; Viegas, D.; Santos, J.L.; Navarrete, M.-C. Refractive index sensing of aqueous media based on plasmonic resonance in tapered optical fibres operating in the 1.5 μm region. *Sens. Actuators B Chem.* **2010**, *146*, 195–198. [CrossRef]
61. Acharya, K.R.; Shapiro, R.; Allen, S.C.; Riordan, J.F.; Vallee, B.L. Crystal structure of human angiogenin reveals the structural basis for its functional divergence from ribonuclease. *Proc. Natl. Acad. Sci. USA* **1994**, *91*, 2915–2919. [CrossRef]
62. Khlebtsov, B.N.; Khlebtsov, N.G. On the measurement of gold nanoparticle sizes by the dynamic light scattering method. *Colloid J.* **2011**, *73*, 118–127. [CrossRef]
63. Capanni, C.; Messori, L.; Orioli, P.; Chiti, F.; Stefani, M.; Ramponi, G.; Taddei, N.; Gabrielli, S. Investigation of the effects of copper ions on protein aggregation using a model system. *Cell. Mol. Life Sci. (CMLS)* **2004**, *61*, 982–991. [CrossRef]
64. Prenesti, E.; Daniele, P.G.; Toso, S. Visible spectrophotometric determination of metal ions: The influence of structure on molar absorptivity value of copper(II) complexes in aqueous solution. *Anal. Chim. Acta* **2002**, *459*, 323–336. [CrossRef]

65. La Mendola, D.; Magri, A.; Santoro, A.M.; Nicoletti, V.G.; Rizzarelli, E. Copper(II) interaction with peptide fragments of histidine-proline-rich glycoprotein: Speciation, stability and binding details. *J. Inorg. Biochem.* **2012**, *111*, 59–69. [CrossRef]
66. Stanyon, H.F.; Cong, X.; Chen, Y.; Shahidullah, N.; Rossetti, G.; Dreyer, J.; Papamokos, G.; Carloni, P.; Viles, J.H. Developing predictive rules for coordination geometry from visible circular dichroism of copper(II) and nickel(II) ions in histidine and amide main-chain complexes. *FEBS J.* **2014**, *281*, 3945–3954. [CrossRef]
67. Hu, G.F. Neomycin inhibits angiogenin-induced angiogenesis. *Proc. Natl. Acad. Sci. USA* **1998**, *95*, 9791–9795. [CrossRef]
68. Liu, J.; Hu, R.; Liu, J.; Zhang, B.; Wang, Y.; Liu, X.; Law, W.-C.; Liu, L.; Ye, L.; Yong, K.-T. Cytotoxicity assessment of functionalized CdSe, CdTe and InP quantum dots in two human cancer cell models. *Mater. Sci. Eng. C* **2015**, *57*, 222–231. [CrossRef]
69. Kalinina, E.V.; Chernov, N.N.; Saprin, A.N. Involvement of thio-, peroxi-, and glutaredoxins in cellular redox-dependent processes. *Biochemistry (Moscow)* **2008**, *73*, 1493–1510. [CrossRef]
70. Salazar-Ramiro, A.; Ramírez-Ortega, D.; Pérez de la Cruz, V.; Hérnandez-Pedro, N.Y.; González-Esquivel, D.F.; Sotelo, J.; Pineda, B. Role of Redox Status in Development of Glioblastoma. *Front. Immunol.* **2016**, *7*. [CrossRef]
71. Lyons, S.M.; Fay, M.M.; Akiyama, Y.; Anderson, P.J.; Ivanov, P. RNA biology of angiogenin: Current state and perspectives. *RNA Biol.* **2017**, *14*, 171–178. [CrossRef]
72. Lee, F.S.; Shapiro, R.; Vallee, B.L. Tight-binding inhibition of angiogenin and ribonuclease A by placental ribonuclease inhibitor. *Biochemistry* **1989**, *28*, 225–230. [CrossRef]
73. Li, L.; Pan, X.Y.; Shu, J.; Jiang, R.; Zhou, Y.J.; Chen, J.X. Ribonuclease inhibitor up-regulation inhibits the growth and induces apoptosis in murine melanoma cells through repression of angiogenin and ILK/PI3K/AKT signaling pathway. *Biochimie* **2014**, *103*, 89–100. [CrossRef]
74. Dos Remedios, C.G.; Chhabra, D.; Kekic, M.; Dedova, I.V.; Tsubakihara, M.; Berry, D.A.; Nosworthy, N.J. Actin binding proteins: Regulation of cytoskeletal microfilaments. *Physiol. Rev.* **2003**, *83*, 433–473. [CrossRef] [PubMed]
75. Pyatibratov, M.G.; Kostyukova, A.S. New insights into the role of angiogenin in actin polymerization. *Int. Rev. Cell Mol. Biol.* **2012**, *295*, 175–198. [CrossRef]
76. Dutta, S.; Bandyopadhyay, C.; Bottero, V.; Veettil, M.V.; Wilson, L.; Pins, M.R.; Johnson, K.E.; Warshall, C.; Chandran, B. Angiogenin interacts with the plasminogen activation system at the cell surface of breast cancer cells to regulate plasmin formation and cell migration. *Mol. Oncol.* **2014**, *8*, 483–507. [CrossRef]
77. Yamasaki, S.; Ivanov, P.; Hu, G.F.; Anderson, P. Angiogenin cleaves tRNA and promotes stress-induced translational repression. *J. Cell Biol.* **2009**, *185*, 35–42. [CrossRef] [PubMed]
78. Saikia, M.; Jobava, R.; Parisien, M.; Putnam, A.; Krokowski, D.; Gao, X.H.; Guan, B.J.; Yuan, Y.; Jankowsky, E.; Feng, Z.; et al. Angiogenin-cleaved tRNA halves interact with cytochrome c, protecting cells from apoptosis during osmotic stress. *Mol. Cell. Biol.* **2014**, *34*, 2450–2463. [CrossRef]
79. Ruggero, D.; Pandolfi, P.P. Does the ribosome translate cancer? *Nat. Rev. Cancer* **2003**, *3*, 179–192. [CrossRef]
80. Xu, Z.-P.; Tsuji, T.; Riordan, J.F.; Hu, G.-F. The nuclear function of angiogenin in endothelial cells is related to rRNA production. *Biochem. Biophys. Res. Commun.* **2002**, *294*, 287–292. [CrossRef]
81. Wei, Y.; Wang, F.; Sang, B.; Xu, Z.; Yang, D. Activation of KRas-ERK1/2 signaling drives the initiation and progression of glioma by suppressing the acetylation of histone H4 at lysine 16. *Life Sci.* **2019**, *225*, 55–63. [CrossRef]
82. Holloway, D.E.; Hares, M.C.; Shapiro, R.; Subramanian, V.; Acharya, K.R. High-Level Expression of Three Members of the Murine Angiogenin Family in Escherichia coli and Purification of the Recombinant Proteins. *Protein Expr. Purif.* **2001**, *22*, 307–317. [CrossRef]
83. Jang, S.-H.; Kang, D.-K.; Chang, S.-I.; Scheraga, H.A.; Shin, H.-C. High level production of bovine angiogenin in E. coli by an efficient refolding procedure. *Biotechnol. Lett.* **2004**, *26*, 1501–1504. [CrossRef]
84. Turkevich, J.; Stevenson, P.C.; Hillier, J. A study of the nucleation and growth processes in the synthesis of colloidal gold. *Discuss. Faraday Soc.* **1951**, *11*. [CrossRef]
85. Navarro, J.R.G.; Werts, M.H.V. Resonant light scattering spectroscopy of gold, silver and gold–silver alloy nanoparticles and optical detection in microfluidic channels. *Analyst* **2013**, *138*, 583–592. [CrossRef]

86. Arciello, M.; Rotilio, G.; Rossi, L. Copper-dependent toxicity in SH-SY5Y neuroblastoma cells involves mitochondrial damage. *Biochem. Biophys. Res. Commun.* **2005**, *327*, 454–459. [CrossRef]
87. Rigiracciolo, D.C.; Scarpelli, A.; Lappano, R.; Pisano, A.; Santolla, M.F.; De Marco, P.; Cirillo, F.; Cappello, A.R.; Dolce, V.; Belfiore, A.; et al. Copper activates HIF-1alpha/GPER/VEGF signalling in cancer cells. *Oncotarget* **2015**, *6*, 34158–34177. [CrossRef]

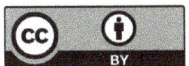
© 2019 by the authors. Licensee MDPI, Basel, Switzerland. This article is an open access article distributed under the terms and conditions of the Creative Commons Attribution (CC BY) license (http://creativecommons.org/licenses/by/4.0/).

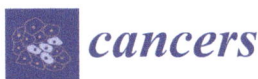

Article

Multi-Drug/Gene NASH Therapy Delivery and Selective Hyperspectral NIR Imaging Using Chirality-Sorted Single-Walled Carbon Nanotubes

Md. Tanvir Hasan [1], Elizabeth Campbell [1], Olga Sizova [2], Veronica Lyle [1], Giridhar Akkaraju [3], D. Lynn Kirkpatrick [4] and Anton V. Naumov [1,*]

1. Department of Physics and Astronomy, Texas Christian University, TCU Box 298840, Fort Worth, TX 76129, USA
2. The University of Texas MD Anderson Cancer Center, 1515 Holcombe Blvd, Houston, TX 77030, USA
3. Department of Biology, Texas Christian University, 2955 South University Drive, Fort Worth, TX 76129, USA
4. Ensysce Biosciences, 3210 Merryfield Row, San Diego, CA 92121, USA
* Correspondence: a.naumov@tcu.edu

Received: 9 July 2019; Accepted: 11 August 2019; Published: 14 August 2019

Abstract: Single-walled carbon nanotubes (SWCNTs) can serve as drug delivery/biological imaging agents, as they exhibit intrinsic fluorescence in the near-infrared, allowing for deeper tissue imaging while providing therapeutic transport. In this work, CoMoCAT (Cobalt Molybdenum Catalyst) SWCNTs, chirality-sorted by aqueous two-phase extraction, are utilized for the first time to deliver a drug/gene combination therapy and image each therapeutic component separately via chirality-specific SWCNT fluorescence. Each of (7,5) and (7,6) sorted SWCNTs were non-covalently loaded with their specific payload: the PI3 kinase inhibitor targeting liver fibrosis or CCR5 siRNA targeting inflammatory pathways with the goal of addressing these processes in nonalcoholic steatohepatitis (NASH), ultimately to prevent its progression to hepatocellular carcinoma. PX-866-(7,5) SWCNTs and siRNA-(7,6) SWCNTs were each imaged via characteristic SWCNT emission at 1024/1120 nm in HepG2 and HeLa cells by hyperspectral fluorescence microscopy. Wavelength-resolved imaging verified the intracellular transport of each SWCNT chirality and drug release. The therapeutic efficacy of each formulation was further demonstrated by the dose-dependent cytotoxicity of SWCNT-bound PX-866 and >90% knockdown of CCR5 expression with SWCNT/siRNA transfection. This study verifies the feasibility of utilizing chirality-sorted SWCNTs for the delivery and component-specific imaging of combination therapies, also suggesting a novel nanotherapeutic approach for addressing the progressions of NASH to hepatocellular carcinoma.

Keywords: single-walled carbon nanotubes; chirality separation; NASH; drug-gene delivery; near IR hyperspectral imaging

1. Introduction

The use of nanomaterials as gene/drug delivery agents has increased significantly over the past few years, owing to their capability of delivering either water-insoluble or unstable drugs or degradable gene therapeutics. Several categories of nanocarriers have been developed/utilized thus far, including quantum dots [1–4], PLGA-PEG (polylactic acid-co-glycolic acid-polyethylene glycol) nanoparticles [5], liposomes [6], self-emulsifying drug delivery systems (SEDDSs) [7], cyclodextrins [8], gold nanoparticles [9], and carbon nanotubes [10,11] as delivery vehicles or diagnostic tools. Among those, single-walled carbon nanotubes (SWCNTs) showed highly promising results for gene/drug delivery coupled with in vitro as well as in vivo imaging [12]. Their quasi-one-dimensional hydrophobic platform aids cellular internalization and the non-covalent or covalent attachment of active agents and targeting moieties [13]. At the same time, the intrinsic photostable fluorescence emission of SWCNTs in NIR (near-infrared) I and II regions with reduced scattering and autofluorescence backgrounds allows imaging through the layers of biological tissue [14,15]. As molecular transporters, SWCNTs can shuttle payloads, including drug molecules [16], proteins [17], DNA [18], and RNA [19] into biological cells and tissues. Functionalized with drugs and targeting agents covalently [20] or non-covalently by π-π stacking [13,21], SWCNTs can provide reduced toxicity [22], greater biological activity [16], accumulation in the liver when formulated [10], and controlled drug release [23]. Due to characteristic NIR SWCNT fluorescent emission, their location can be imaged to confirm the payload delivery. As near-infrared exhibits significantly enhanced tissue penetration and lower scattering, it provides unique promise in the in vivo imaging of shallow targets. Although it has been shown that SWCNTs can be used for the delivery of drugs [11,24], cancer therapeutic siRNA oligos [10,11], and imaging agents [25,26], their capability for multidrug therapy and imaging has been underexplored to date, hampering their advancement to the successful treatment of complex conditions. Additionally, the ability to follow chirally separated SWCNTs by imaging allows one to confirm that each component in multidrug therapies reaches the desired tissue of interest.

SWCNT formulation is known to accumulate in the liver [10], which offers the potential for the treatment of liver diseases including nonalcoholic steatohepatitis (NASH) and its progression into hepatocellular carcinoma (HCC). Thus, in this work, NASH was chosen as a feasible treatment target to demonstrate the imaging/drug delivery capabilities of SWCNTs. NASH is a non-curable condition present in 6–8% of adults in the US. It accounts for a large number of cases of cirrhosis and can progress to HCC, leading to 75% of all liver cancer—the third leading cause of cancer-related deaths. The transformation of NASH into HCC is known to be mediated by fibrosis [27] progressing in over 30% of NASH patients, and inflammatory response with the involvement of a variety of cytokines [28]. Due to the complexity of this condition involving both inflammation and fibrosis, multifactor treatment strategies are required.

Current molecular therapy approaches are often restricted by drug resistance and the inability to target multiple factors [29]. These challenges can be addressed by combination treatments involving multidrug approaches to surmount drug resistance, decrease treatment doses, and affect multiple therapeutic targets. Although effective in treatment [30–32], combination therapies suffer from non-specific toxicity [33,34], difficulties in assessing the adverse effects of each drug separately, and the lack of image-guided capabilities [35]. On the other hand, combination gene [36–38] or drug/gene [39] therapies can circumvent the issue of non-specific toxicity due to the target-specific effects of gene therapeutics while providing effective routes to treatment. However, due to the short lifetime of DNA/RNA oligonucleotides in the body, additional delivery mechanisms are required [40].

Here we explore a therapeutic platform with the capacity to address both inflammation and fibrosis pathways of NASH via combination drug/gene therapy. The therapeutic approach used an siRNA target that has been shown to reduce the inflammatory cytokines that lead to liver fibrosis [41], and a small-molecule PI3 kinase inhibitor, PX-866 [28], that has been shown to reduce tissue fibrosis in vivo. Fibrosis is known to increase the risk of HCC by 25 times [42], as it leads initially to liver cirrhosis and subsequently develops into HCC. In this progression, activated hepatic stellate cells (aHSCs) responsible for fibrosis development are often described as pericytes for angiogenesis and vascular remodeling in the liver [43]. Fibrosis mediated by HSCs is associated with the effects of inflammation, as multiple inflammatory cytokines are known to elicit further activation of HSCs [44]. Although the entire process is not fully understood, fibrotic cytokine release (i.e., TGF-β, sonic hedgehog, and TNF-α) in the course of NASH is believed to contribute to the progression of the latter through the fibrotic stage and cirrhosis to HCC [28]. Therefore, developing delivery and tracking through imaging modules for therapeutic entities that address both fibrosis and inflammation in NASH could be an important step toward mitigating the transformation of NASH into HCC.

Hepatic inflammation can be suppressed by gene therapies interfering with cytokine activation, including several siRNA sequences against the protein. CCR5 (aka RANTES) siRNA is well-known for its anti-inflammatory effects [45–47], and could be a potential key to the reduction of inflammation in the liver. Among effective fibrotic drugs, a PI3 kinase inhibitor, PX-866, was chosen for two reasons: (1) PX-866 was previously shown to reduce fibrosis in the lungs [48]; (2) PX-866 has been evaluated in clinical trials, its safety profile is understood, and it had shown some clinical benefit against solid-tumor cancers [49]. To reduce off-target effects of PX-866 and protect siRNA from enzymatic degradation in the blood, these therapies could benefit from a delivery vehicle that will direct their transport to the liver. Additionally, to allow confirmation of the delivery of each therapeutic entity by the SWCNTs, the capability of image-tracking chiral SWCNTs is advantageous.

In the present work, chiral SWCNTs perform the critical function of delivery/imaging agents capable of protecting siRNA from enzymatic degradation in circulation, and protecting healthy tissue from the off-target effects of PX-866 by focusing this delivery to the liver tissue. While using SWCNTs of one select chirality for the delivery of either siRNA sequence or a drug payload, chirality-specific SWCNT fluorescence [50] in the NIR can be utilized to image the location and delivery pathways of the drug or gene separately.

The goal of this work was to assess the capabilities of SWCNTs for the non-covalent delivery and imaging of combination therapeutics such as PX-866 and siCRR5, each attached to SWCNTs of a particular chirality. The efficacy of each payload was evaluated using hepatocellular carcinoma cells (HepG2) while NIR hyperspectral imaging was used to confirm the location and SWCNT-mediated delivery of each therapeutic separately. Since SWCNTs are produced as a mixture of chiralities, several separation strategies have been developed to isolate single chirality fractions, including gel chromatography [51], density-gradient ultracentrifugation [52], free-solution electrophoresis [53], aqueous two-phase extraction (ATPE) method [54], etc. ATPE is well-known and widely used for its high yield with maximum purity, low-cost surfactants, high production scalability, and availability of instrumentation required for separation in every laboratory. Therefore, in order to develop scalable and affordable combination therapy platforms, in this study single-chirality SWCNTs were separated by a modified ATPE method [54]. We isolated (7,5) and (7,6) chiral SWCNTs from raw CoMoCAT (Cobalt Molybdenum Catalyst) SWCNT samples, as those chiralities exhibit spectrally well-separated emission at 1035 nm and 1130 nm, respectively. NIR hyperspectral imaging was used to separately confirm the internalization of (7,5) and (7,6) chiral nanotubes, ensuring the delivery of drug and gene inside the HepG2 cells. Overall, this work explores the feasibility of using single-chirality SWCNTs as efficient imaging and delivery vehicles. Eventually, the utilization of such chiral SWCNTs may lead to the development of a unique image-guided multimodal therapy addressing several therapeutic targets. Here we particularly explore the possibility of targeting both inflammation and fibrosis, which facilitate the progression of NASH to HCC.

2. Results and Discussion

Since raw SWCNT samples contain nanotubes of different chiralities as well as SWCNT aggregates that are non-emissive and unsuitable for drug delivery, prior to sorting (7,5) and (7,6) chiral nanotubes, raw CoMoCAT SWCNT samples initially underwent aggregate depletion via 180 min centrifugation of sodium deoxycholate (DOC)-dispersed SWCNTs at 21,380× g. This rigorous procedure resulted in the sedimentation of SWCNT aggregates with higher specific gravity than the individually wrapped SWCNTs. In the aqueous two-phase extraction (ATPE) method, centrifuged SWCNTs with constant DOC concentration were combined in a PEG–dextran two-phase system with a variety of sodium dodecyl sulfate (SDS) concentrations, yielding the separation of chiralities from the dextran-enriched bottom to the PEG-enriched top phase. The (7,5) and (7,6) chiral nanotubes were separated at 3 and 4 mg/mL of SDS, respectively allowing a substantial degree of control over top/bottom phase chirality composition, evident from their respective fluorescence and absorbance spectra (Supporting Information Figures S1 and S2) that were pronouncedly different from each other and from the spectra of the parent samples.

Simulation of fluorescence spectra of (7,5) and (7,6) sorted fractions with single SWCNT chirality Lorentzian emission profiles (Figure 1a,b) using the Applied Nanofluorescence Nanospectralyzer fitting routine allows for quantitative assessment of the sample optical properties and composition, yielding calculated excitation–emission maps (Figure 1c,d) and relative abundances (Figure 1e,f). The spectral fitting process used in this work was based mainly on adjusting the expected widths and positions of theoretical fluorescence peaks from a variety of semiconducting SWCNT chiralities to simulate experimental emission spectra collected with four excitation wavelengths (532, 637, 671, and 782 nm), aiming for a perfect match between the simulated and measured spectra (Figure 1a,b).

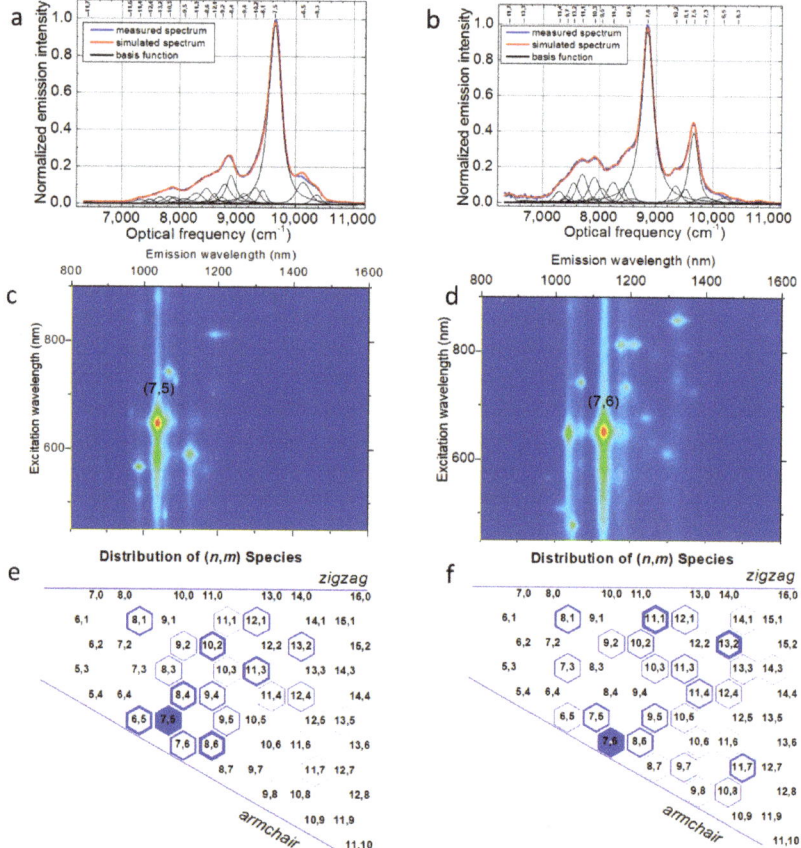

Figure 1. Measured and simulated fluorescence spectra of separated (**a**) (7,5), (**b**) (7,6) chiral single-walled carbon nanotubes (SWCNTs). The corresponding generated photoluminescence–excitation contour plot of (**c**) (7,5), (**d**) (7,6) sorted fractions. Graphene sheet representing the distribution of the emissive species in the respective (**e**) (7,5) and (**f**) (7,6) enriched sorted SWCNT samples. The blue-filled portion of hexagons represent the relative abundance of the species.

Based on the chirality abundances, calculated from the weight of individual chirality contributions to the experimental spectra and reflected in the distribution of (n,m) species (Figure 1e,f), substantial chirality enrichment was achieved in both sorted fractions (either (7,5) or (7,6)), with yields up to 40%. Although not overwhelming, this enrichment left other chiralities with only 1–5% contribution. In order to verify that this degree of separation is sufficient to monitor mainly SWCNTs of a single chirality microscopically, we examined the emission from (7,5) and (7,6) chirally sorted SWCNTs via NIR hyperspectral imaging at particular wavelengths corresponding to (7,3) (990 nm), (7,5) (1024 nm), and (7,6) (1120 nm) SWCNT chirality emission [55]. (7,3) SWCNT emission was dominant in the unsorted sample (Supporting Information Figures S1 and S2) and thus could be a significant contaminant in both fractions. However wavelength-resolved microscopy images show that the (7,5)-sorted fraction exhibited emission only at 1030 nm (Figure 2a–c), corresponding only to (7,5) SWCNTs, whereas the (7,6) fraction only showed observable SWCNT emission at 1130 nm (Figure 2d–f), corresponding to (7,6) SWCNTs. No substantial cross-contamination or contamination from (7,3) SWCNTs was observed. Furthermore, no observable contamination of the sorted sample by other SWCNT chiralities was detected by hyperspectral microscopy as we scanned the emission from 950 to 1350 nm with the step of 10 nm. This indicates that the achieved degree of separation with minor percentages of contaminants of each chirality was sufficient for hyperspectral microscopy imaging.

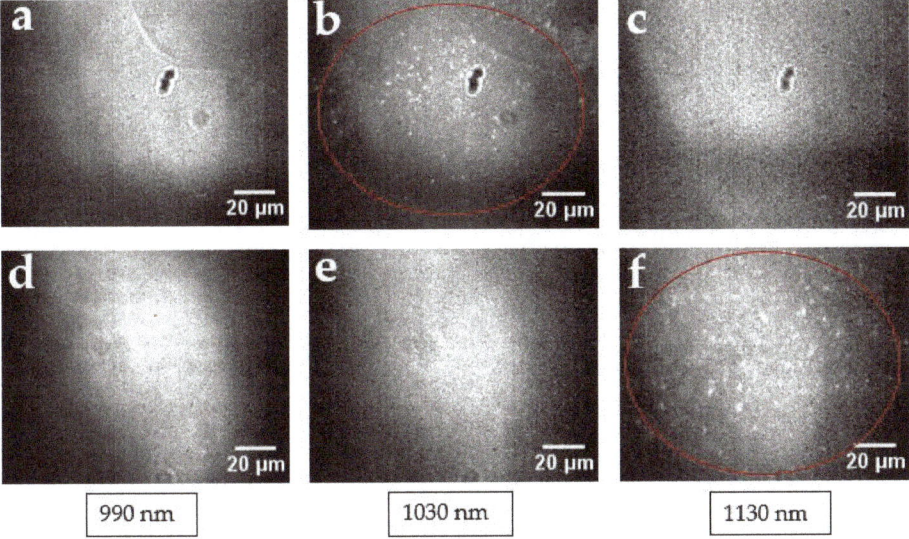

Figure 2. Near-infrared (NIR) hyperspectral images of (7,5) sorted SWCNTs at (**a**) 990, (**b**) 1030, and (**c**) 1130 nm; and (7,6) sorted SWCNTs at (**d**) 990, (**e**) 1030, and (**f**) 1130 nm. SWCNT fluorescence is only observed at the emission wavelengths of the corresponding sorted SWCNTs.

One of the main drawbacks of utilizing chirality-sorted SWCNTs has always been the high toxicity of sorting surfactants. In order to overcome this issue, we performed repeated multi-step centrifugal filtration (washing) with methanol/ethanol/DI water followed by the annealing of sorted SWCNTs at 200 °C for 1 h to remove the additional surfactants from the sorted SWCNTs. The annealed SWCNT samples were cooled down to room temperature before any further processing. The degree of surfactant removal was first verified spectroscopically by comparing the fluorescence spectral features of processed surfactant-purified samples: SWCNTs washed/annealed re-dispersed with EGFR siRNA and the spectra of raw SWCNTs dispersed directly with the same EGFR siRNA (Figure 3a). siRNA was chosen as it complexes non-covalently with SWCNTs and is known to form stable dispersions. Since surfactant wrapping induces observable fluorescence shifts specific to each surfactant [56,57] that are substantially different for bile salts and nucleic acids [58], assessing shifts in the positions of major peaks allows the qualitative removal of surfactant. Here, for the convenience of comparing multiple chirality peaks, we washed/annealed an unsorted SWCNT fraction, but with all the separation surfactants that are regularly present in the sorted samples. Although a starting SWCNT sample which included sorting surfactants (PEG/dextran/SDS) exhibited major emission peaks at ca. 966,

986, 1035, 1130, 1185, and 1265 nm (Figure 3a—black line), upon surfactant removal processing and redispersion with siRNA, major emissive features were observed at 1004, 1046, 1141, 1212, and 1308 nm (Figure 3a—blue line). Substantial shifts in the spectral positions (i.e., 11–18 nm shifts for 986, 1035, and 1130 nm peaks, a 27 nm shift for the 1185 nm peak, and a 43 nm shift for the 1265 nm peak), along with suppression of the 966 feature, indicate a significant change in the dielectric environment of SWCNTs that may have occurred due to the surfactant removal and replacement with siRNA. Furthermore, new peak positions appeared to be close to those of raw SWCNTs dispersed with siRNA (Figure 3a—red curve) that displayed a weak shoulder at 974 nm along with the most prominent emission features at ca. 996, 1041, 1141, 1213, and 1315 nm (comparison of peak positions listed in Supporting Information Figure S3). The processed SWCNTs were re-dispersed, and yielded substantial fluorescence emission with characteristic spectra indicating that the SWCNTs were individualized, while the broadening could arise from only a loose aggregation. Despite the difference in relative peak intensities affected by some aggregation accompanying the process of surfactant washing, substantial surfactant-removal-facilitated shifts of emission peaks toward those of siRNA-dispersed raw SWCNTs suggest a significant degree of surfactant depletion. This may reduce the cytotoxicity of sorted SWCNTs, making them as suitable for biological applications as raw SWCNTs dispersed by siRNA. It was also observed that SWCNTs' characteristic emissions were not affected by thermal annealing, suggesting the preservation of SWCNTs' fluorescence properties due to the thermal annealing at 200 °C for 1 h (Supporting Information Figure S4). Additionally, a comparative fluorescence study was performed between before and after centrifuged washed/annealed SWCNTs + siRNA sample, exhibiting a slight insignificant change of photoluminescence intensity (Supporting Information Figure S5).

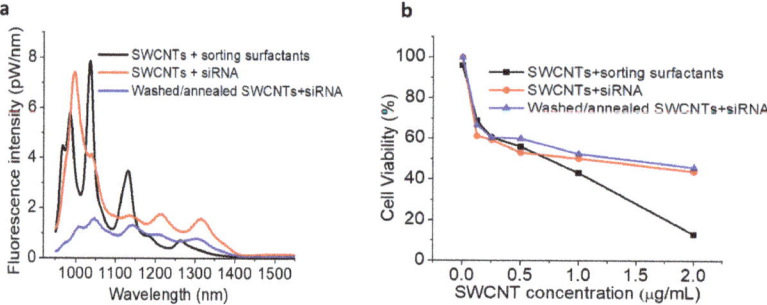

Figure 3. (a) Fluorescence spectra of raw SWCNTs dispersed with sorting surfactants, raw SWCNTs dispersed with siRNA, and SWCNTs washed/annealed for surfactant removal and re-dispersed with siRNA showing similar peak positions for raw SWCNTs dispersed with siRNA and washed/annealed SWCNTs dispersed with siRNA. (b) Cell viability of HepG2 cells subject to SWCNTs dispersed with sorting surfactants, raw SWCNTs dispersed with siRNA, and SWCNTs washed/annealed for surfactant removal and re-dispersed with siRNA.

A MTT cytotoxicity assay of centrifugally filtrated and thermally annealed SWCNTs further helped to assess if any residual surfactants could add to the toxicity profile of the formulation. Confirming the findings derived from spectral position matching, MTT assays showed that washed/annealed SWCNTs had the same or lower cytotoxicity than the raw SWCNTs dispersed in siRNA (Figure 3b). The significantly lowered cell viability found in the assessment of the toxic profile of the parent unsorted SWCNT sample with all separation surfactants presents the benefit of surfactant removal. Although this does not verify complete removal of surfactants, it indicates that washed/annealed SWCNTs are not more toxic than the raw SWCNTs, minimizing the toxicity contribution of sorting surfactants. Further decrease in toxicity of SWCNT/siRNA formulation could be achieved by masking it with DSPE-PEG 5000 [10], which was used for all in vitro studies in this work.

Similar to siRNA, SWCNTs can non-covalently complex with another therapeutic (i.e., PX-866) that was used in this work. Upon ultrasonic processing, raw/unsorted SWCNTs showed a stable dispersion in an aqueous solution of PX-866, as well as distinct fluorescence emission (Figure 4a). Sorted, washed, and annealed SWCNT samples of (7,5) chirality could also be dispersed with PX-866 alone, showing distinct emission features corresponding to (7,5) SWCNTs (Figure 4c). Similarly, with only siRNA dispersion, raw SWCNTs (Figure 4b) and sorted washed/burned SWCNTs ((7,6) chirality) (Figure 4c) also formed stable emissive dispersions. In fact, corresponding fluorescence (Figure 4c) and absorbance (Supporting Information Figure S6a,b) spectra of (7,5) SWCNT/PX-866 and (7,6) SWCNT/siCCR5 fractions still showed the major features of the sorted SWCNT chiralities. Interestingly, PX-866 on its own showed emission in green with 400 nm excitation (Figure 4d) that was quenched when the drug was loaded on the SWCNTs (Supporting Information Figure S7). This feature was used to locate/ensure the delivery of the drug in HepG2 cells as it was released from SWCNTs and the emission was restored.

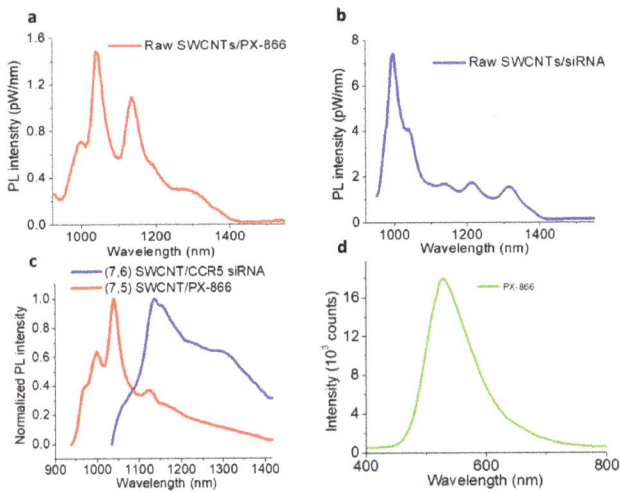

Figure 4. Emission spectra of raw CoMoCAT SWCNTs dispersed with (**a**) PX-866, (**b**) siRNA. Emission spectra of (**c**) (7,5) and (7,6) sorted washed/annealed SWCNTs dispersed with PX-866 and CCR5 siRNA, respectively. (**d**) Visible emission spectrum of PX-866 with 400 nm excitation.

In order to ensure the lower cytotoxicity, improved stability, and in vivo compatibility of the formulations for future studies, both SWCNTs dispersed with PX866 and siCCR5 were additionally coated with DSPE-PEG-5000 (at 1600 µM) via ultrasonic processing. Aggregates that were not fully dispersed were further removed by centrifugal processing at 16,000× g for 5 min, while the excess of siRNA or PX-866, as well as DSPE-PEG-5000, was centrifugally filtered with 100-kDa molecular cutoff filters, leaving only drug or gene/SWCNT complexes in the solution. TEM images of the final samples verify substantial SWCNT coating (Supporting Information Figure S8).

Following successful separation, removal of the sorting surfactants and non-covalent attachment of the drugs and DSPE-PEG-5000, we further assessed the capability of (7,5) and (7,6) SWCNTs to trace the delivery of the drug and gene intracellularly. Since combination therapy is envisioned for NASH, sorted (7,5) and (7,6) SWCNTs complexed with PX-866 and CCR5 siRNA were respectively combined in one suspension in equal proportions based on SWCNT concentrations and introduced to HepG2 cells. After up to 3 h incubation, cells were washed twice with PBS (phosphate-buffered saline) solution to remove any extracellular SWCNTs, and only those that were internalized were imaged. Among 0.5, 1, and 3 h incubation times tested, the highest intracellular emission was assessed at 3 h post transfection which was also found to be one of the optimal time points in the previous works [10,59,60].

However, the efficiency/maximum intracellular emission and cellular uptake may vary with cell types, SWCNT length, and SWCNT functionalization. For example, Sekiyama et al. [61] used oxygen-doped SWCNTs/PEG to perform the intracellular imaging in cultured murine cancer cells (Colon-26) showing no emission/uptake up to 1 day, but started showing/increasing internalization from day 3 to day 7. Additionally, Mao et al. [62] studied the cellular uptake and distribution of collagen-functionalized SWCNTs in bovine articular chondrocytes (BACs), showing longer retention in cells for more than one week. The cellular uptake of SWCNTs was previously hypothesized to occur via nano-spearing of the cell membrane [63,64], explained by needle-like hydrophobic SWCNT structure, while endocytosis [65,66] is currently deemed as a more plausible SWCNT entry pathway and is considered as a major internalization mechanism in the current work.

Herein, in vitro fluorescence imaging was accomplished with custom microscopy setup involving an inverted microscope coupled to two visible (Hamamatsu Image EMCCD) and near-infrared (InGaAs Xenics Xeva) cameras, allowing for filtered emission detection in the visible and spectrally resolved imaging in the near-infrared enabled by a Photon etc. NIR hyperspectral imager. In that configuration, wavelength-resolved images were recorded in the visible range with a lamp and in the NIR with 637 nm laser excitation. This allowed the imaging of SWCNTs specifically at 1030 (Supporting Information Figure S9b) and 1130 nm (Supporting Information Figure S9c), corresponding to the emission wavelengths of sorted chiralities, while PX-866 was imaged in the visible with a 532 nm emission filter. Confirming the sufficient degree of chirality separation, no emission in the NIR was observed outside the aforementioned spectral regions. However, at 1030 and 1130 nm, substantial SWCNT fluorescence was observed within the cells (Supporting Information Figure S10), indicating the successful internalization of both formulations with no emission detected outside the cells. Due to spectrally resolved imaging, no autofluorescence was detected in the non-treatment control. The overlays of the fluorescence images of two chiral SWCNT fractions false-colored in red (for (7,5) SWCNT emission) and blue (for (7,6) SWCNT emission) (Figure 5) verify the capability of tracking each therapeutic separately, as one could pinpoint the internalized SWCNTs or their clusters within HepG2 cells. Additionally, the release of PX-866 could be assessed, as the released drug was no longer quenched by complexation to the SWCNTs: its fluorescence was also observed in the cells and was delocalized from its delivery vehicles while the extracellular PX-866 was removed by washing. PX-866 imaging settings including integration time and excitation lamp intensity were chosen such that they yielded no autofluorescence from non-treatment control cells (Figure 5a). Additionally, the intracellular release of PX-866 was tracked qualitatively with different incubation times (0, 1, 4.5, 12 h) (Supporting Information Figure S11), yielding maximum release at the 3 h time point, also suggesting that 3 h is the best possible incubation time for the intracellular imaging. A separate cellular internalization study was performed in HeLa (cervical cancer) cells, showing a brighter intracellular SWCNT emission (Supporting Information Figure S12) and indicating a substantial uptake capability of SWCNT/siRNA hybrids by several cancer cell lines.

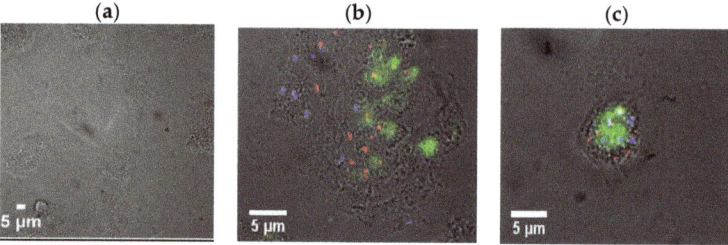

Figure 5. Brightfield/fluorescence overlay images of (**a**) untreated control HepG2 cells and (**b**,**c**) cellular uptake of (7,5) sorted SWCNTs imaged at 1030 nm (red), (7,6) sorted SWCNTs imaged at 1130 nm (blue), and PX-866 imaged at 535 nm (green) after the intracellular release.

The efficacy of the delivered and imaged therapeutics was assessed separately for each drug and gene. The biocompatibility of SWCNTs in DSPE-PEG5000 coating used in these efficacy studies was verified both in HepG2 (Figure 6) and HeLa (Supporting Information Figure S13) cells, indicating that at imaging and treatment concentrations SWCNTs do not exhibit substantial toxicity to several cell lines. Due to the complexity of testing antifibrotic properties of PX-866 in vitro, its efficacy was assessed through the toxic response to HepG2 cancer cells. A comparative MTT cytotoxicity assay was used to assess the toxic effect of PX-866 alone or delivered by the SWCNTs (Figure 6). When formulated with SWCNTs, PX-866 showed more significant cytotoxic (Figure 6) effect, increased by the factor of ~2.8 at 2.5 μg/mL likely due to improved transport with the nanomaterial delivery vehicle, generally known to enhance the efficacy of delivered therapeutics [67–69]. The antifibrotic effect of the drug leads to apparent toxicity that is best analyzed in the cancer cells. The toxicity added by SWCNTs alone cannot be responsible for that increase, as those at 2.5 μg/mL equivalent to 2.5 μg/mL PX-866 concentrations showed only a small toxic response, with cell viability above 80%. For the cytotoxicity testing, the SWCNT/PX-866 conjugation was accomplished using the concentration ratio of 1:1 for SWCNT and PX-866. This yielded a stable SWCNT dispersion via non-covalent complexation with the drug.

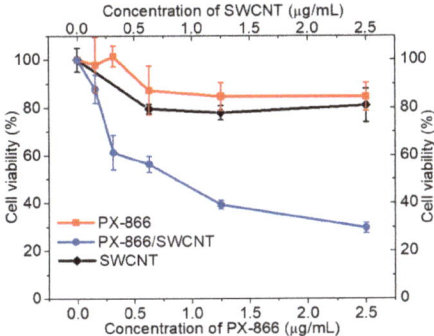

Figure 6. MTT assay cell viability of HepG2 cells treated with either SWCNTs, PX-866, or SWCNT/PX866 conjugates.

The efficacy of SWCNT/siCCR5 formulation was evaluated by assessing the CCR5 siRNA-mediated knockdown in HepG2 cells after 48 h transfection via flow cytometry, as CCR5 is known to be expressed in HepG2 cells [70]. SWCNTs-formulated siRNA transfection showed much lower expression of chemokine receptor type 5 (CCR5) as compared to the natural expression exhibited in the control sample (Figure 7), indicating substantial (over 90%) knockdown above or comparable to that regularly achieved by lyposomally delivered siRNA [18,71,72].

It is evident that SWCNTs also facilitated siRNA transfection, as it does not transfect mammalian cells on its own [73–75]. IgG (immunoglobulin G) antibody was used as isotype control, to help differentiate the non-specific background signal from specific antibody signal. Overall, this study verifies the efficacy of SWCNT/siCCR5 formulation and suggests SWCNTs as a promising gene-silencing carrier for NASH therapeutics.

It is also noteworthy that SWCNTs have the ability to protect the probe (siRNA) from degradation in blood circulation, because: (1) they offer only a small window for nucleases/proteins to degrade siRNA bound to the SWCNT surface; and (2) conjugation of SWCNT/siRNA may form an unusual RNA structure which helps to disguise the siRNA from enzyme binding sites [76]. Additionally, siRNA coating can prevent blood proteins from binding to the SWCNT surface [10], reducing the protein corona formation. The delivered therapeutics were analyzed separately in vitro as the effects of PX-866 would interfere with the determination of protein knockdown. However, in vivo they are expected to perform synergistically against NASH-induced inflammation and fibrosis. The present work shows the potential of chirality-sorted SWCNTs for delivery, separate NIR fluorescence imaging, and increase in the efficacy of combination drug/gene therapy aimed to address inflammation and fibrosis in NASH, which is necessary for the further application of SWCNT-mediated combination therapy for NASH in vivo. Further NASH animal model studies will lead to the direct assessment of the antifibrotic potential of the SWCNT-delivered PX-866 via PCR analysis of TGF-B1, B2 expression, together with the assessment of the synergistic effects of the nanotherapeutics developed here.

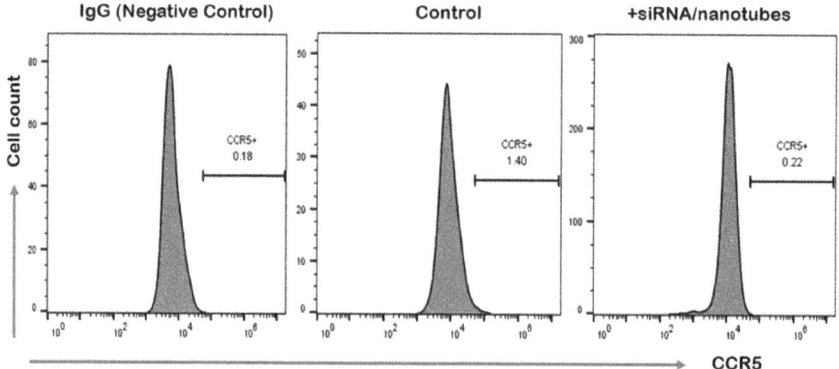

Figure 7. Downregulation of CCR5 in HepG2 cells by siRNA/nanotubes complex. CCR5 expression was detected by flow cytometry after nanotubes-delivered siRNA-mediated knockdown for 48 h. IgG staining was used for isotype control (**left**). Control indicated natural expression of CCR5 in HepG2 cells without any treatment (**middle**) compared to CCR5-targeting siRNA/nanotubes treatment (**right**).

3. Experimental Methods and Procedures

3.1. Sample Preparation

The suspensions of SWCNTs (CoMoCAT, (7,6) chirality, ≥77% carbon as SWCNT) were prepared by dispersing 1.5 mg of SWCNTs in 1 mg/mL sodium deoxycholate (DOC) aqueous solution. The samples were further processed via direct probe ultrasonic treatment (QSonica, Q55) for 60 min at 33 W in an ice bath. The suspension was further centrifuged (Southwest Science, D3024) for 180 min at 21,380× g followed by the removal of SWCNT aggregates into the decant and collecting the supernatant only. The collected SWCNTs were used for the chirality sorting. In order to create two phases, 0.25 g/mL aqueous solution of PEG (MW—6 kDa) and 0.25 g/mL aqueous solution of dextran (MW—75 kDa) were used to produce the stock solution. After that, a ratio of 0.4:0.28:0.28:0.04 (SWCNTs:PEG:dextran:water) was maintained to prepare the final sample for the separation. Sodium dodecyl sulfate (SDS) was added to this final suspension with a variation in concentration from 1 to 7 mg/mL. The targeted (7,5) and (7,6) chiral tubes were separated in the top phase at 3 and 4 mg/mL SDS concentration.

In order to remove sorting surfactants, we performed repeated centrifugal filtration (Amicon Ultra 0.5 mL; 100,000 MWCO filter) using methanol (to condense the samples first) for five times followed by 15 times filtration with ethanol to wash the remainders of the surfactants from the separated SWCNTs. As surfactants were washed through the filter pores, SWCNTs remained on the filter. Washed samples were collected and further processed for thermal annealing at 200 °C for one hour in the mechanical convection oven (precision-18EM laboratory oven). Processed (7,5), (7,6) chiral SWCNTs were then collected and dispersed with PX-866 and CCR5 siRNA (Biolegend, San Diego, CA, USA, Cat#359105) in aqueous suspension, respectively. To assure non-covalent complexation, 0.3 mg/mL of SWCNTs and 0.5 µg/mL of siRNA in nuclease-free water or 0.3 mg/mL of PX-866 in DI water were mixed and subjected to ultrasonic treatment using a Covaris S2 (SN001263) ultrasonic disperser at 70 W for 2 min, which allowed avoidance of contact with the non-sterile probe. Both siRNA and PX-866 were used at concentrations substantially below saturation [10] for SWCNT binding, ensuring maximum loading assumed for PX-866/SWCNT cell viability assays. SWCNTs dispersion with active agents was finally followed by the addition of 1600 µM of DSPE-PEG 5000 (NanoCS, Boston, MA, USA) attached to SWCNTs via additional ultrasonic agitation with Covaris at 50 W for 6 min. SWCNT concentration in the samples was matched via absorption measurements with an extinction coefficient of 31.25 mL mg^{-1}cm^{-1} at 632 nm [10].

Transmission electron microscopy (TEM JEOL JEM-2100) was utilized to observe the morphology of final SWNT formulations. The sample for TEM measurement was prepared on a carbon-coated 200-mesh copper grid under ambient conditions.

3.2. Optical Characterization

Fluorescence and absorbance spectra were measured using an NS2 NanoSpectralyzer (Applied NanoFluorescence, Houston, TX, USA). To measure the photoluminescence of SWCNTs, a 637-nm diode laser excitation was used. The collected fluorescence spectra were simulated using fully integrated Nanospectralyzer GlobalFit software. The software allows for the simulation of experimental SWCNT spectra with individual chirality SWCNT emission peaks for spectra with four excitations, models excitation–emission maps based on those, and extracts relative emissive SWCNT chirality abundances in the sample.

SWCNTs concentration was calculated using the absorbance spectrum similarly to [77,78]:

SWCNTs Concentration (mg/mL) = Absorbance at 632 nm/31.25 mL mg^{-1}cm^{-1}

(Experimental extinction co-efficient).

3.3. Fluorescence Microscopy Measurements

Fluorescence microscopy was performed using an Olympus IX73 fluorescence microscope with 60× (IR-corrected Olympus Plan Apo, Japan) water immersion objective coupled to two detectors: spectrally filtered by 10 filters throughout the visible Hamamatsu Image EMCCD camera, and InGaAs Xenics (Xeva-7870, XEN-000110) coupled to a hyperspectral fluorescence imager (Photon etc., Montreal, QC, Canada) This allowed for spectrally-resolved imaging both in the visible and near-infrared.

3.4. Imaging in the Visible Region

We imaged the green (535 nm) emission of PX-866 in vitro with lamp excitation and (375 ± 25 nm) excitation and (535 ± 20 nm) emission filters by first determining the integration and lamp intensity settings that resulted in zero autofluorescence emission from non-treatment control cells and using the corresponding settings for PX-866 fluorescence imaging.

3.5. Imaging in the NIR Region

SWCNTs fluorescence in hepatocellular carcinoma (HepG2) and HeLa cells was imaged with an InGaAs camera (Xenics Xeva, Belgium) and an NIR hyperspectral imager (Photon etc. IMA-IR^{TM}) with 637 nm (130 mW output power) diode laser excitation. This infrared hyperspectral imager captures full spatial information simultaneously utilizing a Bragg grating imaging filter [79] which collects spectral information successively providing spectrally resolved imaging. Individual SWCNT fluorescence could be resolved for all emissive chiralities using band-pass filtering mode (950–1450 nm), but only particular SWCNT chiralities can be imaged by selecting a specific spectral region. For (7,5) and (7,6) SWCNT chiralities dispersed with PX-866 and CCR5 siRNA, 1030 and 1130 nm filter positions were found optimal. In-vitro control images without SWCNTs were also captured, ensuring no emission in the NIR region.

3.6. Cell Culture

In this work, we used liver hepatocellular carcinoma (HepG2) and HeLa cell lines maintained in a Thermo-Scientific Midi 40 CO_2 Incubator at 37.1 °C with 5% carbon dioxide and 95% air. In order to prepare the glass coverslips for microscopy imaging, they were placed at the bottom of 6-well plates followed by adding cells in the media. SWCNT-carried formulations were added at a concentration of 2 µg/mL in each well after 4 hours of cell attachment to the coverslips. Cells were further washed with 0.5 mL of PBS (phosphate-buffered saline) to remove extracellular SWCNTs, followed by fixing them with 4% paraformaldehyde at room temperature for 30 min. After that, the cell samples were rewashed with 0.5 mL of PBS for the microscopy imaging. Transfection points of 0.5, 1, 3 h were used for imaging, with 2 µg/mL SWCNTs added to each well.

3.7. MTT Assays

In order to assess the cytotoxicity for SWCNT, PX866, and their complex, HepG2 (human hepatocellular carcinoma) and HeLa cells were plated in a 96-well plate at a density of 5000 cells per well (100 µL/well) and kept in an incubator overnight at 37.1 °C while maintaining the CO_2/air ratio of 1:19. After 24 h of incubation, the samples (PX-866, SWCNTs, or SWCNT/PX-866 formulations) were added into each well at concentrations ranging from 0.125 to 2.5 µg/mL. After 24 h of incubation, the medium was replaced by 100 µL of 1 mg/mL thiazolyl blue tetrazolium bromide. The cells were incubated further for 4 h followed by the replacement of MTT (3-(4–dimethylthiazol-2-yl)-2,5-diphenyltetrazolium bromide) with 100 µL of DMSO (dimethyl sulfoxide) in order to solubilize the precipitation. Reduction in MTT influences the metabolic activity of living cells, which can be assessed with absorbance measurements since living cells metabolize the MTT and form a highly absorbing purple colored byproduct known as formazan [80]. We measured the absorbance (essentially the cell viability) of the final sample at 540 nm wavelength using the FLUOstar Omega microplate reader.

3.8. siRNA Transfection

The day before transfection, HepG2 cells were seeded onto 24-well plates in DMEM medium with 10% FBS to give ~30% confluence at the time of transfection. Before the transfection, the culture medium was replaced with fresh DMEM medium supplemented with 15% FBS and the SWCNTs complexed with CCR5 siRNA and DSPE-PEG 5000 as described above were then added to the medium, after which the cells were cultured for 48 h. For transfection efficiency examination, flow cytometry assay was performed at 48 h post-treatment.

3.9. Flow Cytometry

For the flow cytometry of the transfection efficiency experiment, HepG2 cells were washed twice with PBS and harvested by trypsin/EDTA. Following trypsinization, the cells were washed by centrifugation and resuspended in staining buffer (1 × PBS, 2% FBS, 0.5% EDTA, and 0.1% NaN_3). The cell suspension was stained with PE (phycoerythrin)-conjugated human anti-CCR5 antibody (Biolegend, Cat#359105) for 30 min on ice. To test the unspecific antibody binding, IgG (BioLegend, Cat#359105) was used as the isotype control. Flow cytometry was performed using an Accuri C6 plus flow cytometer (BD Biosciences, San Jose, CA, USA), and the data were analyzed using FlowJo software (www.flowjo.com/solutions/flowjo).

3.10. Image Analysis

We utilized ImageJ software to analyze all the images, including the subtraction of the backgrounds and overlays of the bright-field cell images with emission from PX-866 and two sorted SWCNT chiralities (i.e., (7,5), (7,6)) at 1030 and 1130 nm, respectively.

4. Conclusions

In this work, we developed and tested a single-walled carbon nanotube-based drug/gene combination therapeutic platform that allows for the image-tracking of each therapeutic agent. Chirality-sorted SWCNTs emitting at different wavelengths in the NIR were used to selectively track and deliver two therapeutic payloads in vitro: CCR5 siRNA and the small-molecule drug PX-866, targeting inflammation and fibrosis factors that mediate the translation of nonalcoholic steatohepatitis into hepatocellular carcinoma. For that purpose, (7,5) and (7,6) chiral SWCNTs separated from raw CoMoCAT starting material via aqueous two-phase extraction with over ~40% fluorescence-derived purities and cleared from toxic sorting surfactants were individualized by the dispersion and non-covalent complexation with the corresponding drug or gene. Hyperspectral NIR and spectrally-resolved visible fluorescence imaging allowed simultaneous monitoring at 1030 nm emission of (7,5) SWCNTs carrying PX-866 and at 1130 nm emission of (7,6) SWCNTs complexed with CCR5 siRNA internalized in HepG2 cells, as well as the visible 528 nm emission from PX-866 as it was released from the SWCNTs inside the cells. This work demonstrates: (1) the successful delivery of drug/gene therapy with sorted chiral SWCNTs; (2) the potential for locating each therapeutic agent separately through characteristic SWCNT fluorescence; and (3) the improved efficacy of both therapeutics when delivered with SWCNTs with substantially increased effect of SWCNT/PX866 over PX866 alone and high (over 90%) apparent knockdown of CCR5 siRNA when carried by SWCNTs, suggesting a promising potential of these formulations for combination NASH therapy. The emission of individual chiral SWCNTs in the near-infrared with low autofluorescence and high penetration depth could be utilized for multi-gene/drug delivery and imaging in animal models, whereas the high non-targeted liver accumulation of SWCNTs makes them advantageous candidates for liver conditions such as NASH.

Supplementary Materials: The following are available online at http://www.mdpi.com/2072-6694/11/8/1175/s1. Figure S1: Fluorescence and corresponding absorbance spectra of Parent SWCNT sample: raw SWCNTs dispersed with DOC/PEG/Dextran that are used as a starting material for ATPE sorting, bottom phases of ATP system with 3 mg/mL and 4 mg/mL SDS added to sort top phases containing (7,5) and (7,6) chirality-sorted SWCNTs at 3 mg/mL and 4 mg/mL SDS, respectively, Figure S2: Fluorescence and corresponding absorbance spectra of SWCNT collected from top phases containing (7,5) and (7,6) chirality-sorted SWCNTs at 3 mg/mL and 4 mg/mL SDS, respectively, Figure S3: Table describing the peak positions and peak shifts for the following samples: Sample-1: SWCNTs + sorting surfactants; Sample-2: SWCNTs + siRNA; Sample-3: Washed/annealed SWCNTs + siRNA. The oval shaped marker denotes the full restoration of the peak positions after the centrifugal washing/annealing and siRNA dispersion to those of raw SWCNTs dispersed with sRNA, whereas rectangle marker depicts partial but significant peak position recovery after washing/thermal annealing, Figure S4: Fluorescence spectra of untreated (no thermal annealing) SWCNTs/EGFR siRNA formulations, and thermally annealed SWCNTs dispersed with EGFR siRNA, Figure S5: Comparison between the fluorescence spectra of washed/annealed SWCNTs + siRNA before and after the centrifugation, Figure S6: Absorbance spectra of (7,5) SWCNT/PX-866, and (7,6) SWCNTs/CCR5 siRNA, Figure S7: Fluorescence spectra of only PX-866 and PX-866+SWCNT showing the quenching of PX-866 fluorescence after the loading of PX-866 on the SWCNTs, Figure S8: TEM images of the mixture of (7,5) SWCNTs/DSPE-PEG/siCCR5 and (7,6) SWCNTs/DSPE-PEG/PX-866 showing SWCNTs coating (DSPE-PEG-5000, and gene or drug), Figure S9: Fluorescence images of non-treatment control (without SWCNTs), Parent CoMoCat SWCNTs in aqueous dispersion with ATPE surfactants containing SWCNTs of various chiralities imaged at 1030 nm corresponding to (7,5) SWCNT emission, 1130 nm corresponding to (7,6) SWCNT emission, and Fluorescence overlay image of both (7,5) and (7,6) SWCNTs in the sample, Figure S10: Brightfield/fluorescence overlay images of cellular (HepG2 cells) uptake of (7,5) SWCNTs/PX-866 imaged at 1030 nm, (7,6) SWCNTs/siRNA imaged at 1130 nm, and px-866 released from SWCNTs imaged at 535 nm, Figure S11: Brightfield/fluorescence overlay images of cellular (HepG2 cells) uptake and release of px-866 from SWCNTs with 1, 3, 4.5, 12 h incubation time imaged at 535 nm, Figure S12: Brightfield/NIR fluorescence overlay images of cellular (HeLa cells) uptake of SWCNTs/siRNA imaged with 637 nm laser excitation, Figure S13: MTT assay cell viability of HeLa cells treated with SWCNT/siRNA.

Author Contributions: M.T.H. sorted the SWCNT samples using the ATPE method, prepared the samples for the study, performed optical characterization/TEM characterization/cellular imaging, and wrote the draft of the manuscript; E.C. and V.L. assessed the cytotoxicity; O.S. performed the flow cytometry experiment; G.A. prepared the slides for the cellular imaging and supervised the cytotoxicity study; L.K. and A.V.N. edited the manuscript and directed the research project; All authors reviewed the manuscript.

Funding: This work is supported by the TCU Invests in Scholarship grant funding.

Acknowledgments: We would like to thank Jason Strait at Airforce Research Laboratory, Wright-Patterson AFB, OH for his suggestions regarding the nanotubes separation using ATPE method and Bong Lee for the preparation of slides for imaging with HeLa cell lines.

Conflicts of Interest: The authors declare no conflicts of interest.

References

1. Iannazzo, D.; Pistone, A.; Salamò, M.; Galvagno, S.; Romeo, R.; Giofré, S.V.; Branca, C.; Visalli, G.; di Pietro, A. Graphene quantum dots for cancer targeted drug delivery. *Int. J. Pharm.* **2017**, *518*, 185–192. [CrossRef]
2. Bagalkot, V.; Zhang, L.; Levy-Nissenbaum, E.; Jon, S.; Kantoff, P.W.; Langer, R.; Farokhzad, O.C. Quantum Dot–Aptamer Conjugates for Synchronous Cancer Imaging, Therapy, and Sensing of Drug Delivery Based on Bi-Fluorescence Resonance Energy Transfer. *Nano Lett.* **2007**, *7*, 3065–3070. [CrossRef] [PubMed]
3. Guo, W.; Qiu, Z.; Guo, C.; Ding, D.; Li, T.; Wang, F.; Sun, J.; Zheng, N.; Liu, S. Multifunctional Theranostic Agent of $Cu_2(OH)PO_4$ Quantum Dots for Photoacoustic Image-Guided Photothermal/Photodynamic Combination Cancer Therapy. *ACS Appl. Mater. Interfaces* **2017**, *9*, 9348–9358. [CrossRef] [PubMed]
4. Cai, X.; Luo, Y.; Zhang, W.; Du, D.; Lin, Y. pH-Sensitive ZnO Quantum Dots–Doxorubicin Nanoparticles for Lung Cancer Targeted Drug Delivery. *ACS Appl. Mater. Interfaces* **2016**, *8*, 22442–22450. [CrossRef] [PubMed]
5. Cheng, J.; Teply, B.A.; Sherifi, I.; Sung, J.; Luther, G.; Gu, F.X.; Levy-Nissenbaum, E.; Radovic-Moreno, A.F.; Langer, R.; Farokhzad, O.C. Formulation of functionalized PLGA–PEG nanoparticles for in vivo targeted drug delivery. *Biomaterials* **2007**, *28*, 869–876. [CrossRef] [PubMed]
6. Sercombe, L.; Veerati, T.; Moheimani, F.; Wu, S.Y.; Sood, A.K.; Hua, S. Advances and Challenges of Liposome Assisted Drug Delivery. *Front. Pharmacol.* **2015**, *6*, 286. [CrossRef]
7. Neslihan Gursoy, R.; Benita, S. Self-emulsifying drug delivery systems (SEDDS) for improved oral delivery of lipophilic drugs. *Biomed. Pharmacother.* **2004**, *58*, 173–182. [CrossRef]
8. Kanasty, R.; Dorkin, J.R.; Vegas, A.; Anderson, D. Delivery materials for siRNA therapeutics. *Nat. Mater.* **2013**, *12*, 967. [CrossRef]
9. Kim, D.; Jeong, Y.Y.; Jon, S. A Drug-Loaded Aptamer–Gold Nanoparticle Bioconjugate for Combined CT Imaging and Therapy of Prostate Cancer. *ACS Nano* **2010**, *4*, 3689–3696. [CrossRef]
10. Kirkpatrick, D.L.; Weiss, M.; Naumov, A.; Bartholomeusz, G.; Weisman, R.B.; Gliko, O. Carbon Nanotubes: Solution for the Therapeutic Delivery of siRNA? *Materials* **2012**, *5*, 278. [CrossRef]
11. Karimi, M.; Solati, N.; Ghasemi, A.; Estiar, M.A.; Hashemkhani, M.; Kiani, P.; Mohamed, E.; Saeidi, A.; Taheri, M.; Avci, P.; et al. Carbon nanotubes part II: A remarkable carrier for drug and gene delivery. *Expert Opin. Drug Deliv.* **2015**, *12*, 1089–1105. [CrossRef] [PubMed]
12. Liu, Z.; Tabakman, S.; Welsher, K.; Dai, H. Carbon nanotubes in biology and medicine: In vitro and in vivo detection, imaging and drug delivery. *Nano Res.* **2009**, *2*, 85–120. [CrossRef] [PubMed]
13. Pantarotto, D.; Singh, R.; McCarthy, D.; Erhardt, M.; Briand, J.P.; Prato, M.; Kostarelos, K.; Bianco, A. Functionalized Carbon Nanotubes for Plasmid DNA Gene Delivery. *Angew. Chem. Int. Ed.* **2004**, *43*, 5242–5246. [CrossRef] [PubMed]
14. Barone, P.W.; Baik, S.; Heller, D.A.; Strano, M.S. Near-infrared optical sensors based on single-walled carbon nanotubes. *Nat. Mater.* **2004**, *4*, 86. [CrossRef] [PubMed]
15. Welsher, K.; Sherlock, S.P.; Dai, H. Deep-tissue anatomical imaging of mice using carbon nanotube fluorophores in the second near-infrared window. *Proc. Natl. Acad. Sci. USA* **2011**, *108*, 8943–8948. [CrossRef]
16. Bhirde, A.A.; Patel, V.; Gavard, J.; Zhang, G.; Sousa, A.A.; Masedunskas, A.; Leapman, R.D.; Weigert, R.; Gutkind, J.S.; Rusling, J.F. Targeted Killing of Cancer Cells in Vivo and in Vitro with EGF-Directed Carbon Nanotube-Based Drug Delivery. *ACS Nano* **2009**, *3*, 307–316. [CrossRef]
17. Liu, Z.; Fan, A.C.; Rakhra, K.; Sherlock, S.; Goodwin, A.; Chen, X.; Yang, Q.; Felsher, D.W.; Dai, H. Supramolecular Stacking of Doxorubicin on Carbon Nanotubes for in Vivo Cancer Therapy. *Angew. Chem. Int. Ed.* **2009**, *48*, 7668–7672. [CrossRef]
18. Liu, Z.; Winters, M.; Holodniy, M.; Dai, H. siRNA Delivery into Human T Cells and Primary Cells with Carbon-Nanotube Transporters. *Angew. Chem. Int. Ed.* **2007**, *46*, 2023–2027. [CrossRef]
19. Liu, Z.; Sun, X.; Nakayama-Ratchford, N.; Dai, H. Supramolecular Chemistry on Water-Soluble Carbon Nanotubes for Drug Loading and Delivery. *ACS Nano* **2007**, *1*, 50–56. [CrossRef]

20. Bianco, A.; Kostarelos, K.; Prato, M. Applications of carbon nanotubes in drug delivery. *Curr. Opin. Chem. Biol.* **2005**, *9*, 674–679. [CrossRef]
21. Bartholomeusz, G.; Cherukuri, P.; Kingston, J.; Cognet, L.; Lemos, R.; Leeuw, T.K.; Gumbiner-Russo, L.; Weisman, R.B.; Powis, G. In vivo therapeutic silencing of hypoxia-inducible factor 1 alpha (HIF-1α) using single-walled carbon nanotubes noncovalently coated with siRNA. *Nano Res.* **2009**, *2*, 279–291. [CrossRef] [PubMed]
22. Han, Z.J.; Ostriko, K.K.; Tan, C.M.; Tay, B.K.; Peel, S.A. Effect of hydrophilicity of carbon nanotube arrays on the release rate and activity of recombinant human bone morphogenetic protein-2. *Nanotechnology* **2011**, *22*, 295712. [CrossRef] [PubMed]
23. Ji, Z.; Lin, G.; Lu, Q.; Meng, L.; Shen, X.; Dong, L.; Fu, C.; Zhang, X. Targeted therapy of SMMC-7721 liver cancer in vitro and in vivo with carbon nanotubes based drug delivery system. *J. Colloid Interface Sci.* **2012**, *365*, 143–149. [CrossRef] [PubMed]
24. Ohta, T.; Hashida, Y.; Yamashita, F.; Hashida, M. Development of Novel Drug and Gene Delivery Carriers Composed of Single-Walled Carbon Nanotubes and Designed Peptides with PEGylation. *J. Pharm. Sci.* **2016**, *105*, 2815–2824. [CrossRef] [PubMed]
25. De La Zerda, A.; Zavaleta, C.; Keren, S.; Vaithilingam, S.; Bodapati, S.; Liu, Z.; Levi, J.; Smith, B.R.; Ma, T.J.; Oralkan, O.; et al. Carbon nanotubes as photoacoustic molecular imaging agents in living mice. *Nat. Nanotechnol.* **2008**, *3*, 557. [CrossRef] [PubMed]
26. Hernández-Rivera, M.; Zaibaq, N.G.; Wilson, L.J. Toward carbon nanotube-based imaging agents for the clinic. *Biomaterials* **2016**, *101*, 229–240. [CrossRef]
27. Starley, B.Q.; Calcagno, C.J.; Harrison, S.A. Nonalcoholic fatty liver disease and hepatocellular carcinoma: A weighty connection. *Hepatology* **2010**, *51*, 1820–1832. [CrossRef]
28. Sun, B.; Karin, M. Obesity, inflammation, and liver cancer. *J. Hepatol.* **2012**, *56*, 704–713. [CrossRef]
29. Ke, X.; Shen, L. Molecular targeted therapy of cancer: The progress and future prospect. *Front. Lab. Med.* **2017**, *1*, 69–75. [CrossRef]
30. Bang, Y.J.; van Cutsem, E.; Feyereislova, A.; Chung, H.C.; Shen, L.; Sawaki, A.; Lordick, F.; Ohtsu, A.; Omuro, Y.; Satoh, T.; et al. Trastuzumab in combination with chemotherapy versus chemotherapy alone for treatment of HER2-positive advanced gastric or gastro-oesophageal junction cancer (ToGA): A phase 3, open-label, randomised controlled trial. *Lancet* **2010**, *376*, 687–697. [CrossRef]
31. Einhorn, L.H.; Donohue, J. CIs-diamminedichloroplatinum, vinblastine, and bleomycin combination chemotherapy in disseminated testicular cancer. *Ann. Intern. Med.* **1977**, *87*, 293–298. [CrossRef] [PubMed]
32. O'Shaughnessy, J.; Miles, D.; Vukelja, S.; Moiseyenko, V.; Ayoub, J.P.; Cervantes, G.; Fumoleau, P.; Jones, S.; Lui, W.Y.; Mauriac, L.; et al. Superior Survival with Capecitabine Plus Docetaxel Combination Therapy in Anthracycline-Pretreated Patients with Advanced Breast Cancer: Phase III Trial Results. *J. Clin. Oncol.* **2002**, *20*, 2812–2823. [CrossRef] [PubMed]
33. Li, M.C.; Whitmore, W.F., Jr.; Golbey, R.; Grabstald, H. Effects of combined drug therapy on metastatic cancer of the testis. *JAMA* **1960**, *174*, 1291–1299. [CrossRef] [PubMed]
34. Baum, M.; Budzar, A.U.; Cuzick, J.; Forbes, J.; Houghton, J.H.; Klijn, J.G.; Sahmoud, T.; ATAC Trialists' Group. Anastrozole alone or in combination with tamoxifen versus tamoxifen alone for adjuvant treatment of postmenopausal women with early breast cancer: First results of the ATAC randomised trial. *Lancet* **2002**, *359*, 2131–2139.
35. Uematsu, M.; Shioda, A.; Suda, A.; Fukui, T.; Ozeki, Y.; Hama, Y.; Wong, J.R.; Kusano, S. Computed tomography-guided frameless stereotactic radiotherapy for stage I non-small cell lung cancer: A 5-year experience. *Int. J. Radiat. Oncol. Biol. Phys.* **2001**, *51*, 666–670. [CrossRef]
36. Xue, W.; Dahlman, J.E.; Tammela, T.; Khan, O.F.; Sood, S.; Dave, A.; Cai, W.; Chirino, L.M.; Yang, G.R.; Bronson, R.; et al. Small RNA combination therapy for lung cancer. *Proc. Natl. Acad. Sci. USA* **2014**, *111*, E3553–E3561. [CrossRef]
37. Yang, D.; Song, X.; Zhang, J.; Ye, L.; Wang, S.; Che, X.; Wang, J.; Zhang, Z.; Wang, L.; Shi, W. Therapeutic potential of siRNA-mediated combined knockdown of the IAP genes (Livin, XIAP, and Survivin) on human bladder cancer T24 cells. *Acta Biochim. Biophys. Sin.* **2010**, *42*, 137–144. [CrossRef] [PubMed]
38. Han, L.; Zhang, A.L.; Xu, P.; Yue, X.; Yang, Y.; Wang, G.X.; Jia, Z.F.; Pu, P.Y.; Kang, C.S. Combination gene therapy with PTEN and EGFR siRNA suppresses U251 malignant glioma cell growth in vitro and in vivo. *Med. Oncol.* **2010**, *27*, 843–852. [CrossRef] [PubMed]

39. Ganesh, S.; Iyer, A.K.; Weiler, J.; Morrissey, D.V.; Amiji, M.M. Combination of siRNA-directed Gene Silencing with Cisplatin Reverses Drug Resistance in Human Non-small Cell Lung Cancer. *Mol. Ther. Nucleic Acids* **2013**, *2*, e110. [CrossRef]
40. Mendes, R.; Fernandes, A.R.; Baptista, P.V. Gold Nanoparticle Approach to the Selective Delivery of Gene Silencing in Cancer—The Case for Combined Delivery? *Genes* **2017**, *8*, 94. [CrossRef]
41. Seki, E.; de Minicis, S.; Gwak, G.Y.; Kluwe, J.; Inokuchi, S.; Bursill, C.A.; Llovet, J.M.; Brenner, D.A.; Schwabe, R.F. CCR1 and CCR5 promote hepatic fibrosis in mice. *J. Clin. Investig.* **2009**, *119*, 1858–1870. [CrossRef] [PubMed]
42. Guzman, G.; Brunt, E.M.; Petrovic, L.M.; Chejfec, G.; Layden, T.J.; Cotler, S.J. Does Nonalcoholic Fatty Liver Disease Predispose Patients to Hepatocellular Carcinoma in the Absence of Cirrhosis? *Arch. Pathol. Lab. Med.* **2008**, *132*, 1761–1766. [PubMed]
43. Lee, J.S.; Semela, D.; Iredale, J.; Shah, V.H. Sinusoidal remodeling and angiogenesis: A new function for the liver-specific pericyte? *Hepatology* **2007**, *45*, 817–825. [CrossRef] [PubMed]
44. Chen, Y.N.; Hsu, S.L.; Liao, M.Y.; Liu, Y.T.; Lai, C.H.; Chen, J.F.; Nguyen, M.H.T.; Su, Y.H.; Chen, S.T.; Wu, L.C. Ameliorative Effect of Curcumin-Encapsulated Hyaluronic Acid–PLA Nanoparticles on Thioacetamide-Induced Murine Hepatic Fibrosis. *Int. J. Environ. Res. Public Health* **2017**, *14*, 11. [CrossRef]
45. Fallowfield, J.A. Therapeutic targets in liver fibrosis. *Am. J. Physiol. Gastrointest. Liver Physiol.* **2011**, *300*, G709–G715. [CrossRef] [PubMed]
46. Doodes, P.D.; Cao, Y.; Hamel, K.M.; Wang, Y.; Rodeghero, R.; Farkas, B.; Finnegan, A. CCR5 is Involved in Resolution of Inflammation in Proteoglycan-Induced Arthritis. *Arthritis Rheum.* **2009**, *60*, 2945–2953. [CrossRef] [PubMed]
47. Louboutin, J.P.; Chekmasova, A.; Marusich, E.; Agrawal, L.; Strayer, D.S. Role of CCR5 and its ligands in the control of vascular inflammation and leukocyte recruitment required for acute excitotoxic seizure induction and neural damage. *FASEB J.* **2011**, *25*, 737–753. [CrossRef]
48. Le Cras, T.D.; Korfhagen, T.R.; Davidson, C.; Schmidt, S.; Fenchel, M.; Ikegami, M.; Whitsett, J.A.; Hardie, W.D. Inhibition of PI3K by PX-866 Prevents Transforming Growth Factor-α–Induced Pulmonary Fibrosis. *Am. J. Pathol.* **2010**, *176*, 679–686. [CrossRef]
49. Pitz, M.W.; Eisenhauer, E.A.; MacNeil, M.V.; Thiessen, B.; Easaw, J.C.; Macdonald, D.R.; Eisenstat, D.D.; Kakumanu, A.S.; Salim, M.; Chalchal, H.; et al. Phase II study of PX-866 in recurrent glioblastoma. *Neuro Oncol.* **2015**, *17*, 1270–1274. [CrossRef]
50. Bachilo, S.M.; Strano, M.S.; Kittrell, C.; Hauge, R.H.; Smalley, R.E.; Weisman, R.B. Structure-Assigned Optical Spectra of Single-Walled Carbon Nanotubes. *Science* **2002**, *298*, 2361. [CrossRef]
51. Liu, H.; Nishide, D.; Tanaka, T.; Kataura, H. Large-scale single-chirality separation of single-wall carbon nanotubes by simple gel chromatography. *Nat. Commun.* **2011**, *2*, 309. [CrossRef] [PubMed]
52. Arnold, M.S.; Green, A.A.; Hulvat, J.F.; Stupp, S.I.; Hersam, M.C. Sorting carbon nanotubes by electronic structure using density differentiation. *Nat. Nanotechnol.* **2006**, *1*, 60. [CrossRef] [PubMed]
53. Ihara, K.; Endoh, H.; Saito, T.; Nihey, F. Separation of Metallic and Semiconducting Single-Wall Carbon Nanotube Solution by Vertical Electric Field. *J. Phys. Chem. C* **2011**, *115*, 22827–22832. [CrossRef]
54. Fagan, J.A.; Hároz, E.H.; Ihly, R.; Gui, H.; Blackburn, J.L.; Simpson, J.R.; Lam, S.; Walker, A.R.H.; Doorn, S.K.; Zheng, M. Isolation of >1 nm Diameter Single-Wall Carbon Nanotube Species Using Aqueous Two-Phase Extraction. *ACS Nano* **2015**, *9*, 5377–5390. [CrossRef] [PubMed]
55. Weisman, R.B.; Bachilo, S.M. Dependence of Optical Transition Energies on Structure for Single-Walled Carbon Nanotubes in Aqueous Suspension: An Empirical Kataura Plot. *Nano Lett.* **2003**, *3*, 1235–1238. [CrossRef]
56. Lain-Jong, L.; Nicholas, R.J.; Chien-Yen, C.; Darton, R.C.; Baker, S.C. Comparative study of photoluminescence of single-walled carbon nanotubes wrapped with sodium dodecyl sulfate, surfactin and polyvinylpyrrolidone. *Nanotechnology* **2005**, *16*, S202.
57. Park, J.; Yang, H.; Seong, M.J. Comparative study on raman and photoluminescence spectra of carbon nanotubes dispersed in different surfactant solutions. *J. Korean Phys. Soc.* **2012**, *60*, 1301–1304. [CrossRef]
58. Landry, M.P.; Vuković, L.; Kruss, S.; Bisker, G.; Landry, A.M.; Islam, S.; Jain, R.; Schulten, K.; Strano, M.S. Comparative Dynamics and Sequence Dependence of DNA and RNA Binding to Single Walled Carbon Nanotubes. *J. Phys. Chem. C* **2015**, *119*, 10048–10058. [CrossRef] [PubMed]

59. Cheng, J.; Fernando, K.A.S.; Veca, L.M.; Sun, Y.P.; Lamond, A.I.; Lam, Y.W.; Cheng, S.H. Reversible Accumulation of PEGylated Single-Walled Carbon Nanotubes in the Mammalian Nucleus. *ACS Nano* **2008**, *2*, 2085–2094. [CrossRef] [PubMed]
60. Donkor, D.A.; Tang, X.S. Tube length and cell type-dependent cellular responses to ultra-short single-walled carbon nanotube. *Biomaterials* **2014**, *35*, 3121–3131. [CrossRef] [PubMed]
61. Sekiyama, S.; Umezawa, M.; Iizumi, Y.; Ube, T.; Okazaki, T.; Kamimura, M.; Soga, K. Delayed Increase in Near-Infrared Fluorescence in Cultured Murine Cancer Cells Labeled with Oxygen-Doped Single-Walled Carbon Nanotubes. *Langmuir* **2019**, *35*, 831–837.
62. Mao, H.; Kawazoe, N.; Chen, G. Uptake and intracellular distribution of collagen-functionalized single-walled carbon nanotubes. *Biomaterials* **2013**, *34*, 2472–2479.
63. Pantarotto, D.; Briand, J.-P.; Prato, M.; Bianco, A. Translocation of bioactive peptides across cell membranes by carbon nanotubes. *Chem. Commun.* **2004**, *1*, 16–17.
64. Lu, Q.; Moore, J.M.; Huang, G.; Mount, A.S.; Rao, A.M.; Larcom, L.L.; Ke, P.C. RNA Polymer Translocation with Single-Walled Carbon Nanotubes. *Nano Lett.* **2004**, *4*, 2473–2477.
65. Kam, N.W.S.; Liu, Z.; Dai, H. Carbon Nanotubes as Intracellular Transporters for Proteins and DNA: An Investigation of the Uptake Mechanism and Pathway. *Angew. Chem. Int. Ed.* **2006**, *45*, 577–581.
66. Hong, G.; Wu, J.Z.; Robinson, J.T.; Wang, H.; Zhang, B.; Dai, H. Three-dimensional imaging of single nanotube molecule endocytosis on plasmonic substrates. *Nat. Commun.* **2012**, *3*, 700.
67. Li, H.J.; Du, J.Z.; Du, X.J.; Xu, C.F.; Sun, C.Y.; Wang, H.X.; Cao, Z.T.; Yang, X.Z.; Zhu, Y.H.; Nie, S.; et al. Stimuli-responsive clustered nanoparticles for improved tumor penetration and therapeutic efficacy. *Proc. Natl. Acad. Sci. USA* **2016**, *113*, 4164. [CrossRef] [PubMed]
68. van Vlerken, L.E.; Amiji, M.M. Multi-functional polymeric nanoparticles for tumour-targeted drug delivery. *Expert Opin. Drug Deliv.* **2006**, *3*, 205–216. [CrossRef] [PubMed]
69. Wang, A.Z.; Langer, R.; Farokhzad, O.C. Nanoparticle Delivery of Cancer Drugs. *Annu. Rev. Med.* **2012**, *63*, 185–198. [CrossRef] [PubMed]
70. Zhang, T.; Guo, C.J.; Li, Y.; Douglas, S.D.; Qi, X.X.; Song, L.; Ho, W.Z. Interleukin-1beta induces macrophage inflammatory protein-1beta expression in human hepatocytes. *Cell. Immunol.* **2003**, *226*, 45–53. [CrossRef] [PubMed]
71. Kam, N.W.S.; Liu, Z.; Dai, H. Functionalization of Carbon Nanotubes via Cleavable Disulfide Bonds for Efficient Intracellular Delivery of siRNA and Potent Gene Silencing. *J. Am. Chem. Soc.* **2005**, *127*, 12492–12493. [CrossRef] [PubMed]
72. Anderson, T.; Hu, R.; Yang, C.; Yoon, H.S.; Yong, K.T. Pancreatic cancer gene therapy using an siRNA-functionalized single walled carbon nanotubes (SWNTs) nanoplex. *Biomater. Sci.* **2014**, *2*, 1244–1253. [CrossRef]
73. Siu, K.S.; Zhang, Y.; Zheng, X.; Koropatnick, J.; Min, W.P. Non-Covalently Functionalized of Single-Walled Carbon Nanotubes by DSPE-PEG-PEI for SiRNA Delivery. In *SiRNA Delivery Methods: Methods and Protocols*; Shum, K., Rossi, J., Eds.; Springer New York: New York, NY, USA, 2016; pp. 151–163.
74. McNaughton, B.R.; Cronican, J.J.; Thompson, D.B.; Liu, D.R. Mammalian cell penetration, siRNA transfection, and DNA transfection by supercharged proteins. *Proc. Natl. Acad. Sci. USA* **2009**, *106*, 6111. [CrossRef] [PubMed]
75. Lu, J.J.; Langer, R.; Chen, J. A Novel Mechanism Is Involved in Cationic Lipid-Mediated Functional siRNA Delivery. *Mol. Pharm.* **2009**, *6*, 763–771. [CrossRef]
76. Wu, Y.; Phillips, J.A.; Liu, H.; Yang, R.; Tan, W. Carbon Nanotubes Protect DNA Strands during Cellular Delivery. *ACS Nano* **2008**, *2*, 2023–2028. [CrossRef]
77. Jeong, S.H.; Kim, K.K.; Jeong, S.J.; An, K.H.; Lee, S.H.; Lee, Y.H. Optical absorption spectroscopy for determining carbon nanotube concentration in solution. *Synth. Met.* **2007**, *157*, 570–574. [CrossRef]
78. Landi, B.J.; Ruf, H.J.; Evans, C.M.; Cress, C.D.; Raffaelle, R.P. Purity Assessment of Single-Wall Carbon Nanotubes, Using Optical Absorption Spectroscopy. *J. Phys. Chem. B* **2005**, *109*, 9952–9965. [CrossRef] [PubMed]

79. Roxbury, D.; Jena, P.V.; Williams, R.M.; Enyedi, B.; Niethammer, P.; Marcet, S.; Verhaegen, M.; Blais-Ouellette, S.; Heller, D.A. Hyperspectral Microscopy of Near-Infrared Fluorescence Enables 17-Chirality Carbon Nanotube Imaging. *Sci. Rep.* **2015**, *5*, 14167. [CrossRef] [PubMed]
80. Riss, T.L.; Moravec, R.A.; Niles, A.L.; Duellman, S.; Benink, H.A.; Worzella, T.J.; Minor, L. Cell Viability Assays. In *Assay Guidance Manual*; Eli Lilly & Company and the National Center for Advancing Translational Sciences, Bethesda: Rockville, MD, USA, 2013.

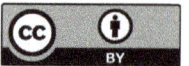

© 2019 by the authors. Licensee MDPI, Basel, Switzerland. This article is an open access article distributed under the terms and conditions of the Creative Commons Attribution (CC BY) license (http://creativecommons.org/licenses/by/4.0/).

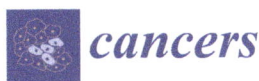

Article

Multifunctional Albumin-Stabilized Gold Nanoclusters for the Reduction of Cancer Stem Cells

Ana Latorre [1], Alfonso Latorre [1], Milagros Castellanos [1], Ciro Rodriguez Diaz [1], Ana Lazaro-Carrillo [2], Tania Aguado [3], Mercedes Lecea [1], Sonia Romero-Pérez [1], Macarena Calero [1,2], José María Sanchez-Puelles [3,*], Ángeles Villanueva [1,2,*] and Álvaro Somoza [1,*]

1. Instituto Madrileño de Estudios Avanzados en Nanociencia (IMDEA Nanociencia) & Nanobiotecnología (IMDEA-Nanociencia), Unidad Asociada al Centro Nacional de Biotecnología (CSIC), 28049 Madrid, Spain
2. Departamento de Biología, Facultad de Ciencias, Universidad Autónoma de Madrid, 28049 Madrid, Spain
3. Centro de Investigaciones Biológicas, Consejo Superior de Investigaciones Científicas, 28040 Madrid, Spain
* Correspondence: jmspuelles@cib.csic.es (J.M.S.-P.); angeles.villanueva@uam.es (Á.V.); alvaro.somoza@imdea.org (Á.S.); Tel.: +34-91299-8856 (Á.S.)

Received: 24 June 2019; Accepted: 9 July 2019; Published: 10 July 2019

Abstract: Controlled delivery of multiple chemotherapeutics can improve the effectiveness of treatments and reduce side effects and relapses. Here in, we used albumin-stabilized gold nanoclusters modified with doxorubicin and SN38 (AuNCs-DS) as combined therapy for cancer. The chemotherapeutics are conjugated to the nanostructures using linkers that release them when exposed to different internal stimuli (Glutathione and pH). This system has shown potent antitumor activity against breast and pancreatic cancer cells. Our studies indicate that the antineoplastic activity observed may be related to the reinforced DNA damage generated by the combination of the drugs. Moreover, this system presented antineoplastic activity against mammospheres, a culturing model for cancer stem cells, leading to an efficient reduction of the number of oncospheres and their size. In summary, the nanostructures reported here are promising carriers for combination therapy against cancer and particularly to cancer stem cells.

Keywords: nanomedicine; drug delivery; stimuli-responsive; DOX; SN38; CSCs

1. Introduction

Besides surgery, chemotherapy is the most common approach to treat cancer. However, this strategy is far from ideal due to the side effects caused by the toxicity of the chemotherapeutics employed. Moreover, multidrug resistance (MDR) [1] is developed when a single drug is administered multiple times, reducing the efficiency of the treatments. To overcome these limitations, chemotherapy is administered as a combination of two or more drugs, which synergistic effect [2] reduces the development of MDR. Furthermore, drug-related toxicity can be reduced due to the lower doses of the individual chemotherapeutic drugs employed in this approach [3]. However, the different solubility, pharmacokinetics, and biodistribution of the therapeutic agents may prevent their accumulation in the required concentrations at the tumor site, reducing their efficacy against the disease [4].

On the other hand, using carriers to deliver drugs has been shown to improve their efficiency and reduce their side effects [5]. This is mainly achieved by evading the reticuloendothelial system, which improves the pharmacokinetic properties of the drugs. In addition, those carriers with a nanometer size larger than 10 nm present an additional advantage due to the enhanced permeability and retention effect (EPR) [6], which leads to preferential accumulation of the delivered drug at the tumor area. Below that size, nanoparticles are quickly eliminated by the kidneys, reducing their interaction with the tumoral area [7]. As a consequence, the efficiency of the treatment may be increased, and the side effects reduced. In this regard, gold nanoclusters stabilized with bovine serum albumin have shown remarkable results in cell culture [8] and animal models [9,10]. This material accumulates efficiently in the tumor area, and therefore it has been used successfully in drug delivery [11,12]. In addition, gold nanoclusters present excellent fluorescent properties, and many reports are focused on exploiting that for imaging purposes [13,14]. The use of serum albumin as a coating for nanostructures provides excellent biochemical and biophysical properties in the in vivo experiments [15]. Furthermore, this coating contains amino and carboxy groups that facilitate the conjugation of different active molecules, such as, small molecule ligands [16], antibodies [17], or drugs [11,12], providing a convenient platform for preparing tailored nanostructures for efficient therapy.

Despite the excellent properties of albumin-stabilized gold nanoclusters, the use of this nanomaterial to deliver more than one drug has not been explored. Even reports on albumin conjugates containing more than one drug are scarce [18]. For these reasons, we decided to prepare a conjugate of albumin-stabilized gold nanoclusters containing two chemotherapeutic drugs for combined therapy.

Particularly, for the functionalization of the albumin-stabilized gold nanoclusters, we selected Doxorubicin (DOX) and SN38. DOX is a first line chemotherapeutic agent widely used in different kind of cancers. It is a hydrophilic molecule that binds topoisomerase II or intercalates in the DNA causing apoptosis [19] or other cell death mechanism depending on DOX concentration [20]. On the other hand, the camptothecin (CPT) analog SN38, is a potent topoisomerase I inhibitor [21], whose use in chemotherapy is limited because of its poor pharmacokinetic and high hydrophobicity [22]. Although the combination of DOX and camptothecins (CPTs) analogs have shown poor results in clinical trials, the pair DOX-CPT has been recently reported as one of the most synergistic combinations when co-delivered as a polymer-drug conjugate [23]. In addition, we envisioned that this combination might also be effective against the tumor-initiating cells, also known as Cancer Stem Cells (CSCs). These cells are a promising target in modern drug discovery programmes [24], since this subpopulation of malignant cells has an optimized DNA repair system, which is responsible for its resistance to therapy. Indeed, the combination of chemotherapeutics has been shown to reduce the population of CSCs [25,26], but this combination of drugs or this nanomaterial [27] has not been reported.

Our results show that the system combining both drugs presents excellent antitumor activity in different cancer cell models, including mammospheres, confirming the promising potential of this nanotherapeutic.

2. Results

2.1. Characterization of Functionalized AuNCs

The albumin-based nanoparticles were prepared by the incubation of BSA with a gold salt and NaOH. This process leads to the formation of the corresponding AuNCs stabilized by BSA. The functionalization of the structure with the drugs requires the introduction of thiols in the structure using iminothiolane. Then, the drugs modified with linkers were added to the nanostructures (Figure 1). In the case of SN38, a linker sensitive to the reductive environment (e.g., GSH) was used. On the other hand, DOX was modified with a different linker sensitive to acidic pHs. Both systems contain a moiety that eases the conjugation with the thiol groups, a disulfide and a maleimide, respectively. Using these derivatives, the AuNCs stabilized by BSA were modified with DOX (AuNCs-D), SN38 (AuNCs-S), or both (AuNCs-DS).

The incorporation of DOX and SN38 on the AuNCs was studied by UV-VIS (Figure S1) after the removal of unbound material. The UV-Vis spectra of AuNCs-D revealed the standard absorption profile of AuNCs and the characteristic band of DOX centered at 495 nm. With AuNCs-S, a band centered at 380 nm corresponding to the absorption of SN38 could be identified. Finally, UV-VIS spectra of AuNCs-DS evidenced the bands corresponding to the three components, indicating that both drugs, DOX and SN38, were efficiently attached to AuNCs. The concentration of the drugs was obtained by interpolating the absorbance measured at 495 nm for DOX and 380 nm for SN38 in the corresponding calibration curve, obtaining 37 µM and 80 µM, respectively. In the case of bi-functionalized nanoclusters AuNCs-DS, the concentrations of DOX and SN38 were 37 µM and 70 µM, respectively.

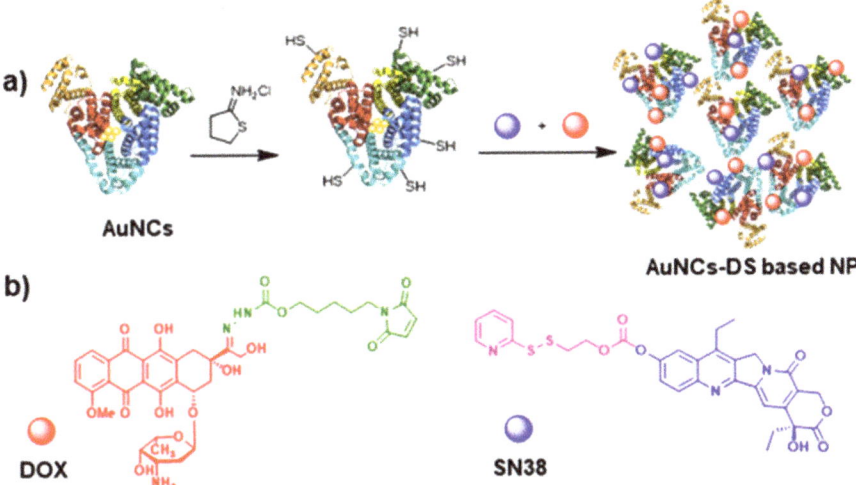

Figure 1. Synthesis of nanoparticles based on AuNCs modified with Doxorubicin (DOX) and SN38. (**a**) Schematic representation of the synthesis of DOX/SN38-AuNCs-based nanoparticles for combined chemotherapy; (**b**) Representation of DOX (red) modified with a pH-sensitive linker (green) and SN38 (blue) modified with a redox-sensitive linker (pink).

The sizes of the structures obtained were studied by dynamic light scattering (DLS) and SEM. DLS measurements of the AuNCs-D revealed the formation of a non-homogeneous material with two nanoparticle size distributions (Figure 2). However, when the hydrophobic SN38 was employed, monodispersed nanoparticles were obtained with an average size of 117.5 nm and a polydispersity index of 0.277. The combined use of DOX and SN38 does not disrupt the formation of monodispersed nanoparticles with an average size of 190.8 nm and a PDI of 0.263. In all cases, the structures obtained presented a globular shape when analyzed by SEM (Figure S2).

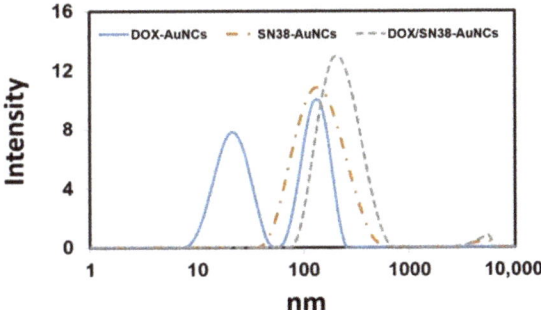

Figure 2. Size of Doxorubicin (DOX)-AuNCs, SN38-AuNCs and DOX/SN38-AuNCs measured by dynamic light scattering (DLS).

Interestingly, the nanoparticles bearing both drugs retained their colloidal stability and size in PBS at least over 15 days (Figure S3). Through this period, DOX remains essentially fully linked to the system, while SN38 is less stable and 62% of the drug is released.

Then, the release of the chemotherapeutics in AuNCs-DS was studied in vitro under the selected triggering conditions. First, DOX release was studied by re-dissolving the nanoparticles in phosphate–citrate buffer at pH = 5. Under these acidic conditions, we observed that the ca. 85% of the total DOX conjugated was released within the first 5 h. Conversely, when the nanoparticles are maintained at pH = 7 the DOX release was not superior to 20%. SN38 release was studied in PBS containing DTT at a concentration of 1 mM, where 80% was released after 48 h. However, when micromolar concentration of DTT was employed, less than 30% was released at the same time (Figure 3a,b, respectively).

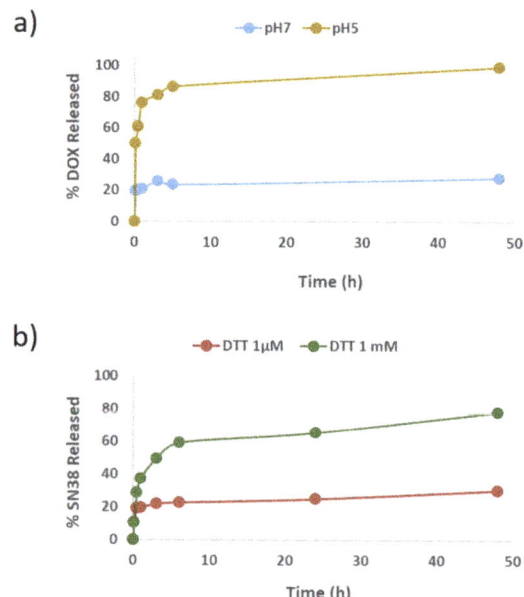

Figure 3. Release profile of Doxorubicin (DOX) and SN38 from AuNCs. (**a**) DOX release profile from AuNCs based nanoparticles in phosphate-citrate buffer (pH = 5 or 7), (**b**) SN38 release profile from AuNCs based nanoparticles in PBS containing 1 mM or 1 µM of DTT.

2.2. Chemotherapeutic Activity of Functionalized AuNCs in MCF7 Cells

In vitro toxicity studies of mono- and bi-functionalized AuNCs were performed in MCF-7 using a constant concentration of AuNCs of 2.6 µM. Cells were exposed to the nanostructures for 24 h, and the cell viability was determined after 48 h. As shown in Figure 4, no significant differences in cell viability were detected in samples exposed to non-functionalized AuNCs compared to untreated samples. This result highlights the excellent biocompatibility of this material. In contrast, mono-functionalized nanoparticles induced a significant reduction in cell survival, being AuNCs-D (70% cell death) more cytotoxic than AuNCs-S (42% cell death). Interestingly, AuNCs functionalized with both chemotherapeutic drugs (AuNCs-DS) exhibited enhanced cytotoxicity. Furthermore, the most active nanostructure (AuNCs-DS) was further assessed at three different times (24 h, 48 h, and 72 h) in three cell lines (MCF7, MDA-MB-231, and Panc-1), revealing similar results (Figure S4).

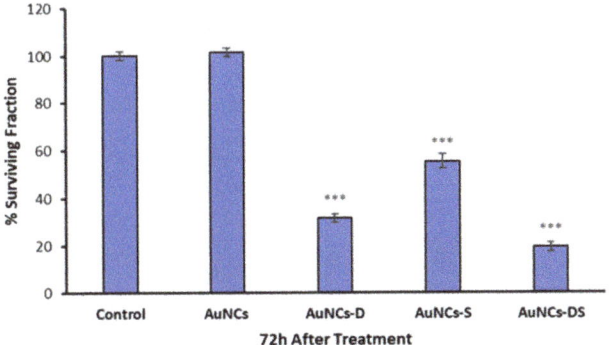

Figure 4. Surviving fraction of MCF-7 cells incubated 24 h with the different AuNCs formulations and evaluated 48 h after by MTT viability assay. Data correspond to mean ± S.D. values from at least six experiments. Statistical analysis was performed using one-way ANOVA Tukey's test (each group vs. Control). *** $p < 0.001$.

The antitumoral activity of the nanostructures in MCF7 was confirmed in the morphological changes produced by the functionalized nanostructures during a neutral red staining assay. Particularly, cells incubated with AuNCs (Figure 5b) showed similar morphology to control cells (Figure 5a). On the contrary, samples incubated with AuNCs-D, or AuNCs-S and AuNCs-DS, showed shrunken cells with condensed or fragmented apoptotic nuclei (Figure 5c–e, respectively).

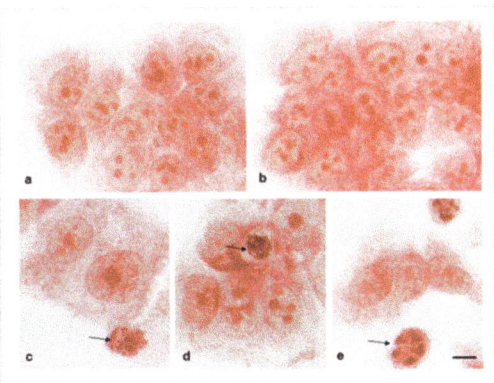

Figure 5. Morphology of MCF-7 cells stained with Neutral Red 48 h after treatment. (**a**) Control cells; (**b–e**) Cells incubated with AuNCs, AuNCs-D, AuNCs-S, and AuNCs-DS, respectively. Arrows indicate nuclei with apoptotic nuclear morphology (chromatin condensation and fragmentation). Scale bar: 10 μm.

The advantage of the bifunctional nanostructure was confirmed by studying cell damage using an inverted microscope. Particularly, the cell density observed when AuNCs-DS was employed (Figure S5d) was lower compared to the other two formulations (Figure S5b,c) and the control (Figure S5a). However, the most prominent change was observed after 9 days, when cells pre-treated with AuNCs-DS did not regrow, and the characteristic microcolonies of MCF-7 cells were no detectable (Figure S5g). On the other hand, when the cells were pre-incubated with AuNCs-D (Figure S5e) or AuNCs-S (Figure S5f), small microcolonies could be visualized, evidencing the superior activity of the bi-functionalized AuNCs. Then, we confirmed that AuNCs were internalized into MCF-7 cells by ICP-MS and confocal microscopy. Particularly, at short times (3–4 h after treatment), AuNCs are clearly detected through its intrinsic fluorescence inside the cells (Figure 6a) and outside the cell membrane (Figure 6b). At longer times (24 h post-treatment), AuNCs fluorescence is sparse, probably due to the expected degradation of the nanoparticle inside the cell, although the presence of Au could be detected by ICP-MS (13 pg/cell). In this period, a substantial fraction of the red fluorescence from DOX co-localizes with blue SN-38 (Figure S6). These results showed that SN38 and DOX can reach the cell nucleus after their release from the nanoparticle, leading to the corresponding cytotoxic effect on the cells.

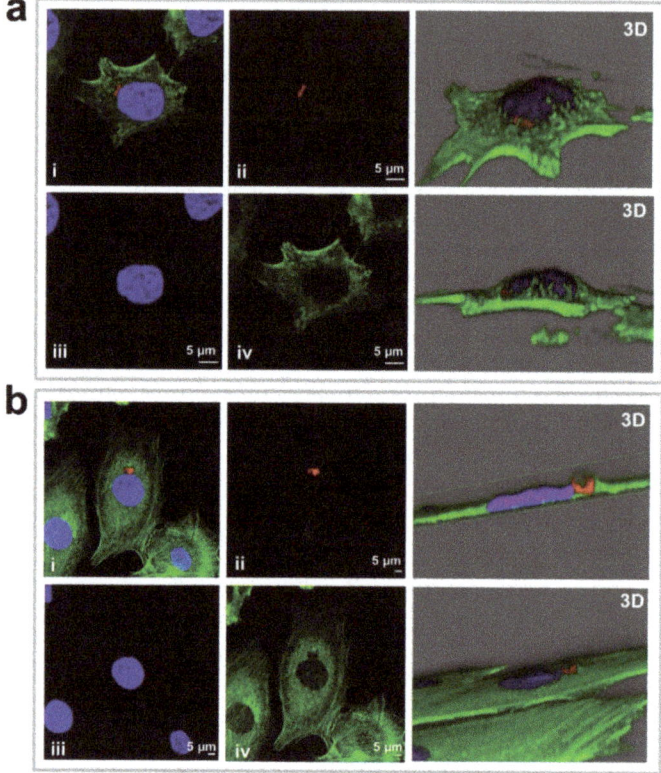

Figure 6. Confocal laser scanning microscope images of AuNCs localization in MCF7 cells after 3–4 h of incubation. Panel **a** shows an example of AuNCs cellular internalization while panel **b** shows AuNCs layered outside, on top of the cells. The left side of the panel corresponds to 2D images (one section or focal plane) for the merge (i), AuNCs in red (ii, Ex.405/Em.680 nm), nucleus with DAPI in blue (iii, Ex.358/Em.461) and actin filaments labeled with Phalloidin in green (iv, Ex.495/Em.519 nm) while the right side shows the 3D reconstructions of those cells.

We further studied the effect of the conjugates through immunofluorescence. Particularly, we assessed their effect on the generation of DNA breaks using antibodies against histone H2AX at serine 139 (γ-H2AX). The fluorescent intensity was higher when the two chemotherapeutics were combined (Figures 7 and S7).

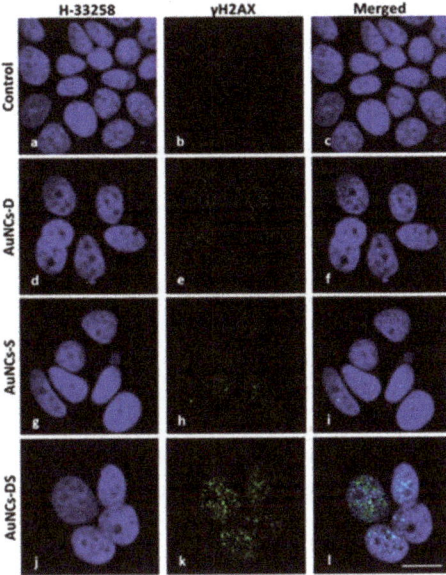

Figure 7. DNA damage study against histone γH2AX. γH2AX fluorescence pattern (green) was observed at the confocal microscope at 48 h after incubation with different AuNCs. MCF-7 cells were fixed and processed for γH2AX immunofluorescence, DNA was counterstained with Hoechst-33258 (blue) and both images were overlapped. (**a**–**c**) Control cells. (**d**–**f**) Cells pre-incubated with AuNCs-D. (**g**–**i**) Cells pre-incubated with AuNCs-S. (**j**–**l**) Cells pre-incubated with AuNCs-DS. Scale bar: 7.5 µm.

2.3. Chemotherapeutic Activity of Functionalized AuNCs in MCF7 Mammospheres

Finally, we evaluated the activity of the bifunctional complex in mammospheres using two concentrations, 0.08 µM (1) and 0.6 µM (2) based on preliminary optimization experiments done with mammospheres. The nanostructure was able to reduce the size of the mammospheres, from 465 µm (control) to 176 and 167 µm (Figure 8 and Figure S8).

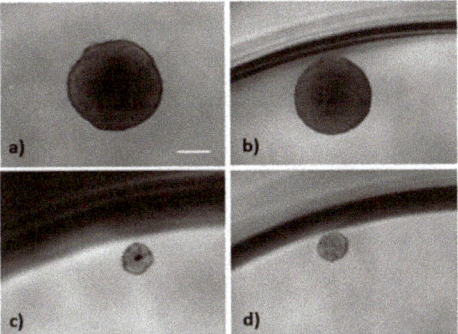

Figure 8. Activity of AuNCs in MCF7 mammospheres. (**a**) Control; (**b**) treated with AuNCs, (**c**) AuNCs-DS-(1), and (**d**) AuNCs-DS-(2), respectively. (1) means 0.08 µM concentration of the bifunctional complex, whereas (2) reflects treatments with the nanoconjugate at 0.6 µM. Scale bar 200 µm.

The surviving fraction of mammospheres was also analyzed by counting the spheres before and after the treatment, and the results show a 24% and 81% reduction when treated at 0.08 µM and 0.6 µM, respectively (Figure 9).

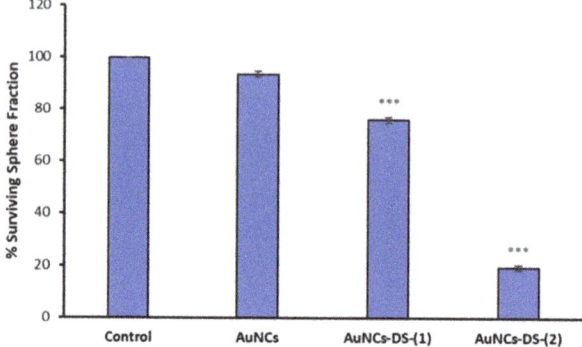

Figure 9. Surviving fraction of mammospheres treated with AuNCs for 7 days. Data correspond to mean ± S.D. values from three experiments. Statistical analysis was performed using one-way ANOVA Tukey's test (each group vs Control). *** $p < 0.0001$.

3. Discussion

Breast cancer is the most frequent malignant tumor among women all over the world, except for non-melanoma skin cancer tumors. They are categorized according to different markers such as histopathology, tumor stage, grade, and receptor/gene expression [28–32]. To assess the potential of our approach to treat this disease, we have focused on two different breast cancer cells: MDA-MB-231 and MCF7. Even though both lines lead to the same kind of tumor, MDA-MB-231 is the "basal" type and triple negative (estrogen receptor (ER), progesterone receptor (PR), and human epidermal receptor 2 (HER2) negative) while MCF7 is "luminal" type and ER and PR positive. Such differences have an effect on their drug sensitivity. For instance, MCF7 presents a higher sensitivity to SN38 and Doxorubicin (DOX) (IC50 0.00790 µM and 0.00984 µM, respectively) compared to MDA-MB-231 (IC50 0.00978 µM and 1.24 µM, respectively) [33]. Those substantial sensitivity differences, along with the distinct clinical prognosis of both cell lines derived tumors, encourage us to choose them as good candidates for testing our therapeutic system. Moreover, in the case of MCF7, we were able to compare the standard 2D-adherent cell cultures to their corresponding mammospheres, which are 3D discrete spherical-shape clusters of cells enriched in CSCs [34].

Furthermore, we tested our system in PANC-1 cell line, which is a well-established model for Pancreatic Ductal Adenocarcinoma (PDAC). PDAC is an orphan disease with a bad prognosis, even when diagnosed early, and its survival rate after 5 years (<5%) has not changed over the last 30 years. In this work, we tested for the first time, to our knowledge, the combination of SN38 and DOX conjugated to AuNCs as a potential therapy against Pancreatic cancer.

The required multifunctional nanostructure was obtained using tailor-made linkers that facilitate the conjugation of the drugs and control their release. Due to the differences in hydrophilicity between SN38 (hydrophobic) and DOX (hydrophilic), their co-delivery using one vehicle is not straightforward [35,36]. In our case, we managed to conjugate DOX and SN38 onto the surface of AuNCs using tailored linkers, which can release the drugs upon specific cell internal stimuli (Figure 1) [37,38]. Particularly, we have exploited the low pH present in the endosomes (pH 5–6) or lysosomes (pH 4–5) [39,40] to trigger the release of DOX. The designed linker [41] contains a pH sensitive imine moiety to control the release of DOX, and a maleimide group to ease its conjugation with the previously sulfhydryl-activated AuNCs. The introduction of thiol moieties on the surface of AuNCs is easily carried out in one step and provides a convenient way to modify the structure with the drugs further. On the other hand, the high concentration of glutathione (1–10 mM) in the cytoplasm provides the required reducing environment to trigger the release SN38 [42,43]. Here, the linker employed contains a disulfide-based self-immolative moiety and a 2-mercaptopyridyl leaving group to ease the conjugation with the sulfhydryl-activated AuNCs [44]. The conjugation of one drug (AuNCs-D and AuNCs-S) or two (AuNCs-DS) onto AuNCs using these linkers was achieved just by mixing the components in a single step. Hence, this methodology provides an easy and efficient way of preparing multidrug delivery systems. Since the chemical transformations employed in developing this system are robust and widely used, integrating other drugs should be possible, enabling the exploration of other chemotherapeutic combinations. Also, the linkers employed allow the release of the drugs with no modification, ensuring that they reach their corresponding targets in their most active form. Using different linkers on the same nanostructure for the controlled release of therapeutic agents is scarce and to the best of our knowledge has not been employed to prepare BSA-stabilized AuNCs.

Interestingly, the conjugation of the drugs onto AuNCs induced a rapid formation of nanoparticles due to the self-assembly of drug loaded AuNCs [45]. This rearrangement is driven by the interactions between hydrophobic BSA domains, and the SN38 [46]. Dynamic light scattering measurements of the AuNCs-D revealed the formation of a non-homogeneous material with two nanoparticle size distributions (Figure 2), while the use of the hydrophobic SN38 monodispersed nanoparticles were obtained. The combined use of DOX and SN38 does not disrupt the formation of monodispersed nanoparticles, which were surprisingly stable in PBS for at least 15 days. SEM micrographs showed globular structures as found in other albumin-based nanoparticles (Figure S2) [47]. It is noteworthy that albumin-stabilized AuNCs based nanoparticles could accumulate better in tumor tissues due to their higher size compared with AuNCs ($\leq$10 nm), since blood vessels of tumor tissues are larger than 10 nm [48].

Since DOX and SN38 were conjugated using respective sensitive linkers to pH and reductive environment, the drug release was investigated using different conditions (Figure 3). The DOX was efficiently released when the pH was reduced to 5 using a citrate-based buffer and SN38 when exposed at 1 mM of dithiothreitol (DTT).

The antitumoral effect of the nanostructures was assessed in MCF7 cells, where the three systems showed antitumoral activity. The best inhibition was obtained with the construction that carries the two chemotherapeutics (AuNCs-DS) (Figure 4). This combined system was also tested in additional breast cancer (MDA-MB-231) and pancreatic cancer (Panc-1) cell lines at different times after treatment (24 h, 48 h, and 72 h), showing similar results and highlighting the potential of the approach and its efficacy compared with the results obtained with the free drugs (Figure S4).

These results are in agreement with previous studies, where DOX and SN38 induced senescence, mitotic catastrophe, apoptosis, or necrosis, depending on the dose of the drugs [20,49]. In our case, MCF-7 cells undergoing apoptosis after treatment with mono- and bi-functional AuNCs.

It is known that DOX and SN38 are inducers of DNA damage and activate the DNA damage response (DDR) [50]. For this reason, we wonder if the superior activity of AuCNs-DS was related to the DNA damage generated by the structures. In this regard, it is well known that the phosphorylation of histone H2AX at serine 139 (γ-H2AX) is the most sensitive marker to examine DNA damage (double-stranded breaks, DSBs) in cells exposed to ionizing radiation or DNA-damaging chemotherapeutic agents. These phosphorylation events are easily detected as nuclear foci by specific antibodies to the phosphorylated form of H2AX (γ-H2AX), and the foci formation has been extensively used as a marker of DSB formation [51].

Since mono- or bi-functionalized gold nanoclusters need to be internalized by cells and, subsequently, chemotherapeutic drugs must enter to cell nuclei to induce cell damage, we performed an analysis of DNA double-strand breaks in MCF-7 cells to detect phosphorylation of H2AX by immunofluorescence techniques following the treatment with different loaded AuNCs. As seen in Figure 7, γ-H2AX fluorescence signals were detected in both, AuNCs-D and AuNCs-S, although the fluorescent intensity in cells treated with bi-functionalized AuNCs was significantly higher. This result suggests that the enhanced activity observed in the bifunctional nanostructures might be due to increased DNA damage generated by the combination of the two drugs at the nuclei. In addition, optical microscopy studies revealed that the AuNCs-DS induces higher morphological damage after 48 h and prevents the generation of colonies after 9 days, compared to the other formulations (Figures S7 and S8).

To further assess the therapeutic potential of this nanostructure, we decided to test it against mammospheres. These spherical structures resemble better the tumor environment, compared with standard 2D cell culture [52], and what is more, is an excellent model to test therapeutics against cancer stem cells (CSCs). CSCs are small cell populations with self-renewing and high tumorigenic capabilities, which is responsible for drug resistance and relapses [53,54]. This kind of cell is present in a vast variety of tumors [55,56] such as glioblastomas [57] or breast cancer [58].

Standard chemotherapeutics do not remove this subpopulation of a tumor, due to their inherent drug resistance and its efficient DNA repair system [59] For these reasons, we believe that our nanoconjugated system might be useful to control this CSCs population due to its inherent efficiency in the generation of DNA damage, as shown in Figure 7 and S7.

We assessed the activity of AuNCs-DS at different concentrations in MCF7 cells. We selected two concentrations 0.08 µM (1) and 0.6 µM (2) for the mammosphere experiments based on this data and preliminary experiments with mammospheres. The high potency of the conjugates obliged us to use these concentrations in the mammosphere assay model to prevent the complete elimination of the spheres after 7 days of treatment. At the selected concentrations, we observed a significant variation on the size of the mammospheres, which are reduced from an average diameter of 465 µm (control) to 176 and 167 µm (Figure 8 and S8).

We also analysed the surviving fraction of mammospheres by counting the spheres before and after the treatment, and the results show a 24% and 81% reduction when treated at 0.08 µM and 0.6 µM, respectively (Figure 8).

4. Materials and Methods

4.1. Synthesis of AuNCs

To a solution of BSA (1 mL, 50 mg/mL) at 37 °C, hydrogen tetrachloroaurate (III) hydrate (HAuCl$_4$) (1 mL, 10 mM) was added at 37 °C and stirred for 2 min. Then, 100 µL of NaOH 1M was added, and the mixture was stirred for 24 h. AuNCs were purified using an exclusion column NAP-10 of Sephadex-G25 according to the specifications of the distributor.

4.2. Sulfhydryl Activation of AuNCs

To a solution of AuNCs (1 mL, 20 µM) in PBS (pH = 7.8), a solution 6.5 mM of 2-iminothiolane hydrochloride (77 µL) was added and incubated at room temperature for 16 h. The product was purified using an exclusion column NAP-10 of Sephadex-G25 according to the specifications of the distributor.

4.3. Functionalization of AuNCs

To synthesize AuNCs-D, 100 µL of a solution of modified DOX (3) (1 mM) in DMF was added to 1 mL of a solution of sulfhydryl-activated AuNCs (20 µM) in PBS (pH = 7.8) and stirred at room temperature for 16 h. Then, AuNCs-D were purified using a NAP-10 column. AuNCs-S were prepared as above by using 150 µL of a solution of modified SN38 (6) (1 mM) in DMF. The synthesis of AuNCs-DS was carried out using the same procedure by adding 100 µL of a solution of modified DOX (3) (1 mM) in DMF, immediately followed by the addition of 100 µL of a solution of modified SN38 (6) (1 mM) in DMF.

4.4. Quantification of Drug Functionalization

The drug functionalization was determined using UV-Vis spectroscopy. In brief, the absorption of DOX (490 nm) and SN38 (380 nm) of the corresponding formulations were measured, and the concentration quantified by interpolation from a calibration curve.

Drug loading was calculated by following the formula:

$$\text{Drug Loading(weight \%)} = \frac{\text{weight of drug in nanoparticles}}{\text{total weight of nanoparticles}} \times 100$$

4.5. Dynamic Light Scattering Measurements

Dynamic light scattering (DLS) measurements were performed at 25 °C at a 173° scattering angle using disposable microcuvettes. The Z-Average hydrodynamic diameter and polydispersity index (PDI) were obtained by three cumulative analyses of 100 µL of the corresponding formulation of AuNCs (20 µM).

4.6. Scanning Electron Microscopy

One drop of a solution of corresponding functionalize AuNCs was deposited over a silica wafer and air-dried during 16 h. Then, the samples were observed using a Carl Zeiss AURIGA scanning electron microscope (Zeiss, Jana, Germany).

4.7. In Vitro Doxorubicin (DOX)/SN38 Release

DOX release profile was evaluated using fluorescence spectrophotometry. 1 mL of a solution of DOX-AuNCs in saline citrate buffer at pH = 7 or 5 were incubated at 37 °C. At different time intervals, 100 µL of this solution were withdrawn and treated with 100 µL of a 2% ZnSO4 solution in H20/MeOH (1:1). After vigorous stirring, this mixture was centrifuged at 13200 rpm for 10 min, and the fluorescence of the DOX released analyzed by fluorescence from the supernatant (λ_{exc} = 495 nm, λ_{em} = 590 nm). SN38 release profile was evaluated using a similar protocol. In this case, 1 mL of a solution of SN38-AuNCs in PBS at pH = 7.4 containing dithiothreitol at 1 µM or 1 mM of concentration was incubated, and the SN38 released analyzed by fluorescence from the supernatant (λ_{exc} = 370 nm, λ_{em} = 550 nm).

4.8. Cell Culture

Human breast adenocarcinoma (MCF-7 and MDA-MB-231) and human pancreatic adenocarcinoma (Panc-1) cells were obtained from American Type Culture Collection (ATCC)®. Both cell lines were grown as monolayer cultures in Dulbecco's modified Eagle's medium (DMEM) supplemented with 10% (v/v) fetal bovine serum (FBS), 1% L-Glutamine, 50 U/mL penicillin, and 50 µg/mL streptomycin and incubated at standard conditions (37 °C, 5% CO_2).

4.9. Neutral Red Staining

MCF-7 cells grown on coverslips in 24-well plates and incubated for 24 h with the nanostructures were fixed in cold methanol for 5 min and then stained with 0.5% neutral red for 2 min. Coverslips were washed with distilled water, air-dried, mounted in DePeX and examined by light microscopy.

4.10. Cytotoxicity Assays

4.10.1. MTT Tetrazolium Reduction Assay

Cells were incubated with the nanostructures (AuNCs concentration of 2.6 µM) in complete cell culture media for 24 h. After incubation, the culture medium was removed, and samples were washed three times with phosphate-buffered saline (PBS, pH 7.4) and cells were incubated 48 h after treatment.

Then, toxicity was assessed by MTT (dimethylthiazolyl-diphenyl-tetrazolium bromide) colorimetric assay. Briefly, the culture medium was replaced with DMEM containing MTT (5 mg/mL). Five hundred microliters of this MTT solution (50 µg/mL MTT in culture medium) was added to each culture dish and cells were incubated for 4 h at 37 °C. Then, MTT was removed by aspiration and reduced formazan crystals were dissolved with 500 µL of dimethylsulfoxide and the absorbance measured at 540 nm using a microplate reader. Cell survival was expressed as the percentage of absorption of treated cells in comparison with control cells. Besides, experiments with AuNCs non-functionalized were also performed, to exclude a possible cytotoxic effect exercised by gold nanoclusters per se. Data corresponded to mean values ± standard deviation from at least five different experiments.

4.10.2. Resazurin Reduction Assay

Breast Cancer (MCF7 and MDA-MB-231) and pancreatic cancer (Panc-1) cell lines were seeded (40,000 cells/well, 24 h prior treatment) in 24 well plates and incubated in standard conditions. Then, the cells were incubated with the nanostructures using a constant concentration of AuNCs (2.6 µM) or the free drugs (1.1 µM DOX or 2.4 µM SN38) for 24 h. After incubation, the culture medium was removed, and cells were washed twice with PBS (pH = 7.4). Toxicity was measured 24, 48, and 72 h after treatment, using the resazurin assay following the manufacturer's protocol. Briefly, the cell culture medium was replaced with fresh culture medium containing 1% of resazurin solution (1 mg/mL in PBS), and cells were incubated for 3 h more at 37 °C, 5% CO_2. Fluorescence from 100 µL of the culture media was measured using a microplate reader ((λexc = 550 nm, λem = 590 nm). Cell viability was expressed as a percentage of fluorescence of treated cells and compared with the control. Data corresponded to mean values ± standard deviation from at least three different experiments

4.11. *Inductively Coupled Plasma Mass Spectrometry (ICP-MS)*

MCF7 cells treated with 2.3 µM AuNCs for 24 h were harvested and quantified, prior digestion O/N in aqua regia and subsequent dilution in pure water. After that, the quantity of Au^+ in the sample was determined by ICP-MS and relativized per cell unit.

4.12. *Live Cell Imaging*

Cells were incubated with the nanostructures for 48 h, washed three times with PBS, and maintained in culture medium for 9 days, and the culture medium was changed every 2–3 days. Untreated control, as well as cells incubated with AuNCs without a drug, were also visualized. Cells were imaged daily under a differential interference contrast (DIC) inverted microscope (Leica DMI 6000B) equipped with a Leica DFC420 C digital camera (Leica Microsystems, Heerbrugg, Switzerland).

4.13. *Subcellular Localization*

4.13.1. AuNCs at Short Times (3–4 h after Treatment)

MCF7 cells grown in 24 well plates with glass coverslips were treated with 50 µM AuNCs during 3–4 h and fixed afterward with 4% paraformaldehyde for 15 min/RT. Fixed cells were subsequently permeabilized and labeled for 20 minutes/RT in darkness with a mix containing Saponin 0.25% (Sigma, Saint Louis, MO, USA), DAPI (diluted 1:300 from a 1 mg/mL stock solution, Sigma), Phalloidin (diluted 1:250 from a 1 mg/mL stock solution, Sigma), and FBS 5% in PBS buffer. After washing 3 times with PBS, coverslips were mounted onto slides using Fluoroshield medium (Sigma) and visualized by confocal microscopy (Confocal multispectral Leica TCS SP8 system). Data acquisition was performed with Leica software LAS X and images were prepared with ImageJ (https://imagej.nih.gov/ij/). To avoid possible artifacts due to the crosstalk between the red and the blue channels, the blue signal was subtracted from the red 2D images using ImageJ processing.

4.13.2. AuNCs-DS at Long Times (24 h after Treatment)

Internalization of bifunctionalized AuNCs into MCF-7 cells were visualized by confocal microscopy. Cells grown on coverslips were incubated for 24 h with AuNCs-DS, washed three times with culture medium without FBS, and visualized under differential interference contrast (DIC) microscopy and confocal fluorescence microscopy using a multispectral Leica TCS SP5 confocal microscope, operating with 405 Diode (UV) and DPSS (561, visible) laser lines.

4.14. Microscopic Detection of DNA Damage

MCF-7 cells grown on glass coverslips and incubated with the different AuNCs for 24 h were immunostained for histone phosphorylated H2AX (γ-H2AX) at 48 h after treatments. Cells were fixed with formaldehyde in PBS (1:10 v/v) for 20 min, washed three times for 5 min with PBS, and then permeabilized with 0.5% Triton X-100 in PBS for 5 min. After incubation with a blocking solution (5% bovine serum albumin, 5% FBS, 0.02% Triton X-100 in PBS) at room temperature for 30 min, cells were washed three times with PBS. Then, cells were incubated with primary monoclonal mouse anti-γ-H2AX antibody (Merck Millipore, Darmstadt, Germany) diluted 1:100 at 37 °C in a wet chamber for 1 h. After three washes with PBS, incubation with secondary antibody (Alexa Fluor® 488 goat anti-mouse, Life Technologies (Waltham, MA, USA) was identical to that of the first one and so were final washings. Finally, DNA was counterstained by addition of Hoechst-33258 (0.05 mg/mL in distilled water) for 5 min, and the sample was mounted with ProLong Gold antifade reagent. Immunofluorescence images were captured using a laser scanning confocal microscope using a multispectral Leica TCS SP5 confocal microscope (Leica, Wetzlar, Germany), operating with 405 nm (argon–UV) and 488 nm (argon) laser lines. All images were taken with a photomultiplier value (PTM) of 1029.

4.15. Mammosphere Culture

Single-cell suspensions of MCF-7 cell line were plated in P96 well plates at 10 cells per well in DMEM/F-12 medium supplemented with GlutaMAX, B27 (Gibco: Thermo Fisher, Waltham, MA, USA), 10 ng/mL epidermal growth factor (EGF: Invitrogen) and 10 ng/mL basic fibroblast growth factor (bFGF: Millipore, Burlington, MA, USA) and they were maintained at 37 °C in 5% CO_2. At day 10, the number of wells with mammospheres were counted and then nanostructures were added. The final proportion of living spheres were quantified at day 17.

4.16. Statistical Analysis

For statistical calculations, one-way ANOVA Tukey's test and the R (R Foundation for Statistical Computing, Vienna, Austria) were used. p values < 0.05 (*), <0.01 (**), and < 0.001 (***) were considered as statistically significant.

5. Conclusions

Toxicity and side effects are serious drawbacks that hinder the use of the chemotherapeutics to treat tumors. Furthermore, the development of drug resistance contributes to a great extent to the failure of current treatments. In this regard, the combination of two or more agents allows a reduction in the number of individual components, decreasing their toxicity and preventing the development of resistance by tumor cells. However, the rapid clearance and the low accumulation of the drugs in the tumor are drawbacks that must be solved. In this sense, nanomedicine tries to tackle these problems using nanostructures capable of delivering drugs more efficiently and safely.

In this work, we have demonstrated that bovine serum stabilized AuNCs can be used as safety carriers of two chemotherapeutics such as DOX and SN38. We have used tailored linkers to functionalize the AuNCs with the drugs, which render in the spontaneous formation of nanoparticles with a diameter below 200 nm. It is worth mentioning that the chemistry employed is robust and the system could be adapted to other drug combinations. Two internal cell stimulus controls the release of the drugs.

In particular, DOX is released at low pHs, such as that found in the endosomes and lysosomes. The release of SN38 takes place in a reducing environment equivalent to the one present in the cytoplasm. AuNCs have not shown toxicity in MCF-7 cells. However, AuNCs-D and AuNCs-S evidenced a reduction in cancer cell viability. Remarkably, this activity was enhanced when we used bi-functional nanoparticles (AuNCs-DS). This particular cytotoxic activity might be of interest to reduce CSCs subpopulation, which is involved in metastasis and recurrences. The immunofluorescent studies carried out suggest that the superior activity of the bi-functional nanostructure might be due to the prominent DNA damage generated. Interestingly, our system is also active in the reduction of the size and number of mammospheres, a model of CSC.

Supplementary Materials: The following are available online at http://www.mdpi.com/2072-6694/11/7/969/s1, Supplementary Materials and Methods: Synthesis of Intermediates and Pro-Drugs, Figure S1: UV-Vis spectra of AuNCs, and AuNCs modified with DOX (AuNCs-D), SN38 (AuNCs-S) and both DOX and SN38 (AuNCs-DS), Figure S2: SEM pictures of modified AuNCs. (a) AuNCs-D, (b) AuNCs-S and (c) AuNCs-DS, Figure S3: Stability study in PBS of AuNCs-DS over time stored at room temperature. Mean ± SD, $n = 3$, Figure S4: Surviving fraction of breast cancer MCF-7, MDA-MB-231 and pancreatic cancer Panc-1 cells incubated 24 h with AuNCs and AuNCs-DS or the free unmodified drugs and evaluated at different times a) 24 h; b) 48 h; and c, d) 72 h after treatment by resazurin viability assay, Figure S5: MCF-7 cell density recorded under Differential Interference Contrast (DIC) microscopy 48 h after incubation in control (untreated) cells (a) or incubated with AuNCs-D (b), AuNCs-S (c) and AuNCs-DS (d), Cells 9 days after incubation with AuNCs-D (e), AuNCs-S (f) and AuNCs-DS (g), Figure S6: Confocal laser scanning microscope images of subcellular localization of AuNCs-DS after 24 h incubation, Figure S7: Foci detected by γH2AX immunofluorescence analysed with ImageJ software, Figure S8: Size of mammospheres treated with AuNCs-DS at 0.08 µM (1) and 0.6 µM (2) for 7 days.

Author Contributions: Á.S. and A.L. (Alfonso Latorre) designed the experiments; A.L. (Alfonso Latorre), A.L. (Ana Latorre), M.L., S.R.-P., C.R.D. and M.C. (Milagros Castellanos) performed the synthesis and characterization of nanostructures; A.L. (Ana Latorre), M.C. (Milagros Castellanos), A.L.-C., Á.V. and M.C. (Macarena Calero) performed the 2-D cell culture experiments; T.A. and J.M.S.-P. carry out the 3-D culture experiment; Á.S., A.L. (Alfonso Latorre) and A.L. (Ana Latorre) wrote the paper.

Funding: This research was funded by the Spanish Ministry of Economy and Competitiveness (CTQ2016-78454-C2-2-R, SAF2014-56763-R, and SAF2017-87305-R), Comunidad de Madrid (S2013/MIT-2850), Asociación Española Contra el Cáncer, and IMDEA Nanociencia IMDEA Nanociencia acknowledges support from the 'Severo Ochoa' Programme for Centres of Excellence in R&D (MINECO, Grant SEV-2016-0686).

Acknowledgments: The authors recognize the valuable contribution of Sylvia Gutiérrez (Confocal Microscopy, Centro Nacional de Biotecnología, CNB-CSIC, Madrid).

Conflicts of Interest: The authors declare no conflict of interest.

References

1. Persidis, A. Cancer multidrug resistance. *Nat. Biotechnol.* **1999**, *17*, 94–95. [CrossRef] [PubMed]
2. Greco, F.; Vicent, M.J. Combination therapy: Opportunities and challenges for polymer–drug conjugates as anticancer nanomedicines. *Adv. Drug Deliv. Rev.* **2009**, *61*, 1203–1213. [CrossRef] [PubMed]
3. Parhi, P.; Mohanty, C.; Sahoo, S.K. Nanotechnology-based combinational drug delivery: An emerging approach for cancer therapy. *Drug Discov. Today* **2012**, *17*, 1044–1052. [CrossRef] [PubMed]
4. Miao, L.; Guo, S.; Lin, C.M.; Liu, Q.; Huang, L. Nanoformulations for combination or cascade anticancer therapy. *Adv. Drug Deliv. Rev.* **2017**, *115*, 3–22. [CrossRef] [PubMed]
5. Fan, W.; Yung, B.; Huang, P.; Chen, X. Nanotechnology for Multimodal Synergistic Cancer Therapy. *Chem. Rev.* **2017**, *117*, 13566–13638. [CrossRef] [PubMed]
6. Stylianopoulos, T. EPR-effect: Utilizing size-dependent nanoparticle delivery to solid tumors. *Ther. Deliv.* **2013**, *4*, 421–423. [CrossRef] [PubMed]
7. Hoshyar, N.; Gray, S.; Han, H.; Bao, G. The effect of nanoparticle size on in vivo pharmacokinetics and cellular interaction. *Nanomedicine* **2016**, *11*, 673–692. [CrossRef] [PubMed]
8. Khandelia, R.; Bhandari, S.; Pan, U.N.; Ghosh, S.S.; Chattopadhyay, A. Gold Nanocluster Embedded Albumin Nanoparticles for Two-Photon Imaging of Cancer Cells Accompanying Drug Delivery. *Small* **2015**, *11*, 4075–4081. [CrossRef]

9. Chen, J.; Chen, Q.; Liang, C.; Yang, Z.; Zhang, L.; Yi, X.; Dong, Z.; Chao, Y.; Chen, Y.; Liu, Z. Albumin-templated biomineralizing growth of composite nanoparticles as smart nano-theranostics for enhanced radiotherapy of tumors. *Nanoscale* **2017**, *9*, 14826–14835. [CrossRef]
10. Ding, C.; Xu, Y.; Zhao, Y.; Zhong, H.; Luo, X. Fabrication of BSA@AuNC-Based Nanostructures for Cell Fluoresce Imaging and Target Drug Delivery. *ACS Appl. Mater. Interfaces* **2018**, *10*, 8947–8954. [CrossRef]
11. Chen, H.; Li, B.; Ren, X.; Li, S.; Ma, Y.; Cui, S.; Gu, Y. Multifunctional near-infrared-emitting nano-conjugates based on gold clusters for tumor imaging and therapy. *Biomaterials* **2012**, *33*, 8461–8476. [CrossRef] [PubMed]
12. Chen, T.; Xu, S.; Zhao, T.; Zhu, L.; Wei, D.; Li, Y.; Zhang, H.; Zhao, C. Gold Nanocluster-Conjugated Amphiphilic Block Copolymer for Tumor-Targeted Drug Delivery. *ACS Appl. Mater. Interfaces* **2012**, *4*, 5766–5774. [CrossRef] [PubMed]
13. Wu, X.; He, X.; Wang, K.; Xie, C.; Zhou, B.; Qing, Z. Ultrasmall near-infrared gold nanoclusters for tumor fluorescence imaging in vivo. *Nanoscale* **2010**, *2*, 2244–2249. [CrossRef] [PubMed]
14. Retnakumari, A.; Setua, S.; Menon, D.; Ravindran, P.; Muhammed, H.; Pradeep, T.; Nair, S.; Koyakutty, M. Molecular-receptor-specific, non-toxic, near-infrared-emitting Au cluster-protein nanoconjugates for targeted cancer imaging. *Nanotechnology* **2010**, *21*, 055103. [CrossRef] [PubMed]
15. Sleep, D. Albumin and its application in drug delivery. *Expert Opin. Drug Deliv.* **2015**, *12*, 793–812. [CrossRef] [PubMed]
16. Qiao, J.; Mu, X.; Qi, L.; Deng, J.; Mao, L. Folic acid-functionalized fluorescent gold nanoclusters with polymers as linkers for cancer cell imaging. *Chem. Commun.* **2013**, *49*, 8030–8032. [CrossRef] [PubMed]
17. Wang, Y.; Chen, J.; Irudayaraj, J. Nuclear targeting dynamics of gold nanoclusters for enhanced therapy of HER2 + breast cancer. *ACS Nano* **2011**, *5*, 9718–9725. [CrossRef]
18. Qi, J.; Zhang, Y.; Gou, Y.; Lee, P.; Wang, J.; Chen, S.; Zhou, Z.; Wu, X.; Yang, F.; Liang, H. Multidrug Delivery Systems Based on Human Serum Albumin for Combination Therapy with Three Anticancer Agents. *Mol. Pharm.* **2016**, *13*, 3098–3105. [CrossRef]
19. Tacar, O.; Sriamornsak, P.; Dass, C.R. Doxorubicin: An update on anticancer molecular action, toxicity and novel drug delivery systems. *J. Pharm. Pharmacol.* **2013**, *65*, 157–170. [CrossRef]
20. Eom, Y.-W.; Kim, M.A.; Park, S.S.; Goo, M.J.; Kwon, H.J.; Sohn, S.; Kim, W.-H.; Yoon, G.; Choi, K.S. Two distinct modes of cell death induced by doxorubicin: Apoptosis and cell death through mitotic catastrophe accompanied by senescence-like phenotype. *Oncogene* **2005**, *24*, 4765–4777. [CrossRef]
21. Al-kasspooles, M.F.; Williamson, S.K.; Henry, D.; Howell, J.; Niu, F.; Decedue, C.J.; Roby, K.F. Preclinical antitumor activity of a nanoparticulate SN38. *Investig. New Drugs* **2013**, *31*, 871–880. [CrossRef] [PubMed]
22. Bala, V.; Rao, S.; Boyd, B.J.; Prestidge, C.A. Prodrug and nanomedicine approaches for the delivery of the camptothecin analogue SN38. *J. Control. Release* **2013**, *172*, 48–61. [CrossRef] [PubMed]
23. Camacho, K.M.; Kumar, S.; Menegatti, S.; Vogus, D.R.; Anselmo, A.C.; Mitragotri, S. Synergistic antitumor activity of camptothecin–doxorubicin combinations and their conjugates with hyaluronic acid. *J. Control. Release* **2015**, *210*, 198–207. [CrossRef] [PubMed]
24. Pattabiraman, D.R.; Weinberg, R.A. Tackling the cancer stem cells—What challenges do they pose? *Nat. Rev. Drug Discov.* **2014**, *13*, 497–512. [CrossRef] [PubMed]
25. Yu, Z.; Zhao, G.; Li, P.; Li, Y.; Zhou, G.; Chen, Y.; Xie, G. Temozolomide in combination with metformin act synergistically to inhibit proliferation and expansion of glioma stem-like cells. *Oncol. Lett.* **2016**, *11*, 2792–2800. [CrossRef] [PubMed]
26. Kim, Y.J.; Siegler, E.L.; Siriwon, N.; Wang, P. Therapeutic strategies for targeting cancer stem cells. *J. Cancer Metastasis Treat.* **2016**, *2*, 233. [CrossRef]
27. Qin, W.; Huang, G.; Chen, Z.; Zhang, Y. Nanomaterials in targeting cancer stem cells for cancer therapy. *Front. Pharmacol.* **2017**, *8*, 1–15. [CrossRef]
28. Totsuka, K.; Makioka, Y.; Iizumi, K.; Takahashi, K.; Oshima, Y.; Kikuchi, H.; Kubohara, Y. Halogen-Substituted Derivatives of Dictyostelium Differentiation-Inducing Factor-1 Suppress Serum-Induced Cell Migration of Human Breast Cancer MDA-MB-231 Cells in Vitro. *Biomolecules* **2019**, *9*, 256. [CrossRef]
29. Hwang, S.-Y.; Park, S.; Kwon, Y. Recent therapeutic trends and promising targets in triple negative breast cancer. *Pharmacol. Ther.* **2019**, *199*, 30–57. [CrossRef]
30. Engebraaten, O.; Vollan, H.K.M.; Børresen-Dale, A.-L. Triple-Negative Breast Cancer and the Need for New Therapeutic Targets. *Am. J. Pathol.* **2013**, *183*, 1064–1074. [CrossRef]

31. Jiao, Q.; Wu, A.; Shao, G.; Peng, H.; Wang, M.; Ji, S.; Liu, P.; Zhang, J. The latest progress in research on triple negative breast cancer (TNBC): Risk factors, possible therapeutic targets and prognostic markers. *J. Thorac. Dis.* **2014**, *6*, 1329–1335. [PubMed]
32. Abubakar, M.; Sung, H.; Devi, B.C.R.; Guida, J.; Tang, T.S.; Pfeiffer, R.M.; Yang, X.R. Breast cancer risk factors, survival and recurrence, and tumor molecular subtype: Analysis of 3012 women from an indigenous Asian population. *Breast Cancer Res.* **2018**, *20*, 114. [CrossRef] [PubMed]
33. Yang, W.; Soares, J.; Greninger, P.; Edelman, E.J.; Lightfoot, H.; Forbes, S.; Bindal, N.; Beare, D.; Smith, J.A.; Thompson, I.R.; et al. Genomics of Drug Sensitivity in Cancer (GDSC): A resource for therapeutic biomarker discovery in cancer cells. *Nucleic Acids Res.* **2012**, *41*, D955–D961. [CrossRef] [PubMed]
34. Ponti, D.; Costa, A.; Zaffaroni, N.; Pratesi, G.; Petrangolini, G.; Coradini, D.; Pilotti, S.; Pierotti, M.A.; Daidone, M.G. Isolation and In vitro Propagation of Tumorigenic Breast Cancer Cells with Stem/Progenitor Cell Properties. *Cancer Res.* **2005**, *65*, 5506–5511. [CrossRef] [PubMed]
35. Wang, H.; Zhao, Y.; Wu, Y.; Hu, Y.; Nan, K.; Nie, G.; Chen, H. Enhanced anti-tumor efficacy by co-delivery of doxorubicin and paclitaxel with amphiphilic methoxy PEG-PLGA copolymer nanoparticles. *Biomaterials* **2011**, *32*, 8281–8290. [CrossRef] [PubMed]
36. Huang, F.; You, M.; Chen, T.; Zhu, G.; Liang, H.; Tan, W. Self-assembled hybrid nanoparticles for targeted co-delivery of two drugs into cancer cells. *Chem. Commun.* **2014**, *50*, 3103–3105. [CrossRef] [PubMed]
37. Liu, M.; Du, H.; Zhang, W.; Zhai, G. Internal stimuli-responsive nanocarriers for drug delivery: Design strategies and applications. *Mater. Sci. Eng. C* **2017**, *71*, 1267–1280. [CrossRef] [PubMed]
38. Mura, S.; Nicolas, J.; Couvreur, P. Stimuli-responsive nanocarriers for drug delivery. *Nat. Mater.* **2013**, *12*, 991–1003. [CrossRef]
39. He, X.; Li, J.; An, S.; Jiang, C. pH-sensitive drug-delivery systems for tumor targeting. *Ther. Deliv.* **2013**, *4*, 1499–1510. [CrossRef]
40. Liu, Y.; Wang, W.; Yang, J.; Zhou, C.; Sun, J. pH-sensitive polymeric micelles triggered drug release for extracellular and intracellular drug targeting delivery. *Asian J. Pharm. Sci.* **2013**, *8*, 159–167. [CrossRef]
41. Kratz, F.; Warnecke, A.; Scheuermann, K.; Stockmar, C.; Schwab, J.; Lazar, P.; Drückes, P.; Esser, N.; Drevs, J.; Rognan, D.; et al. Probing the Cysteine-34 Position of Endogenous Serum Albumin with Thiol-Binding Doxorubicin Derivatives. Improved Efficacy of an Acid-Sensitive Doxorubicin Derivative with Specific Albumin-Binding Properties Compared to That of the Parent Compound. *J. Med. Chem.* **2002**, *45*, 5523–5533. [CrossRef]
42. Latorre, A.; Somoza, A. Glutathione-Triggered Drug Release from Nanostructures. *Curr. Top. Med. Chem.* **2015**, *14*, 2662–2671. [CrossRef]
43. Latorre, A.; Posch, C.; Garcimartín, Y.; Celli, A.; Sanlorenzo, M.; Vujic, I.; Ma, J.; Zekhtser, M.; Rappersberger, K.; Ortiz-Urda, S.; et al. DNA and aptamer stabilized gold nanoparticles for targeted delivery of anticancer therapeutics. *Nanoscale* **2014**, *6*, 7436–7442. [CrossRef] [PubMed]
44. Latorre, A.; Couleaud, P.; Aires, A.; Cortajarena, A.L.; Somoza, Á. Multifunctionalization of magnetic nanoparticles for controlled drug release: A general approach. *Eur. J. Med. Chem.* **2014**, *82*, 355–362. [CrossRef]
45. Chen, Q.; Wang, X.; Wang, C.; Feng, L.; Li, Y.; Liu, Z. Drug-Induced Self-Assembly of Modified Albumins as Nano-theranostics for Tumor-Targeted Combination Therapy. *ACS Nano* **2015**, *9*, 5223–5233. [CrossRef] [PubMed]
46. Ding, D.; Tang, X.; Cao, X.; Wu, J.; Yuan, A.; Qiao, Q.; Pan, J.; Hu, Y. Novel Self-assembly Endows Human Serum Albumin Nanoparticles with an Enhanced Antitumor Efficacy. *AAPS Pharmscitech* **2014**, *15*, 213–222. [CrossRef] [PubMed]
47. Yu, Z.; Yu, M.; Zhang, Z.; Hong, G.; Xiong, Q. Bovine serum albumin nanoparticles as controlled release carrier for local drug delivery to the inner ear. *Nanoscale Res. Lett.* **2014**, *9*, 343. [CrossRef]
48. Danhier, F.; Danhier, P.; De Saedeleer, C.J.; Fruytier, A.-C.; Schleich, N.; Des Rieux, A.; Sonveaux, P.; Gallez, B.; Préat, V. Paclitaxel-loaded micelles enhance transvascular permeability and retention of nanomedicines in tumors. *Int. J. Pharm.* **2015**, *479*, 399–407. [CrossRef]
49. Hu, T.; Chung, Y.M.; Guan, M.; Ma, M.; Ma, J.; Berek, J.S.; Hu, M.C.T. Reprogramming ovarian and breast cancer cells into non-cancerous cells by low-dose metformin or SN-38 through FOXO3 activation. *Sci. Rep.* **2015**, *4*, 5810. [CrossRef]

50. Matt, S.; Hofmann, T.G. The DNA damage-induced cell death response: A roadmap to kill cancer cells. *Cell. Mol. Life Sci.* **2016**, *73*, 2829–2850. [CrossRef]
51. Sharma, A.; Singh, K.; Almasan, A. *Histone H2AX Phosphorylation: A Marker for DNA Damage*; Humana Press: Totowa, NJ, USA, 2012; Volume 531, pp. 613–626, ISBN 978-1-61-7799-976.
52. Bielecka, Z.F.; Maliszewska-Olejniczak, K.; Safir, I.J.; Szczylik, C.; Czarnecka, A.M. Three-dimensional cell culture model utilization in cancer stem cell research. *Biol. Rev.* **2017**, *92*, 1505–1520. [CrossRef] [PubMed]
53. Choi, H.S.; Kim, D.-A.; Chung, H.; Park, I.H.; Kim, B.H.; Oh, E.-S.; Kang, D.-H. Screening of breast cancer stem cell inhibitors using a protein kinase inhibitor library. *Cancer Cell Int.* **2017**, *17*, 25. [CrossRef] [PubMed]
54. Liu, M.; Shen, S.; Wen, D.; Li, M.; Li, T.; Chen, X.; Gu, Z.; Mo, R. Hierarchical Nanoassemblies-Assisted Combinational Delivery of Cytotoxic Protein and Antibiotic for Cancer Treatment. *Nano Lett.* **2018**, *18*, 2294–2303. [CrossRef] [PubMed]
55. Batlle, E.; Clevers, H. Cancer stem cells revisited. *Nat. Med.* **2017**, *23*, 1124–1134. [CrossRef] [PubMed]
56. Papaccio, F.; Paino, F.; Regad, T.; Papaccio, G.; Desiderio, V.; Tirino, V. Concise Review: Cancer Cells, Cancer Stem Cells, and Mesenchymal Stem Cells: Influence in Cancer Development. *Stem Cells Trans. Med.* **2017**, *6*, 2115–2125. [CrossRef]
57. Bradshaw, A.; Wickremsekera, A.; Tan, S.T.; Peng, L.; Davis, P.F.; Itinteang, T. Cancer Stem Cell Hierarchy in Glioblastoma Multiforme. *Front. Surg.* **2016**, *3*, 1–15. [CrossRef] [PubMed]
58. Bozorgi, A.; Khazaei, M.; Khazaei, M.R. New Findings on Breast Cancer Stem Cells: A Review. *J. Breast Cancer* **2015**, *18*, 303–312. [CrossRef]
59. Maugeri-Sacca, M.; Bartucci, M.; de Maria, R. DNA Damage Repair Pathways in Cancer Stem Cells. *Mol. Cancer Ther.* **2012**, *11*, 1627–1636. [CrossRef]

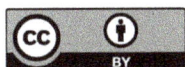

© 2019 by the authors. Licensee MDPI, Basel, Switzerland. This article is an open access article distributed under the terms and conditions of the Creative Commons Attribution (CC BY) license (http://creativecommons.org/licenses/by/4.0/).

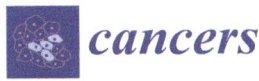

Article

The Delivery Strategy of Paclitaxel Nanostructured Lipid Carrier Coated with Platelet Membrane

Ki-Hyun Bang [1,†], Young-Guk Na [1,†], Hyun Wook Huh [1], Sung-Joo Hwang [2], Min-Soo Kim [3], Minki Kim [1], Hong-Ki Lee [1,*] and Cheong-Weon Cho [1,*]

1. College of Pharmacy, Chungnam National University, Daejeon 34134, Korea; robotkr@nate.com (K.-H.B.); youngguk@cnu.ac.kr (Y.-G.N.); hhw3573@nate.com (H.W.H.); zkzkang@naver.com (M.K.)
2. College of Pharmacy and Yonsei Institute of Pharmaceutical Sciences, Yonsei University, 162-1 Songdo-dong, Yeonsu-gu, Incheon 406-840, Korea; sjh11@yonsei.ac.kr
3. College of Pharmacy, Pusan National University, 63 Busandaehak-ro, Geumjeong-gu, Busan 609-735, Korea; minsookim@pusan.ac.kr
* Correspondence: dvmlhk@gmail.com (H.-K.L.); chocw@cnu.ac.kr (C.-W.C.); Tel.: +82-42-821-5934 (H.-K.L. & C.-W.C.); Fax: +82-42-823-6566 (H.-K.L. & C.-W.C.)
† These authors contributed equally.

Received: 2 May 2019; Accepted: 10 June 2019; Published: 11 June 2019

Abstract: Strategies for the development of anticancer drug delivery systems have undergone a dramatic transformation in the last few decades. Lipid-based drug delivery systems, such as a nanostructured lipid carrier (NLC), are one of the systems emerging to improve the outcomes of tumor treatments. However, NLC can act as an intruder and cause an immune response. To overcome this limitation, biomimicry technology was introduced to decorate the surface of the nanoparticles with various cell membrane proteins. Here, we designed paclitaxel (PT)-loaded nanostructured lipid carrier (PT-NLC) with platelet (PLT) membrane protein because PLT is involved with angiogenesis and interaction of circulating tumor cells. After PLT was isolated from blood using the gravity-gradient method and it was used for coating PT-NLC. Spherical PT-NLC and platelet membrane coated PT-NLC (P-PT-NLC) were successfully fabricated with high encapsulation efficiency (EE) (99.98%) and small particle size (less than 200 nm). The successful coating of PT-NLC with a PLT membrane was confirmed by the identification of CD41 based on transmission electron microscopy (TEM), western blot assay and enzyme-linked immunosorbent assay (ELISA) data. Moreover, the stronger affinity of P-PT-NLC than that of PT-NLC toward tumor cells was observed. In vitro cell study, the PLT coated nanoparticles successfully displayed the anti-tumor effect to SK-OV-3 cells. In summary, the biomimicry carrier system P-PT-NLC has an affinity and targeting ability for tumor cells.

Keywords: nanostructured lipid carrier; platelet membrane; biomimicry; paclitaxel

1. Introduction

Paclitaxel (PT) is a microtubule inhibitor that promotes polymerization and prohibits dissociation of microtubules. PT has been widely used in the treatment of solid tumors, including breast, ovarian and lung cancers. In particular, PT is the front-line pharmaceutical in ovarian cancer chemotherapy, which is the seventh most common cancer worldwide, with an incidence estimated at around 6.3 per 100,000 women globally [1,2]. Patients with ovarian cancer have a low survival rate [3–5]. However, platinum and PT combination chemotherapy is now considered the standard treatment for those with newly diagnosed ovarian cancer, showing excellent response rates ranging from 60% to 70% [6,7].

Despite this, the low solubility of PT and efflux by p-glycoprotein impair its clinical efficacy [8–10]. In addition, its use has been limited by significant side effects, including myelosuppression, neutropenia and hypersensitivity [2,11], with neutropenia becoming more profound at higher doses and over longer infusion times. Taxol®, the commercial formulation, includes the Cremophor® EL, which caused the side effects. Hypersensitivity is characterized by dyspnea, hypotension and urticaria, all of which are most likely caused by polyoxyl 35 castor oil (Cremophor® EL). During its development, the ortotaxel, PT analogous, showed 50% oral bioavailability, but also had significant, toxic side effects [12]. Its clinical use is limited by reasons of the low bioavailability and adverse effects caused by Cremophor® EL [13].

To overcome these side effects, the development of an alternative drug delivery system for PT is needed. There have been several approaches to developing a PT delivery system, including liposome, emulsion and nanoparticles [9,14,15]. Among these, solid lipid nanoparticles (SLNs) were developed as an alternative drug delivery system (DDS) for liposome emulsion and polymeric nanoparticles [16]. SLNs for antitumor drugs improved the tumor-specific targeting and bioavailability, and showed profound cytotoxicity to multidrug resistant cancer cells [17]. However, the issues such as low drug loading capacity, crystallization of the lipid matrix and drug expulsion have limited the clinical use of SLN.

Nanostructured lipid carrier (NLC) was introduced as an alternative carrier of SLNs [18]. NLC, a type of nanoparticle, is a second-generation lipid nanoparticle composed of both solid and liquid lipids. Using this mixture, NLC has an intense solid state but does not crystallize, allowing higher drug loading [19]. Nanoparticles also possess several limitations to applied clinical use. They may be acted on as a foreign substance, causing an immune response. Although these responses, including immunostimulation and immunosuppression, may be either desirable or undesirable, they may also cause safety concerns [20,21]. Consistent with this, nanoparticles have the potential for elimination by the reticuloendothelial system (RES), which limits the effectiveness of drug delivery to target sites. Further, non-targeted nanoparticles, which exhibit an enhanced permeability and retention (EPR) effect, may cause the unwanted side effect. To overcome these limitations, biomimicry technology was introduced to decorate the surface of the nanoparticles with various cell membrane proteins [22,23].

Platelets (PLTs) are anuclear fragments and small circulating cells in whole blood. They are involved with thrombosis and hemostasis processes, responding to vascular damage and contributing to clot formation. PLTs, also, are involved with angiogenesis and cancer triggers and interact with circulating tumor cells. It has been recognized that the aggregation between PLT and tumor cells correlates with the tumor metastasis. The mechanism of aggregation of platelets surrounding tumor cells includes biomolecular binding such as P-selectin [24] and structure-based capture [25]. Recently, several investigations have shown that tumor-specific targeting can be attained through biomimicry using PLT membrane proteins [22,25,26]. The camouflage using a PLT membrane possesses versatile characteristics. It has been reported that PLT membrane-coated nanoparticles have reduced macrophage cellular uptake and lack particle-induced complement activation [27]. Moreover, the PLT membrane-coated nanoparticles showed a specific affinity to tumor tissues and damaged vasculatures [28].

Therefore, the objective of this study was to fabricate a PT-loaded NLC (PT-NLC) coated with PLTs to overcome the known limitations and increase the anticancer effects.

2. Results

2.1. Screening of Liquid Lipid, Solid Lipid and Surfactant

The solubility profile of PT in a lipid matrix plays a key role in encapsulation efficiency (EE) and loading capacity (LC) of NLC. In this study, a solubility profile of PT in liquid, solid lipids and surfactant solutions was evaluated.

PT is a lipophilic drug, which have poor water solubility, with a log P value of 3.0. Figure 1a displays the solubility of PT in various liquid lipids. While semisynthetic modified oils (Capryols, Capmuls, Lauroglycols, and Labrafils) showed high solubility, unmodified dietary oils such as oleic acid and olive oil showed low solubility (0.42 ± 0.04 and 0.43 ± 0.06 mg/mL, respectively). In addition, nanoparticles with unmodified dietary oils showed poor emulsification properties. Capryol 90 (propylene glycol monocaprylate) showed the highest solubility (75.72 ± 15.58 mg/mL). High solubility of PT in Capryol 90 might be due to its natural self-emulsifying property [29]; thus, Capryol 90 was selected as the liquid lipid. Figure 1b displays the solubility of PT in various solid lipids. The solubility of PT was high in the following order; Compritol 888 ATO, glyceryl monostearate (GMS) and Gelucire 44/14 (6.7 ± 1.1, 5.3 ± 1.1 and 5.0 ± 0.6 mg/gm, respectively), compared with other solid lipids. The solubility of PT in 1% surfactants solutions is shown in Figure 1c. While tween 80 and poloxamer 188 showed low solubility (3.5 ± 1.6 and 1.0 ± 0.9 µg/mL, respectively), Cremophor® EL, span 85 and transcutol-HP showed high PT solubility (33.70 ± 5.38, 32.66 ± 9.22 and 31.69 ± 0.64 µg/mL, respectively) compared with other surfactant solutions.

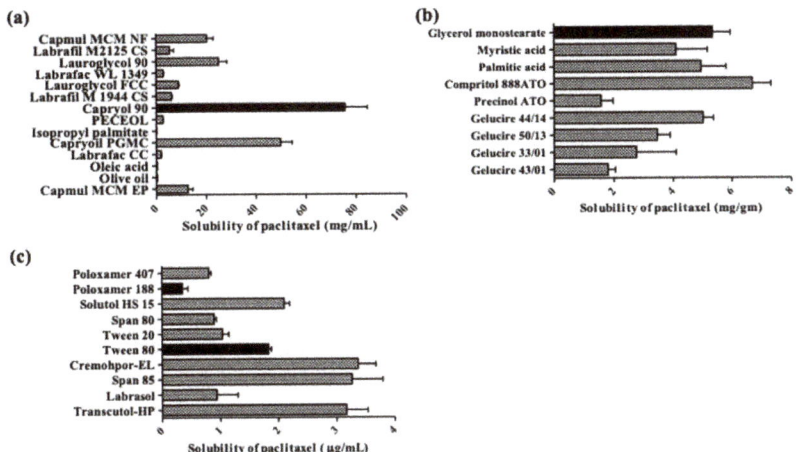

Figure 1. Solubility profiles of paclitaxel (PT) in lipids or surfactants. (**a**), liquid lipids; (**b**), solid lipids; (**c**), 1% surfactant solutions. Black bar represents the liquid, solid lipids and surfactants for PT-nanostructured lipid carrier (NLC).

2.2. Physicochemical Properties

2.2.1. Particle Size, Polydispersity Index (PDI), Zeta Potential (ZP), EE and LC

The various compositions of formulations of PT-NLC and their physicochemical properties, including particle sizes, PDI, ZP, EE and LC are listed in Table 1a,b, respectively. The final concentration of PT in formulations was fixed at 5 mg/10 mL. For changes in GMS and Capryol 90 ratio (Table 1b), code 4 showed the smallest particle size (115.2 ± 3.9 nm). Code 1 showed a high LC value (3.44 ± 0.01%) and the lowest ZP value (2.24 ± 0.5 mV) compared with the others. ZP is a key factor for characterizing the surface charge of colloids and the stability of the colloidal system. Particles for which the ZP is close to zero tend to be aggregated [30,31]. Based on the ZP values, code 1 was unstable compared with code 4 (−15.00 ± 0.9 mV). In previous studies, nanoparticles with small size tend to accumulate in tumors; this is known as the enhanced permeability and retention (EPR) effect [22,32]. It is expected that small NLCs (particle size < 200 nm) will have increased target specificity for tumor sites. Thus, the fixed ratio of GMS and Capryol 90 (2:1) was used. Next, the total lipid amount was altered and the formulations characterized (Table 1b). The particle size was increased in proportion to the increase in the total lipid amount. However, code 1 and 2 showed the particle size values above 200 nm despite the low volume of total lipid. Thus, the fixed amount of total lipid (210 mg) was used for fabrication of formulation. When the poloxamer 188 or Tween 80 was individually used as a surfactant, the particle size of the formulation was 161.8 or 259.8 nm, respectively. Herein, the code 4 showed the smallest particle size.

Table 1. Various compositions for PT-NLCs (a) and their physicochemical properties (b) ($n = 3$).

(a) Various Compositions for PT-NLCs

Code	GMS (mg)	Capryol 90 (mg)	PT (mg)	% of Poloxamer 188 in 10 mL	% of Tween 80 in 10 mL
1	70	70	5	0.5	1
2	120	60	5	0.5	1
3	140	70	5	1	0.5
4	140	70	5	0.5	1
5	160	80	5	0.5	1
6	180	90	5	0.5	1
7	210	70	5	0.5	1
8	280	70	5	0.5	1

(b) Physicochemical Properties

Code	Particle Size (nm)	PDI	EE (%)	LC (%)	ZP (mV)
1	279.2 ± 10.4	0.308 ± 0.012	99.79 ± 0.18	3.44 ± 0.01	2.24 ± 0.51
2	266.5 ± 46.8	0.360 ± 0.011	99.94 ± 0.03	2.70 ± 0.03	−22.70 ± 1.46
3	161.3 ± 0.9	0.311 ± 0.301	99.62 ± 0.05	2.25 ± 0.01	−16.40 ± 0.82
4	115.2 ± 3.9	0.284 ± 0.015	99.98 ± 0.01	2.33 ± 0.01	−15.00 ± 0.93
5	123.0 ± 0.9	0.352 ± 0.022	99.95 ± 0.02	2.04 ± 0.01	−30.60 ± 0.31
6	164.4 ± 12.2	0.321 ± 0.017	99.94 ± 0.05	1.82 ± 0.02	−29.40 ± 1.59
7	158.6 ± 9.8	0.297 ± 0.012	99.96 ± 0.06	1.75 ± 0.01	−25.33 ± 0.62
8	2599.4 ± 392.7	0.220 ± 0.150	99.51 ± 0.03	1.40 ± 0.01	−31.43 ± 0.54

P-PT-NLC was fabricated via a sonication method. The particle size and ZP of P-PT-NLC were 171 ± 0.31 nm and −8.0 ± 0.77 mV, respectively. After the coating of the PLT membrane, the particle size of P-PT-NLC increased compared with that of PT-NLC, but it was smaller than that of PLT fragments (Figure 2a). In addition, when the PLT membrane protein was coated to PT-NLC, ZP decreased to be similar to PLT fragments (Figure 2b). Changes in the particle size and ZP of P-PT-NLC indicated successful coating with PLT membrane [33].

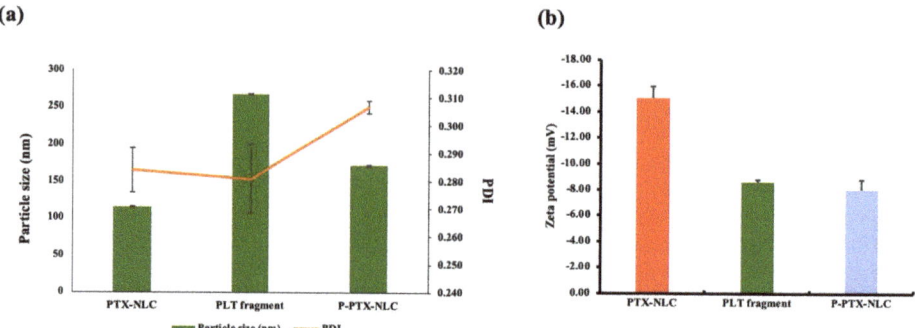

Figure 2. The physicochemical characterizations. (**a**), particle size and polydispersity index (PDI); (**b**), zeta potential of PT-NLC, PLT and P-PT-NLC ($n = 3$, mean ± standard deviation (SD)).

2.2.2. Differential Scanning Calorimetry (DSC) and Powder X-ray Diffraction (PXRD) Analysis

In general, DSC analysis is used to evaluate the melting behavior or crystallization of nanoparticles. [34,35]. Figure 3a shows the DSC diagram of excipients, PT, lyophilized NLC with or without mannitol and physical mixture with or without mannitol. The melting point of mannitol, poloxamer 188 and GMS were 167 °C, 58 °C and 60 °C, respectively. PT showed two different peaks: endothermal (220 °C) and exothermal (240 °C). In thermograms of PT-NLC formulations, the peak of

PT and excipients was decreased. The decreased PT peak of PT-NLC indicates the encapsulation of PT in the lipid matrix [36].

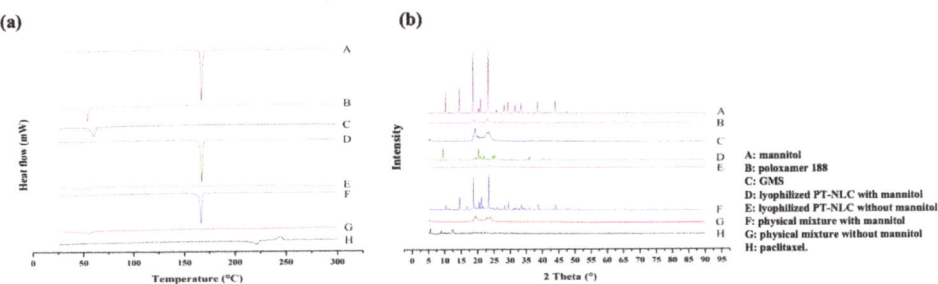

Figure 3. Differential scanning calorimetry (**a**) and powder X-ray diffraction (**b**) analysis.

Figure 3b shows PXRD analysis of PT and NLC. PT powder showed a few diffraction peaks at 5.5°, 7.8°, 10.1° and 12.6°. Many crystalline diffraction patterns of PT indicate that PT had crystallinity. Broad peaks were displayed at 19.2° and 24.2° for poloxamer 188, and 19.8° and 24.1° for GMS. These patterns were not displayed in lyophilized NLC without mannitol, but the physical mixture without mannitol showed a PT peak, suggesting that PT was encapsulated in PT-NLC in an amorphous form [37].

2.2.3. Transmission Electron Microscopy (TEM) Analysis

To confirm the shape and PLT coating on nanoparticles, TEM analysis was conducted with negative staining of uranyl acetate. PT-NLC and P-PT-NLC in Figure 4 show that the nanoparticle morphology of PT-NLC (Figure 4a) and P-PT-NLC (Figure 4b) was spherical.

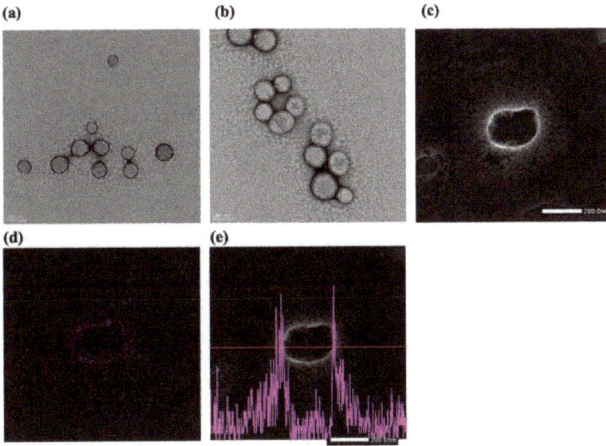

Figure 4. Transmission electron microscopy images of PT-NLC (**a**) and P-PT-NLC (**b**). scanning transmission electron microscopy-energy dispersive X-ray spectroscopy (STEM-EDS) image (**c**), EDS mapping image of uranium elements (**d**) and STEM-EDS line analysis (**e**) of P-PT-NLC.

To evaluate the elemental distribution and composition of P-PT-NLC, EDS mapping and spectra were used (Figure 4). PLT membrane coating was confirmed using scanning transmission electron microscopy-energy dispersive X-ray spectroscopy (STEM-EDS). Figure 4c,d shows the STEM image and EDS mapping of uranium (U) for P-PT-NLC. P-PT-NLC showed a spherical shape with the shell stained by uranyl acetate. In addition, STEM-EDS line analysis showed PLT coating on P-PT-NLC (Figure 4e), indicating that P-PT-NLC was successfully coated with PLT membrane [38,39].

2.3. Western Blot Assay and Enzyme-Linked Immunosorbent Assay (ELISA) of CD41

PLT, PLT fragment, blank-NLC, PT-NLC and P-PT-NLC were separated with 10% polyacrylamide gel stained by coomassie brilliant blue (CBB), and then western blot assay was used to identify the CD41 on P-PT-NLC. CD41, a part of the integrin αIIb, plays a key role in PLT adhesion [40]. CD41 (131 kDa) was detected in PLT, PLT fragment and P-PT-NLC, except for blank-NLC and PT-NLC (Figure 5a, More details can be found in Figure S1), indicating that CD41 protein successfully coated P-PT-NLC.

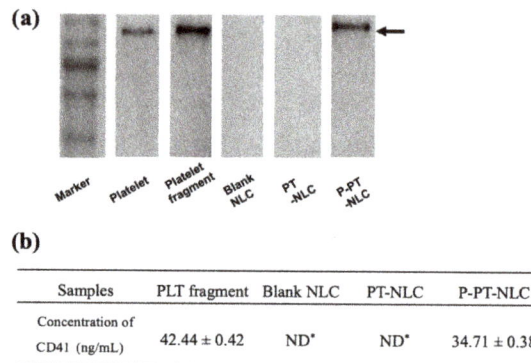

Figure 5. Identification of integrin αIIb (CD41) on P-PT-NLC. (**a**), western blot analysis; (**b**), enzyme-linked immunosorbent assay (ELISA) analysis ($n = 3$, mean ± SD). ND*, not detected. Black arrow indicates the CD41 band (131 kDa).

To quantify CD41 in the formulations, rat PLT membrane glycoprotein 2B3A/CD41$^+$CD61$^+$ ELISA kit was used. CD41 was detected and quantified in PLT and P-PT-NLC (Figure 5b). The amount of CD41 in P-PT-NLC decreased compared to that in PLT. P-PT-NLC yields using two different analytical methods were calculated and the yields of P-PT-NLC using western blot assay and ELISA were 81.72 ± 0.85 and 79.23 ± 1.08%, respectively.

2.4. In Vitro Cell Experiments

Following this, a confocal laser scanning microscopy (CLSM) study was performed to determine the presence of CD41 on P-PT-NLC. To assess the attachment abilities of nanoparticles to tumor cells, a CLSM study was conducted with PT-NLC and P-PT-NLC on SK-OV-3 cells. CLSM images of PT-NLC and P-PT-NLC are shown in Figure 6. In Figure 6b, CD41 on the surface of P-PT-NLC was detected on SK-OV-3 cells. By contrast, CD41 was not detected in PT-NLC (Figure 6a). In merging the images of P-PT-NLC, CD41 (green fluorescence) was co-localized in 4′,6-diamidino-2-phenylindole (DAPI) (blue fluorescence) and rhodamine–phalloidin (red fluorescence) staining sites. This indicates that P-PT-NLC was attached to SK-OV-3 cancer cells and that CD41 on P-PT-NLC possesses a high tumor-cell affinity [33,40,41].

The cytotoxic effects of PT, blank-NLC, PT-NLC and P-PT-NLC at 24 and 48 h were evaluated with SK-OV-3 cells (Figure 7). Blank-NLC consisted of an equivalent lipid concentration of PT-NLC and P-PT-NLC. In the 0.1–7.5 µg/mL concentration range, all formulations were more toxic compared with blank-NLC after 24 h. The cell viability of blank-NLC at 10 µg/mL was 71.56 ± 10.12%; therefore, the excipient of NLC showed cytotoxicity to SK-OV-3 cells (Figure 7a). At 10 µg/mL, the cell viability of PT (, PT-NLC (47.52 ± 5.10%) and P-PT-NLC (47.07 ± 4.95%) were less than that of blank-NLC (79.07 ± 5.24%) at 48 h post-incubation. PT-NLC and P-PT-NLC were significantly more toxic than PT ($p < 0.01$)

at all concentration ranges, but no significant difference was observed between PT-NLC and P-PT-NLC (Figure 7b), indicating that the release profile of PT-NLC and P-PT-NLC was a sustained release.

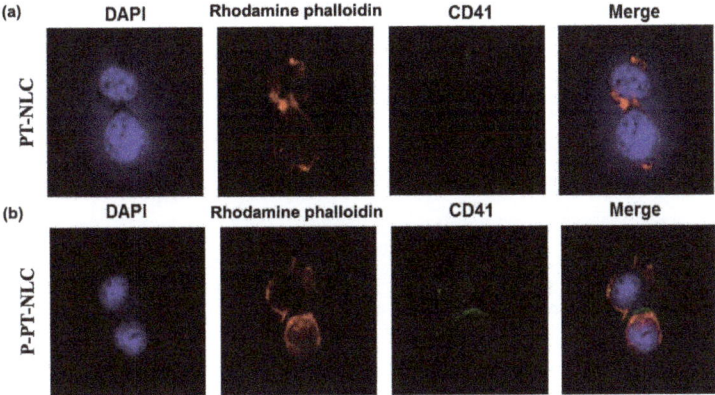

Figure 6. Confocal fluorescent microscopy images. (**a**), PT-NLC; (**b**), P-PT-NLC. After treatment with PT-NLC and P-PT-NLC, SK-OV-3 cell was stained with 4′,6-diamidino-2-phenylindole (DAPI), rhodamine–phalloidin and integrin αIIb Alexa Fluor® 488 antibody (1:100) (blue= nuclear, red = F-actin, green = CD41).

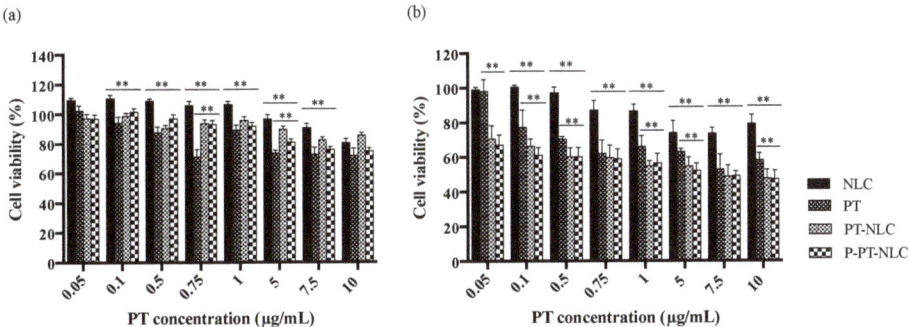

Figure 7. Cytotoxicity assay of PT, PT-NLC and P-PT-NLC in SK-OV-3 cells after 24 h (**a**) and 48 h (**b**). ** $p < 0.01$ (multiple t-tests).

2.5. Biodistribution Study

Following administration of PT, PT-NLC and P-PT-NLC, PT concentration was continuously eliminated in the kidney. However, in PT-NLC and P-PT-NLC, PT concentration increased to 8 h and was eliminated at 24 h; therefore, it seems to accumulate in the kidney, while the PT concentration was reduced at 24 h (Figure 8a). This indicates that PT-NLC and P-PT-NLC were sufficiently eliminated from the kidney. PT-NLC and P-PT-NLC accumulated in the liver at higher levels compared to PT (Figure 8b). This issue could be explained by the reticuloendothelial system (RES) or liver Kupffer cells uptake [9,42]. When particle size is between 50 and 200 nm, nanoparticles tend to accumulate in the liver by RES. This indicates that nanoparticles with a diameter of 50–200 nm were caught by the RES, resulting in sustained release [23,43]. PT-NLC and P-PT-NLC tended to accumulate in the liver more than PT, but PT-NLC and P-PT-NLC appeared to be eliminated from the liver over time. This means that as the nanoparticles are taken up by the RES, they are slowly released over time. Moreover, it has been reported that the liver was one of the major organs for the physiological clearance of PLT [44]. To clarify this issue, additional liver toxicity studies should be conducted for PT-NLC and P-PT-NLC.

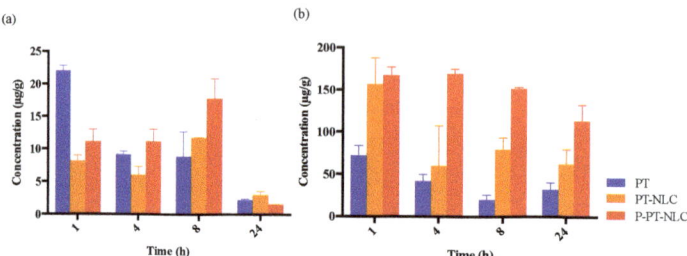

Figure 8. Biodistribution at the 10 mg/kg dose of PT, PT-NLC and P-PT-NLC in kidney (**a**) and liver (**b**) at 1, 4, 8 and 24 h. Each column represents the mean ± SD (n = 2).

3. Discussion

In this study, PT-NLC was fabricated considering the EE and the particle size. Composition of PT NLC with the highest EE value and the optimal particle size (less 200 nm) [45] was selected for the fabrication of P-PT-NLC. Compritol 888ATO showed the highest solubility as a solid lipid; however, PT-NLC with Compritol 888ATO showed the excessive solidification during the fabrication. Thus, GMS was selected as the solid lipid. Surfactant, which has low drug solubility, affects the association between the drug and lipid matrix and materializes drugs in the lipid core. Surfactant use with NLC leads to drug distribution in the core rather than the exterior of the NLC [29,46]. Thus, non-ionic surfactant provides the steric hindrance and static repulsion for particles [32]. Previously, we successfully fabricated the NLC-loaded ticagrelor using the poloxamer 188 and Tween 80 as surfactants [47]. In addition, the previous study suggested that using Poloxamer 188 (1%), a steric stabilizer, with Tween 80 (2%) as a surfactant, in the manufacture of NLC could provide a stable NLC with a particle size below 100 nm [48]. Thus, Tween 80 and poloxamer 188 were selected as surfactant and co-surfactant with a ratio of 2:1, respectively.

To confirm whether PT was encapsulated in NLC, DSC and PXRD patterns were conducted with NLC and its ingredients (Figure 3). When PT-NLC was freeze-dried with the lyophilizing agent, mannitol, the PT peak decreased. However, the mannitol peak was still high; therefore, blank NLC and PT-NLC were lyophilized without mannitol to remove its effect on the DSC and PXRD patterns. The PT peak was decreased in freeze-dried PT-NLC. However, the physical mixture still had a PT peak, indicating that the crystallites of PT were not detected in lyophilized PT-NLC without mannitol and that PT was encapsulated successfully in the lipid matrix.

When P-PT-NLC was fabricated with PT-NLC and PLT by sonication, particle size increased by around 50 nm and ZP was similar to PLT fragment. It is reported that the size of nanoparticles coated with PLT was about 20 nm larger than the bare nanoparticles in previous studies [22,49,50]. Moreover, it is stated that the ZP of nanoparticles coated with PLT was similar to that of the surface charge of PLT in accordance with the previous investigation. P-PT-NLC with increased size and charged to the same level as a PLT fragment means that P-PT-NLC was coated with PLT.

The shapes of PT-NLC and P-PT-NLC were inspected and confirmed by TEM (Figure 4). Nanoparticles were spherical and the particle size was similar compared with electrophoretic light scattering (ELS) data. In addition, PT-NLC and P-PT-NLC were negatively stained with uranyl acetate, which can bind to surfaces of the phosphate moiety of lipid structures by ionic interaction [51]. The PLT membrane was composed of phospholipid, so uranyl acetate could interact with the PLT membrane. Using this interaction between the PLT membrane and uranyl acetate, STEM/EDS analysis was utilized to confirm the PLT membrane coating in P-PT-NLC. In the STEM image (Figure 4c), PLT membrane on P-PT-NLC was shown as a white line from uranyl acetate, indicating that uranium may be present on the PLT membrane. The intensity of uranium was investigated using EDS mapping (Figure 4d) and line analysis (Figure 4e), and PLT coating in P-PT-NLC was confirmed, with strong uranium intensity, on the surface of P-PT-NLC.

Before the western blot assay, sodium dodecyl sulfate–polyacrylamide gel electrophoresis (SDS-PAGE) was used to separate various proteins from PLT fragments and to identify PLT membranes in P-PT-NLC. The SDS-PAGE patterns of PLT and PLT fragments were consistent with that reported in a previous study [30]. In the western blot assay, the PLT marker (CD41) was detected in P-PT-NLC, suggesting that PT-NLC was successfully coated with the PLT fragment. In summary, the PLT membrane proteins were successfully translocated to PT-NLC. However, PLT pattern intensity in P-PT-NLC was lower compared with PLT and PLT fragments, possibly due to the purification of P-PT-NLC. Because of this step, PLT pattern intensity was decreased compared with PLT fragment. Similar result was obtained by ELISA.

The affinity of P-PT-NLC for SK-OV-3 cells was confirmed by CLSM (Figure 6). It has been reported that PLTs play a role in the survival, migration and growth of tumor cells [52,53]. In fact, anticoagulants have been shown to reduce tumor growth, metastasis and angiogenesis [54,55]. In this experiment, CD41 was used as a PLT maker. When P-PT-NLC was treated with SK-OV-3 cells, CD41 was observed on the surface of SK-OV-3 cells. However, no CD41 was detected with PT-NLC. CD41 was co-localized on the cytoplasm rather than the nuclei, indicating that P-PT-NLC was bound to the surface of tumor cells and that PLT coated particles might be used to target tumor cells.

Cytotoxicity to ovarian cancer cells was confirmed by MTT assay (Figure 7). Blank NLC did not show cytotoxicity at all concentrations because cell viability exceeded 80%. However, PT, PT-NLC and P-PT-NLC showed cytotoxicity to SK-OV-3 cells. After 48 h of incubation, low doses of PT-NLC and P-PT-NLC produced cytotoxic effects, while PT did not. In addition, the cytotoxic effects of PT-NLC and P-PT-NLC were superior compared with PT, suggesting that PT-NLC and P-PT-NLC produce a profound in vitro cytotoxic effect in ovarian cancer cells.

An in vivo biodistribution study of PTC-NLC and P-PT-NLC showed late elimination from the kidney and liver (Figure 8). In the kidney, nanoparticles seemed to accumulate at an early stage after i.v. injection. However, similar amounts of nanoparticles and PT remained in kidney at 24 h. The nanoparticles coated with PLT were found to be distributed to the kidney at the similar level of the bare nanoparticles after 24 h administrations, as has previously been investigated [50]. In the liver, however, formulations accumulated up to 24 h after i.v. injection. It may be that nanoparticles accumulate by RES in the liver causing hepatoxicity. However, nanoparticles were also excreted from the liver over the study period, indicating that nanoparticles were slowly released into systemic circulation. Therefore, hepatotoxicity analyses of PT-NLC and P-PT-NLC are needed to determine liver toxicity.

4. Materials and Methods

4.1. Chemicals and Reagents

PT and docetaxel (internal standard, IS) were gifted by Korea United Pharm, Inc. (Seoul, Korea). Isopropyl palmitate, palmitic, myristic and stearic acid were purchased from Daejung Chemical (Cheongwon, Korea). Tween 80, Tween 20, GMS, oleic acid, Span 85 and 80, phosphoric acid and mannitol were obtained Samchun Chemical (Pyungtaek, Korea). Capmul® MCM-NF and -EP were purchased from Abitec Corporation (Columbus, OH, USA). Gelucire 44/14, 33/01, 43/01, 50/13, Capryol™ PGMC, Compritol® 888 ATO, Capryol 90, Labrafac™ WL 1349 and CC, Labrasol, Cremophor® EL, Labrafil® M 2125 CS, Peceol, Lauroglycol 90, Transcutol® HP, Lauroglycol™ FCC, precirol ATO, and Labrafil® M 1944 CS were obtained by Gattefossé (Saint Priest, Cedex, France). Poloxamer 188, 407 and Solutol® HS-15 were obtained from BASF (Ludwigshafen, Germany). Dimethyl sulfoxide (DMSO), DAPI, 3-(4,5-dimethylthoazol-2yl)-2,5-diphenyl-2H-tetrazolium bromide (MTT) and rhodamine–phalloidin were obtained from Sigma-Aldrich (St. Louis, MO, USA). SK-OV-3 cells, an ovarian cancer cell line, were obtained from the Korean Cell Line Bank (Seoul, Korea). High-performance liquid chromatography (HPLC)-grade methanol (MeOH) and acetonitrile (ACN) were obtained from JT Baker (Phillipsburg, NJ, USA).

4.2. Screening of Liquid Lipid, Solid Lipid and Surfactant

PT solubility in liquid lipids, solid lipids and surfactant solutions was evaluated for screening of liquid, solid lipid and surfactant. To evaluate the PT solubility in solid lipids, briefly, 1 g of various solid lipids was weighed to glass vials and boiled in a water. PT was added until the saturation of PT in the solid lipid. The amount of PT dissolved in solid lipids was considered as its solid lipid solubility. To evaluate the PT solubilities in liquid lipids and surfactants, excess amount of PT was added to 0.5 mL of various oils and 1% (w/v) surfactants and mixed at 1000 rpm for 72 h. After the centrifugation (15,000× g for 10 min), the supernatant was diluted with ACN and PT solubility was evaluated using a HPLC with an ultraviolet (UV) detector. All samples were performed in triplicate.

4.3. PT-NLC Preparation

PT-NLC was fabricated using the hot melt emulsification and sonication methods. In each experiment, liquid (Capryol 90®) and solid lipid (GMS) were mixed in a 75 °C water bath. Five milligrams of PT were added to the melted lipids and mixed. Heated Tween 80 and poloxamer 188 were added and homogenized at 15,000 rpm for 1 min. They were sonicated with 108 W of amplitude for 10 min. After the cooling, formulations were freeze-dried with or without mannitol by lyophilizer (FD-1000, EYELA, Tokyo, Japan). Blank-NLC was fabricated without PT.

4.4. P-PT-NLC Preparation

PLTs were isolated using the gravity-gradient method as previously described [26], with slight modification. Briefly, whole blood was collected in anticoagulated tubes with sodium citrate from rat jugular veins. PLTs with the number of 10^8–10^9 cell/mL were used and the number of PLTs was measured by an automated blood counter. Whole blood samples were centrifuged at 200 g for 10 min and supernatant was collected, and this was centrifuged at 110× g for 6 min to discard red and white blood cells, after which the supernatants were collected in a tube. This was centrifuged at 1500× g for 15 min to separate the PLT pellet. Pellet was washed three times with phosphate-buffered saline (PBS) containing protease inhibitor (Thermo Scientific, Waltham, MA, USA). The final number of PLT was 10^3–10^4 cell/mL for P-PT-NLC fabrication.

A preselected PT-NLC formulation was used to prepare P-PT-NLC. Two hundred microliters of PLT concentrate were added to 10 mL of PT-NLC, which was then sonicated using Vibra-Cell (amplitude 80 W, 3 min, turned on for 5 s and off for 2 s per cycle). P-PT-NLC was then placed in an ice bath for cooling and used for the characterization study.

4.5. Physicochemical Properties of Formulations

4.5.1. Evaluation of Particle Size, PDI and ZP

Various formulations (code 1–8) were prepared by increasing the solid lipid (GMS) amount in fixing liquid lipid, increasing the total lipid amount in fixing the ratio between solid lipid and liquid lipid, and changing the surfactant ratio.

Physiochemical parameters, including the particle sizes and PDIs of various PT-NLC formulations were measured using a laser scattering analyzer (ELS-8000, Otsuka Electronics, Osaka, Japan). ZPs of different PT-NLC nanoparticles were assessed using a Zetasizer Nano Z (Malvern Panalytical Ltd., Malvern, UK).

4.5.2. DSC and PXRD Analysis

To evaluate the thermal characteristics of formulations and change of crystallinity of ingredients in PT-NLC, DSC and PXRD analysis were performed using a DSC N-650 thermal analyzer (Scinco, Seoul, Korea) and D/Max-2200 Ultima/PC (Rigaku, Tokyo, Japan) with Ni filtered Cu-Kα (40 kV, 40 mA). For DSC analysis, briefly, samples were heated from 25 °C to 300 °C at a heating rate of 10 °C/min using an aluminum pan under nitrogen gas flow. PXRD analysis was conducted from 5° to 60° with a step size of 0.02 °/s.

4.5.3. TEM Analysis

Morphology of PT-NLC and P-PT-NLC were evaluated using a JEM 2100F field emission electron microscope (JEOL Ltd., Tokyo, Japan) at 200 kV. In addition, STEM-EDS analysis was performed. Samples were placed on a 200 mesh copper grid and washed with distilled water. Then, they were negatively stained with 2% uranyl acetate (Agar Scientific Ltd., Stansted, UK).

4.5.4. EE and LC Determination

The PT content of samples was diluted with ACN and determined by HPLC. Sample EE and LC were evaluated using an ultrafiltration method. Two hundred microliters of sample were added to the chambers of the centrifuge tube in an Amicon filter (10 kDA, Millipore, Billerica, MA, USA), which was centrifuged at 14,000× g for 30 min at 4 °C. The pellet was diluted with ACN to measure the free PT of formulations by the HPLC system. EE and LC were determined as follows:

$$\text{EE (\%)} = \frac{\text{Total amount of PT} - \text{Amount of free PT}}{\text{Total amount of PT}} \times 100 \quad (1)$$

$$\text{LC (\%)} = \frac{\text{Total amount of PT in NLC}}{\text{Total amount of lipids} + \text{Total amount of PT in NLC}} \times 100 \quad (2)$$

4.6. Characterization of PLT Membrane Protein Coated NLC (P-PT-NLC)

To evaluate the PLT coating, PLT membrane protein integrin αIIb (CD41) was identified and quantified using electrophoresis, western blot and enzyme-linked immunosorbent assay (ELISA). For all methods, the degree of PLT coating was assessed as relative intensity:

$$\text{Relative intensity (\%)} = \frac{\text{Intensity of P} - \text{PT} - \text{NLC}}{\text{Intensity of PLT}} \times 100 \quad (3)$$

4.6.1. Western Blot

Samples were added in loading buffer (Biosesang Inc., Sungnam, Korea) and heated to 100 °C for 10 min. Samples were loaded on 10% polyacrylamide gel and separated at 100 V for 120 min. Samples on gels were transferred to a polyvinylidene difluoride (PVDF) membrane at 80 V for 180 min. Membranes were blocked with 5% bovine serum albumin at room temperature for 1 h. Then, membranes were incubated with integrin αIIb horseradish peroxidase (HRP) antibody (1:1000 dilution; Santa Cruz Biotechnology, Inc., Dallas, TX, USA) at room temperature overnight. They were treated with ECL® prime western blotting detection reagent (GE Healthcare Bio-Sciences, Pittsburgh, PA, USA). CD41 (131k Da) band was detected using the Fusion SL2 chemiluminescent imaging system (Vilber Lourmat, Marne-la-Vallée Cedex, France). P-PT-NLC yield was measured by comparing the CD41 band intensity of PLT fragment and P-PT-NLC.

4.6.2. ELISA

To quantify CD41, rat PLT membrane glycoprotein 2B3A/CD41+CD61+ELISA kit was used (MyBioSource, Inc., San Diego, CA, USA). Briefly, 50 µL of sample were placed in each well and 100 µL of HRP-conjugate reagent were added. After the incubation at 37 °C for 60 min under dark conditions, plate was washed three times with wash solution. Each 50 µL of chromogen solution A and B was added to each well. The plate was incubated under dark conditions at 37 °C for 15 min. After the addition of stop solution, the optical density was measured using a microplate reader (Sunrise, Tecan,

Männedorf, Switzerland) at 450 nm within 15 min. P-PT-NLC yield was measured by comparing the CD41 value of PLT fragment and P-PT-NLC.

4.6.3. CLSM Analysis

SK-OV-3 (10^6 cell) was preincubated overnight and samples was added to the cells. Integrin αIIb Alexa Fluor® 488 antibody (1:100 dilution; Santa Cruz Biotechnology, Dallas, TX, USA) was treated for 3 h. Then, cells were washed three times with PBS and stained with DAPI and rhodamine–phalloidin. Fluorescence images were analyzed using a super resolution confocal laser scanning microscope (LSM880 with Airyscan; Carl Zeiss, Oberkochen, Germany)

4.7. Cytotoxicity Study

Human ovarian cancer cell line SK-OV-3 was cultured with Dulbecco's modified eagle medium (DMEM) supplemented with 10% fetal bovine serum (FBS), 100 µg/mL of streptomycin and 100 U/mL of penicillin at 37 °C in a humidified incubator supplied with 5% CO_2 atmosphere.

The cytotoxicity of formulations against SK-OV-3 cells was determined using MTT assay. Cells (5×10^4 cells/well) were prepared and various concentrations of PT, blank-NLC, PT-NLC and P-PT-NLC (0.01–10 µg/mL) were added to cells. Blank-NLC consisted of an equivalent lipid concentration of PT-NLC and P-PT-NLC. At 24 and 48 h post-incubation, 30 µL of MTT solution (5 mg/mL) was added and the plate was incubated for 3 h. Mediums on the plate were discarded and DMSO was added to each well. The absorbance was measured with a microplate reader (Sunrise, Tecan, Austria) at 560 nm. Cell viability was calculated as:

$$\text{Cell viability (\%)} = \frac{OD_{test}}{OD_{control}} \times 100 \qquad (4)$$

where OD_{test} is the absorbance of the cells treated with PT and $OD_{control}$ is the absorbance intensity of the cells incubated with 0.1% DMSO in DMEM medium.

4.8. Biodistribution Study

Male Sprague–Dawley rats (age: 7–8 weeks; body weight: 400–420 g) were provided by Samtako (Osan, Korea) for the biodistribution study. Rats were housed at 22 °C with a 12-h light–dark cycle and given free access to food and water. The rats were acclimated for 1 week prior to the experiments. All procedures were approved by the Local Ethical Committee of Chungnam National University (Protocol No. CNU-00911).

Animals were randomly divided into three groups (8 animals for each group): group A (PT), group B (PT-NLC) or group C (P-PT-NLC). Before the injection of formulations, animals were fasted for 12 h. PT as a control was dissolved in Cremophor® EL and ethanol (1:1, *w/w*) and diluted with normal saline. Freeze-dried PT-NLC and P-PT-NLC were prepared to dilute with normal saline. Animals in groups A, B and C received PT, PT-NLC or P-PT-NLC, respectively, via IV to the tail vein at a dose of 10 mg/kg. After the injection, animals were killed by CO_2 at 1, 4, 8 or 24 h (2 animals for each time point), and organs (kidneys and livers) were collected.

For the preparations of samples, 2 mL of 0.15 M NaCl solution and 2 g of kidney were homogenized at 15,000 rpm for 10 min using a homogenizer. For liver samples, 5 g of liver and 5 mL of distilled water were homogenized at 15,000 rpm for 10 min. Then, 25 µL of IS solution (5 µg/mL of docetaxel in ACN) was added to 100 µL of tissue sample. After the addition of 1 mL ACN, samples were vortexed and shaken for 2 min. Samples were centrifuged for 10 min at 15,000× *g* and 900 µL of organic layer was collected and evaporated with nitrogen gas. Evaporated samples were reconstituted with 50 µL of distilled water and ACN mixture (1:1). After the centrifugation (15,000× *g* for 10 min), 40 µL of supernatant was injected into the HPLC system.

4.9. HPLC Condition

Agilent 1100 HPLC system (Santa Clara, CA, USA) with a UV detector was used for HPLC analysis of PT. Kinetex® C18 column (4.6 × 250 mm, 100 Å, 5 µm; Phenomenex, Torrance, CA, USA) was used and the mobile phase was consisted of ACN and 0.1% phosphoric acid buffer (45:55%, v/v). The flow rate and column temperature were 1.3 mL/min and 30 °C. The injection volume was 20 µL and UV detection of PT was performed at 227 nm.

For the biodistribution study, the mobile phase of ACN and 0.1% phosphoric acid buffer (55:45%, v/v) was used and the injection volume was 40 µL.

4.10. Data and Statistical Analysis

Data was evaluated using a *t*-test to determine the significant differences among groups. Data was expressed as mean ± standard deviation (SD). All analysis was conducted using a GraphPad Prism (Graph-Pad Software, CA, USA). Western blot data were evaluated using Image J software (National Institutes of Health, Bethesda, MD, USA).

5. Conclusions

Herein, the P-PT-NLC was fabricated to avoid an immune response and target tumor cells. PT-NLC was successfully fabricated using hot melt emulsification and sonication methods. In addition, the PLT membrane protein was successfully coated using a sonication method. Spherical PT-NLC and P-PT-NLC were fabricated with high EE (99.98%) and small particle size (less than 200 nm). Based on TEM, western blot assay and ELISA data, the P-PT-NLC was enclosed by CD41, a PLT membrane protein. Moreover, we confirmed the affinity of P-PT-NLC for tumor cells. PT-NLC and P-PT-NLC showed the cytotoxic effect to SK-OV-3 cells. In a biodistribution study, NLC formulation was distributed to both the liver and kidney. In summary, P-PT-NLC has an affinity and targeting ability for tumor cells. This might be due to PLTs, which play a key role in various physiologic and pathologic processes. Biomimicry carrier systems, especially PLT membrane coating, promise new drug delivery platforms.

Supplementary Materials: The following are available online at http://www.mdpi.com/2072-6694/11/6/807/s1, Figure S1: The whole membrane with all molecular weight markers on the western blot.

Author Contributions: Conceptualization, K.-H.B., M.-S.K. and S.-J.H.; methodology, K.-H.B. and Y.-G.N.; software, H.W.H.; formal analysis, K.-H.B., M.K.; writing—original draft preparation, H.-K.L.; writing—review and editing, H.-K.L.; supervision, C.-W.C. On the other hand, results in this study have been published as a student thesis (K.-H.B.) by Chungnam National University.

Funding: This work was supported by the Basic Science Research Program (2016R1A2B4011294) through the National Research Foundation of Korea (NRF) funded by the Ministry of Education, Science and Technology.

Conflicts of Interest: The authors declare no conflict of interest.

References

1. Kampan, N.C.; Madondo, M.T.; McNally, O.M.; Quinn, M.; Plebanski, M. Paclitaxel and its evolving role in the management of ovarian cancer. *Biomed. Res. Int.* **2015**, 413076. [CrossRef] [PubMed]
2. Kumar, S.; Mahdi, H.; Bryant, C.; Shah, J.P.; Garg, G.; Munkarah, A. Clinical trials and progress with paclitaxel in ovarian cancer. *Int. J. Womens Health* **2010**, *2*, 411–427. [CrossRef] [PubMed]
3. Shao, Y.; Li, H.; Du, R.; Meng, J.; Yang, G. Involvement of non-coding RNAs in chemotherapy resistance of ovarian cancer. *J. Cancer.* **2018**, *9*, 1966–1972. [CrossRef] [PubMed]
4. Prat, J.; Oncology, F.C.O.G. Staging classification for cancer of the ovary, fallopian tube, and peritoneum. *Int. J. Gynaecol. Obstet.* **2014**, *124*, 1–5. [CrossRef] [PubMed]
5. Lawrie, T.A.; Winter-Roach, B.A.; Heus, P.; Kitchener, H.C. Adjuvant (post-surgery) chemotherapy for early stage epithelial ovarian cancer. *Cochrane Database Syst. Rev.* **2015**, CD004706. [CrossRef]

6. Einzig, A.I.; Wiernik, P.H.; Sasloff, J.; Runowicz, C.D.; Goldberg, G.L. Phase II study and long-term follow-up of patients treated with taxol for advanced ovarian adenocarcinoma. *J. Clin. Oncol.* **1992**, *10*, 1748–1753. [CrossRef]
7. Thigpen, J.T.; Blessing, J.A.; Ball, H.; Hummel, S.J.; Barrett, R.J. Phase II trial of paclitaxel in patients with progressive ovarian carcinoma after platinum-based chemotherapy: A Gynecologic Oncology Group study. *J. Clin. Oncol.* **1994**, *12*, 1748–1753. [CrossRef]
8. Han, S.M.; Baek, J.S.; Kim, M.S.; Hwang, S.J.; Cho, C.W. Surface modification of paclitaxel-loaded liposomes using d-alpha-tocopheryl polyethylene glycol 1000 succinate: Enhanced cellular uptake and cytotoxicity in multidrug resistant breast cancer cells. *Chem. Phys. Lipids.* **2018**, *213*, 39–47. [CrossRef]
9. Zhang, C.; Qu, G.; Sun, Y.; Wu, X.; Yao, Z.; Guo, Q.; Ding, Q.; Yuan, S.; Shen, Z.; Ping, Q.; et al. Pharmacokinetics, biodistribution, efficacy and safety of N-octyl-O-sulfate chitosan micelles loaded with paclitaxel. *Biomaterials* **2008**, *29*, 1233–1241. [CrossRef]
10. Patel, K.; Patil, A.; Mehta, M.; Gota, V.; Vavia, P. Oral delivery of paclitaxel nanocrystal (PNC) with a dual Pgp-CYP3A4 inhibitor: Preparation, characterization and antitumor activity. *Int. J. Pharm.* **2014**, *472*, 214–223. [CrossRef]
11. Gligorov, J.; Lotz, J.P. Preclinical pharmacology of the taxanes: Implications of the differences. *Oncologist* **2004**, *9* (Suppl. 2), 3–8. [CrossRef]
12. Sharma, S.; Verma, A.; Teja, B.V.; Shukla, P.; Mishra, P.R. Development of stabilized Paclitaxel nanocrystals: In-vitro and in-vivo efficacy studies. *Eur. J. Pharm. Sci.* **2015**, *69*, 51–60. [CrossRef] [PubMed]
13. Baek, J.S.; Cho, C.W. Controlled release and reversal of multidrug resistance by co-encapsulation of paclitaxel and verapamil in solid lipid nanoparticles. *Int. J. Pharm.* **2015**, *478*, 617–624. [CrossRef] [PubMed]
14. Sofias, A.M.; Dunne, M.; Storm, G.; Allen, C. The battle of "nano" paclitaxel. *Adv. Drug Deliv. Rev.* **2017**, *122*, 20–30. [CrossRef] [PubMed]
15. Kim, C.H.; Lee, S.G.; Kang, M.J.; Lee, S.; Choi, Y.W. Surface modification of lipid-based nanocarriers for cancer cell-specific drug targeting. *J. Pharm. Investig.* **2017**, *47*, 203–227. [CrossRef]
16. Pardeike, J.; Hommoss, A.; Muller, R.H. Lipid nanoparticles (SLN, NLC) in cosmetic and pharmaceutical dermal products. *Int. J. Pharm.* **2009**, *366*, 170–184. [CrossRef] [PubMed]
17. Joshi, M.D.; Muller, R.H. Lipid nanoparticles for parenteral delivery of actives. *Eur. J. Pharm. Biopharm.* **2009**, *71*, 161–172. [CrossRef]
18. Gupta, B.; Yong, C.S.; Kim, J.O. Solid matrix-based lipid nanoplatforms as carriers for combinational therapeutics in cancer. *J. Pharm. Investig.* **2017**, *47*, 461–473. [CrossRef]
19. Emami, J.; Rezazadeh, M.; Varshosaz, J.; Tabbakhian, M.; Aslani, A. Formulation of LDL targeted nanostructured lipid carriers loaded with paclitaxel: A detailed study of preparation, freeze drying condition, and in vitro cytotoxicity. *J. Nanomater.* **2012**, *2012*, 1–10. [CrossRef]
20. Zolnik, B.S.; Gonzalez-Fernandez, A.; Sadrieh, N.; Dobrovolskaia, M.A. Nanoparticles and the immune system. *Endocrinology* **2010**, *151*, 458–465. [CrossRef]
21. Le, Q.-V.; Choi, J.; Oh, Y.-K. Nano delivery systems and cancer immunotherapy. *J. Pharm. Investig.* **2018**, *48*, 527–539. [CrossRef]
22. Rao, L.; Bu, L.-L.; Meng, Q.-F.; Cai, B.; Deng, W.-W.; Li, A.; Li, K.; Guo, S.-S.; Zhang, W.-F.; Liu, W.; et al. Antitumor Platelet-Mimicking Magnetic Nanoparticles. *Adv. Funct. Mater.* **2017**, *27*, 1604774. [CrossRef]
23. Hu, H.; Liu, D.; Zhao, X.; Qiao, M.; Chen, D. Preparation, characterization, cellular uptake and evaluation in vivo of solid lipid nanoparticles loaded with cucurbitacin B. *Drug Dev. Ind. Pharm.* **2013**, *39*, 770–779. [CrossRef] [PubMed]
24. Borsig, L.; Wong, R.; Feramisco, J.; Nadeau, D.R.; Varki, N.M.; Varki, A. Heparin and cancer revisited: Mechanistic connections involving platelets, P-selectin, carcinoma mucins, and tumor metastasis. *Proc. Natl. Acad. Sci. USA* **2001**, *98*, 3352–3357. [CrossRef] [PubMed]
25. Labelle, M.; Begum, S.; Hynes, R.O. Platelets guide the formation of early metastatic niches. *Proc. Natl. Acad. Sci. USA* **2014**, *111*, E3053–3061. [CrossRef] [PubMed]
26. Goubran, H.A.; Stakiw, J.; Radosevic, M.; Burnouf, T. Platelet-cancer interactions. *Semin. Thromb. Hemost.* **2014**, *40*, 296–305. [PubMed]
27. Hu, C.M.; Fang, R.H.; Wang, K.C.; Luk, B.T.; Thamphiwatana, S.; Dehaini, D.; Nguyen, P.; Angsantikul, P.; Wen, C.H.; Kroll, A.V.; et al. Nanoparticle biointerfacing by platelet membrane cloaking. *Nature* **2015**, *526*, 118–121. [CrossRef]

28. Hu, Q.; Sun, W.; Qian, C.; Wang, C.; Bomba, H.N.; Gu, Z. Anticancer Platelet-Mimicking Nanovehicles. *Adv. Mater.* **2015**, *27*, 7043–7050. [CrossRef]
29. Shete, H.; Patravale, V. Long chain lipid based tamoxifen NLC. Part I: Preformulation studies, formulation development and physicochemical characterization. *Int. J. Pharm.* **2013**, *454*, 573–583. [CrossRef]
30. Donovan, L.E.; Dammer, E.B.; Duong, D.M.; Hanfelt, J.J.; Levey, A.I.; Seyfried, N.T.; Lah, J.J. Exploring the potential of the platelet membrane proteome as a source of peripheral biomarkers for alzheimer's disease. *Alzheimer Res. Ther.* **2013**, *5*, 32. [CrossRef]
31. Honary, S.; Zahir, F. Effect of Zeta Potential on the Properties of Nano-Drug Delivery Systems—A Review (Part 1). *Trop. J. Pharm. Res.* **2013**, *12*, 255–264.
32. Olerile, L.D.; Liu, Y.; Zhang, B.; Wang, T.; Mu, S.; Zhang, J.; Selotlegeng, L.; Zhang, N. Near-infrared mediated quantum dots and paclitaxel co-loaded nanostructured lipid carriers for cancer theragnostic. *Colloids Surf. B Biointerfaces* **2017**, *150*, 121–130. [CrossRef] [PubMed]
33. Wei, X.; Ying, M.; Dehaini, D.; Su, Y.; Kroll, A.V.; Zhou, J.; Gao, W.; Fang, R.H.; Chien, S.; Zhang, L. Nanoparticle functionalization with platelet membrane enables multifactored biological targeting and detection of atherosclerosis. *ACS Nano* **2018**, *12*, 109–116. [CrossRef] [PubMed]
34. Demetzos, C. Differential Scanning Calorimetry (DSC): A tool to study the thermal behavior of lipid bilayers and liposomal stability. *J. Liposome Res.* **2008**, *18*, 159–173. [CrossRef] [PubMed]
35. Shen, J.; Bi, J.; Tian, H.; Jin, Y.; Wang, Y.; Yang, X.; Yang, Z.; Kou, J.; Li, F. Preparation and evaluation of a self-nanoemulsifying drug delivery system loaded with Akebia saponin D-phospholipid complex. *Int. J. Nanomed.* **2016**, *11*, 4919–4929.
36. Kassem, A.A.; Abd El-Alim, S.H.; Basha, M.; Salama, A. Phospholipid complex enriched micelles: A novel drug delivery approach for promoting the antidiabetic effect of repaglinide. *Eur. J. Pharm. Sci.* **2017**, *99*, 75–84. [CrossRef]
37. Tao, L.; Jiang, J.; Gao, Y.; Wu, C.; Liu, Y. Biodegradable Alginate-Chitosan Hollow Nanospheres for Codelivery of Doxorubicin and Paclitaxel for the Effect of Human Lung Cancer A549 Cells. *Biomed. Res. Int.* **2018**, 4607945. [CrossRef]
38. Xu, J.; He, F.; Gai, S.; Zhang, S.; Li, L.; Yang, P. Nitrogen-enriched, double-shelled carbon/layered double hydroxide hollow microspheres for excellent electrochemical performance. *Nanoscale* **2014**, *6*, 10887–10895. [CrossRef]
39. Bao, H.; Wang, L.; Li, C.; Luo, J. Structural Characterization and Identification of Graphdiyne and Graphdiyne-Based Materials. *ACS Appl. Mater. Interfaces* **2018**, *11*, 2717–2729. [CrossRef]
40. Dehaini, D.; Wei, X.; Fang, R.H.; Masson, S.; Angsantikul, P.; Luk, B.T.; Zhang, Y.; Ying, M.; Jiang, Y.; Kroll, A.V.; et al. Erythrocyte-platelet hybrid membrane coating for enhanced nanoparticle functionalization. *Adv. Mater.* **2017**, *29*, 1606209. [CrossRef]
41. Danhier, F.; Vroman, B.; Lecouturier, N.; Crokart, N.; Pourcelle, V.; Freichels, H.; Jerome, C.; Marchand-Brynaert, J.; Feron, O.; Preat, V. Targeting of tumor endothelium by RGD-grafted PLGA-nanoparticles loaded with paclitaxel. *J. Control. Release* **2009**, *140*, 166–173. [CrossRef] [PubMed]
42. Gao, W.; Chen, Y.; Thompson, D.H.; Park, K.; Li, T. Impact of surfactant treatment of paclitaxel nanocrystals on biodistribution and tumor accumulation in tumor-bearing mice. *J. Control. Release* **2016**, *237*, 168–176. [CrossRef] [PubMed]
43. Jia, Y.; Ji, J.; Wang, F.; Shi, L.; Yu, J.; Wang, D. Formulation, characterization, and in vitro/vivo studies of aclacinomycin A-loaded solid lipid nanoparticles. *Drug Deliv.* **2016**, *23*, 1317–1325. [PubMed]
44. Grozovsky, R.; Hoffmeister, K.M.; Falet, H. Novel clearance mechanisms of platelets. *Curr. Opin. Hematol.* **2010**, *17*, 585–589. [CrossRef] [PubMed]
45. Kobayashi, H.; Watanabe, R.; Choyke, P.L. Improving conventional enhanced permeability and retention (EPR) Effects; What is the appropriate target? *Theranostics* **2014**, *4*, 81–89. [CrossRef] [PubMed]
46. Lu, Y.; Wang, Z.H.; Li, T.; McNally, H.; Park, K.; Sturek, M. Development and evaluation of transferrin-stabilized paclitaxel nanocrystal formulation. *J. Control. Release* **2014**, *176*, 76–85. [CrossRef]
47. Son, G.H.; Na, Y.G.; Huh, H.W.; Wang, M.; Kim, M.K.; Han, M.G.; Byeon, J.J.; Lee, H.K.; Cho, C.W. Systemic design and evaluation of ticagrelor-loaded nanostructured lipid carriers for enhancing bioavailability and antiplatelet activity. *Pharmaceutics* **2019**, *11*. [CrossRef]
48. Patel, K.; Padhye, S.; Nagarsenker, M. Duloxetine HCl lipid nanoparticles: Preparation, characterization, and dosage form design. *AAPS PharmSciTech* **2012**, *13*, 125–133. [CrossRef]

49. Wei, X.; Gao, J.; Fang, R.H.; Luk, B.T.; Kroll, A.V.; Dehaini, D.; Zhou, J.; Kim, H.W.; Gao, W.; Lu, W.; et al. Nanoparticles camouflaged in platelet membrane coating as an antibody decoy for the treatment of immune thrombocytopenia. *Biomaterials* **2016**, *111*, 116–123. [CrossRef]
50. He, Y.; Li, R.; Liang, J.; Zhu, Y.; Zhang, S.; Zheng, Z.; Qin, J.; Pang, Z.; Wang, J. Drug targeting through platelet membrane-coated nanoparticles for the treatment of rheumatoid arthritis. *Nano Res.* **2018**, *11*, 6086–6101. [CrossRef]
51. Asadi, J.; Ferguson, S.; Raja, H.; Hacker, C.; Marius, P.; Ward, R.; Pliotas, C.; Naismith, J.; Lucocq, J. Enhanced imaging of lipid rich nanoparticles embedded in methylcellulose films for transmission electron microscopy using mixtures of heavy metals. *Micron* **2017**, *99*, 40–48. [CrossRef] [PubMed]
52. Takagi, S.; Sato, S.; Oh-hara, T.; Takami, M.; Koike, S.; Fujita, N. Platelets promote tumor growth and metastasis via direct interaction between Aggrus/podoplanin and CLEC-2. *PLoS ONE* **2013**, *8*, e73609. [CrossRef] [PubMed]
53. Lou, X.L.; Sun, J.; Gong, S.Q.; Yu, X.F.; Gong, R.; Deng, H. Interaction between circulating cancer cells and platelets: Clinical implication. *Chinese J. Cancer Res.* **2015**, *27*, 450–460.
54. Bobek, V.; Kovarik, J. Antitumor and antimetastatic effect of warfarin and heparins. *Biomed. Pharmacother.* **2004**, *58*, 213–219. [CrossRef] [PubMed]
55. Smorenburg, S.M.; Van Noorden, C.J. The complex effects of heparins on cancer progression and metastasis in experimental studies. *Pharmacol. Rev.* **2001**, *53*, 93–105. [PubMed]

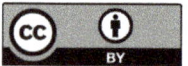

© 2019 by the authors. Licensee MDPI, Basel, Switzerland. This article is an open access article distributed under the terms and conditions of the Creative Commons Attribution (CC BY) license (http://creativecommons.org/licenses/by/4.0/).

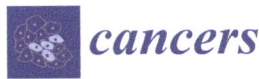

Article

A Multifunctional Graphene Oxide Platform for Targeting Cancer

Nikola Bugárová [1,*], Zdenko Špitálsky [1], Matej Mičušík [1], Michal Bodík [2], Peter Šiffalovič [2], Martina Koneracká [3], Vlasta Závišová [3], Martina Kubovčíková [3], Ivana Kajanová [4], Miriam Zaťovičová [4], Silvia Pastoreková [4], Miroslav Šlouf [5], Eva Majková [2] and Mária Omastová [1,*]

1. Polymer Institute, SAS, Dúbravská cesta 9, 845 41 Bratislava, Slovakia; zdeno.spitalsky@savba.sk (Z.Š.); matej.micusik@savba.sk (M.M.)
2. Institute of Physics, SAS, Dúbravská cesta 9, 845 11 Bratislava, Slovakia; michal.bodik@savba.sk (M.B.); peter.siffalovic@savba.sk (P.Š.); eva.majkova@savba.sk (E.M.)
3. Institute of Experimental Physics, SAS, Watsonova 47, 040 01 Košice, Slovakia; konerack@saske.sk (M.K.); zavisova@saske.sk (V.Z.); kubovcikova@saske.sk (M.K.)
4. Institute of Virology, Biomedical Research Center, SAS, Dúbravská cesta 9, 845 11 Bratislava, Slovakia; viruivvi@savba.sk (I.K.); viruzato@savba.sk (M.Z.); virusipa@savba.sk (S.P.)
5. Institute of Macromolecular Chemistry AS CR, Heyrovského nám. 2, 162 06 Prague 6, Czech Republic; slouf@imc.cas.cz
* Correspondence: nikola.bugarova@savba.sk (N.B.); maria.omastova@savba.sk (M.O.)

Received: 10 April 2019; Accepted: 25 May 2019; Published: 29 May 2019

Abstract: Diagnosis of oncological diseases remains at the forefront of current medical research. Carbonic Anhydrase IX (CA IX) is a cell surface hypoxia-inducible enzyme functionally involved in adaptation to acidosis that is expressed in aggressive tumors; hence, it can be used as a tumor biomarker. Herein, we propose a nanoscale graphene oxide (GO) platform functionalized with magnetic nanoparticles and a monoclonal antibody specific to the CA IX marker. The GO platforms were prepared by a modified Hummers and Offeman method from exfoliated graphite after several centrifugation and ultrasonication cycles. The magnetic nanoparticles were prepared by a chemical precipitation method and subsequently modified. Basic characterization of GO, such as the degree of oxidation, nanoparticle size and exfoliation, were determined by physical and chemical analysis, including X-ray photoelectron spectroscopy (XPS), transmission electron microscopy (TEM), energy dispersive X-ray analysis (EDX), and atomic force microscopy (AFM). In addition, the size and properties of the poly-L-lysine-modified magnetic nanoparticles were characterized. The antibody specific to CA IX was linked via an amidic bond to the poly-L-lysine modified magnetic nanoparticles, which were conjugated to GO platform again via an amidic bond. The prepared GO-based platform with magnetic nanoparticles combined with a biosensing antibody element was used for a hypoxic cancer cell targeting study based on immunofluorescence.

Keywords: graphene oxide; magnetic nanoparticles; monoclonal antibodies; tumor targeting

1. Introduction

Recently, carbon-based nanoparticles have attracted a great amount of attention due to their interesting surface properties and ability to act as a platform for modification with various substances, including inorganic nanoparticles, drugs and ligands. Carbon nanotubes, quantum dots [1], nanoporous graphene [2], but mainly graphene and derivative graphene oxide [3], have frequently been used as new tools for targeting cancer. Graphene, with its numerous exceptional properties, has a wide range of applications in different fields, as has been described by a number of research groups [4–9].

Graphene, as a single atomic layer of graphite, was the first available two-dimensional crystal, with a large surface area and delocalized π electrons, and is hydrophobic, lipophilic [10] and a good electrical and thermal conductor [3,11,12]. Oxidized graphene, i.e., graphene oxide (GO), can be prepared in large quantities [13] through oxidation and exfoliation of bulk graphite, e.g., by a modified Hummers method [14]. GO, which is covered by oxygen functional groups, is hydrophilic, and the oxygen functional groups ensure its reactivity and covalent surface modification. GO contains oxygenated aliphatic regions (–OH) and (–O–) located above and below each layer, while the carboxylic groups are usually located at the edges of GO sheets. The hydrophilicity of GO is a useful property in bioapplications, and numerous different functionalizations with various molecules have been reported [15,16] for the use of modified GO in biosensors, drug carriers or tissue engineering. However, we should not forget about the possible cytotoxicity of GO, which was mentioned in vivo [17] and somewhat more in in vitro applications. Factors affecting the cytotoxic effects of GO have been described, such as the lateral dimension, the thickness of the nanolayers, the functional group, and especially the concentration [7,18–20].

In particular, the hydrophilic character of GO permits the production of reliable, highly sensitive and ultrafast targeted platforms. The size tunability of GO nanosheets from several microns down to less than 100 nm is also important for preparing GO nanosheets that are small enough to penetrate biological barriers, including those of tumor tissue [18,21]. This type of nanoparticle also enables the combination of diagnosis with therapy (theranostics) [22–24]. Photothermal therapy with a combination of treatments has resulted from the functionalization of GO with inorganic nanoparticles, other nanostructures or polymers to create composites [25,26]. The most widespread and facile method of functionalization is amidation. Shan et al. prepared modified GO with poly-L-lysine (PLL) through a covalent amide bond. The same bond used for functionalization of the gold electrode by PLL-functionalized GO [27]. The carboxylic acid groups (–COOH) of GO can interact with the amine groups of the nanostructures or nanoparticles that are being attached to create amide bonds. This process occurs in two steps in the presence of activators, namely, either 1-ethyl-3-(3-dimethylaminopropyl) carbodiimide (EDC) or N–ethyl–N'–(3–dimethylaminopropyl) carbodiimide hydrochloride (EDAC) and N–hydroxysuccinimide (NHS) [27–29]. The first step involves activation of the carboxyl group of GO and the formation of a stable active ester. The second step is a reaction between the active ester and an amine group on the attaching nanostructure, forming a covalent bond between GO and the nanoparticle [30]. Another important modification method is esterification. The esterification reaction involves a reaction between the –COOH groups localized on the edges of GO and CH_2OH–terminated functional groups. For example, the grafting of poly(3-hexylthiophene) (P3HT) onto the GO surface was performed by esterification [31].

The key role of a GO-linked modifier is its selective transportation to the target cell or tissue, where the compound can be preferentially administered. Spherical magnetite nanoparticles (MNps) prepared by a coprecipitation method with ferric and ferrous salts in an alkaline aqueous medium [32] have great potential for use in oncological medicine due to their biocompatibility and facile synthesis. They can easily be tuned and functionalized for specific applications [30,33–35]. MNps have been coated by an amino acid polymer, poly-L-lysine, to improve their biocompatibility [36,37]. The importance of the amino acid L-lysine lies in the fact that it helps in the production of antibodies, is utilized by numerous hormones and enzymes and is necessary for tissue repair.

The bioconjugation of nanoparticles to proteins is critically important for a number of applications in life science research, diagnostics, and therapeutics [38]. Antibody molecules possess a number of functional groups suitable for modification or conjugation purposes. Monoclonal antibodies (MAb), antibodies made by identical immune cells that are all clones of a unique parent cell, are able to react specifically with tumor-associated antigens [39]. Consequently, the presence of MAb can increase the targeting properties of graphene oxide platforms. In particular, MAb M75 recognizes a linear epitope region of the enzyme carbonic anhydrase IX (CA IX). This enzyme is frequently expressed in human carcinomas because of its strong induction by tumor hypoxia, and it is absent from the corresponding normal tissue [40,41]. CA IX facilitates survival of cancer cells in hostile tumor microenvironment and contributes to their metastatic propensity. Due to its epitope specificity to CA IX, MAb M75 does not exhibit any cross-reactivity with other known members of the carbonic anhydrase family, which all lack similar regions [42]. Antibody-labeled GO has been used to detect cancer or, more generally, to detect proteins. An antibody-GO complex was used as a recognition element, which enabled rapid screening of aflatoxin B_1 (AFB_1) in a lateral flow system; the anti-AFB_1 monoclonal antibody was prepared by Yu et al. [43]. Another study demonstrated the modification of screen-printed carbon electrodes by assembling graphene oxide to obtain electrochemical immunosensors with immobilized antibodies specific to mucin 1, which is a well-known tumor marker for a variety of malignant tumors [44]. Efforts to detect or target CA IX have been mostly focused on development of diverse nanoparticles decorated by inhibitors of Carbonic anhydrases with modifications conferring selectivity towards CA IX and/or other cell surface isoforms [45–48]. These approaches require access to active site of the enzyme, whereas the antibodies can bind CA IX even in an inactive state. In vitro tests were conducted at this stage of the research. Here we demonstrate that our approach, based on GO platforms decorated with MNps and M75 MAb can selectively bind cells expressing CA IX and thus can represent a promising tool for cancer imaging.

In this work, the preparation of a new type of GO-based platform containing magnetic nanoparticles and monoclonal antibodies is reported, with the aim of creating nanocarriers that are able to target hypoxia-inducing cancer cells. The combination of a MAb specific to CA IX and GO as a nanocarrier combined with magnetic nanoparticles is a novel and original approach for targeting CA IX-positive cancer cells. Magnetic nanoparticles immobilized with the MAb M75 were used and bound to the GO platform. These antibodies, which are specific to the hypoxia-induced extracellular enzyme CA IX, are one of the best intrinsic markers. The topology of the produced GO platform was examined using transmission electron microscopy (TEM) and atomic force microscopy (AFM), while its structure and surface properties were confirmed by X-ray photoelectron spectroscopy (XPS). AFM is a suitable technique rapidly screening the attached nanoparticles. As a result, the GO functionalization with poly-L-lysine-modified magnetic nanoparticles functionalized with MAb was validated by AFM. Additionally, TEM, immunofluorescence, viability, and flow cytometry tests were performed on the functionalized GO platforms.

2. Results

For our study, it was necessary to prepare GO platforms in the form of monolayers with particle sizes below 500 nm for further functionalization. The GO platforms were prepared by a modified Hummer and Offerman reaction. Obtained GO particles were washed with deionized water and hydrogen peroxide led to a brown suspension, and multiple cycles alternating between centrifugation and sonication were utilized. The centrifugation speed, duration, and number of cycles enabled the selection of different size distributions of the GO platforms. The purity and degree of GO oxidation were characterized by XPS method, while the morphologies and particle size of the GO platforms were examined by AFM and TEM.

2.1. Preparation and Functionalization of Graphene Oxide

X-ray photoelectron spectroscopy (XPS) was used to confirm the structural and chemical composition of the prepared graphene oxide platforms. First, the original graphite powder (G5) used for GO production was characterized. G5 showed only slight oxidation with no other contaminates on its surface (Table 1). GO product showed some traces of surface contamination by sulfur, potassium and chloride from the reaction procedure. Aluminum from the substrates was also detected since the samples for XPS measurements were prepared by drop casting a GO solution onto aluminum foil. Figure 1b clearly demonstrates the formation of carbon-oxygen bonds (C–O at ca 287 eV, C = O at ca 288 eV and OC = O at ca 289 eV) on the surface of the prepared GO, which was accessible for further modification. After modification with MNps and MAb C1s spectra of GO-MNps-MAb and

GO-EDC-MNps-MAb are not differ much from the original GO, which indicates that the surface of GO is not fully covered. This could be very important for further potential application as drug delivery since there is still space to attach various active substances on the GO platform.

Table 1. X-ray photoelectron spectroscopy analysis of graphite, GO and purified GO.

Sample	Surface Chemical Composition [at. %]					
	C1s	O1s	S2p	N1s	Fe2p	K 2s/Cl2p/Al2p/P2p/Si2s/Na1s/Br3d
Graphite G5	90.2	9.8	—	—	—	—/—/—/—/—/—/—
GO	61.7	33.7	1.9	0.9	—	0.5/0.4/1.0/—/—/—/—
MNPs	29.6	41.2	0.8	6.8	19.7	—/—/—/—/—/1.0/1.0
MNps-MAb	32.7	39.7	—	4.3	12.0	0.1/3.4/—/2.2/0.3/5.3/—
GO-MNps-MAb	69.2	26.6	0.6	1.0	0.2	—/0.6/1.4/—/0.1/0.3/—
GO-MNps-EDC-MAb	62.5	32.8	0.8	0.7	0.2	—/0.6/2.4/—/—/0.1/—
Purified GO	70.8	28.2	0.2	0.1	—	—/—/0.9/—/—/—/—

*XPS = X-ray photoelectron spectroscopy; G5 = Graphite powder; GO = graphene oxide; MNps = magnetic nanoparticles; MNps-MAb = magnetic nanoparticles modified antibodies; GO-MNps-MAb = graphene oxide platforms with magnetic nanoparticles modified antibodies; GO-MNps-EDC-MAb = graphene oxide platforms with magnetic nanoparticles modified antibodies in the presence of 1–ethyl-3–(3-dimethylaminopropyl) carbodiimide.

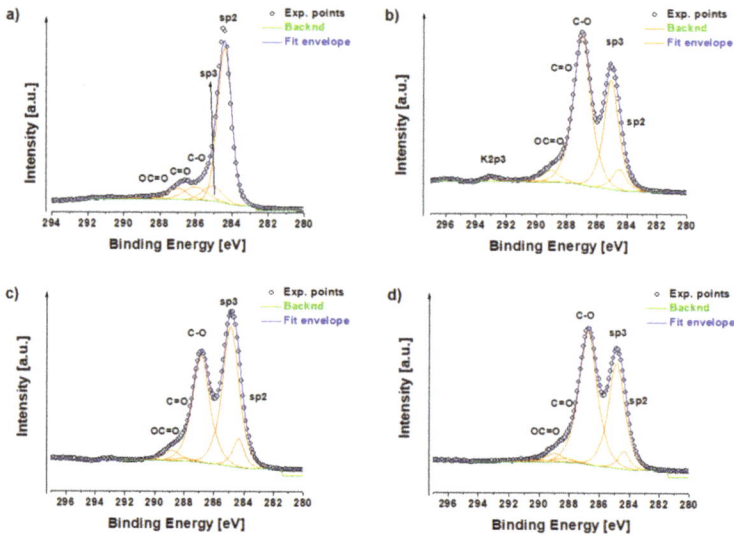

Figure 1. X-ray photoelectron spectroscopy C1s region spectra of (a) graphite powder; (b) graphene oxide; (c) graphene oxide platforms with magnetic nanoparticles modified antibodies (GO-MNps-MAb) and (d) graphene oxide platforms with magnetic nanoparticles modified antibodies in the presence of 1–ethyl-3–(3-dimethylaminopropyl) carbodiimide (GO-MNps-EDC-MAb).

We have discussed the surface chemistry of modified iron nanoparticles in a previous paper [36]. Fe_3O_4 can be written as Fe_2O_3:FeO (Fe III: Fe II) in a 2:1 ratio and exhibits contributions of these two iron valence states [49]. Fe_2O_3 possesses satellite features at ca. 719 eV and FeO at ca. 716 eV. In Fe_3O_4 the satellite feature is not visibly resolved because of the contributions of both of them (Fe III, Fe II) [50]. Figure 2a shows the comparison of the Fe2p region of MNps (Fe_3O_4-PLL), MNps-MAb, GO-MNps-MAb and GO-EDC-MNps-MAb. In the case of MNps there is a clearly visible Fe III satellite peak at ca. 719 eV, what indicates a Fe^{3+}-rich surface. After MAb modification the Fe2p spectrum remained almost the same, with a similar Fe^{3+}-rich surface. This implies that the MAb is binding through the PLL on the surface of MNps. When attached to the surface of GO, Fe2p peaks exhibit in both cases (GO-MNps-MAb and GO-EDC-MNps-MAb) a strong signal at ca. 716 eV corresponding to the Fe II satellite. This indicates that MNps interact with GO platform through the iron oxide nanoparticles and that Fe^{3+} is interacting with GO resulting in a partial reduction of iron. As it was shown in [36] iron oxide nanoparticles are most probably interacting with the carboxylate groups of GO leading to the chemisorption of MNps onto the GO surface.

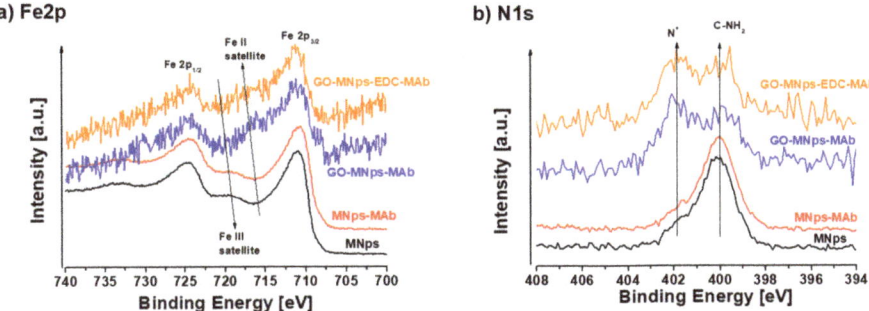

Figure 2. X-ray photoelectron spectroscopy of (**a**) Fe2p region and (**b**) of N1s region of magnetic nanoparticles (MNps), magnetic nanoparticles modified antibodies (MNps-MAb), graphene oxide platforms with magnetic nanoparticles modified antibodies (GO-MNps-MAb) and graphene oxide platforms with magnetic nanoparticles modified antibodies in the presence of 1–ethyl–3–(3–dimethylaminopropyl) carbodiimide (GO-MNps-EDC-MAb) (spectra are autoscaled).

In Figure 2b showing the N1s spectra, the detected signal at ca. 400 eV corresponds to C-N bonds like C-N-, C-NH-, C-NH$_2$ and the one at ca. 402 eV it corresponds to some quaternized nitrogen labeled as N$^+$ (XPS knowledge database of Avantage 5.9911, Thermo Fisher Scientific, Loughborough, UK). In the case of MNps it is a confirmation of PLL on the surface, there is almost no change after MAb attachment, but after attachment to the GO platform C–N and N$^+$ with some proportional increase of N$^+$ is still detected, indicating that the active NH$_3^+$ group of M75 is accessible on the surface.

After this surface chemistry study, we decided to try additional purification of the initial GO platform and get rid of the relatively high (ca 2 at. %) amount of sulfur (S2p peak centered at 168.9 eV corresponding to SO$_3$). This contamination comes from the sulfuric acid used during the GO preparation process. The presence of SO$_3$ could be detrimental for the biocompatibility [10]; therefore, in the next step, this contaminant was successfully removed. After further purification with H$_2$O$_2$ and deionized water, the sulfur content decreased from 1.9 to 0.2 at. % (Table 1), as is obvious from comparison of the S2p peaks in Figure 3. For further reactions this purified GO was used.

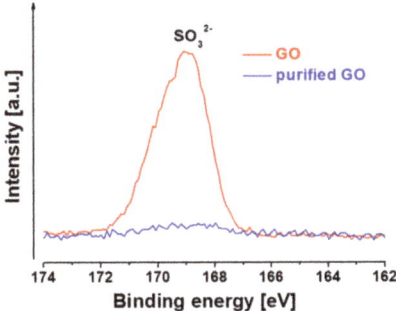

Figure 3. X-ray photoelectron spectroscopy S2p region spectra of graphene oxide (red) and purified graphene oxide (blue).

The samples for AFM measurements were deposited by a modified Langmuir–Schaefer deposition method to obtain a thin monolayer film suitable for imaging. The preparation of a GO monolayer was described in our previous article [51,52]. A representative AFM image of the GO monolayer deposited on the Si substrate and the corresponding size distribution of the GO platforms are shown in Figure 4a,b, respectively. The prepared solution of GO was composed of approximately 90% GO monolayer platforms. The size distribution confirmed that 90% of all GO platforms had a lateral size smaller than 500 nm. The average lateral size of the GO platforms was 302 ± 183 nm. The heights analyzing of the AFM scan in Figure 4a is depicted in Figure 4c, showing the amount of monolayers and multilayers. The first peak at 1.81 nm with a peak width 0.67 nm corresponds to the substrate roughness value. The peak of monolayers is located at 2.95 nm with a peak width of 0.78 nm. The bilayers are detected at 4 nm with a width of 0.82 nm, so they are again 1 nm higher. The amount of trilayers is very small. Peak area for monolayers is 0.67863 nm^2 and 0.05997 nm^2 for bilayers, respectively. This analysis indicated that monolayers represent 91.8% in the prepared unmodified GO solution.

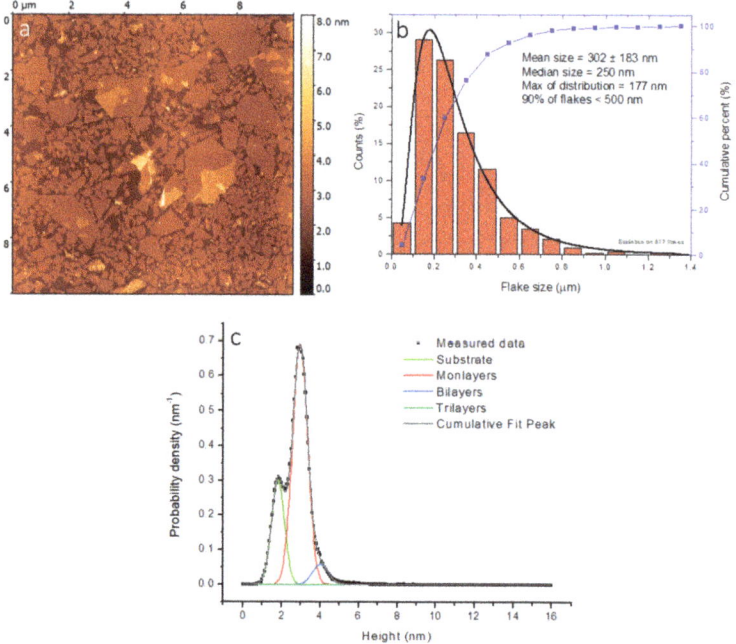

Figure 4. Purified graphene oxide: (**a**) atomic force microscopy (AFM) image, (**b**) size distribution of the graphene oxide platforms and (**c**) height analysis of AFM scan. The analysis of AFM scans was done by program Gwyddion [52] The size distribution was obtained manually.

The stability of purified GO was examined by Zeta potential, with the results shown in Table 2. The general dividing line between a stable and non-stable suspension is usually taken as 30 or −30 mV and particles that have zeta potentials outside these limits are normally considered stable. According to values above ±30 mV, the sample is considered stable [53,54]. In the case of GO prepared by us, it is stable in the pH range of 4–11.

Table 2. Zeta potential analysis of purified graphene oxide.

pH	2	3	4	5	6,5	8	9	10	11
GO	−12	−15.8	−39.3	−35.3	−41.3	−46.3	−44.4	−42.8	−44.9

The GO prepared and purified of the sulfur residues was modified by MNps in the next step. The reaction described in the experimental section formed amide bonds between the hydroxyl groups of the GO surface and the amine groups of the poly-L-lysine shell on the MNps in the presence of EDC and sulfo-NHS. Hermanson has extensively reviewed the use of zero-length cross-linkers, to which EDC, NHS, and sulfo-NHS belong [55]. Their universal application to the conjugation of nanoparticles and biological substances has widely been used in a variety of systems. The conjugation of the GO platforms containing carboxylate groups with the MNps containing amine groups was thoroughly examined. Several reaction pathways were followed to determine the optimum ratio of GO, MNps, EDC and sulfo-NHS. Generally, EDC reacts with the carboxylates on the GO surface to form O-acylisourea as an intermediate reactive ester. The active EDC ester reacts with sulfo-NHS to form a sulfo-NHS ester intermediate, which rapidly reacts with the amines located on the MNps. We chose sulfo-NHS due to its hydrophilic properties and better reaction yield compared to that for the EDC linker alone [55].

Initial reactions to verify the correct ratio of the binding linkers to GO as well as the ratio of GO to nanoparticles were performed on poly-L-lysine modified MNps. The ratio of GO:MNps was varied from 1:1 to 10:1. The formation of amide bonds between the hydroxyl groups of GO and the amino groups of poly-L-lysine on the MNps ensured that only unbound platforms were removed by washing with deionized water, while a magnet was set up. Bound MNps on the GO remained loosely dispersed in solution after washing. AFM was used for screening the GO surface modification with the MNps. At a high 1:1 ratio of GO:MNps, large MNps agglomerates were found on the GO surface. At a ratio of 10:1, a number of the GO platforms remained unmodified in suspension. Experimentally, the optimal ratio was 3:1. Figure 5 shows the evidence for the MNps on the GO platforms on the Si substrate for the abovementioned ratio of 3:1. The same ratio of 3:1 was used to functionalize the GO platform with MNps modified with MAb. The MNps modified with MAb were prepared in solution with and without the EDC binding agent.

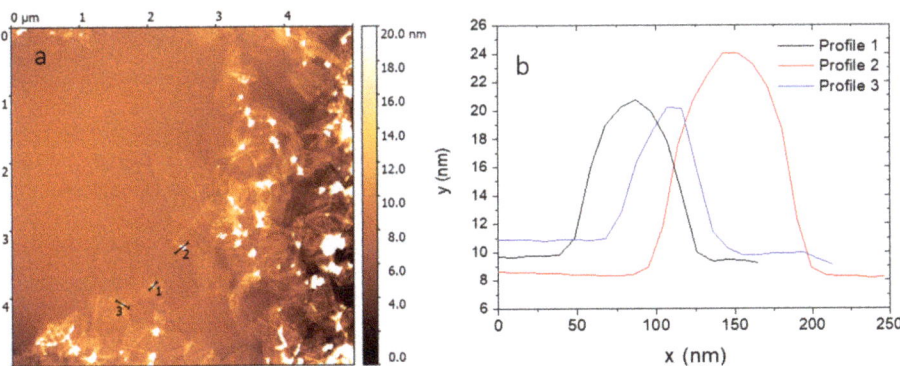

Figure 5. Modified graphene oxide platforms by magnetic nanoparticles: (**a**) atomic force microscopy (AFM) image, and (**b**) selected height profiles across the magnetic nanoparticles.

2.2. Synthesis of Modified GO with MNps and MAb

The GO functionalized platform was studied by TEM, but the initial elemental composition and crystalline structure of the prepared MNps were verified by the same method. The particles were visualized by bright field imaging (Figure 6a). Their selected area electron diffraction pattern (SAED, Figure 6a, upper left corner) was converted into a 1D-pattern and compared with the calculated powder X-ray diffraction pattern of magnetite (PXRD, Figure 6b). The perfect agreement between the experimental SAED pattern and the theoretical magnetite PXRD pattern proved that the prepared nanoparticles exhibited a magnetite structure (Figure 6b). This was further confirmed by the energy dispersive X-ray analysis (EDX) spectra (Figure 6c), which contained only the peaks corresponding to the supporting carbon-coated copper grid (peaks of C and Cu) and the peaks corresponding to the prepared iron oxide nanoparticles (peaks of Fe and O).

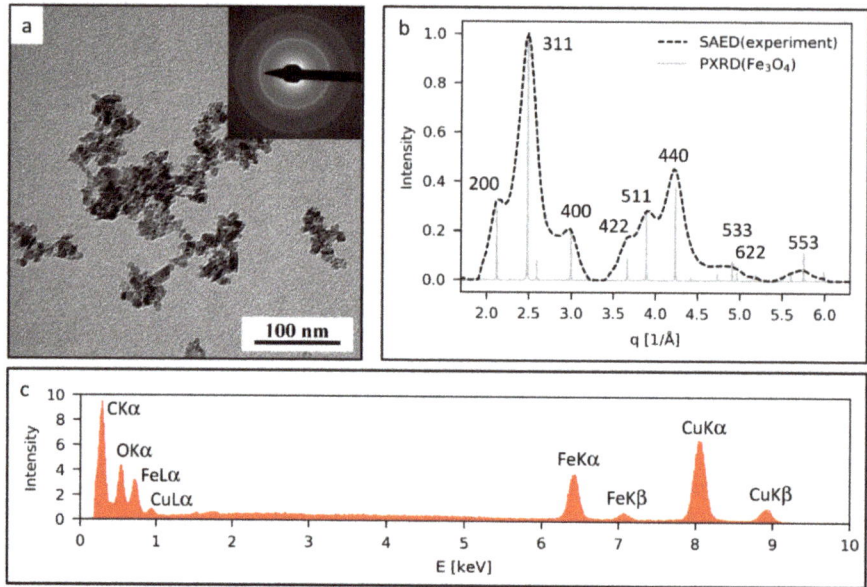

Figure 6. Transmission electron microscopy (TEM) analysis of the prepared magnetic nanoparticles (MNps): (**a**) TEM micrograph with corresponding selected area electron diffraction pattern (TEM/SAED) diffraction pattern, (**b**) comparison of the experimental TEM/SAED diffraction pattern with the theoretically calculated diffraction pattern of magnetite and (**c**) the energy dispersive X-ray analysis (TEM/EDX) spectrum of the MNps.

The morphology of purified GO was examined by transmission electron microscopy (TEM). The representative micrographs of the purified GO in Figure 7a,b show a smooth platform surface with occasional folds. Functionalization of the platforms by magnetic nanoparticles could be clearly observed in the TEM images due to the high contrast of the attached nanoparticles, as illustrated in Figure 7c,d. Notably, some of the visualized platforms were quite large, with sizes >500 nm. The existence of these large platforms was in agreement with the AFM results (Figure 4). However, the majority of the nanoparticles exhibited dimensions well below 500 nm.

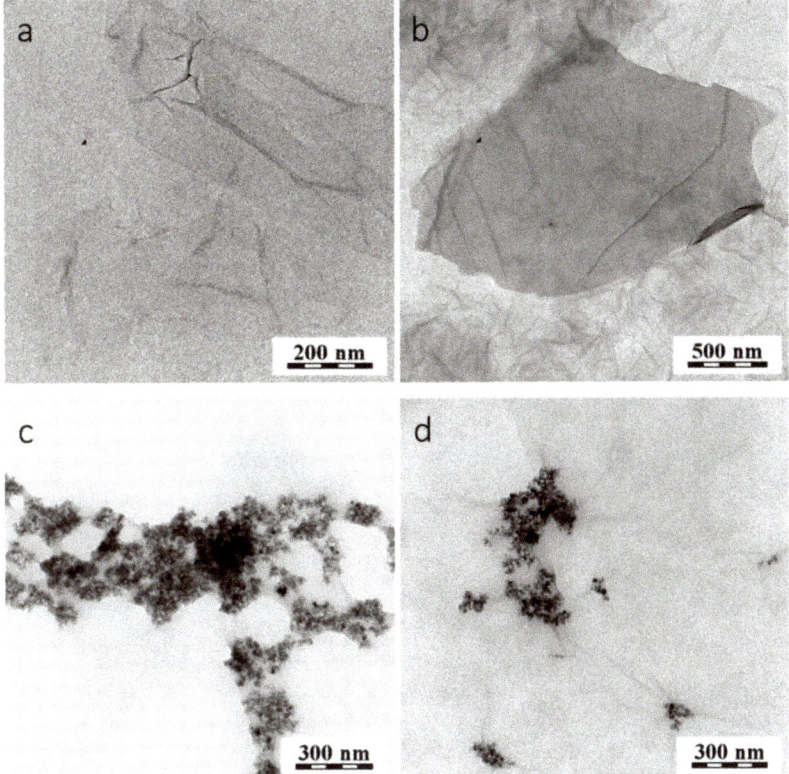

Figure 7. Transmission electron microscopy (TEM) micrographs of the (**a**,**b**) pure GO platforms; (**c**) graphene oxide platforms with magnetic nanoparticles modified antibodies (GO-MNps-MAb), and (**d**) graphene oxide platforms with magnetic nanoparticles modified antibodies in the presence of 1–ethyl–3–(3–dimethylaminopropyl) carbodiimide (GO-MNps-EDC-MAb).

Magnetic nanoparticles with MAbs were prepared with and without the EDC coupling agent. The sample of conjugated nanoparticles prepared by reaction with EDC was labeled MNps-EDC-MAb, and the sample without the EDC binding agent was labeled MNps-MAb. The hydrodynamic size (100 nm) of the MNps without the MAbs can serve as a guide for locating the MNps. During GO modification, aggregates of the MNps were formed. In Figure 6c, comparatively more aggregates were present when compared with the platform shown in Figure 6d. Spherical MNps with a diameter of approximately 30–40 nm after being coating with poly-L-lysine resulted in smaller aggregates with fewer particles only in the case of GO-MNps-EDC-MAb. Notably, the MNps with MAbs were bound to the GO surface and remained attached to the surface even after several purification reactions.

2.3. Cell Viability Assay

Before all experiments with conjugation of magnetic nanoparticles and monoclonal antibodies to GO were done, a viability assay of cell lines in the environment with GO was performed during 5 days, as described in previous work [56], where application of GO as a low-toxicity platform for the next functionalization and was demonstrated.

To control the toxicity of the prepared GO-platform functionalized with MNps and MAbs specific to CA IX, viability tests were performed to estimate the cytotoxicity or cytostatic effects. Pure medium without GO-MNps-MAb and GO-MNps-EDC-MAb was used as a control for both cell type and each sample type. The cell line B16 CA IX was B16-F0 mouse melanoma cells permanently transfected with the full-length CA IX cDNA. The mock-transfected cells, meaning without the CA IX enzyme, is labelled as B16-neo. The charts in Figure 8 show the results obtained during the five-day toxicity measurement with standard deviations. All experiments were performed in triplicates. Effect of the GO-MNps-MAb and GO-MNps-EDC-MAb on cell viability of cancer cell line B16-F0 at various periods of incubation was evaluated by CellTiter-Blue assay (CTB, Promega, Madison, WI, USA). First measurement was performed immediately after the establishment of the cell culture. The CTB fluorescence value of the control cells measured at the start of the experiment was set as 1. The CTB values of treated B16-neo and B16 CA IX cells were normalized to the non-treated control. Fluorescence measurement was performed after incubating for 24, 48, 72, and 120 h.

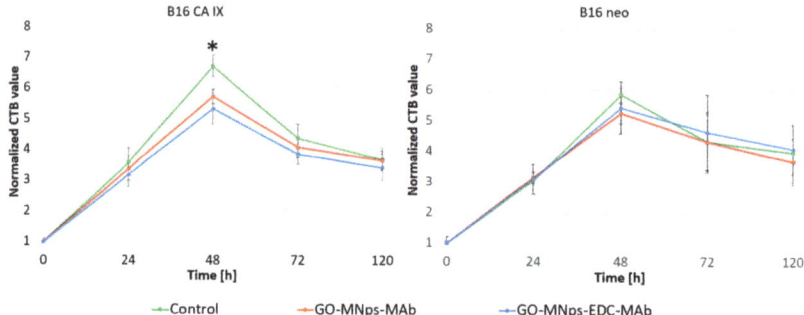

Figure 8. Viability testing of graphene oxide platforms with magnetic nanoparticles modified antibodies (GO-MNps-MAb) and graphene oxide platforms with magnetic nanoparticles modified antibodies in the presence of 1–ethyl–3–(3–dimethylaminopropyl) carbodiimide (GO-MNps-EDC-MAb) was performed on mouse melanoma cells (B16). Cell line was permanently transfected with full-length carbonic anhydrase IX (CA IX) cDNA. Control cell line was used (neo) without transfected CA IX cDNA. A significant difference in viability of B16 CA IX cells between the control and samples after 48 h cultivation is marked by *.

According to the trends indicated by the controls in B16-neo cell line, there was no cytotoxicity from the GO-MNps-MAb and GO-MNps-EDC-MAb in comparison to the control sample. The apparent behavior similarity of B16-F0 cells with CA IX and B16-neo cells without CA IX enzyme is the implication that both cell types come from a single cell line. But there is slight cytostatic effect specific only to B16 cells with CA IX (B16 CA IX) from both functionalized GO platforms (GO-MNps-MAb and GO-MNps-EDC-MAb), detected with the reduced trend at the graph in comparison to the control sample. This was also confirmed by statistical analysis using the Student's t-test, where a significant difference between control and samples was obtained for a B16 CA IX cells after 48 h. However, this finding can be seen as a positive result or added value. Prepared platforms have the task of specifically targeting cells, which is also indirectly confirmed in this case. By looking at the significant difference in cells with CA IX enzyme and we do not observe this difference for neo cells, it is possible to speak about specific uptake/binding of functionalized platform to cells even in viability assay.

2.4. Immunofluorescence Assay

The immunofluorescence assay can confirm the presence of modified GO platforms and bound magnetic nanoparticles with antibodies in cells. Besides that, the immunofluorescence indirectly validated the binding of the MNps with MAbs onto the GO. The GO itself is not able to produce the green fluorescence of a positive response. The positive signal was due to the secondary anti-mouse Alexa Fluor® 488 antibody (Thermo Fisher Scientific, Loughborough, UK) bound to MAb M75. The MAb is specific to extracellular antigen CA IX, and free antibody M75 is not able to internalize into the cells at 37 °C [40].

In order to verify the specific binding of the modified GO platform, the B16 CA IX cells and no enzyme B16-neo were used for the assay. Cells without enzyme CA IX represent the negative control. There were differences between the neo cells and the cells expressing CA IX. In the negative control (B16-neo cells) in either case of exposure to samples (GO-MNps-MAb and GO-MNps-EDC-MAb) with secondary antibody, no or only a minimal signal at 488 nm was observed. In contrast, B16 CA IX cells, contain sufficient secondary antibody signal in both cases (Figure 9a,c) around their nuclei. This signifies a specific binding of the primary antibody with magnetic nanoparticles bound to GO platform to cells with CA IX. For cells exposed to the GO-MNps-MAb sample in Figure 9a, green signal aggregates were observed at multiple places. In the case of the GO-MNps-EDC-MAb sample, smaller aggregates were observed and also smaller points characterizing individual modified GO platforms could be identified. For this reason, the GO-MNps-EDC-MAb sample is presented with a two-fold approach as shown in Figure 9c,d. The GO-MNps-EDC-MAb sample, which was prepared in solution with the binding agent EDC, showed more intense fluorescence. These results were supported by another experiment that quantified the binding of functionalized GO platforms to live cells with CA IX enzyme. Figure 9 shows a positive signal detected on the surface of as well as in the cells. This evidence for cellular internalization of functionalized GO platforms (GO-MNps-MAb and GO-MNps-EDC-MAb) indicated an interesting phenomenon. While the free antibodies could not penetrate the cell membranes, the antibodies conjugated to the MNps and GO could pass through the membranes and accumulate within the cells. The described phenomenon would be helpful in later studies on drug uptake in certain cell types and intracellular localization.

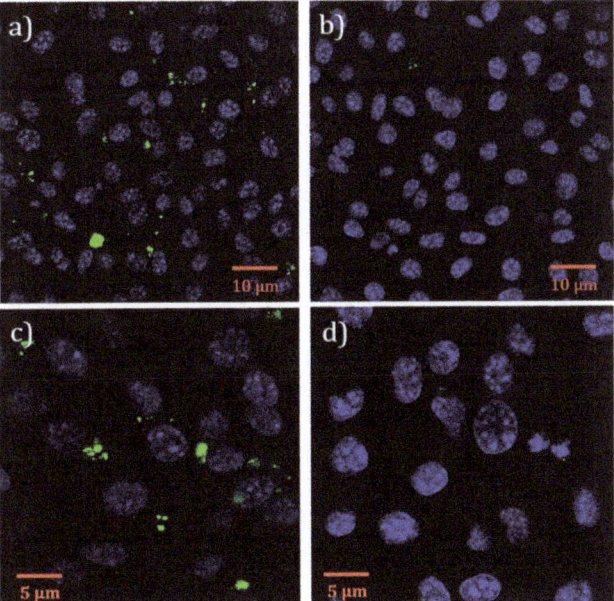

Figure 9. Immunofluorescence of graphene oxide platforms with magnetic nanoparticles modified antibodies (GO-MNps-MAb) into the B16 cells. Sample GO-MNps-MAb was examined in (**a**) B16 cells with carbonic anhydrase IX (CA IX) and (**b**) B16-neo cells without CA IX. Sample with the binding agent graphene oxide platforms with magnetic nanoparticles modified antibodies in the presence of 1–ethyl–3–(3–dimethylaminopropyl) carbodiimide (GO-MNps-EDC-MAb) were examined in the same cell types: (**c**) B16 CA IX and (**d**) B16-neo cells.

2.5. Flow Cytometry

Using flow cytometry it is possible to quantify the specific binding of functionalized GO platform to carbonic anhydrase IX. The measured cell line was MDCK line with (MDCK CA IX) and without (MDCK neo) CA IX enzyme. Table 3 presents results of binding for negative controls and samples. There were done two negative controls. Unmodified GO platforms in the first row and cells labeled only with secondary antibody anti-mouse Alexa Fluor® 488 (marked as A488, Thermo Fisher Scientific, Loughborough, UK) in the second row of the table.

Table 3. Flow cytometry analysis of specific binding to CA IX cells.

No.	Sample	MDCK Cell Line	
		CA IX [%]	Neo [%]
1	GO, neg. control	1.12	1.43
2	A488, neg. control	0.10	0.03
3	GO-MNps-MAb	22.16	6.07
4	GO-MNps-EDC-MAb	48.63	6.01

MDCK = Madin-Darby Canine Kidney cells; CA IX = cells with carbonic anhydrase IX; Neo = cells without carbonic anhydrase IX; GO = graphene oxide; A488 = Alexa Fluor® 488; GO-MNps-MAb = graphene oxide platforms with magnetic nanoparticles modified antibodies; GO-MNps-EDC-MAb = graphene oxide platforms with magnetic nanoparticles modified antibodies in the presence of 1–ethyl–3–(3–dimethylaminopropyl) carbodiimide.

As shown in line 2 in Table 3, the anti-mouse antibody alone did not demonstrate cell binding. From the results in row 1 in Table 3, there is proof of interaction between GO and fluorescent labeled anti-mouse antibody. If there is some low interaction between GO and secondary anti-mouse antibody Alexa Fluor® 488, nevertheless it is not able to produce non-specific binding to any cell line, what is shown by low presence of GO as negative control in cells. The examined samples were functionalized GO platforms with magnetic nanoparticles modified antibodies, designated GO-MNps-MAb and GO-MNps-EDC-MAb. The difference between these samples is in the preparation of modified nanoparticles with monoclonal antibodies. In the GO-MNps-MAb sample, the EDC binding agent was not used for modification, as opposed to the GO-MNps-EDC-MAb sample, which has so far shown better results. Otherwise, it was not even after a cytometric analysis that confirmed these findings. In Figure 10, graphs comparing both samples. The GO-MNps-EDC-MAb sample is more positive for MDCK CA IX cells, which corresponds to the shift to right on x-axis of the magenta-stained peak for MDCK CA IX cells. Also, the 4th row of the table correlates with the graph where 48% of all living cells in population contained at least one functionalized platform. In the case of MDCK neo cells, only 6% of the live cells were positive and contained at least one platform. This corresponds to the specific binding of the functionalized GO to CA IX-positive cells.

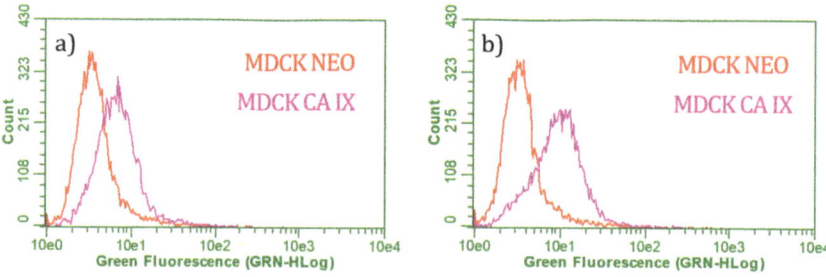

Figure 10. Cytometric analysis of (**a**) graphene oxide platforms with magnetic nanoparticles modified antibodies (GO-MNps-MAb) and (**b**) graphene oxide platforms with magnetic nanoparticles modified antibodies in the presence of 1–ethyl–3–(3–dimethylaminopropyl) carbodiimide (GO-MNps-EDC-MAb) samples.

The hydrophilic character and better reactivity caused by the oxygen-containing functional groups indicated the potential biological and medical use of GO in targeted therapy. Our study demonstrated the functionality of the prepared multifunctional GO platforms conjugated with MNps and MAb. The specificity of MAb to CA IX remained unchanged even after conjugation to the MNps, and the GO platform was targeted into the cancer cells. The results present a new possibility for the use of GO in cancer therapy with minimal side effects.

3. Discussion

Recent technological advances and new possibilities for the application of graphene-based sensors in biomedicine open up new possibilities for cancer detection. The intention was to use graphene oxide (GO) as a platform for developing a new type of a promising tool for cancer imaging. With the purpose of such functionalization, we have prepared GO platforms using a modified Hummer and Offerman reaction. A modified Hummer's method was used for example, for the preparation of nanographene, which was after PEGylation was used for the delivery of the insoluble camptothecin (CPT) analogue, SN38 [19,57]. Graphene oxide platforms were modified by magnetic nanoparticles and monoclonal antibodies. For this study, it was necessary to prepare GO platforms in the form of monolayers with particle sizes below 500 nm for further functionalization. Seabra et al. have reviewed the behaviour of GO in terms of cytotoxicity [19]. They described the relationship with its thickness (number of layers), size, concentration, time of exposure, method of functionalization, and it also depends on the cell line on which the GO toxicity is investigated. More times the comparison of graphene, GO and reduced GO is mentioned, when GO has the least toxicity due to its hydrophilic character caused by functional groups [17,19]. Likewise, GO with a surface containing COOH groups and NH_2 groups [58,59] have shown less toxicity than non-functionalized [19,57]. However, the GO toxicity phenomenon is still not sufficiently investigated and therefore the claims cannot be generalized. For this reason, we performed cytotoxicity tests on the B16-F0 cell line after functionalization, with no toxicity. GO modification with magnetic nanoparticles and a monoclonal antibody specific to the CA IX marker is new approach and combination of nanomaterials and antibody. The specificity of this MAbs for tumor cells plays an essential role in the preparation of a nanoparticle modified by magnetic nanoparticles and monoclonal antibodies. Differences between B16 CA IX cells and neo cells without CA IX enzyme confirm specific binding of functionalized GO platform to cancer marker cells. Targeting functionalized GO nanoparticles to tumor cells at this stage of research represents a vision of possibilities to visualize cancer cells in vitro for now and in vivo at later stages of research.

Rationale for the exploitation of CA IX as a target for cancer imaging stems from an increasing number of studies demonstrating that its expression pattern is tightly related to cancer. Meta-analysis of studies encompassing more than 24,000 patients revealed strongly significant associations between CA IX expression evaluated by immunohistochemistry and all endpoints: overall survival, disease-free survival, loco-regional control, disease-specific survival, metastasis-free survival, and progression-free survival [60]. Subgroup analyses showed similar associations in the majority of tumor sites and types. The results showed that patients having tumors with high CA IX expression have higher risk of disease progression, and development of metastases, independent of tumor type or site.

Actually, transcription of CA IX is strongly induced by hypoxia and the protein is also functionally involved in cancer progression due to regulation of pH, control of cell adhesion and invasion, facilitation of glycolytic metabolism and metastatic dissemination as supported by data from suppression of CA IX in diverse cancer models [61]. Since hypoxia as well as acidosis are microenvironmental stresses linked to aggressive cancer behavior, visualization of regions where cancer cells are exposed and adapted to these stresses offers opportunity to predict prognosis and therapy outcome. In this context, it is meaningful to use CA IX for targeting cancer via detection of hypoxic/acidic tumors. In addition to classical means of imaging tumors with CA IX via radiolabeled antibodies, the literature describes several nanoparticle-based approaches. Except one study using silica nanoparticles coated with the anti-CA IX MAb M75 [62], all other studies exploited carbonic anhydrase inhibitors. As CA inhibitors are principally acting towards diverse CA isoforms due to similarities in their active sites, selectivity to CA IX was conferred by diverse carriers [45], gold nanoparticles [46], pH-responsive nanoparticles [47], polymer-based photodynamic nanoinhibitor particles [48]. However, the approaches using inhibitors principally differ from the approach using monoclonal antibodies. Inhibitors are expected to access and bind to the catalytic site of the enzymatically active CA IX, whereas the MAb directed to the N-terminal region of CA IX, such as M75, can access and bind CA IX outside of the catalytic site and thus the binding does not depend on the activity of the enzyme and is highly specific. This might be particularly important in tumor tissues where CA IX is present on the surface of acutely hypoxic cells (due to induction by hypoxia) as well as of post-hypoxic and/or acidic cells (due to high protein stability) that already underwent adaptation to hypoxia and acidosis and have aggressive properties, thus broadening the clinically meaningful area of tumor targeting. The data presented here suggest that this approach is viable and deserves further development.

4. Experimental Section

4.1. Materials

Graphite (particle size 5 μm, SGL Carbon GmbH, Meitingen, Germany), 1–ethyl–3–(3–dimethylaminopropyl) carbodiimide (EDC, 98+%, ACROS Organics part of Thermo Fisher Scientific, Geel, Belgium), sulfo-NHS (N-hydroxysulfosuccinimide, 98+%, ACROS Organics part of Thermo Fisher Scientific, Geel, Belgium), phosphate buffered saline (PBS) tablets (100 mL, Biotechnology grade, VWR™, part of Avantor, Bridgeport, NJ, USA) and TWEEN® 20 (Sigma-Aldrich Co., St. Louis, MO, USA) were used as received. All chemicals used for graphite oxidation were of 97% analytical grade purity and were used as received. Magnetic nanoparticles coated with poly-L-lysine (MNps), with a hydrodynamic size of 27–33 nm, and magnetic nanoparticles coated with poly-L-lysine and conjugated with monoclonal antibody M75 (MNps-MAb and MNps-EDC-MAb) were prepared and synthesized as described in a previous report [37].

4.2. Preparation of Graphene Oxide

Graphene oxide (GO) was prepared from graphite by a modified Hummers and Offeman method [14]. The exfoliation was performed by numerous repetitions of mixing, sonication and centrifugation with a Sigma 3–30 K centrifuge (Sigma Centrifuges, Newtown, UK) at 10,000× g for 40 min. The prepared solution had a GO concentration of approximately 10 mg/mL.

4.3. Modification of the Graphene Oxide Surface with Magnetic Nanoparticles

A PBS solution and TWEEN® 20 (Sigma-Aldrich Co., St. Louis, MO, USA) were mixed with the GO solution. A solution of EDC and sulfo-NHS was added to the GO solution at a weight ratio of 1:1. A suspension of the magnetic nanoparticles coated with poly-L-lysine was added dropwise into the reaction mixture. The weight ratio of GO to MNps was 3:1. The reaction mixture was placed in an ultrasound bath for two hours. The GO platforms modified with MNps were separated in the reaction vessel with a magnet and purified several times with deionized water. The prepared platform was labelled GO-MNps.

4.4. Synthesis of GO-MNps-MAb and GO-MNps-EDC-MAb

Two kinds of MNps conjugated with MAb were employed for GO modification. The first one was prepared by reaction with a binding agent, EDC, and labeled MNps-EDC-MAb, the second, without the EDC binding agent, was labeled MNps-MAb. The detailed preparation procedure was described in a previous report [37].

In brief, magnetite nanoparticles were precipitated from an aqueous solution of Fe^{2+} and Fe^{3+} ions upon gradual addition of ammonium hydroxide. The formed precipitate was washed with ultrapure water and agitated with an immersed sonicator probe (Model 450, BRANSON, Danbury, CT,

USA) for 5 min at a power of 280 W in a water bath. Then, the suspension of nanoparticles was mixed with a PLL solution (0.1%) at the theoretical PLL: Fe_3O_4 weight ratio of 1 and again sonicated in an ice bath. Next, the samples were ultracentrifuged at 44,000 g for 2 h at 4 °C. The sediment was carefully redispersed in ultrapure water and collected to form the PLL-MNps sample with magnetite and PLL concentrations of 18.5 and 3.6 mg/mL, respectively. The modified nanoparticles were subsequently incubated with an added MAb solution, with and without EDC, in PBS. After incubating for 24 h, the nanoparticles were centrifuged and washed to ensure that the unbound MAb was removed. The GO particles were later modified with both types of MNps as described in Section 2.3, and the samples were labeled GO-MNps-MAb and GO-MNps-EDC-MAb.

4.5. Characterization Techniques

AFM images of the GO platforms were obtained with a MultiMode 8 microscope (Bruker, Billerica, MA, USA). The measurements were performed in the ScanAsyst mode in air. The AFM tips used for the measurements were ScanAsyst-Air probes (Bruker, Billerica, MA, USA). The XPS measurements were performed using a Thermo Scientific K-Alpha XPS system (Thermo Fisher Scientific, Loughborough, UK) equipped with a microfocused monochromatic Al Kα X-ray source (1 486.6 eV). The Zeta potential (Malvern, Houston, TX USA) was measured at Zetasizer Nano-ZS for purified G0 in the pH range from 2 to 11. pH was adjusted with KOH solution and controlled by pH/mV/Temperature BENCH METER (Hanna Instruments Czech s.r.o., Prague, Czech Republic). TEM micrographs of the platforms were obtained with a Tecnai G2 Spirit Twin 12 transmission electron microscope (FEI, Prague, Czech Republic). A small droplet (2 µL) of a suspension containing the magnetic nanoparticles (concentration ca. 5 mg/mL) or the platforms with and/or without the nanoparticles (concentration ca. 1 mg/mL) was deposited onto a commercial carbon-coated copper grid for TEM and left to equilibrate (8 min). Then, the excess solution was removed by touching the bottom of the grid to a small piece of filter paper (the fast drying method, which minimizes possible drying artifacts). The dried samples were observed in the transmission electron microscope using bright field imaging at 120 kV. Moreover, the magnetic nanoparticles were also analyzed by energy dispersive analysis of X-rays (EDX, to confirm their elemental composition) and by selected area electron diffraction (SAED, to confirm their expected magnetite crystalline structure). The SAED diffraction pattern was compared with the calculated powder X-ray diffraction pattern (PXRD) of magnetite, as described in a previous report [63].

4.6. Cell Viability Assay

The cytotoxicity or cytostatic effect evaluation of the modified GO-MNps-MAb and GO-MNps-EDC-MAb was performed on B16 mouse melanoma cells permanently transfected with the full-length CA IX cDNA (B16 CA IX), and mock-transfected cells B16-neo. The CellTiter-Blue (CTB) viability assay (Promega, Madison, WI, USA) was used. Testing was performed according to the instructions provided by the manufacturer. The cells were incubated in 96-well plates for 24 h cell at 37 °C. The measurements were performed immediately after the establishment of the cell culture, and the following values were measured after 24, 48, 72 and 120 h. The CTB fluorescence value of the control cells measured at the start of the experiment was set as 1. The CTB values of treated cells were normalized to their non-treated control. Each measurement was performed after the direct addition of 20 µL of the CellTiter-Blue solution to the wells and incubation for 4 h at 37 °C. The fluorescence was recorded with a 530 nm/590 nm (excitation/emission) filter set using a Synergy HT microplate reader (Bio-Tek, Winooski, VT, USA). The samples were run in triplicate for each concentration of the GO-MNps-MAb and GO-MNps-EDC-MAb.

4.7. Immunofluorescence Assay

The B16 mouse melanoma cell line with (B16 CA IX) and without (B16-neo) CA IX was plated (300,000 cells per Petri dish) on sterile glass coverslips 24 h before the experiment. The live cells were incubated at 4 °C for 30 min with GO-MNps-MAb and GO-MNps-EDC-MAb diluted in culture medium to characterize the uptake of MAb by the extracellular enzyme CA IX. The cells were then washed to remove unbound platforms and transferred to incubate at 37 °C for 3 h to allow endocytosis. The washing was repeated again to remove unbound GO nanoparticles and antibodies. The presence of conjugated M75 was visualized in cells fixed in ice-cold methanol at −20 °C for 5 min using an anti-mouse Alexa Fluor® 488 (Thermo Fisher Scientific, Loughborough, UK) conjugated secondary antibody. Finally, the cells were mounted onto slides and analyzed by confocal laser-scanning microscopy (CLSM) on a Zeiss LSM 510 Meta instrument (Heidelberg, Germany).

4.8. Flow Cytometry Assay

Madin-Darby Canine Kidney cells with CAIX (MDCK CAIX) and without enzyme (MDCK neo) were used for cytometric analysis of the functionalized GO platform by magnetic nanoparticles and conjugated M75 antibodies. Cells were established at 35,000/cm2. GO platform samples were pre-incubated with anti-mouse Alexa Fluor® 488 antibody diluted 1:1000, 1 h at 37 °C on an orbital stirrer. After the cells adhered to the surface of the plate, preincubated 1:4 GO platforms samples were added to the culture media. The cells were then incubated overnight at 37 °C. Subsequently, the culture media were removed; the cells were washed three times with PBS solution and released with trypsin. The cell suspensions were then washed with Verzene (cell centrifugation was 5 min at 400 g) and analyzed by Guava EasyCyte plus flow cytometry (Millipore, Burlington, MA, USA) using a 525/30 nm filter. Data was evaluated using Cytosoft 5.2 software (Millipore, Burlington, MA, USA) with Guava ExpressPro.

5. Conclusions

Graphene oxide platforms were prepared with a mean size of 302 ± 183 nm, as determined by AFM. The GO was purified to remove sulfur. The surface composition of the prepared GO was characterized by XPS; additionally, the oxidation state and ratio of C:O were determined by XPS. TEM micrographs that confirmed the smooth surface of the GO platforms and the attachment of the magnetic nanoparticle onto the GO surface. A ratio of 3:1 for GO:MNps was chosen for further functionalization of the GO by MAb. After performing toxicological assays at B16-F0 cell line, no cytotoxicity effect of the multifunctional GO platforms were ascertained. However, there was a significant cytostatic effect for B16 CA IX cells after 48 h. The immunofluorescence test indirectly confirmed the bonding between graphene oxide and the magnetic nanoparticles conjugated to the monoclonal antibody. The selectivity of the GO-MNps-MAb and GO-MNps-EDC-MAb platforms toward tumor cell targeting was demonstrated; therefore, the potential use of GO-MNps-EDC-MAb in tumor treatment was indicated. The GO-MNps-EDC-MAb sample prepared with an EDC binding agent showed better results in the immunofluorescence assay. As an initial step, this study provides promising evidence of tumor targeting with broad potential for visualization and future tumor treatment.

Author Contributions: N.B. designed the GO modification experiments under the supervision of M.O. M.M. characterized the prepared materials by XPS and evaluated the obtained results. GO was prepared by Z.Š. M.B. investigated prepared GO by AFM method under supervision of P.Š. and E.M. M.K. and V.Z. prepared magnetic nanoparticles, which were modified by M.K. M.Š. characterized magnetic nanoparticles and GO platforms by transmission electron microscopy and energy dispersive X-ray analysis. The toxicity testing of the prepared GO-platform and Immunofluorescence was done by M.Z. and N.B., and cytometry measurement by I.K. under supervision of S.P. M.O. and N.B. wrote the main part of the paper. Discussion was written by S.P. and M.O.

Funding: This research was funded by the Slovak Research and Development Agency under contract Nos. APVV-14–0120 and APVV-15-0641 and by Science Grant Agency VEGA project Nos. 2/0010/18 and 2/033/19 (Slovakia). Electron microscopy at the Institute of Macromolecular Chemistry was supported by projects TE01020118 (Technology Agency of the CR) and POLYMAT LO1507 (Ministry of Education, Youth and Sports of the CR, program NPU I).

Conflicts of Interest: The authors declare no conflict of interest.

References

1. Pardo, J.; Peng, Z.; Leblanc, R.; Pardo, J.; Peng, Z.; Leblanc, R.M. Cancer Targeting and Drug Delivery Using Carbon-Based Quantum Dots and Nanotubes. *Molecules* **2018**, *23*, 378. [CrossRef]
2. Moreno, C.; Vilas-Varela, M.; Kretz, B.; Garcia-Lekue, A.; Costache, M.V.; Paradinas, M.; Panighel, M.; Ceballos, G.; Valenzuela, S.O.; Peña, D.; et al. Bottom-up synthesis of multifunctional nanoporous graphene. *Science* **2018**, *360*, 199–203. [CrossRef]
3. Geim, A.K.; Novoselov, K.S. The rise of graphene. *Nat. Mater.* **2007**, *6*, 183–191. [CrossRef]
4. Ghany, N.A.A.; Elsherif, S.A.; Handal, H.T. Revolution of Graphene for different applications: State-of-the-art. *Surfaces Interfaces* **2017**, *9*, 93–106. [CrossRef]
5. Ubani, C.A.; Ibrahim, M.A.; Teridi, M.A.M.; Sopian, K.; Ali, J.; Chaudhary, K.T. Application of graphene in dye and quantum dots sensitized solar cell. *Sol. Energy* **2016**, *137*, 531–550. [CrossRef]
6. Hu, Y.; Sun, X. Chemically Functionalized Graphene and Their Applications in Electrochemical Energy Conversion and Storage. In *Advances in Graphene Science*; Aliofkhazraei, M., Ed.; InTechOpen: London, UK, 2013; pp. 161–189. ISBN 978-953-51-1182-5.
7. Koyakutty, M.; Sasidharan, A.; Nair, S. Biomedical Applications of Graphene: Opportunities and Challenges. In *Graphene: Synthesis, Properties, and Phenomena*; Rao, C.N.R., Sood, A.K., Eds.; Wiley-VCH Verlag GmbH & Co. KGaA.: Weinheim, Germany, 2012; pp. 373–408. ISBN 9783527332588.
8. Potts, J.R.; Dreyer, D.R.; Bielawski, C.W.; Ruoff, R.S. Graphene-based polymer nanocomposites. *Polymer (Guildf)* **2011**, *52*, 5–25. [CrossRef]
9. Gao, W. The chemistry of graphene oxide. *Graphene Oxide Reduct. Recipes Spectrosc. Appl.* **2015**, *39*, 61–95. [CrossRef]
10. Novoselov, K.S.; Fal'ko, V.I.; Colombo, L.; Gellert, P.R.; Schwab, M.G.; Kim, K. A roadmap for graphene. *Nature* **2012**, *490*, 192–200. [CrossRef] [PubMed]
11. Han, W.; Kawakami, R.K.; Gmitra, M.; Fabian, J. Graphene spintronics. *Nat. Nanotechnol.* **2014**, *9*, 794–807. [CrossRef]
12. Novoselov, K.S.; Geim, A.K.; Morozov, S.V.; Jiang, D.; Zhang, Y.; Dubonos, S.V.; Grigorieva, I.V.; Firsov, A.A. Electric field effect in atomically thin carbon films. *Science* **2004**, *306*, 666–669. [CrossRef]
13. Kostiuk, D.; Bodik, M.; Siffalovic, P.; Jergel, M.; Halahovets, Y.; Hodas, M.; Pelletta, M.; Pelach, M.; Hulman, M.; Spitalsky, Z.; et al. Reliable determination of the few-layer graphene oxide thickness using Raman spectroscopy. *J. Raman Spectrosc.* **2016**, *47*, 391–394. [CrossRef]
14. Hummers, W.S.; Offeman, R.E. Preparation of Graphitic Oxide. *J. Am. Chem. Soc.* **1958**, *80*, 1339. [CrossRef]
15. Shin, S.R.; Li, Y.-C.; Jang, H.L.; Khoshakhlagh, P.; Akbari, M.; Nasajpour, A.; Zhang, Y.S.; Tamayol, A.; Khademhosseini, A.; Ryon, S.; et al. Graphene-based materials for tissue engineering. *Adv. Drug Deliv. Rev.* **2016**, *105*, 255–274. [CrossRef] [PubMed]
16. Goenka, S.; Sant, V.; Sant, S. Graphene-based nanomaterials for drug delivery and tissue engineering. *J. Control. Release* **2014**, *173*, 75–88. [CrossRef] [PubMed]
17. Yang, K.; Gong, H.; Shi, X.; Wan, J.; Zhang, Y.; Liu, Z. In vivo biodistribution and toxicology of functionalized nano-graphene oxide in mice after oral and intraperitoneal administration. *Biomaterials* **2013**, *34*, 2787–2795. [CrossRef]
18. Rao, C.N.R.; Sood, A.K. *Graphene: Synthesis, Properties, and Phenomena*; Rao, C.N.R., Sood, A.K., Eds.; First Edit.; Wiley-VCH Verlag GmbH and Co. KGaA.: Weinheim, Germany, 2012; ISBN 9783527332588.
19. Seabra, A.B.; Paula, A.J.; De Lima, R.; Alves, O.L.; Durán, N. Nanotoxicity of graphene and graphene oxide. *Chem. Res. Toxicol.* **2014**, *27*, 159–168. [CrossRef]
20. Ferrari, A.C.; Bonaccorso, F.; Falko, V.; Novoselov, K.S.; Roche, S.; Bøggild, P.; Borini, S.; Koppens, F.; Palermo, V.; Pugno, N.; et al. Science and technology roadmap for graphene, related two-dimensional crystals, and hybrid systems. *Nanoscale* **2014**, *7*, 4598–4810. [CrossRef]
21. Zhang, Y.; Nayak, T.R.; Hong, H.; Cai, W. Graphene: A versatile nanoplatform for biomedical applications. *Nanoscale* **2012**, *4*, 3833–3842. [CrossRef]
22. Shen, H.; Zhang, L.; Liu, M.; Zhang, Z. Biomedical applications of graphene. *Theranostics* **2012**, *2*, 283–294. [CrossRef]
23. Xie, J.; Lee, S.; Chen, X. Nanoparticle-based theranostic agents. *Adv. Drug Deliv. Rev.* **2010**, *62*, 1064–1079. [CrossRef]

24. Lonkar, S.P.; Deshmukh, Y.S.; Abdala, A.A. Recent advances in chemical modifications of graphene. *Nano Res.* **2015**, *8*, 1039–1074. [CrossRef]
25. Chen, Y.; Su, Y.; Hu, S.; Chen, S. Functionalized graphene nanocomposites for enhancing photothermal therapy in tumor treatment. *Adv. Drug Deliv. Rev.* **2016**, *105*, 190–204. [CrossRef]
26. Yang, Y.; Asiri, A.M.; Tang, Z.; Du, D.; Lin, Y. Graphene based materials for biomedical applications. *Mater. Today* **2013**, *16*, 365–373. [CrossRef]
27. Shan, C.; Yang, H.; Han, D.; Zhang, Q.; Ivaska, A.; Niu, L. Water-soluble graphene covalently functionalized by biocompatible poly-L-lysine. *Langmuir* **2009**, *25*, 12030–12033. [CrossRef]
28. Shen, J.; Shi, M.; Ma, H.; Yan, B.; Li, N.; Hu, Y.; Ye, M. Synthesis of hydrophilic and organophilic chemically modified graphene oxide sheets. *J. Colloid Interface Sci.* **2010**, *352*, 366–370. [CrossRef] [PubMed]
29. Li, N.; Jiang, H.-L.; Wang, X.-L.; Wang, X.; Xu, G.-J.; Zhang, B.-B.; Wang, L.-J.; Zhao, R.-S.; Lin, J.-M. Recent advances in graphene-based magnetic composites for magnetic solid-phase extraction. *TrAC Trends Anal. Chem.* **2018**, *102*, 60–74. [CrossRef]
30. Chen, W.; Yi, P.; Zhang, Y.; Zhang, L.; Deng, Z.; Zhang, Z. Composites of Aminodextran-Coated Fe3O4 Nanoparticles and Graphene Oxide for Cellular Magnetic Resonance Imaging. *ACS Appl. Mater. Interfaces* **2011**, *3*, 4085–4091. [CrossRef]
31. Yu, D.; Yang, Y.; Durstock, M.; Baek, J.-B.; Dai, L. Soluble P3HT-Grafted Graphene for Efficient Bilayer–Heterojunction Photovoltaic Devices. *ACS Nano* **2010**, *4*, 5633–5640. [CrossRef]
32. Závišová, V.; Koneracká, M.; Múčková, M.; Kopčanský, P.; Tomašovičová, N.; Lancz, G.; Timko, M.; Pätoprstá, B.; Bartoš, P.; Fabián, M. Synthesis and characterization of polymeric nanospheres loaded with the anticancer drug paclitaxel and magnetic particles. *J. Magn. Magn. Mater.* **2009**, *321*, 1613–1616. [CrossRef]
33. Antal, I.; Kubovcikova, M.; Zavisova, V.; Koneracka, M.; Pechanova, O.; Barta, A.; Cebova, M.; Antal, V.; Diko, P.; Zduriencikova, M.; et al. Magnetic poly(d,l-lactide) nanoparticles loaded with aliskiren: A promising tool for hypertension treatment. *J. Magn. Magn. Mater.* **2015**, *380*, 280–284. [CrossRef]
34. Koneracká, M.; Antošová, A.; Závišová, V.; Gažová, Z.; Lancz, G.; Juríková, A.; Tomašovčová, N.; Kováč, J.; Fabián, M.; Kopčanský, P. Preparation and characterization of albumin containing magnetic fluid as potential drug for amyloid diseases treatment. *Phys. Procedia* **2010**, *9*, 254–257. [CrossRef]
35. He, F.; Fan, J.; Ma, D.; Zhang, L.; Leung, C.; Chan, H.L. The attachment of Fe3O4 nanoparticles to graphene oxide by covalent bonding. *Carbon N. Y.* **2010**, *48*, 3139–3144. [CrossRef]
36. Antal, I.; Koneracka, M.; Kubovcikova, M.; Zavisova, V.; Khmara, I.; Jelenska, L.; Vidlickova, I.; Pastorekova, S.; Zatovicova, M.; Bugarova, N.; et al. D,L-Lysine functionalized Fe3O4 nanoparticles for detection of cancer cells. *Colloids Surfaces B Biointerfaces* **2018**, *163*, 236–245. [CrossRef]
37. Khmara, I.; Koneracka, M.; Kubovcikova, M.; Zavisova, V.; Antal, I.; Csach, K.; Kopcansky, P.; Vidlickova, I.; Csaderova, L.; Pastorekova, S.; et al. Preparation of poly-L-lysine functionalized magnetic nanoparticles and their influence on viability of cancer cells. *J. Magn. Magn. Mater.* **2017**, *427*, 114–121. [CrossRef]
38. Tabish, T.; Pranjol, M.; Horsell, D.; Rahat, A.; Whatmore, J.; Winyard, P.; Zhang, S.; Tabish, T.A.; Pranjol, M.Z.I.; Horsell, D.W.; et al. Graphene Oxide-Based Targeting of Extracellular Cathepsin D and Cathepsin L As A Novel Anti-Metastatic Enzyme Cancer Therapy. *Cancers (Basel)* **2019**, *11*, 319. [CrossRef]
39. Zatovicova, M.; Jelenska, L.; Hulikova, A.; Ditte, P.; Ditte, Z.; Csaderova, L.; Svastova, E.; Schmalix, W.; Boettger, V.; Bevan, P.; et al. Monoclonal antibody G250 targeting CA IX: Binding specificity, internalization and therapeutic effects in a non-renal cancer model. *Int. J. Oncol.* **2014**, *45*, 2455–2467. [CrossRef]
40. Zatovicova, M.; Jelenska, L.; Hulikova, A.; Csaderova, L.; Ditte, Z.; Ditte, P.; Goliasova, T.; Pastorek, J.; Pastorekova, S. Carbonic Anhydrase IX as an Anticancer Therapy Target: Preclinical Evaluation of Internalizing Monoclonal Antibody Directed to Catalytic Domain. *Curr. Pharm. Des.* **2010**, *16*, 3255–3263. [CrossRef]
41. Pastoreková, S.; Zaťovičová, M.; Pastorek, J. Cancer-associated carbonic anhydrases and their inhibition. *Curr. Pharm. Des.* **2008**, *14*, 685–698. [CrossRef]
42. Chrastina, A.; Závada, J.; Parkkila, S.; Kaluz, Š.; Kaluzová, M.; Rajčáni, J.; Pastorek, J.; Pastoreková, S. Biodistribution and pharmacokinetics of 125I-labeled monoclonal antibody M75 specific for carbonic anhydrase IX, an intrinsic marker of hypoxia, in nude mice xenografted with human colorectal carcinoma. *Int. J. Cancer* **2003**, *105*, 873–881. [CrossRef]
43. Yu, L.; Li, P.; Ding, X.; Zhang, Q. Graphene oxide and carboxylated graphene oxide: Viable two-dimensional nanolabels for lateral flow immunoassays. *Talanta* **2017**, *165*, 167–175. [CrossRef]

44. Rauf, S.; Mishra, G.K.; Azhar, J.; Mishra, R.K.; Goud, K.Y.; Nawaz, M.A.H.; Marty, J.L.; Hayat, A. Carboxylic group riched graphene oxide based disposable electrochemical immunosensor for cancer biomarker detection. *Anal. Biochem.* **2018**, *545*, 13–19. [CrossRef]
45. Tatiparti, K.; Sau, S.; Gawde, K.A.; Iyer, A.K. Copper-free 'click' chemistry-based synthesis and characterization of carbonic anhydrase-IX anchored albumin-paclitaxel nanoparticles for targeting tumor hypoxia. *Int. J. Mol. Sci.* **2018**, *19*, 838. [CrossRef]
46. Shabana, A.M.; Mondal, U.K.; Alam, M.R.; Spoon, T.; Ross, C.A.; Madesh, M.; Supuran, C.T.; Ilies, M.A. PH-Sensitive Multiligand Gold Nanoplatform Targeting Carbonic Anhydrase IX Enhances the Delivery of Doxorubicin to Hypoxic Tumor Spheroids and Overcomes the Hypoxia-Induced Chemoresistance. *ACS Appl. Mater. Interfaces* **2018**, *10*, 17792–17808. [CrossRef]
47. Liu, S.; Luo, X.; Liu, S.; Xu, P.; Wang, J.; Hu, Y. Acetazolamide-Loaded pH-Responsive Nanoparticles Alleviating Tumor Acidosis to Enhance Chemotherapy Effects. *Macromol. Biosci.* **2019**, *19*, 1–11. [CrossRef]
48. Jiang, Y.; Li, J.; Zeng, Z.; Xie, C.; Lyu, Y.; Pu, K. Organic Photodynamic Nanoinhibitor for Synergistic Cancer Therapy. *Angew. Chemie Int. Ed.* **2019**. [CrossRef]
49. Yamashita, T.; Hayes, P. Analysis of XPS spectra of Fe2+ and Fe3+ ions in oxide materials. *Appl. Surf. Sci.* **2008**, *254*, 2441–2449. [CrossRef]
50. Fujii, T.; de Groot, F.M.F.; Sawatzky, G.A.; Voogt, F.C.; Hibma, T.; Okada, K. In situ XPS analysis of various iron oxide films grown by NO_2-assisted molecular-beam epitaxy. *Phys. Rev. B* **1999**, *59*, 3195–3202. [CrossRef]
51. Bodik, M.; Zahoranova, A.; Micusik, M.; Bugarova, N.; Spitalsky, Z.; Omastova, M.; Majkova, E.; Jergel, M.; Siffalovic, P. Fast low-temperature plasma reduction of monolayer graphene oxide at atmospheric pressure. *Nanotechnology* **2017**, *28*, 145601. [CrossRef]
52. Nečas, D.; Klapetek, P. Gwyddion: An open-source software for SPM data analysis. *Open Phys.* **2012**, *10*, 181–188. [CrossRef]
53. Kadu, P.J.; Kushare, S.S.; Thacker, D.D.; Gattani, S.G. Enhancement of oral bioavailability of atorvastatin calcium by self-emulsifying drug delivery systems (SEDDS). *Pharm. Dev. Technol.* **2011**, *16*, 65–74. [CrossRef]
54. Malvern Instruments Ltd. Stabilita Suspenzí a Disperzí—Proč Jsou Parametry jako Velikost Částic, Zeta Potenciál a Reologické Vlastnosti tak Důležité? *Chemagazín* **2011**, *21*, 14–16.
55. Hermanson, G.T. *Bioconjugate Technicques, 3rd Edition*; Audet, J., Preap, M., Eds.; Third edit.; Elsevier Inc.: Amsterdam, The Netherlands, 2013; ISBN 9780123822390.
56. Sohová, M.E.; Bodík, M.; Siffalovic, P.; Bugarova, N.; Zaťovičová, M.; Hianik, T.; Omastová, M.; Majkova, E. Label-Free Tracking of Nanosized Graphene Oxide Cellular Uptake by Confocal Raman Microscopy. *Analyst* **2018**, *143*, 3686–3692. [CrossRef]
57. Liu, Z.; Robinson, J.T.; Sun, X.; Dai, H. PEGylated Nanographene Oxide for Delivery of Water-Insoluble Cancer Drugs. *J. Am. Chem. Soc.* **2008**, *130*, 10876–10877. [CrossRef]
58. Sasidharan, A.; Panchakarla, L.S.; Chandran, P.; Menon, D.; Nair, S.; Rao, C.N.R.; Koyakutty, M. Differential nano-bio interactions and toxicity effects of pristine versus functionalized graphene. *Nanoscale* **2011**, *3*, 2461–2464. [CrossRef]
59. Singh, S.K.; Singh, M.K.; Kulkarni, P.P.; Sonkar, V.K.; Grácio, J.J.A.; Dash, D. Amine-Modified Graphene: Thrombo-Protective Safer Alternative to Graphene Oxide for Biomedical. *ACS Nano* **2012**, *6*, 2731–2740. [CrossRef] [PubMed]
60. Van Kuijk, S.J.A.; Yaromina, A.; Houben, R.; Niemans, R.; Lambin, P.; Dubois, L.J. Prognostic Significance of Carbonic Anhydrase IX Expression in Cancer Patients: A Meta-Analysis. *Front. Oncol.* **2016**, *6*, 69. [CrossRef]
61. Pastorekova, S.; Gillies, R.J. The role of carbonic anhydrase IX in cancer development: Links to hypoxia, acidosis and beyond. *Cancer Metastasis Rev.* **2019**, (in press). [CrossRef]
62. Tokárová, V.; Pittermannová, A.; Král, V.; Řezáčová, P.; Štěpánek, F. Feasibility and constraints of particle targeting using the antigen-antibody interaction. *Nanoscale* **2013**, *5*, 11490–11498. [CrossRef] [PubMed]
63. Kostiv, U.; Patsula, V.; Šlouf, M.; Pongrac, I.M.; Škokić, S.; Radmilović, M.D.; Pavičić, I.; Vrček, I.V.; Gajović, S.; Horák, D. Physico-chemical characteristics, biocompatibility, and MRI applicability of novel monodisperse PEG-modified magnetic Fe3O4 &SiO 2 core–shell nanoparticles. *RSC Adv.* **2017**, *7*, 8786–8797. [CrossRef]

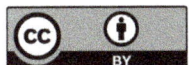

© 2019 by the authors. Licensee MDPI, Basel, Switzerland. This article is an open access article distributed under the terms and conditions of the Creative Commons Attribution (CC BY) license (http://creativecommons.org/licenses/by/4.0/).

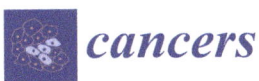

Article

In Vivo Evaluation of Dual-Targeted Nanoparticles Encapsulating Paclitaxel and Everolimus

Loujin Houdaihed, James Christopher Evans and Christine Allen *

Leslie Dan Faculty of Pharmacy, University of Toronto, Toronto, ON M5S 3M2, Canada; loujin.houdaihed@mail.utoronto.ca (L.H.); james.evans@utoronto.ca (J.C.E.)
* Correspondence: cj.allen@utoronto.ca

Received: 23 April 2019; Accepted: 23 May 2019; Published: 29 May 2019

Abstract: A synergistic combination of paclitaxel (PTX) and everolimus (EVER) can allow for lower drug doses, reducing the toxicities associated with PTX, while maintaining therapeutic efficacy. Polymeric nanoparticles (NPs) of high stability provide opportunities to modify the toxicity profile of the drugs by ensuring their delivery to the tumor site at the synergistic ratio while limiting systemic drug exposure and the toxicities that result. The goal of the current study is to evaluate the in vivo fate of human epidermal factor receptor 2 (HER2) and epidermal growth factor receptor (EGFR) dual-targeted PTX+EVER-loaded NPs (Dual-NPs) in an MDA-MB-231-H2N breast cancer (BC) tumor-bearing mouse model. The pharmacokinetic parameters, plasma area under the curve (AUC) and half-life ($t_{1/2}z$) were found to be 20-fold and 3 to 4-fold higher, respectively, for the drugs when administered in the Dual-NPs in comparison to the free-drug combination (i.e., PTX+EVER) at an equivalent dose of PTX. While maintaining anti-tumor efficacy, the levels of body weight loss were significantly lower ($p < 0.0001$) and the overall degree of neurotoxicity was reduced with Dual-NPs treatment in comparison to the free-drug combination when administered at an equivalent dose of PTX. This study suggests that Dual-NPs present a promising platform for the delivery of the PTX and EVER combination with the potential to reduce severe PTX-induced toxicities and in turn, improve quality of life for patients with BC.

Keywords: nanoparticles; drug combination; paclitaxel; everolimus; dual-targeting; breast cancer

1. Introduction

Paclitaxel (PTX)-induced toxicities continue to be one of the main challenges associated with the use of this agent. PTX has several dose-limiting adverse effects including neutropenia and neurotoxicity. Additionally, the commercial formulation of PTX (Taxol) has been associated with severe hypersensitivity reactions, mainly caused by the excipients used for drug solubilization (i.e., ethanol and Cremophor EL) [1].

Over the years, drug-combinations have emerged as one promising avenue for the treatment of cancer. We can take advantage of the synergistic effects of drug-combinations with the administration of doses that are much lower than the maximum tolerated doses (MTDs) of the drugs. This can lead to a reduction in systemic toxicity, while improving or at least maintaining the desired therapeutic effect [2–5].

The combination of the chemotherapeutic agent PTX, and the mammalian target of rapamycin (mTOR) inhibitor everolimus (EVER) has previously been shown to have pronounced synergistic effects in breast cancer (BC) cells in vitro [6]. Despite the potential of this drug combination, only modest efficacy was seen in clinical studies conducted to date—with no significant improvements with respect to toxicity (e.g., NCT00876395 and NCT00915603) [7,8]. This outcome may be attributed to the distinct pharmacokinetic profiles of the drugs, and the administration of agents at their MTDs or standard doses, thereby preventing the delivery of the drugs to the tumor at the optimal synergistic ratio, which hampers the potential synergistic effects.

Recent advances in cancer nanomedicines provide unique opportunities to modify the toxicity profile of the drugs by increasing their delivery to the target site while limiting systemic drug exposure and the toxicities that result. Vyxeos® (Jazz Pharmaceuticals, Dublin, Ireland) is a promising "two-in-one" formulation that includes liposomes that co-encapsulate the combination of cytarabine and daunorubicin at a synergistic molar ratio of 5:1. Vyxeos was approved in 2017 by the FDA for treating patients with high risk acute myeloid leukemia (AML) [9]. In a Phase III clinical trial (NCT01696084), Vyxeos demonstrated good tolerability and significant improvements in the overall survival of patients compared to the free-drug combination in patients with AML [10].

We have developed and characterized PTX+EVER-loaded NPs composed of poly (ethylene glycol)-*b*-poly(lactide-co-glycolide) copolymer (mPEG$_{5000}$-*b*-PLGA$_{15,800}$, 50:50 LA/GA). The NPs are actively targeted to human epidermal factor receptor 2 (HER2) and epidermal growth factor receptor (EGFR), using HER2-targeted trastuzumab (TmAb) and EGFR-targeted Panitumumab (PmAb) Fab fragments, to deliver the drug combination to BC cells (Scheme 1, Table 1) [11].

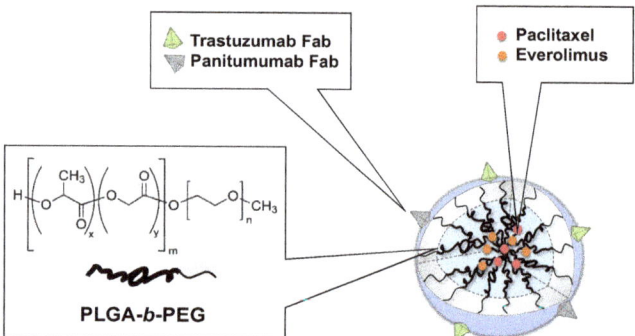

Scheme 1. Graphical schematic depicting the composition of dual-targeted paclitaxel (PTX)+everolimus (EVER)-loaded nanoparticles (Dual-NPs). Adapted with permission from "Loujin Houdaihed, James C. Evans, Christine Allen. Codelivery of Paclitaxel and Everolimus at the Optimal Synergistic Ratio: A Promising Solution for the Treatment of Breast Cancer. *Molecular Pharmaceutics*. **2018**, 15(9): 3672-3681". Copyright © (2018), American Chemical Society.

Table 1. Drug loading, size, and surface charge of dual-targeted paclitaxel (PTX)+everolimus (EVER)-loaded nanoparticles (Dual-NPs).

Formulation	PTX:EVER LC (wt%) [a]	PTX (mg/mL)	EVER (mg/mL)	PTX:EVER Molar Ratio	Size (nm)	Zeta Potential (mV)
Dual-NPs	5.6 ± 1.1	1.2 ± 0.2	0.5 ± 0.1	1:0.37	101.3 ± 6.3	−11.3 ± 2.1

[a] LC% = Loading content.

Active targeting has been widely utilized to increase the cellular internalization of anticancer therapies into cancer cells, with a goal towards improving therapeutic effects [12]. HER2 is overexpressed in 15–25% of breast cancer (BC) [13], whereas EGFR is found in 15–20% of BC and in up to 60% of basal triple-negative BC. Importantly, up to 35% of HER2+ BC co-expresses EGFR [14]. In addition, patients with tumors co-expressing both receptors demonstrate the shortest survival times when compared to those with tumors positive for only one of the receptors [14]. Taken together, HER2 and EGFR represent two attractive complementary targets for the design of a therapy against HER2+/EGFR+ BC.

The current study builds on the promising results seen with Dual-NPs in vitro and examines the pharmacokinetics and biodistribution profiles of PTX and EVER when administered in the Dual-NPs compared with the free-drug combination in a relevant animal model of BC. Furthermore, the therapeutic effect of PTX and EVER administered in Dual-NPs was evaluated in mice bearing MDA-MB-231-H2N BC tumors which co-express HER2 and EGFR (HER2$_{mod}$/EGFR$_{mod}$). Additionally, the safety profile of Dual-NPs relative to the free-drug combination was evaluated by examining neurotoxicity and hemotoxicity post administration. This study demonstrates that Dual-NPs have high stability in vivo and, subsequently, result in significant improvements with regard to safety compared to the free-drug combination in the MDA-MB-231-H2N BC tumor-bearing mouse model.

2. Results

2.1. Preparation and Characterization of Dual-NPs

PTX and EVER were co-encapsulated at the optimal synergistic ratio within poly(ethylene glycol)-*b*-poly(lactide-*co*-glycolide) (mPEG$_{5000}$-*b*-PLGA$_{15,800}$, 50:50 LA/GA) polymeric nanoparticles. TmAb(Fab) and PmAb(Fab) were prepared, purified and conjugated to the surface of PTX+EVER-loaded NPs via amine coupling. The physicochemical characteristics of the Dual-NP are summarized in Table 1.

2.2. Pharmacokinetic Study

Healthy BALB/c female mice were given a single intravenous injection of either the free PTX+EVER combination or Dual-NPs at a PTX-equivalent dose of 15 mg/kg and EVER-equivalent dose of 7.5 mg/kg (at a molar ratio of 1:0.5). The levels of PTX and EVER were measured in the plasma at various timepoints (Figure 1A) and the pharmacokinetic parameters of each group were calculated using non-compartmental analysis (Table 2). Both, PTX and EVER encapsulated in Dual-NPs exhibited slower clearance from the plasma compared to the free-drug combination. While PTX and EVER in Dual-NPs were detectable in the plasma for up to 48 h and 24 h post-administration, respectively, free PTX and EVER were last detected in the plasma 12 h and 6 h post-administration, respectively. The area under the curve (AUC) for both PTX and EVER in Dual-NPs was approximately 20-fold higher than that of the free drug. The maximum plasma concentrations (C_{max}) of PTX and EVER were 7-fold and 9-fold higher for Dual-NPs than for the free drugs, respectively. Furthermore, the half-life ($t_{1/2}z$) was approximately 3 and 4 times greater for PTX and EVER, respectively, in Dual-NPs than for the free drugs. Analysis of the PTX:EVER molar ratio in the plasma revealed that Dual-NPs maintained the ratio of 1:0.5 for 24 h after administration (Figure 1B). This molar ratio had been found to be synergistic in in vitro studies conducted by our group [6]. The total drug concentrations found in plasma for mice administered the Dual-NPs reflect NP encapsulated and released drug. However, the rapid elimination of the free drugs from the circulation indicates that the majority of the PTX and EVER measured in the plasma are likely encapsulated within the NPs.

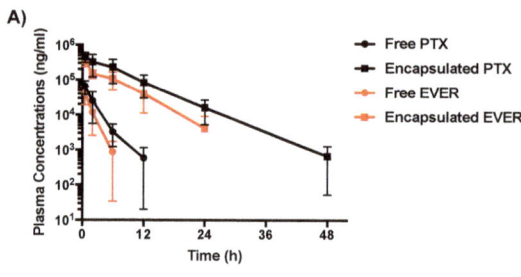

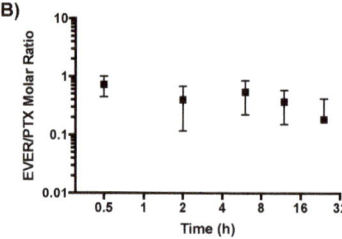

Figure 1. (**A**) Plasma concentrations of paclitaxel (PTX) and everolimus (EVER) after single intravenous administration of dual-targeted PTX+EVER-loaded nanoparticles (Dual-NPs) or free PTX+EVER combination to healthy BALB/c female mice at a PTX-equivalent dose of 15 mg/kg and EVER-equivalent dose of 7.5 mg/kg. (**B**) EVER:PTX molar ratio of drugs released from Dual-NPs in the plasma. ($n = 5$).

Table 2. Pharmacokinetics parameters for the plasma concentrations of paclitaxel (PTX) and everolimus (EVER) after a single intravenous administration of dual-targeted PTX+EVER-loaded nanoparticles (Dual-NPs) versus free PTX+EVER combination to healthy BALB/c female mice.

Treatment		C_{max} (µg/mL)	$T_{1/2}z$ (h)	AUC_{0-t} (µg h mL^{-1})	$AUC_{0-inf.}$ (µg h mL^{-1})	CL_{tot} (mL h kg^{-1})	V_d (mL kg^{-1})
Free Combination	PTX	64.91	1.88	170.49 [a]	172.09	81.35	222.52
	EVER	38.41	1.02	83.6 [b]	84.88	88.35	131.73
Dual-NPs	PTX	458.03	5.17	3666.65 [c]	3671.59	3.81	28.47
	EVER	351.25	3.78	1792.52 [d]	1814.83	4.13	22.85

C_{max} = the maximum plasma concentration; $t_{1/2}z$ = half-life at the terminal phase; AUC = area under the curve; CL_{tot} = total body clearance; V_d = volume of distribution. [a] $AUC_{0-12\,h}$, [b] $AUC_{0-6\,h}$, [c] $AUC_{0-48\,h}$, [d] $AUC_{0-24\,h}$. ($n = 5$).

2.3. Biodistribution Study

Evaluation of the biodistribution of PTX+EVER (as a free-drug combination versus encapsulated within Dual-NPs) in tumor-bearing mice was performed at 2, 6, 24 and 48 h after administration. At 24 h post-administration, the Dual-NPs group showed a 2-fold increase in the tumor PTX accumulation compared to the levels detected in the free PTX+EVER group ($p = 0.27$, Figure 2). At 48 h post-administration, PTX was still detected in the tumor in the Dual-NPs group, however, PTX levels were below the limit of detection in the tumor in the free PTX+EVER group.

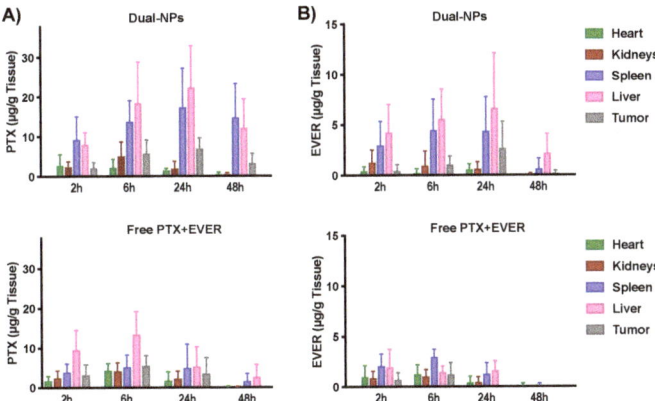

Figure 2. Tissue distribution of (**A**) paclitaxel (PTX) and (**B**) everolimus (EVER) in female Nonobese diabetic/severe combined immunodeficiency (NOD/SCID) mice bearing MDA-MB-231-H2N BC xenografts (HER2$_{mod}$/EGFR$_{mod}$) after single intravenous administration of dual-targeted PTX+EVER-loaded nanoparticles (Dual-NPs) or free PTX+EVER combination at a PTX-equivalent dose of 15 mg/kg and EVER-equivalent dose of 7.5 mg/kg. (n = 5).

EVER accumulated in the tumor in the Dual-NPs group in a time dependent manner, achieving peak concentrations at 24 h, with values decreasing by 48 h. For EVER in the free PTX+EVER group, the drug levels in the tumor were below the limit of detection at 24 h and 48 h after administration. Importantly, the molar ratio of PTX:EVER that accumulated in the tumor in the Dual-NPs group at 24 h was 1:0.38 which remains close to the optimal synergistic ratio (1:0.5) found in vitro [6]. On the other hand, the optimal synergistic ratio of PTX:EVER was not seen in the tumor for the free PTX+EVER group at any time point. Overall, the levels of PTX and EVER seen in the tumors in mice treated with the Dual-NPs were higher relative to the levels seen for the free PTX+EVER group at 24 h and 48 h. However, at the earlier timepoints (2 and 6 h) the drug concentrations were comparable between the two groups.

Comparable levels of PTX and EVER were found to accumulate in the hearts and kidneys of mice in the Dual-NPs and free PTX+EVER groups. Differential accumulation of PTX and EVER following administration in Dual-NPs and free PTX+EVER occurred mainly in the spleen and liver. A 2–5 fold and 2–7 fold increase in liver and spleen uptake of PTX was seen in the Dual-NPs group relative to the free-drug combination group, while a 2–4 fold and 2–6 fold increase was noted in liver and spleen uptake of EVER, respectively, for the Dual-NPs group compared with the free-drug combination group. This outcome can be attributed to the clearance of the NPs via the mononuclear phagocyte system (MPS), which is one of the main elimination pathways for NPs [15].

2.4. Efficacy Studies

Tumor growth in NOD/SCID mice bearing subcutaneous (s.c.) MDA-MB-231-H2N BC tumors was inhibited following the administration of free PTX+EVER and Dual-NPs. Dual-NPs were associated with enhanced antitumor activity in comparison with the free-drug combination. The extent of tumor growth inhibition was significantly different at day 55 (p = 0.001) and day 65 (p = 0.0003) post initiation of treatment in the Dual-NPs group relative to the free-drug combination group (Figure 3A). In addition, the degree of body weight loss was significantly reduced in mice treated with the Dual-NPs compared with those receiving the same dose of the free PTX+EVER combination (p < 0.0001) (Figure 4). As shown in Figure 3B, Kaplan-Meier survival analysis revealed that the Dual-NPs resulted in comparable overall survival to that obtained with the free-drug combination. Median survival was 79 days for mice receiving Dual-NPs, and 76 days for those receiving the free PTX+EVER.

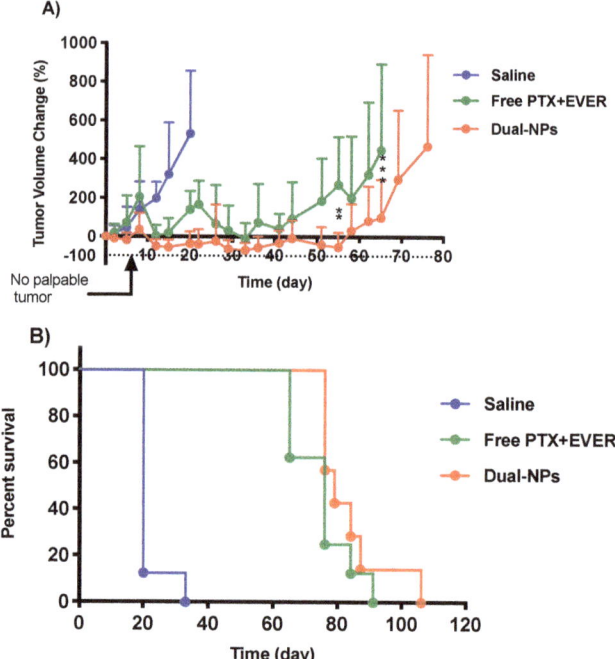

Figure 3. (**A**) Tumor growth inhibition of saline (blue), free paclitaxel and everolimus (PTX+EVER) (green), and dual-targeted PTX+EVER-loaded nanoparticles (Dual-NPs) (red) in female NOD/SCID mice bearing MDA-MB-231-H2N BC xenografts (HER2$_{mod}$/EGFR$_{mod}$) after intravenous administration of treatments at a PTX-equivalent dose of 15 mg/kg and EVER-equivalent dose of 7.5 mg/kg once a week for eight consecutive weeks. Data represent mean ± SD ($n = 8$). Two-way analysis of variance (ANOVA) was conducted where ** and *** indicate $p = 0.001$ and $p = 0.0003$, respectively. (**B**) Kaplan-Meier survival analysis.

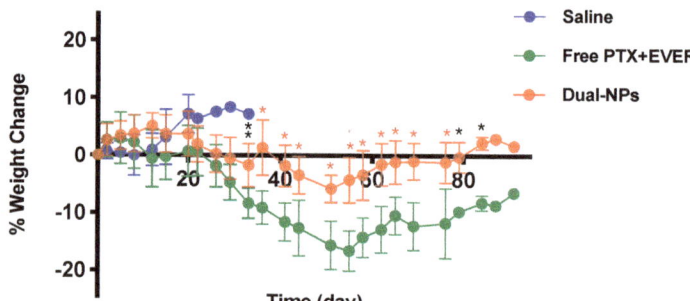

Figure 4. Animal body weight change in mice receiving saline (blue), free paclitaxel and everolimus (PTX+EVER) (green), and dual-targeted PTX+EVER-loaded nanoparticles (Dual-NPs) (red) from the first day of treatment to the ethical endpoint. Data represent mean ± SD ($n = 8$). Two-way analysis of variance (ANOVA) was conducted where *, **, and * indicate $p < 0.04$, $p = 0.004$, and $p < 0.0001$, respectively.

2.5. Toxicity Studies

Neurotoxicity was evaluated using histological examination of the sciatic nerve sections removed two to three days after the sixth weekly injection of saline, Dual-NPs, or free PTX+EVER (i.e., at the low dose of PTX (8 mg/kg, molar ratio of PTX:EVER of 1:0.5) (Figure 5, left panel). Mice in the Dual-NPs treatment group were found to have fewer degenerative myelinated fibers in contrast to mice treated with the free-drug combination. Only very slight degenerative changes were seen in sections of the sciatic nerve from two of nine mice in the Dual-NPs group. On the other hand, in the free-drug combination group, four out of nine mice showed very slight degenerative changes and one mouse showed slight degenerative changes in their sciatic nerve sections. Degenerative changes consisted of vesicular degeneration, while axonal swelling was not identified in any of the examined nerve sections.

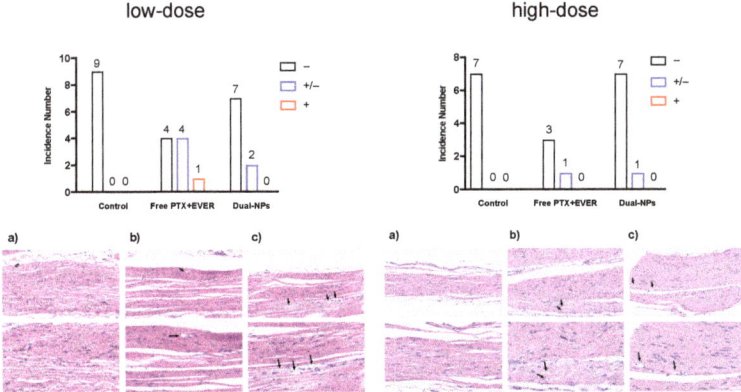

Figure 5. Degenerating myelinated nerve fibers (arrow) were examined in the sciatic nerve after staining with haematoxylin and eosin (H & E) two to three days after weekly injections for six weeks with saline (**a**), dual-targeted PTX+EVER-loaded nanoparticles (Dual-NPs) (**b**), and Free paclitaxel and everolimus (PTX+EVER) (**c**) at a PTX-equivalent dose of 8 mg/kg (left panel) or 15 mg/kg (right panel). Magnification, 20X (upper) and 40X (lower). A semi-quantitative scoring system was used in the evaluation of histologic sections of the sciatic nerve blinded as to the group. The scoring system addresses degenerative changes to myelinated nerve fibers (axonal swelling and vesicular degeneration). Several histologic sections, cut in a longitudinal plane, were examined from each sample. As previously described [16], the degenerating myelinated fiber score was defined as follows: −, no degenerative changes; +/−, very slight degree of degenerative changes (scattered, single fibers affected); +, slight degree of degenerative changes (scattered small groups of degenerative myelinated fibers).

The same study was repeated using a higher dose of PTX (15 mg/kg, molar ratio of PTX:EVER of 1:0.5) (Figure 5, right panel). Most sections of the sciatic nerve from mice in the Dual-NPs and free-drug combination groups were histologically unremarkable. Very slight degenerative changes, characterized by vesicular degeneration in a single nerve fiber or very few scattered individual fibers, were seen in the sections of the sciatic nerve from one mouse in the Dual-NPs group and one mouse in the free PTX+EVER group. Due to technical difficulties and incidence of death in the free PTX+EVER group early in the study, the number of sciatic nerve sections tested in the free PTX+EVER group was less than those in the Dual-NPs group, which makes further interpretation of the results difficult.

Blood samples from mice receiving the high-dose of PTX were evaluated for hemotoxicity and a complete blood count (CBC) analysis was performed using VetScan HM5 v2.2 (Abaxis, Union City, CA, USA). Considering the marked increase in Dual-NPs accumulation in the liver and spleen relative to free PTX+EVER, blood samples were also analyzed for biochemistry markers looking mainly for cues of liver and spleen toxicity.

For red blood cell count (RBC), hemoglobin concentration (HGB), hematocrit (HCT) and the mean corpuscular cell volume (MCV), values for all groups were within normal levels. Interestingly, the level of neutrophils in mice in all groups was comparable but below the lower normal limit. This outcome was previously seen by Nemzek and colleagues and was attributed to the strain of mice and sampling site used. It was found that in BALB/c mice, when blood is collected from the heart through cardiac puncture, neutrophil levels drop due to the reduced peripheral vascular resistance to the flow of blood cells [17,18]. Overall, there was no evidence of hemotoxicity in all groups (Figure 6).

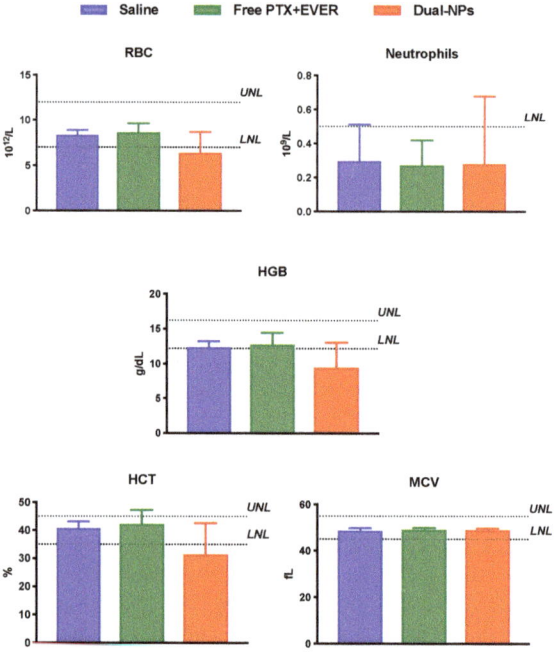

Figure 6. Red blood cell count (RBC), neutrophil count, hemoglobin concentration (HGB), hematocrit (HCT) and the mean corpuscular cell volume (MCV) in mice 2–3 days after receiving saline (blue), free paclitaxel and everolimus (PTX+EVER) (green), and dual-targeted PTX+EVER-loaded nanoparticles (Dual-NPs) (red) weekly for six weeks at a PTX-equivalent dose of 15 mg/kg. Data represent mean ± SD (n = 5–8).

Alkaline phosphatase (ALP) values (elevated in the blood most commonly by liver or bone disorders) and blood urea nitrogen (BUN) values (elevated in liver and kidney disorders) were within normal limits in all groups. Alanine aminotransferase (ALT) values (elevated with high specificity in liver disorders) were within normal limits in the saline and Dual-NPs groups, while mice in the free PTX+EVER group showed ALT levels higher than the upper limit. This increase in ALT levels, however, was not statistically significant relative to the saline and the Dual-NP groups (Figure 7). Therefore, there was no indication of liver toxicity in all groups. These results were further confirmed by the histopathological examination of formalin-embedded sections of the liver and spleen in all groups, which demonstrated normal histological appearance and no appreciable degeneration was observed (Figure 8).

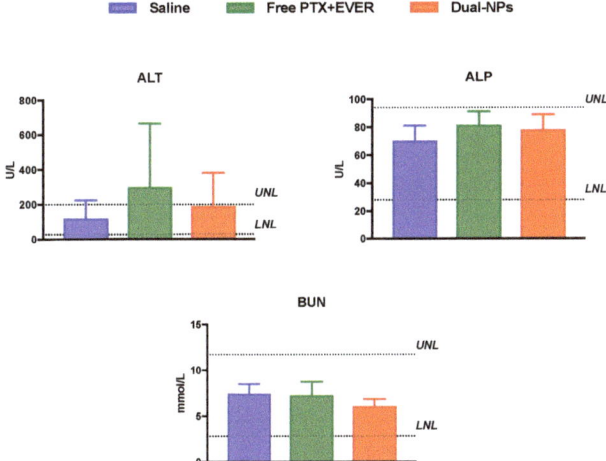

Figure 7. Alanine aminotransferase (ALT), alkaline phosphatase (ALP), and blood urea nitrogen (BUN) in mice 2–3 days after receiving saline (blue), free paclitaxel and everolimus (PTX+EVER) (green), and dual-targeted PTX+EVER-loaded nanoparticles (Dual-NPs) (red) weekly for 6 weeks at a PTX-equivalent dose of 15 mg/kg. Data represent mean ± SD (n = 5–8).

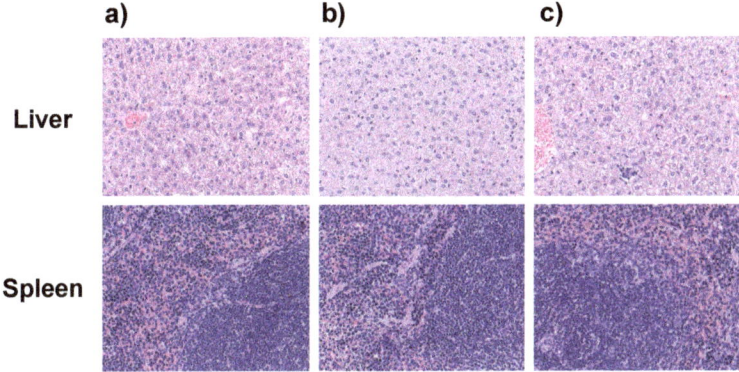

Figure 8. Cross-sections of the liver (upper) and spleen (lower) after staining with haematoxylin and eosin (H & E) 2–3 days after weekly injections for 6 weeks with saline (**a**), dual-targeted PTX+EVER-loaded nanoparticles (Dual-NPs) (**b**), and free paclitaxel and everolimus (PTX+EVER) (**c**) at a PTX-equivalent dose of 15 mg/kg. Magnification, 20X (n = 5–8).

To evaluate the kidney function, serum creatinine (SCR) levels were also quantified. SCR values in all groups were reported to be <18 µM/L. The low levels of SCR, along with the normal levels of blood urea nitrogen (BUN), negate the presence of kidney disorders—usually associated with high SCR levels—in all groups.

3. Discussion

Previously, the Dual-NPs demonstrated good stability in vitro with less than 50% PTX and EVER released after 72 h of incubation in BSA-supplemented media at 37 °C [11]. In the current study, PTX and EVER in Dual-NPs exhibited prolonged blood circulation whereas the free-drug combination showed rapid clearance. Consequently, the C_{max}, AUCs, and half-lives of the drugs were significantly higher when administered in Dual-NPs in comparison to the free drug combination. In addition, the Dual-NPs maintained the synergistic molar ratio of PTX:EVER in the plasma for up to 24 h after administration. These results indicate that the Dual-NPs retained their stability in the blood circulation, which is essential for the successful co-delivery of PTX and EVER (at the optimal synergistic ratio) to the tumor site.

The stability of the Dual-NPs may be attributed mainly to their low drug to material ratio or drug loading level (i.e., 5.6% w/w). We have previously found that the drug to material ratio can significantly impact the stability of NPs. Dynamic light scattering (DLS) was used to measure the size of different untargeted NPs composed of mPEG$_{5000}$-b-PLGA$_{15,800}$ at different drug (i.e., PTX+EVER) to material ratios (6.5%, 8.9%, 11.7%, 15.3% and 16.1% w/w) to monitor their stability for 48 h (data not shown). Formulations with high drug to material ratios of 16.1% and 15.3%, significantly aggregated forming large clusters that could be seen with the naked eye within 6 h, indicating the low stability of the NPs. With drug to material ratios of 11.7% and 8.9%, aggregation of the NPs began after 24 h, leading to an increase in hydrodynamic diameter of about 40% and 70% of the initial size, respectively. On the other hand, with a drug to material ratio of 6.5%, the NPs maintained their initial size for 48 h at room temperature and this size was also maintained when the NPs were incubated in cell culture media containing 10% FBS at 37 °C. Therefore, the untargeted NP formulation with the lowest drug loading level (6.5%) was used for the development of Dual-NPs. The conjugation of the targeting moieties to the surface of the NPs resulted in a reduction in drug loading from 6.5% to 5.6% (w/w). Other studies have confirmed our findings and demonstrated that PLGA NPs with lower drug to material ratios are often associated with a higher degree of stability [19–21].

The development of a polymeric NP formulation that physically encapsulates a taxane (paclitaxel or docetaxel) and is stable in vivo has proven to be challenging [22–24]. Cynviloq (Genexol-PM) is the first block copolymer micelle (BCM) drug formulation approved for human use for treating different types of cancer including metastatic BC. Cynviloq is composed of the copolymer methoxy-PEG-b-poly(D,L-lactide) (mPEG-b-PDLLA) and has a drug loading level of 16% (w/w). In preclinical studies conducted in mice, the plasma AUC for PTX was 30% lower with Cynviloq than with Taxol despite the higher injected dose (50 mg/kg versus 20 mg/kg for Cynviloq and Taxol, respectively) [23]. The rapid release of PTX from the micelles after administration was attributed to the kinetic instability of this formulation [25].

Administration of PTX and EVER in the Dual-NPs resulted in only marginal improvements in tumor growth inhibition and survival in MDA-MB-231-H2N tumor-bearing mice relative to the free-drug combination. The Dual-NP formulation was compared to free PTX+EVER at chemically equivalent doses of both drugs. One may expect that a greater degree of antitumor efficacy could be achieved for the Dual-NP formulation if a higher dose had been administered. Given the good toxicity profile observed for this formulation, it is also likely that higher doses of the formulation could be safely administered. However, the low drug loading level of 5.6% (w/w) in the formulation limits the maximum dose of drug that can be administered (i.e., 15 mg/kg). Therefore, there must be a balance between high drug loading and sufficient in vivo stability in the design of the NP formulation to allow for superior antitumor effects.

Empty Dual-NPs are unlikely to have any toxic or therapeutic effects. PEG-b-PLGA is a biocompatible copolymer which has a long history of safe use in pre-clinical and clinical studies [26–28]. Fab fragments, unlike full antibodies, lack the fragment crystallizable region (Fc) and the growth-inhibitory properties of the full antibody responsible for the toxicities associated with the full antibody [29].

Importantly, as previously shown by other groups, active targeting of a NP formulation may not result in an increase in their tumor accumulation. In some cases, the accumulation of NPs at the tumor site, even with active targeting moieties at the surface of the NPs, can be mainly attributed to the enhanced permeability and retention (EPR) effect (passive targeting) [30,31]. There is great heterogeneity associated with the EPR effect. As a result, the accumulation of NPs can vary significantly in the same or different tumor types [32,33].

Peripheral neuropathy remains a persistent distressing side effect to patients receiving conventional PTX, interfering with their daily activities and negatively affecting their quality of life. Symptoms include numbness, tingling, burning, muscles weakness and cramping. This toxicity is seen in 70–90% of patients receiving conventional PTX, and even after discontinuation of therapy, it takes several months for symptoms of neuropathy to resolve [34,35]. With PTX becoming a key component of the standard treatment for BC in the adjuvant and metastatic setting, stopping or reducing drug administration due to neuropathy is undesirable as it can have significant implications on treatment outcomes [36].

Importantly, in the present study, neurotoxicity was found to be reduced with the administration of the drugs in the Dual-NPs relative to the free-drug combination. In addition, the formulation showed superior tolerability to free PTX+EVER in terms of body weight loss. This outcome could be attributed to the prolonged retention of the drugs within Dual-NPs in the blood circulation, enabling effective exploitation of the EPR effect which leads to selective tumor accumulation and, subsequently, reduced systemic drug exposure and associated toxicities [37]. In addition, the use of polymeric NPs composed of the biocompatible polymer PEG-b-PLGA, which has a good safety profile allowed for the elimination of the small-molecule surfactant Cremophor EL, which has been associated with PTX-induced neurotoxicity [1].

4. Methods

4.1. Tumor Cells

The human BC cell line, MDA-MB-231-H2N, was provided by Dr. Raymond Reilly (University of Toronto, ON). The cells were cultured in Dulbecco's Modified Eagle Medium/Nutrient Mixture F-12) (DMEM/F12) with 10% fetal bovine serum (FBS) at 37 °C in 5% CO_2 and 90% relative humidity. The medium was supplemented with penicillin/streptomycin solution to 1% of final volume. Based on previous assessments of HER2 and EGFR expression by radioligand binding assays, MDA-MB-231-H2N has moderate HER2 (4.5×10^5 receptors/cell) and EGFR expression (4.8×10^5 receptors/cell) [38]. Based on these receptor densities, the cell line was designated as $HER2_{mod}/EGFR_{mod}$.

4.2. Animals and Tumor Model

Four-week old, healthy, female BALB/c mice were purchased from Charles River Laboratories (Wilmington, MA, USA) for the pharmacokinetics and toxicity studies. Four-week old, female NOD/SCID mice were purchased from an in-house breeding facility for the biodistribution studies and from Charles River Laboratories for the efficacy studies. Animal studies were conducted following protocols approved by University of Toronto's Animal Care Committee (approval No. 20012011, 7 August 2017).

4.3. Preparation of Dual-NPs

PTX+EVER-loaded NPs were prepared as previously described [6]. Briefly, PTX, EVER, $mPEG_{5000}$-b-$PLGA_{15,800}$ and COOH-PEG-b-PLGA (at ~1% of total polymer weight) were dissolved in acetone. Under magnetic stirring, following complete dissolution, the organic phase was added drop-wise to deionized water. The mixture was left under vacuum overnight at RT to evaporate the organic phase. The formulation was filtered and purified by ultrafiltration (3500 g for 10 min at RT) using ultracentrifugal filter units (Nominal molecular weight limit (NMWL) of 100 kDa) (Millipore Canada Ltd., Etobicoke, Canada). The HER2-targeted trastuzumab (TmAb) and EGFR-targeted panitumumab (PmAb) Fab fragments were generated by digestion of TmAb and PmAb IgG using immobilized papain following a well-established method [39]. The purity and identity of the Fab fragments were confirmed by sodium dodecyl sulfate polyacrylamide gel electrophoresis (SDS-PAGE) and size exclusion high performance liquid chromatography (SEC-HPLC). The Fab fragments were conjugated to previously prepared PTX+EVER-loaded NPs using the amine coupling method similar to that described by

Gao et al. [40]. Briefly, the NP suspension was incubated with N-Hydroxysuccinimide (NHS) (100 mM) and N-Ethyl-N'-(3-dimethylaminopropyl)carbodiimide (EDC) (400 mM) (Sigma-Aldrich, Etobicoke, Canada) for 15 min at RT. The resulting NHS-activated NPs were incubated with TmAb Fab fragments to prepare T-NPs, or a 1:1 mix of TmAb and PmAb Fab fragments (5 mg/mL in PBS, pH 7) for 1 h at RT. The resulting suspension of the dual-targeted PTX+EVER-loaded NPs (Dual-NPs) was purified by ultrafiltration (3500 g for 10 min at RT) using ultracentrifugal filter units (NMWL of 100 kDa). The purification of Dual-NPs was repeated three times. The amount of Fab fragment conjugated to the NPs' surface, was quantified using the Bradford assay, and found to be approximately 13 μg Fab per 1 mg of NPs (resulting in a ligand density of ca. 12 ligands per NP).

4.4. Pharmacokinetic Study

Healthy BALB/c female mice were injected intravenously (i.v.) via the tail vein with either the free PTX+EVER combination or the Dual-NP formulation at a PTX-equivalent dose of 15 mg/kg and EVER-equivalent dose of 7.5 mg/kg (i.e., PTX to EVER molar ratio of 1:0.5). The free-drug combination was dissolved in a 1:1 mixture of Cremophor EL and anhydrous ethanol. The resulting yellow viscous mixture was then diluted with saline and vortexed for 20 s to obtain a clear solution of the drugs. Mice were sacrificed by cardiac puncture under anesthesia at selected time points post-administration. Blood was collected using heparinized tubes and centrifuged at 15,000 rpm for 10 min at 4 °C to isolate plasma. Plasma was stored at −80 °C prior to analysis. Acetonitrile was added to the plasma at a 2:1 (v/v) ratio and the mixture was centrifuged for 10 min at 5000 g at 4 °C to precipitate the protein content of plasma. Supernatant was collected and the drugs were extracted by liquid-liquid extraction using t-butylmethylether (TBME). The organic phase was collected and evaporated under nitrogen before resuspending in the mobile phase (acetonitrile and water, 1:1 v/v).

PTX and EVER were quantified using HPLC as previously reported [6]. In brief, PTX and EVER were measured by isocratic reverse-phase HPLC analysis (Agilent) using a C18 column. Acetonitrile and water (50:50 v/v) or methanol, water, trifluoroacetic acid (95:4.9:0.1 v/v) were used as mobile phases for PTX and EVER, respectively, at a flow rate of 1.0 mL/min. A diode array detector was set at wavelengths of 227 nm and 279 nm for detection of PTX and EVER, respectively (Agilent, CA, USA). The extraction efficiencies were 86% and 81%, the limit of detection (LOD) was 0.1 μg/mL and 0.05 μg/mL (at a signal to noise ratio of ≥3), and the limit of quantification (LOQ) was 0.4 μg/mL and 0.1 μg/mL for PTX and EVER, respectively.

Non-compartmental analysis was used to calculate all pharmacokinetic parameters as previously reported [41]. The half-life at the terminal phase ($t_{1/2}z$) was calculated by dividing 0.693 by the slope of the terminal phase (k). The AUC_{0-t} was calculated using the linear trapezoidal rule where t is the time of the last measurable concentration. AUC_{t-inf} was calculated by dividing the last detected concentration by the slope of the terminal phase (k). The clearance (Cl) was estimated by the equation Cl = dose/AUC_{0-inf}, and the volume of distribution (V_d) by V_d = dose/(AUC_{0-t} K).

4.5. Tumor Inoculation

MDA-MB-231-H2N tumor-bearing female NOD/SCID mice were used for the biodistribution and efficacy studies. 1.0×10^6 MDA-MB-231-H2N cells suspended in a 100 μL mixture of culture medium and Matrigel (1:1 v/v) were injected subcutaneously in the right hind limb of mice. When the tumor size reached 5–8 mm in diameter, mice were randomly allocated to the treatment or control groups.

4.6. Biodistribution Study

NOD/SCID female mice bearing MDA-MB-231-H2N tumors were injected i.v. into the tail vein with either free PTX+EVER or Dual-NPs at a PTX-equivalent dose of 15 mg/kg and EVER-equivalent dose of 7.5 mg/kg (PTX:EVER at a molar ratio of 1:0.5). At selected time points post-administration, mice were sacrificed and tumors, spleens, livers, hearts and kidneys were collected and stored at −80 °C. Organs obtained were homogenised in 0.9% NaCl and the resulting homogenate was extracted and quantified using the methods described above for plasma. The extraction efficiencies were 80% and 76% for PTX and EVER, respectively. The LOD was 0.2 µg/mL (at a signal to noise ratio of ≥3) for both drugs, and the LOQ was 0.5 µg/mL and 0.4 µg/mL for PTX and EVER, respectively. Data were analyzed using the Student's t test, and p-values < 0.05 were considered statistically significant.

4.7. Efficacy Studies

NOD/SCID female mice bearing MDA-MB-231-H2N tumors received either saline, free PTX+EVER, or Dual-NPs as an i.v. dose administered weekly for eight consecutive weeks at a PTX-equivalent dose of 15 mg/kg and EVER-equivalent dose of 7.5 mg/kg (PTX: EVER at a molar ratio of 1:0.5). Tumor growth was monitored by caliper measurements of tumor width (w) and length (l). Tumor volume was determined using the formula $v = \pi/6 * l * (w^2)$, while drug toxicity was determined by monitoring changes in animal behavior and body weight. Groups were excluded from the tumor volume efficacy study when the first mouse in each group reached the ethical endpoint. Statistical significance was calculated by the two-way ANOVA (analysis of variance) test.

Mice were sacrificed and removed from the survival study when they reached the ethical endpoint—if any of the following was observed: hunched or abnormal posture; weight loss exceeding 20% of normal body weight; tumor mass compromising normal behavior, ambulation, limited food and water intake; failure to groom (piloerection). Survival data were plotted using Kaplan-Meier survival analysis, and statistical significance was determined using the log-rank test.

4.8. Toxicity Studies

Four-week old, healthy, female BALB/c mice were given the following weekly treatments via i.v. tail vein injection: Dual-NPs, free PTX+EVER at a PTX-equivalent dose of 8 mg/kg (low-dose study) or 15 mg/kg (high-dose study) (PTX:EVER at a molar ratio of 1:0.5). The control group received weekly injections of saline for six consecutive weeks. Mice were sacrificed two to three days after receiving the last injection and the severity of neurotoxicity was examined using light microscopy. Segments of the sciatic nerve were embedded in formalin. Sections of 4 µm in thickness were stained with haematoxylin and eosin (H & E) before examination under light microscopy by a veterinary pathologist blinded to the groups to determine the degenerative changes in the myelinated nerve fibers.

For mice receiving the higher dose of the drugs, blood was collected into heparinized tubes for biochemistry analysis and in Ethylenediaminetetraacetic acid (EDTA) tubes for complete blood count analysis (CBC). Blood biochemical markers were measured using the VetScan VS2 (Abaxis, Union City, CA, USA) Comprehensive Diagnostic Profile, while CBC analysis was conducted using the VetScan HM5 v2.2 hematology analyzer. Mice in this group were also evaluated for liver and spleen toxicity by histopathological examination of formalin-embedded sections of the liver and spleen. Data were analyzed using the Student's t test, and p-values < 0.05 were considered statistically significant.

5. Conclusions

While maintaining therapeutic efficacy, Dual-NPs were successful in improving the toxicity profile of PTX relative to the free-drug combination. In addition to showing preliminary evidence of reducing neurotoxicity, Dual-NPs were significantly more tolerable than the free-drug combination with regards to body weight loss when administered at the same dose. Considering the severe toxicities associated with conventional PTX (Taxol), especially at this time when the overall survival rates for BC have improved; the development of well-tolerated medicines should be prioritized alongside the search for curative measures.

Author Contributions: Investigation: L.H.; project administration: J.C.E.; supervision: C.A.; writing—original draft preparation: L.H.; writing—review and editing: J.C.E., C.A.

Funding: L.H. is the recipient of the CIHR Doctoral Research Award and the Centre for Pharmaceutical Oncology Scholarship. C.A. acknowledges research support from CIHR (Grant MOP325013).

Acknowledgments: LH acknowledges Giovanna Rocha De Medeiros Schver for assistance with analysis of the pharmacokinetics data.

Conflicts of Interest: The authors have no conflict of interest to declare.

References

1. Gelderblom, H.; Verweij, J.; Nooter, K.; Sparreboom, A. Cremophor EL: The drawbacks and advantages of vehicle selection for drug formulation. *Eur. J. Cancer* **2001**, *37*, 1590–1598. [CrossRef]
2. Hidalgoa, M.; Sánchez-Morenob, C.; Pascual-Teresa, S. Flavonoid–flavonoid interaction and its effect on their antioxidant activity. *Food Chem.* **2010**, *121*, 691–696. [CrossRef]
3. Chou, T.; Talalay, P. Quantitative Dose-effect relationships: The combined effects of multiple drug or enzyme inhibitors. *Adv. Enzym. Regul.* **1984**, *22*, 27–55. [CrossRef]
4. Mignani, S.; Bryszewska, M.; Klajnert-Maculewicz, B.; Zablocka, M.; Majoral, J.P. Advances in combination therapies based on nanoparticles for efficacious cancer treatment: An analytical report. *Biomacromolecules* **2015**, *16*, 1–27. [CrossRef] [PubMed]
5. Jadia, R.; Scandore, C.; Rai, P. Nanoparticles for Effective Combination Therapy of Cancer. *Int. J. Nanotechnol. Nanomed.* 2016, 1. Available online: http://www.opastonline.com/wp-content/uploads/2016/10/nanoparticles-for-effective-combination-therapy-of-cancer-ijnn-16-003.pdf. (accessed on 12 November 2017).
6. Houdaihed, L.; Evans, J.C.; Allen, C. Codelivery of Paclitaxel and Everolimus at the Optimal Synergistic Ratio: A Promising Solution for the Treatment of Breast Cancer. *Mol. Pharm.* **2018**, *15*, 3672–3681. [CrossRef] [PubMed]
7. Gonzalez-Angulo, A.M.; Akcakanat, A.; Liu, S.; Green, M.C.; Murray, J.L.; Chen, H.; Palla, S.L.; Koenig, K.B.; Brewster, A.M.; Valero, V.; et al. Open-label randomized clinical trial of standard neoadjuvant chemotherapy with paclitaxel followed by FEC versus the combination of paclitaxel and everolimus followed by FEC in women with triple receptor-negative breast cancer. *Ann. Oncol.* **2014**, *25*, 1122–1127. [CrossRef] [PubMed]
8. Campone, M.; Levy, V.; Bourbouloux, E.; Berton Rigaud, D.; Bootle, D.; Dutreix, C.; Zoellner, U.; Shand, N.; Calvo, F.; Raymond, E. Safety and pharmacokinetics of paclitaxel and the oral mTOR inhibitor everolimus in advanced solid tumours. *Br. J. Cancer* **2009**, *100*, 315–321. [CrossRef] [PubMed]
9. Approved Drugs—FDA Approves Liposome-Encapsulated Combination of Daunorubicin-Cytarabine for Adults with Some Types of Poor Prognosis AML. Available online: https://www.fda.gov/Drugs/InformationOnDrugs/ApprovedDrugs/ucm569950.htm (accessed on 23 October 2017).
10. Lancet, J.E.; Uy, G.L.; Cortes, J.E.; Newell, L.F.; Lin, T.L.; Ritchie, E.K.; Stuart, R.K.; Strickland, S.A.; Hogge, D.; Solomon, S.R.; et al. Final results of a phase III randomized trial of CPX-351 versus 7+3 in older patients with newly diagnosed high risk (secondary) AML. *J. Clin. Oncol.* **2016**, *34*. [CrossRef]
11. Houdaihed, L.; Evans, J.; Allen, C. Dual-Targeted Delivery of Nanoparticles Encapsulating Paclitaxel and Everolimus: A Novel Strategy to Overcome Breast Cancer Receptor Heterogeneity. **2019**, under review.
12. Van der Meel, R.; Vehmeijer, L.J.C.; Kok, R.J.; Storm, G.; van Gaal, E.V.B. Ligand-targeted particulate nanomedicines undergoing clinical evaluation: Current status. *Adv. Drug Deliv. Rev.* **2013**, *65*, 1284–1298. [CrossRef] [PubMed]
13. Lux, M.; Nabieva, N.; Hartkopf, A.D.; Huober, J.; Volz, B.; Taran, F.-A.; Overkamp, F.; Kolberg, H.-C.; Hadji, P.; Tesch, H.; et al. Therapy Landscape in Patients with Metastatic HER2-Positive Breast Cancer: Data from the PRAEGNANT Real-World Breast Cancer Registry. *Cancers* **2019**, *11*, 10. [CrossRef] [PubMed]
14. DiGiovanna, M.P.; Stern, D.F.; Edgerton, S.M.; Whalen, S.G.; Moore, D.; Thor, A.D. Relationship of epidermal growth factor receptor expression to ErbB-2 signaling activity and prognosis in breast cancer patients. *J. Clin. Oncol.* **2005**, *23*, 1152–1160. [CrossRef] [PubMed]
15. Owens, D.E.; Peppas, N.A. Opsonization, biodistribution, and pharmacokinetics of polymeric nanoparticles. *Int. J. Pharm.* **2006**, *307*, 93–102. [CrossRef] [PubMed]
16. Hamaguchi, T.; Matsumura, Y.; Suzuki, M.; Shimizu, K.; Goda, R.; Nakamura, I.; Nakatomi, I.; Yokoyama, M.; Kataoka, K.; Kakizoe, T. NK105, a paclitaxel-incorporating micellar nanoparticle formulation, can extend in vivo antitumour activity and reduce the neurotoxicity of paclitaxel. *Br. J. Cancer* **2005**, *92*, 1240–1246. [CrossRef] [PubMed]

17. Remick, D.; Nemzek, J.A.; Bolgos, G.L.; Williams, B.A.; Remick, D.G. Differences in normal values for murine white blood cell counts and other hematological parameters based on sampling site. *Inflamm. Res.* **2001**, *50*, 523–527.
18. Quimby, F.H.; Goff, L.G. Effect of Source of Blood Sample on Total White Cell Count of the Rat. *Am. J. Physiol.* **1952**, *170*, 196–200. [CrossRef] [PubMed]
19. Musacchio, T.; Laquintana, V.; Latrofa, A.; Trapani, G.; Torchilin, V. PEG-PE micelles loaded with paclitaxel and surface-modified by a PBR-ligand: Synergistic anticancer effect. *Mol. Pharm.* **2009**, *6*, 468–479. [CrossRef]
20. Abouzeid, A.H.; Patel, N.R.; Torchilin, V.P. Polyethylene glycol-phosphatidylethanolamine (PEG-PE)/vitamin e micelles for co-delivery of paclitaxel and curcumin to overcome multi-drug resistance in ovarian cancer. *Int. J. Pharm.* **2014**, *464*, 178–184. [CrossRef]
21. Averineni, R.; Shavi, G.V.; Gurram, A.K.; Deshpande, P.B.; Arumugam, K.; Maliyakkal, N.; Meka, S.R.; Nayanabhirama, U. PLGA 50:50 nanoparticles of paclitaxel: Development, in vitro anti-tumor activity in BT-549 cells and in vivo evaluation. *Bull. Mater. Sci.* **2010**, *35*, 319–326. [CrossRef]
22. Hrkach, J.; Von Hoff, D.; Mukkaram Ali, M.; Andrianova, E.; Auer, J.; Campbell, T.; De Witt, D.; Figa, M.; Figueiredo, M.; Horhota, A.; et al. Preclinical Development and Clinical Translation of a PSMA-Targeted Docetaxel Nanoparticle with a Differentiated Pharmacological Profile. *Sci. Transl. Med.* **2012**, *4*, 128ra39. [CrossRef]
23. Kim, S.C.; Kima, D.W.; Shima, Y.H.; Banga, J.S.; Oh, H.S.; Kim, S.W.; Seoa, M.H. In vivo evaluation of polymeric micellar paclitaxel formulation: Toxicity and efficacy. *J. Control Release* **2001**, *72*, 191–202. [CrossRef]
24. Chen, H.; Kim, S.W.; He, W.; Wang, H.F.; Low, P.S.; Park, K.; Cheng, J.X. Fast release of lipophilic agents from circulating PEG-PDLLA micelles revealed by in vivo Forster resonance energy transfer imaging. *Langmuir* **2008**, *24*, 5213–5217. [CrossRef] [PubMed]
25. Kim, T.Y.; Kim, D.W.; Chung, J.Y.; Shin, S.G.; Kim, S.C.; Heo, D.S.; Kim, N.K.; Bang, Y.J. Phase I and pharmacokinetic study of Genexol-PM, a Cremophor-free, polymeric micelle-formulated paclitaxel, in patients with advanced malignancies. *Clin. Cancer Res.* **2004**, *10*, 3708–3716. [CrossRef] [PubMed]
26. Beletsi, A.; Panagi, Z.; Avgoustakis, K. Biodistribution properties of nanoparticles based on mixtures of PLGA with PLGA-PEG diblock copolymers. *Int. J. Pharm.* **2005**, *298*, 233–241. [CrossRef] [PubMed]
27. Koopaei, M.N.; Khoshayand, M.R.; Mostafavi, S.H.; Amini, M.; Khorramizadeh, M.R.; Tehrani, M.J.; Atyabi, F.; Dinarvanda, R. Docetaxel Loaded PEG-PLGA Nanoparticles: Optimized Drug Loading, In-vitro Cytotoxicity and In-vivo Antitumor Effect. *Iran. J. Pharm. Res.* **2014**, *13*, 819–833.
28. Rezvantalab, S.; Drude, N.I.; Moraveji, M.K.; Güvener, N.; Koons, E.K.; Shi, Y.; Lammers, T.; Kiessling, F. PLGA-based nanoparticles in cancer treatment. *Front. Pharmacol.* **2018**, *9*, 1260. [CrossRef] [PubMed]
29. Neve, R.M.; Nielsen, U.B.; Kirpotin, D.B.; Poul, M.; Marks, J.D.; Benz, C.C. Biological Effects of Anti-ErbB2 Single Chain Antibodies Selected for Internalizing Function. *Biochem. Biophys. Res. Commun.* **2001**, *280*, 274–279. [CrossRef]
30. Kirpotin, D.B.; Drummond, D.C.; Shao, Y.; Shalaby, M.R.; Hong, K.; Nielsen, U.B.; Marks, J.D.; Benz, C.C.; Park, J.W. Antibody targeting of long-circulating lipidic nanoparticles does not increase tumor localization but does increase internalization in animal models. *Cancer Res.* **2006**, *66*, 6732–6740. [CrossRef]
31. Carstens, M.G.; de Jonga, P.; van Nostrum, C.F.; Kemmink, J.; Verrijk, R.; de Leede, L.; Crommelin, D.; Hennink, W.E. The effect of core composition in biodegradable oligomeric micelles as taxane formulations. *Eur. J. Pharm. Biopharm.* **2008**, *68*, 596–606. [CrossRef]
32. Harrington, K.J.; Mohammadtaghi, S.; Uster, P.S.; Glass, D.; Peters, A.M.; Vile, R.G.; Stewart, J.S. Effective Targeting of Solid Tumors in Patients With Locally Advanced Cancers by Radiolabeled Pegylated Liposomes Effective Targeting of Solid Tumors in Patients With Locally Advanced Cancers by Radiolabeled Pegylated Liposomes. *Clin. Cancer Res.* **2001**, *7*, 243–254.
33. Maeda, H. Toward a full understanding of the EPR effect in primary and metastatic tumors as well as issues related to its heterogeneity. *Adv. Drug Deliv. Rev.* **2015**, *91*, 3–6. [CrossRef] [PubMed]
34. Starobova, H.; Vetter, I.; Vetter, I. Pathophysiology of Chemotherapy-Induced Peripheral Neuropathy. *Front. Mol. Neurosci.* **2017**, *10*, 1–21. [CrossRef] [PubMed]
35. Scripture, C.D.; Figg, W.D.; Sparreboom, A. Peripheral Neuropathy Induced by Paclitaxel: Recent Insights and Future Perspectives. *Curr. Neuropharmacol.* **2006**, *4*, 165–172. [CrossRef] [PubMed]

36. Waseem, A.; Rao, R.R.; Agarwal, A.; Saha, R.; Bajpai, P.; Qureshi, S.; Mittal, A. Incidence of Neuropathy with Weekly Paclitaxel and Role of Oral Glutamine Supplementation for Prevention of Paclitaxel Induced Peripheral Neuropathy Randomized Controlled Trial. *Indian J. Med. Paediatr. Oncol.* **2018**, *39*, 339–348.
37. Houdaihed, L.; Evans, J.C.; Allen, C. Overcoming the Road Blocks: Advancement of Block Copolymer Micelles for Cancer Therapy in the Clinic. *Mol. Pharm.* **2017**, *14*, 2503–2517. [CrossRef] [PubMed]
38. Razumienko, E.; Dryden, L.; Scollard, D.; Reilly, R.M. MicroSPECT/CT Imaging of Co-Expressed HER2 and EGFR on Subcutaneous Human Tumor Xenografts in Athymic Mice Using 111In-Labeled Bispecific Radioimmunoconjugates. *Breast Cancer Res. Treat.* **2013**, *138*, 709–718. [CrossRef] [PubMed]
39. Hoang, B.; Reilly, R.M.; Allen, C. Block Copolymer Micelles Target Auger Electron Radiotherapy to the Nucleus of HER2-Positive Breast Cancer Cells. *Biomacromolecules* **2012**, *13*, 455–465. [CrossRef]
40. Gao, J.; Kou, G.; Wang, H.; Chen, H.; Li, B.; Lu, Y.; Zhang, D.; Wang, S.; Hou, S.; Qian, W.; et al. PE38KDEL-loaded anti-HER2 nanoparticles inhibit breast tumor progression with reduced toxicity and immunogenicity. *Breast Cancer Res. Treat.* **2009**, *115*, 29–41. [CrossRef]
41. Sparreboom, A.; van Tellingen, O.; Nooijen, W.J.; Beijnen, J.H. Nonlinear Pharmacokinetics of Paclitaxel in Mice Results from the Pharmaceutical Vehicle Cremophor EL. *Cancer Res.* **1996**, *56*, 2112–2115.

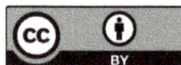

© 2019 by the authors. Licensee MDPI, Basel, Switzerland. This article is an open access article distributed under the terms and conditions of the Creative Commons Attribution (CC BY) license (http://creativecommons.org/licenses/by/4.0/).

MDPI
St. Alban-Anlage 66
4052 Basel
Switzerland
Tel. +41 61 683 77 34
Fax +41 61 302 89 18
www.mdpi.com

Cancers Editorial Office
E-mail: cancers@mdpi.com
www.mdpi.com/journal/cancers

www.ingramcontent.com/pod-product-compliance
Lightning Source LLC
LaVergne TN
LVHW070128100526
838202LV00016B/2247